FORENSIC DNA ANALYSIS

Technological Development and Innovative Applications

FORENSIC DNA ANALYSIS

Technological Development and Innovative Applications

Edited by
Elena Pilli, PhD
Andrea Berti, PhD

AAP | APPLE
ACADEMIC
PRESS

First edition published 2021

Apple Academic Press Inc.
1265 Goldenrod Circle, NE,
Palm Bay, FL 32905 USA
4164 Lakeshore Road, Burlington,
ON, L7L 1A4 Canada

CRC Press
6000 Broken Sound Parkway NW,
Suite 300, Boca Raton, FL 33487-2742 USA
2 Park Square, Milton Park,
Abingdon, Oxon, OX14 4RN UK

First issued in paperback 2021

Library and Archives Canada Cataloguing in Publication

Title: Forensic DNA analysis : technological development and innovative applications / edited by Elena Pilli, PhD, Andrea Berti, PhD.

Other titles: Forensic DNA analysis (Boca Raton, Fla.)

Names: Pilli, Elena, editor. | Berti, Andrea, editor.

Description: Includes bibliographical references and index.

Identifiers: Canadiana (print) 2020031436X | Canadiana (ebook) 20200314440 | ISBN 9781771889056 (hardcover) | ISBN 9781003043027 (ebook)

Subjects: LCSH: DNA—Analysis. | LCSH: Forensic genetics.

Classification: LCC RA1057.5 .F67 2021 | DDC 614/.12—dc23

Library of Congress Cataloging-in-Publication Data

Names: Pilli, Elena, editor. | Berti, Andrea, editor.

Title: Forensic DNA analysis : technological development and innovative applications / edited by Elena Pilli, Andrea Berti.

Other titles: Forensic DNA analysis (Pilli)

Description: Palm Bay, FL : Apple Academic Press, 2021. | Includes bibliographical references and index. | Summary: "Forensic DNA Analysis: Technological Development and Innovative Applications provides a fascinating overview of new and innovative technologies and current applications in forensic genetics. Edited by two forensic experts with many years of forensic crime experience with the Italian police and with prestigious academic universities, the volume takes an interdisciplinary perspective. It presents an introduction to genome polymorphisms, discusses forensic genetic markers, presents a variety of new methods and techniques in forensic genetics, and looks at a selection of new technological innovations and inventions now available from commercial vendors. Key features: Examines the genome polymorphisms and forensic identity markers Presents new scientific and technological developments in forensic genetics Describes the sequencing technology in forensic science in depth Presents the different fields of application of the new sequencing technology Highlights the importance of physical and molecular methods to solve forensic anthropology issues Looks at forensic genetics issues in criminal justice, ancestry, wildlife, entomology, etc. The book is an important resource for scientists, researchers, and other experts in the field who will find it of interest for its exhaustive discussion of the most important technological innovations in forensic genetics. For those newer to the field, the volume will be an invaluable reference guide to the forensic world"-- Provided by publisher.

Identifiers: LCCN 2020037573 (print) | LCCN 2020037574 (ebook) | ISBN 9781771889056 (hardcover) | ISBN 9781003043027 (ebook)

Subjects: MESH: Forensic Genetics--methods | Sequence Analysis, DNA--methods | DNA--analysis | Genotyping Techniques--methods

Classification: LCC RA1057.55 (print) | LCC RA1057.55 (ebook) | NLM W 750 | DDC 614/.1--dc23

LC record available at https://lccn.loc.gov/2020037573

LC ebook record available at https://lccn.loc.gov/2020037574

ISBN: 978-1-77188-905-6 (hbk)
ISBN: 978-1-77463-758-6 (pbk)
ISBN: 978-1-00304-302-7 (ebk)

About the Editors

Elena Pilli, PhD, is a Professor of Forensic Anthropologist at University of Florence, Italy. She is also Captain on leave from the Italian Military Police "Carabinieri" at the Forensic Scientific Centre in Rome, Italy. An expert in analysis of DNA extracted from highly degraded samples, such as human and animal bones and teeth and human and animal hair, she concentrates her research activity on next-generation sequencing technology. Dr. Pilli was involved in several important cold cases of national interest, and she was also in charge of the identification of the Fallen at the Fosse Ardeatine (a mass grave national case) and of the identification of human remains of Strage di Bologna (terroristic attack occurred in 1980). The author of approximately 40 publications in national and international scientific peer-reviewed journals and author of several book chapters, she was recognized for her scientific research for a Science Breakthrough of the Year. She is a reviewer of international journals, such as *PLos One, BMC Genetics, Scientific Reports, Forensic Science International,* and *Australian Journal of Forensic Science.* Her PhD was earned in biology, anthropology, and primatology and her 2nd level master degree in Forensic Science.

Andrea Berti, PhD, is a Forensic Biologist and Lgt. Colonel of the Italian Military Police "Carabinieri" at the Forensic Scientific Centre in Rome, Italy. He has been working in a forensic DNA laboratory since 1997 and has been the Technical Manager of the Forensic Biology Unit since 2010 (accredited ISO:IEC 17025 since 2012). The biology unit works on approximately 1,400 crime cases each year that occur in central and southern Italy, handling about 3,000 items of forensic evidence and performing 20,000 DNA analyses each year. The unit also employs NGS technology for forensic applications. Dr. Berti is certified as a BPA analyst and internal auditor for QA in forensics. He is a member of many professional organizations and is co-author of more than 40 articles published in forensic journals. Since 1999, Dr. Berti has been a trainer to the Italian military academy for forensic crime scene investigation and DNA analysis. He is also involved in managing the Italian DNA database as a CODIS supervisor.

Contents

Contributors

Jorge Amigo
Grupo de Medicina Xenómica (GMX), Faculty of Medicine, University of Santiago de Compostela, Galicia, Spain

Roberta Aversa
Menarini Silicon Biosystems Spa, 40013 Castel Maggiore (BO), Italy

Pedro A. Barrio Caballero
Instituto Nacional de Toxicología y Ciencias Forense, José Echegaray 4, 28232 Madrid, Spain

Alejandro Blanco-Verea
Grupo de Xenética Cardiovascular, Instituto de Investigación Sanitaria de Santiago, Complexo Hospitalario Universitario de Santiago de Compostela, 15706 Santiago de Compostela, Spain

Maria Brion
Grupo de Xenética Cardiovascular, Instituto de Investigación Sanitaria de Santiago, Complexo Hospitalario Universitario de Santiago de Compostela, 15706 Santiago de Compostela, Spain

Ozlem Bulbul
Institute of Forensic Sciences, Istanbul University—Cerrahpasa, Istanbul, Turkey

Elisa Castoldi
Molecular Biology and Genetics Unit, Carabinieri Scientific Investigation Department, 43100 Parma, Italy
LABANOF, Laboratorio di Antropologia e Odontologia Forense, Sezione di Medicina Legale, Dipartimento di Scienze Biomediche per la Salute, Università Degli Studi di Milano, 20133 Milan, Italy

Cristina Cattaneo
LABANOF, Laboratorio di Antropologia e Odontologia Forense, Sezione di Medicina Legale, Dipartimento di Scienze Biomediche per la Salute, Università Degli Studi di Milano, 20133 Milan, Italy

Elaine Y. Y. Cheung
Forensic Genetics Unit, Institute of Forensic Sciences, Faculty of Medicine, University of Santiago de Compostela, Galicia, Spain
National Centre for Forensic Studies, Faculty of Science and Technology, University of Canberra, ACT 2617, Australia

Bianca Maria Ciminelli
Department of Biology, University of Rome Tor Vergata, Via della Ricerca Scientifica 1, 00133 Rome, Italy

Manuel Crespillo Márquez
Instituto Nacional de Toxicología y Ciencias Forense, Carrer de la Mercè 1, 08071 Barcelona, Spain

Fulvio Cruciani
Department of Biology and Biotechnology, Sapienza University of Rome, Piazzale A. Moro 5, 00185, Rome, Italy

Runa Daniel
Office of the Chief Forensic Scientist, Victoria Police Forensic Services Centre, Macleod, VIC 3085, Australia

Eugenia D'Atanasio
Institute of Molecular Biology and Pathology, National Research Council,
Piazzale A. Moro 5, 00185 Rome, Italy

Maria de la Puente
Forensic Genetics Unit, Institute of Forensic Sciences, Faculty of Medicine,
University of Santiago de Compostela, Galicia, Spain
Institute of Legal Medicine, Innsbruck Medical University, Innsbruck, Austria

Laura Dodd
Foster + Freeman Ltd, Vale Park, Evesham, Worcestershire, United Kingdom, WR11 1TD

Francesca Fontana
Menarini Silicon Biosystems Spa, 40013 Castel Maggiore (BO), Italy

Luisa Garofalo
Istituto Zooprofilattico Sperimentale delle Regioni Lazio e Toscana "M. Aleandri,"
Centro di Referenza Nazionale per la Medicina Forense Veterinaria, Viale Europa 30,
58100 Grosseto, Italy

Katherine B. Gettings
US Department of Commerce, National Institute of Standards and Technology,
Biomolecular Measurement Division, 100 Bureau Drive, Mail Stop 8314, Gaithersburg,
MD 20899, USA

Leonor Gusmão
DNA Diagnostic Laboratory, State University of Rio de Janeiro, Pavilhão Haroldo Lisboa da Cunha,
São Francisco Xavier, 524-Maracanã, 20550-900 Rio de Janeiro, Brazil

Tobias Hampshire
ParaDNA, LGC Ltd, Queens Road, Teddington, Middlesex TW11 0LY, United Kingdom

SallyAnn Harbison
Institute of Environmental Science and Research Ltd., Private Bag 92021, Auckland 1142, New Zealand

Cydne L. Holt
Verogen Inc., 11111 Flintkote Ave, San Diego, CA 92121, USA

Rohaizah I. James
Promega Corporation, 2800 Woods Hollow Road, Madison, WI 53711, USA

Kenneth K. Kidd
Department of Genetics, Yale University, New Haven, CT 06520-8005, USA

Simonetta Lambiase
Department of Public health, Experimental and Forensic Medicine, Pavia University, 27100 Pavia, Italy

Maria Victoria Lareu
Forensic Genetics Unit, Institute of Forensic Sciences, Faculty of Medicine,
University of Santiago de Compostela, Galicia, Spain

Rita Lorenzini
Istituto Zooprofilattico Sperimentale delle Regioni Lazio e Toscana "M. Aleandri,"
Centro di Referenza Nazionale per la Medicina Forense Veterinaria, Viale Europa 30, 58100 Grosseto, Italy

Nicolò Manaresi
Menarini Silicon Biosystems Spa, 40013 Castel Maggiore (BO), Italy

Dennis McNevin
Centre for Forensic Science, School of Mathematical and Physical Sciences (MaPS),
Faculty of Science, University of Technology Sydney, Ultimo, NSW 2007, Australia

Gianni Medoro
Menarini Silicon Biosystems Spa, 40013 Castel Maggiore (BO), Italy

Andrea Novelletto
Department of Biology, University of Rome Tor Vergata, Via della Ricerca Scientifica 1, 00133 Rome, Italy

Carolina Núñez Domingo
Instituto Nacional de Toxicología y Ciencias Forense, Carrer de la Mercè 1, 08071 Barcelona, Spain

Nicola J. Oldroyd Clark
Verogen Inc., 11111 Flintkote Ave, San Diego, CA 92121, USA

Vânia Pereira
Section of Forensic Genetics, Department of Forensic Medicine, Faculty of Health and Medical Sciences,
University of Copenhagen, Frederik V's Vej, 11, DK-2100 Copenhagen

Christopher Phillips
Forensic Genetics Unit, Institute of Forensic Sciences, Faculty of Medicine,
University of Santiago de Compostela, Galicia, Spain

Elena Pilli
Molecular Anthropology and Forensic Unit, Laboratory of Anthropology, Department of Biology,
University of Florence, 50122 Firenze, Italy
Molecular Biology and Genetics Unit, Carabinieri Scientific Investigation Department, 00191 Roma, Italy

Daniele Podini
Department of Forensic Sciences, George Washington University, 2100 Foxhall Road NW,
Washington, DC 20007, USA

Stephanie Regan
Kauai Police Department, 3990 Kaana Street, Suite 200, Lihue, HI 96766, United States

Richard F. Selden
Ande Corporation 266 Second Avenue Waltham, Massachusetts 02451

Aaron M. Tarone
Department of Entomology, Texas A&M University, College Station, TX 77843-2475, USA

Beniamino Trombetta
Department of Biology and Biotechnology, Sapienza University of Rome,
Piazzale A. Moro 5, 00185, Rome, Italy

Rosemary Turingan Witkowski
Ande Corporation 266 Second Avenue Waltham, Massachusetts 02451

Debora Vergani
Dipartimento di Scienze Biochimiche, Sperimentali e Cliniche "Mario Serio,"
Università degli Studi di Firenze, Viale Morgagni 50, 50134 Firenze, Italy

Silvia Zoppis
Florida International University, International Forensic Research Institute, 11200 SW 8th St.,
Miami, Florida 33199.

Abbreviations

AAAD	Abdominal Aortic Aneurysm and Dissection
ACMG	American College of Medical Genetics and Genomics
AIMs	Ancestry Informative Markers
AP	Apurinic/Apyrimidinic
ARVC	Arrhythmogenic Right Ventricular Cardiomyopathy
AUC	Area Under the Curve
BAM	Binary Alignment Map
BGC	Biased Gene Conversion
BMI	Body Mass Index
BrS	Brugada Syndrome
CBP LSSD	Customs and Border Protection Laboratories and Scientific Services Directorate
cDNA	Complementary DNA
CE	Capillary Electrophoresis
CEATS	Camp Ethan Allen Training Site
CITES	Convention on International Trade in Endangered Species of Wild Fauna and Flora
CMOS	Complementary Metal–Oxide Semiconductor
CNVs	Copy Number Variant
CODIS	Combined DNA Index System
COI	Cytochrome Oxidase I
CPVT	Catecholaminergic Polymorphic Ventricular Tachycardia
CR	Control Region
CRS	Cambridge Reference Sequence
rCRS	Revised Cambridge Reference Sequence
dbSNP	Single-Nucleotide Polymorphism Database
DCM	Dilated Cardiomyopathy
ddNTPs	Dideoxyribonucleotide Triphosphates
DEP	Dielectrophoresis
DNM	*de novo* Mutation
dNTPs	Deoxyribonucleotide Triphosphates
DSBs	Double-Strand Breaks
DTT	Dithiothreitol
DVI	Disaster Victim Identification

EGDP	Estonian Biocentre Genome Diversity Panel
emPCR	Emulsion PCR
EMPOP	European DNA Profiling Group Mitochondrial DNA Population Database
eQTL	Expression Quantitative Trait Loci
ESS	European Standard Set
EVCs	External Visible Characteristics
ExAC	Exome Aggregation Consortium
FACS	Fluorescence-Activated Cell Sorting
FMA	Forensic Molecular Anthropologist
GA	Genome Analyzer
gDNA	Genomic DNA
GHEP-ISFG	Spanish and Portuguese Speaking Working Group of the International Society for Forensic Genetics
GWAS	Genome-Wide Association Study
HCM	Hypertrophic Cardiomyopathy
HGDP-CEPH	Human Genome Diversity Project—Center d'Étude du Polymorphisme Human HGDP–CEPH
HGP	Human Genome Project
HID	Human Identification
HR	Homologous Recombination
HR	Human Remains
HVS-I	Hypervariable Segment I
HVS-II	Hypervariable Segment II
IGSR	International Genome Sample Resource
IISNP	Identity-Informative SNP
ILS	Internal Lane Standard
Indels	Insertions/Deletions
ISFET	Ion-Sensitive Field-Effect Transistor
ISFG	International Society for Forensic Genetics
ISP	Ion Sphere Particle
IUPAC	International Union of Pure and Applied Chemistry
KPD	Kauai Police Department
LCM	Laser-Capture Microdissection
LD	Linkage Disequilibrium
LHP	Length Heteroplasmy
LINE1	Long Interspersed Nuclear Element 1
LISNP	Lineage Informative SNP
LQTS	Long QT Syndrome

LRs	Likelihood Ratios
MC1R	Melanocortin-1 Receptor Gene
mCNVs	Multiallelic Copy Number Variants
MFS	Marfan Syndrome
MHL	Minimal Haplotype Loci
MPB	Male Pattern Baldness
MPS	Massively Parallel Sequencing
mRNA	Messenger RNA
mtDNA	Mitochondrial DNA
mtGenome	Mitochondrial Genome
NDIS	National DNA Index System
NGS	Next Generation Sequencing
NRY	Nonrecombining Region on the Y Chromosome
OCME	Office of the Chief Medical Examiner
PARs	Pseudoautosomal Regions
PCA	Principal Component Analysis
PCR	Polymerase Chain Reaction
PD	Power of Discrimination
PE	Paired-End
PGM	Personal Genome Machine™
PHP	Point Heteroplasmy
PISNP	Phenotype Informative SNP
PMI	*Post Mortem* Interval
PSVs	Paralogous Sequence Variants
QC	Quality Control
QI	Quality Indicator
qPCR	Quantitative PCR
RFLP	Restriction Fragment Length Polymorphism
RM	Rapidly Mutating
RMP	Random Match Probability
RNA-Seq	RNA Sequencing
SADS	Sudden Arrhythmic Death Syndrome
SAK	Sexual Assault Kit
SAM	Sequence Alignment Map
SBE	Single-Base Extension
SBS	Sequencing by Synthesis
SCD	Sudden Cardiac Death
SD	Segmental Duplications
SGDP	Simons Foundation Genome Diversity Project

SMRT	Single-Molecule Real Time
SMS	Single-Molecule Sequencing
SNPs	Single Nucleotide Polymorphisms
SNSs	Single-Nucleotide Substitutions
SQTS	Short QT Syndrome
STRs	Short Tandem Repeats
SVs	Structural Variants
SWGDAM	Scientific Working Group on DNA Analysis Methods
TAAD	Thoracic Aortic Aneurysm and Dissection
TGFβ	Transforming Growth Factor β
TMRCA	Time of Their Most Recent Common Ancestor
TSS	Torrent Server Suite™
TVC	Torrent Variant Caller
UAS	Universal Analysis Software
UEPs	Unique Event Polymorphisms
VCF	Variant Call Format
VF	Ventricular Fibrillation
VNTRs	Variable Number of Tandem Repeats
VSMC	Vascular Smooth Muscle Cell
VT	Ventricular Tachycardia
WES	Whole Exome Sequencing
WGS	Whole Genome Sequencing
YHRD	Y-Chromosome STR Haplotype Reference Database
ZMW	Zero-Mode Waveguide

Foreword

The forensic analysis of biological material today plays a significant role in both the criminal justice system in helping resolve medical–legal matters and in a humanitarian capacity via the identification of human remains in mass fatality and missing people investigations. About 10 years or so ago the field of forensic genetics was in a bit of a lull in that, seemingly, the ability to recover DNA suitable for short tandem repeats typing from a variety of sample types, whether degraded or not and whether present in large quantities or not, was routine. However, this period of relative calm changed when important reliability issues were raised in court about the interpretation of complex mixtures, the case-contextual information surrounding an obtained DNA profile, and whether low-template DNA analysis was fit for purpose. More recently, significant technological developments such as massively parallel sequencing (MPS) and Rapid-DNA, and technical advances such as SNP typing for individualization, ancestry, and external visible traits are in the process of revolutionizing forensic genomics practice. Forensic genetics is no longer only principally concerned with case disposition but is equally involved in the provision of forensic intelligence to its customers. Many of these recent developments are covered in the various chapters of this book.

One of the main challenges for forensic scientists and other interested parties within the criminal justice community is how to keep up with all of the changes taking place. The printed word whether in physical or digital form still plays a significant role in that regard. Technical papers serve to communicate recent research data to specialists, but the individual contents are, of necessity, typically narrow and address a particular problem. Books, such as the present one, permit authors to provide general overviews of their subjects from their own perspective and, as such, are expected to appeal to a broader audience. The latter task, therefore, requires a careful choice of authors and, as readers will discover, the Editors of the present volume (Elena Pilli and Andrea Berti, both of whom are experienced forensic scientists with the Carabinieri Forensic Laboratory in Rome) have selected authors up to the task.

The book's aim is to provide an overview of new technologies and current applications in forensic genetics. It accomplishes this with chapters on genome structure and DNA polymorphisms and the different classes of biomarker types that have current forensic utility. Novel technologies and techniques in forensic genomics are addressed by authors on topics including MPS, phenotypic traits and biogeographical ancestry. Pleasingly, the book recognizes that human forensic geneticists do not operate in a vacuum and are not the only people who deal with biological material and hence chapters on forensic anthropology, entomology, wildlife forensics, and molecular autopsy of sudden cardiac death are included. Uniquely, a voice is given to a number of commercial vendors with scientific descriptions of their innovative technologies.

Prospective readers who would benefit from reading the book, or chapters therein, include forensic geneticists and other forensic specialists who desire up-to-date reviews on the state of the art in forensic genomics, criminal justice professionals including trial attorneys, and educators and their students.

Jack Ballantyne
University of Central Florida, Orlando, FL, USA

Introduction

The enormous potential of the genetic analysis as a crime-solving tool comes from the assumption that no two people are genetically identical, with the exception of monozygotic twins, and the genetic patrimony of an individual remains unchanged for life (with the exception to serious pathological conditions). The ability of identifying people from their biological material lies in the fact that an extremely minor part of the human genome contains regions that vary between individuals. This interindividual genetic variability is located in the so-called polymorphic DNA regions, defined as the occurrence of alternative forms (alleles) at a locus in different individuals.

DNA fingerprinting or DNA typing was first described in 1985 by Alec Jeffreys, father of forensic genetics and an english geneticist. He found that certain regions of DNA contained DNA sequence that were repeated over and over again next to each other. In addition, he discovered that the number of repeated units, apparently without a specific biological function, could differ from individual to individual. By developing a technique to examine the length variation of these DNA sequences, Jeffreys made the human identification assay possible, and allowed to associate to each individual a genetic profile that identifies him/her in a unique way. This technique was first adopted in an english immigration case, and, immediately after, to solve a double homicide case. Alec Jeffrey's markers were highly variable between individuals but to produce a DNA profile required a great deal of labor, time, and expertise associated with long repeat units, unsuitable to be analyzed in degraded samples, and the need to have relevant amount of DNA, not always available in forensic traces. Subsequently, a better solution including a high power of discrimination and a rapid analysis speed has been achieved with short tandem repeats (STR) DNA markers analyzed via polymerase chain reaction (PCR) technique. The short sizes of STRs permitted that they can be examined by multiple STRs in the same DNA test (multiplexing), producing highly discriminating results and successfully measuring sample mixtures and biological samples containing degraded DNA molecules.

Since it was first used, DNA testing has improved, and the advent of DNA technology has resulted in the increased ability to perform human identity testing in order to determine the crime perpetrator and deliver him/her to justice, and exonerate the innocent.

The recent technological and scientific development in the field of forensic biology is leading to expand the informative potential toward new goals. In particular, the development lines regarding analytical methods concern both the improvement of the analytical performance of the procedures and instruments used for DNA typing until now, and primarily the introduction of new technologies such as, for example, next generation sequencing (NGS) technology or Rapid DNA. The progression from Sanger-type sequencing to NGS has made a significant impact in the field of forensic science, not only in human health areas. The advent of NGS technology is also revolutionizing forensic genetics field. These new technologies provide clear advantages regarding high-throughput due to an extensive multiplexing capacity and parallel sequencing of millions of molecules (multiple parallel sequencing, MPS), allowing a faster and more informative analysis of the genomic material in a sample. The advance of NGS technologies has allowed us to considerably increase the number and type (STRs and SNPs) of polymorphic DNA regions that can be analyzed simultaneously, detect rare polymorphisms, and provide useful information for the analysis of complex mixtures. Not only a DNA profile with STR markers can be obtained, but also ancestry and phenotyping can be determined by the use of SNPs. Besides autosomal DNA, also mtDNA can be analyzed with NGS, and the discrimination power can be increased by sequencing whole mitochondrial genome in one run. The type of tissue or body fluid, the chronological age of a person, and differentiation between identical twins is possible by analyzing DNA methylation using NGS systems. Especially from degraded samples significantly more information can be obtained with NGS than with the conventional techniques. In addition, also nonhuman forensic genetics is expanding to more and more biological areas due to the increasing emergence of forensic cases based on nonhuman genetic material, and the possibility to analyze also complex samples (i.e., commingled samples with DNA from more than one contributor/species) via NGS.

A further innovation in forensic genetics is represented by Rapid DNA. Unlike traditional DNA analysis, which can take weeks, Rapid DNA analysis processes DNA samples in less than 2 h. This is a fully automated (hands free) process of developing a CODIS Core Loci STR profile from a reference sample buccal swab. The "swab in-profile out" process consists of automated extraction, amplification, separation, detection, and allele calling without human intervention. In certain scenarios, this extremely fascinating technology could revolutionize the workflow of a forensic investigation because this Rapid DNA system could be operable in the field and maximize the impact of DNA identification for law enforcement, disaster victim identification and military applications.

We are witnessing a period of enormous change. Molecular biology techniques have rapidly advanced in recent years and keep on moving ahead at a staggering speed, mainly in the area of sequencing. To date, the information that can be obtained from a biological trace collected at the crime scene has surprisingly increased. Everything at once, it is a bit of the philosophy that accompanies not only the forensic sciences but also the daily life of each of us today. The real challenge that awaits each of us and the forensic scientific community is to properly regulate and manage this amount of available data.

This book examines the recent technological and scientific development, focusing on novelties in forensic genetics; allowing companies that wanted to participate in the project to present their innovations and future vision. The book has been divided into four primary sections covering an introduction to genome polymorphisms, forensic genetic markers, novelties in forensic genetics, and finally company innovations.

In the Introduction to Genome Polymorphisms section, the two presented chapters provide some basic and general information on DNA structure and polymorphisms. The Forensic Genetic Markers section includes Chapters 3–6. The first chapter of this section displays an overview of current forensic identity markers, STRs, and SNPs, the most common forensic DNA analysis methods used today. Chapters 4 and 5 focus on Y- and X-chromosome markers, technology for typing them and the role of these markers in forensic contexts. Finally, the last chapter of this section discusses the application of mitochondrial DNA as a tool in forensic field, covering the processes involved in classical analysis, highlighting the importance of the work areas separation, and touching on the use of the NGS technology to sequence whole mtDNA genome and provide more information to forensic investigations. The Novelties in Forensic Genetics section is comprised of Chapters 7 to 14.

This section is the longest one and focuses on the recent technological and scientific development in forensic genetic field. The section begins with a detailed review on sequencing technology in forensic science focusing on the next generation sequencing. Chapter 7 goes into the sequencing technology (first-, second- and third-generation sequencing), focusing on the second-generation sequencing, describing the technology and the sample preparation and showing the use of NGS in forensics. The second to last paragraph of this chapter covers the data analysis, and the last one cover forensic considerations. Chapter 8 provides information on externally visible characteristics. After an initial introduction, the chapter discusses the pigmentation and relative informative markers, age estimation, and other externally visible characteristics such as craniofacial features, height, baldness, and hair structure. Chapter 9 covers ancestry origin and discusses what is needed for ancestry inference in forensics, methods for estimating ancestry of an individual, and interpreting results from ancestry inference analysis. Because the adoption of ancestry analysis in forensic laboratories requires a change in the approach used for population data analysis, and the production of a specific database for the use in a forensic laboratory is not easy task, Chapter 10 focuses on the evaluation of population and marker composition of major online whole-genome variant database in order to use them in forensic data analysis. Subsequently, Chapter 11 covers forensic anthropology, showing the importance of specialized figures to analyze bone, teeth, and hair samples, and of a joint approach between physical and molecular anthropologists to aid forensic investigations. Starting from physical anthropology techniques used to assist the police by providing biological profiles to ascertain identities, Chapter 11 focuses on DNA recovered from human remains (forensic molecular anthropology) and its analysis. Both factors influencing the success of DNA profiling such as, for example, contaminating DNA, and PCR inhibitors, and the choice of which skeletal elements to sample, are discussed. Finally, the chapter provides information on the DNA analysis from skeletal remains and molecular solutions to forensic anthropology issues such as species identification, sex identification, age at death, and etc. Chapter 12 goes into the molecular autopsy, defining what sudden cardiac death is, explaining the importance of *post-mortem* evaluation, and the recent development of molecular approach via NGS technology in identifying genetic predisposition. Chapter 13 focuses on genetic markers and techniques mostly used in wildlife forensics. The authors show the most frequent queries posed during the investigations of crimes against animal and mention the methods for the statistical treatment of genetic data obtained. Chapter 14 covers forensic entomology. This chapter summarizes the application of forensic entomology in the medical–legal field with emphasis on genetic identification, which is also the least used approach in investigations. The contents of this chapter are intended to give a general overview of how different insects may be used in forensic entomology as a means to assist geneticists in understanding how to aid or augment current applications.

Finally, the last section of this book that includes Chapters 15–19 focuses on innovations of the companies that wanted to participate to the project. Promega, LGC Ltd (ParaDNA technology), Silicon Biosystem (DEPArray™), ANDE Corporation (Rapid DNA), and Verogen show their solutions for a forensic world and the future perspectives.

PART I
Introduction to Genome Polymorphisms

CHAPTER 1

DNA Polymorphisms and Genome Structure: Different Scales of Variation in the Human Genome

ANDREA NOVELLETTO*, and BIANCA MARIA CIMINELLI

Department of Biology, University of Rome Tor Vergata, Via della Ricerca Scientifica 1, 00133 Rome, Italy

Corresponding author. E-mail: novelletto@bio.uniroma2.it

ABSTRACT

Modern human genetic diversity is the result of mutation, selection, migration, admixture, isolation, and drift. In the latest years, hundreds of thousands of human genomes have been sequenced. We briefly discuss the main findings concerning the occurrence of three classes of variations, that is, single-nucleotide polymorphisms, short tandem repeats, and structural variants as reported in seminal works, and provide a short guide to browsers and databases to query these variants' features. We discuss some key aspects of genetic variation as far as the molecular bases, quantitative impact, and population distribution are concerned. The availability of these immense catalogs is only the first step to work out the effects of interindividual differences in functional elements encoded in the genome.

1.1 INTRODUCTION

Modern human genetic diversity is the result of the emergence of new variants by mutation, demographic history of humanity as a whole, and selective effects that have acted to adapt different populations to their environments. Extant patterns of diversity at the global level are now considered mainly the legacy of an Out of Africa model for the evolution and dispersal of anatomically modern humans. On top of this, more local processes, such as migration, admixture, adaptation, isolation, and drift, have molded the genome pools of local human groups, generating a kaleidoscopic distribution of variants across space.

Human genetic diversity has been long explored at the protein level, characterizing individuals and populations for electrophoretically or serologically detectable variants (Cavalli-Sforza et al., 1994). In just few decades of DNA sequencing, the milestone where approximately 0.1% of living humans will have had their genomes resequenced to some degree is being reached, whereas resequencing of the genomes of our ancestors and other hominins is reshaping our understanding of human history (Shendure et al., 2017). This has produced catalogs of genetic variants that are growing at a thrilling pace and are freely available to the scientific community. These variations can be of several types, from simple substitutions that do not affect sequence length, to those that result in minor length differences, to those that affect multiple genes and multiple chromosomes (Kitts et al., 2014). In this chapter, we discuss some key aspects of genetic variation as far as the molecular bases, quantitative impact, and population distribution are concerned. The immense bibliography produced on these issues in recent years prevents any comprehensive presentation of the works, and references in the text should be all considered illustrative. As recent as they can be, we gave preference to seminal reviews, and the reader will find therein indications for a wealth of additional readings.

Sequence variation is of scientific interest to a variety of disciplines. Population geneticists analyze genetic diversity to work out phenomena as diverse as the descent of human groups (including the introgression with archaic hominins [Sankararaman et al., 2014]), and the effects, duration, and intensity of natural selection on different portions of the genome, possibly in response to specific environmental conditions (Itan et al., 2010; Brown 2012; Yi et al., 2010; Hancock et al., 2011; Perry 2014). Genetic mapping of Mendelian traits in humans could only be pursued by linking specific traits to genetic variations spontaneously present in segregating pedigrees (Strachan and Read, 2011). Historically, the need for an advancement in mapping human genes has been a main driver for improving the description of genetic variation in all parts of the genome. Additionally, the investigation of relationships between variation and phenotype leveraged the available catalogs of variants in at least three main lines: to analyze the association between variant alleles and phenotypes in cohorts of unrelated cases and controls, according to the so-called Genome-wide Association Study (GWAS) approach (Altshuler et al., 2008; Mackay et al., 2009; Rosenberg et al., 2010); to obtain a compilation of coding variants by sequencing of massive numbers of exomes (Lek et al., 2016); to establish precise relationships between the presence of specific variant alleles and the level of expression of genes in a large array of tissues (GTEx Consortium 2017).

Progress in the description of DNA variation has been heavily dependent on the scaling up of the power of typing technologies (including genotyping arrays, exome capture, and massive parallel sequencing). However, its impact on everyday practice would have been minor without a parallel development of proper and easily accessible and searchable catalogs. Different databases have been implemented, each tailored on the specific features of different types of variants. These have been now integrated into genome browsers that allow the visualization of the occurrence and organization of variants onto the genome reference sequence (see Table 1.1).

The main leap forward toward a genome-wide description of variation at the level of DNA sequence has been produced by the 1000 Genome Project (1KGP), launched to discover, genotype, and provide accurate haplotype information on all forms of human DNA polymorphism in multiple human populations. Specifically, the goal was to characterize over 95% of variants that have allele frequency of 1% or higher (the classical definition of polymorphism) in each of five major population groups (populations with ancestry from Europe, East Asia, South Asia, West Africa, and the Americas) (The 1000 Genomes Project Consortium 2010). During its performance, the Project has grown both in the number of populations (and hence subjects) and depth of sequencing, reaching 2504 subjects at a mean depth of 7.4× (The 1000 Genomes Project Consortium 2015). The results were reported separately for molecularly distinct sources of genetic variation. In the rest of this text we will keep this distinction, referring mainly to the results of this study.

1.2   SINGLE-NUCLEOTIDE POLYMORPHISMS (SNPs)

An SNP is a variation, typically of a single base position in DNA, in which the less common form (allele) has a frequency of at least 1% in the population (see above). Indeed, the acronym SNP has now been extended also to variants that have been observed in a single instance (singletons), variants consisting in change of more nucleotides in a row, and variants consisting in the presence/absence of one or a few nucleotides (small indels). The majority of SNPs are biallelic, that is, there is only a reference and an alternative base at the variable position. Only multiple mutational hits can generate SNPs

TABLE 1.1 An Initial List of Browsers and Searchable Databases on Human Genetic Variation

Acronym	URL	Short Description
Browsers		
NCBI Genome data viewer	https://www.ncbi.nlm.nih.gov/genome/gdv/	The NCBI Genome Data Viewer (GDV) is a genome browser supporting the exploration and analysis of eukaryotic RefSeq genome assemblies. It allows users to visualize different types of sequence-associated data in a genomic context.
Ensembl	http://www.ensembl.org/index.html	Ensembl is a genome browser for vertebrate genomes that supports research in comparative genomics, evolution, sequence variation, and transcriptional regulation. Ensembl annotate genes, computes multiple alignments, predicts regulatory functions, and collects disease data.
UCSC Genome browser	http://genome-euro.ucsc.edu/cgi-bin/hgGateway?redirect=manual	The UCSC genome browser provides a rapid and reliable display of any requested portion of genomes at any scale, together with dozens of aligned annotation tracks.
gnomAD	https://gnomad.broadinstitute.org/	The Genome Aggregation Database (gnomAD) is a coalition of investigators seeking to aggregate and harmonize exome and genome sequencing data from a variety of large-scale sequencing projects, and to make summary data available for the wider scientific community.
Databases		
SNP		
dbSNP	https://www.ncbi.nlm.nih.gov/snp	The Single-Nucleotide Polymorphism database is a public domain archive for a broad collection of simple genetic polymorphisms. This collection includes single-base nucleotide substitutions, small-scale multibase deletions or insertions (also called deletion and insertion polymorphisms or DIPs), and retroposable element insertions and microsatellite repeat variations.
STR		
STRCAT	http://strcat.teamerlich.org/	A catalog of STR variation using over 1000 individuals from the 1000 Genomes Project.

TABLE 1.1 *(Continued)*

Acronym	URL	Short Description
STRBase	https://strbase.nist.gov/index.htm https://strbase.nist.gov/ly_strs.htm	Facts and sequence information on each STR system, population data, commonly used multiplex STR systems, PCR primers and conditions, and a review of various technologies for analysis of STR alleles are included in this database.
SV		
DGV	http://dgv.tcag.ca/dgv/app/home	A curated catalog of human genomic structural variation.
DBVAR	https://www.ncbi.nlm.nih.gov/dbvar	NCBI database for structural variation.
DECIPHER	https://decipher.sanger.ac.uk/	DECIPHER (DatabasE of genomiC varIation and Phenotype in Humans using Ensembl Resources) is an interactive web-based database that incorporates a suite of tools designed to aid the interpretation of genomic variants.
mtDNA		
EMPOP mtDNA database	https://empop.online/	The EMPOP database aims at the collection, quality control, and searchable presentation of mtDNA haplotypes from all over the world.
MITOMAP	https://www.mitomap.org// MITOMAP	MITOMAP reports published data on human mitochondrial DNA variation.
Y chromosome		
YHRD	https://yhrd.org/	Generates reliable Y-STR haplotype frequency estimates for Y-STR haplotypes to be used in the quantitative assessment of matches in forensic and kinship casework. Assessment of male population stratification among worldwide populations as far as reflected by Y-STR and Y-SNP.
Other		
ALFRED	https://alfred.med.yale.edu/alfred/index.asp	ALFRED is a resource of gene frequency data on human populations.
ALLST*R	http://allstr.de/allstr/home.seam	The ALLST*R database contains data of a huge number of allele frequencies for different autosomal markers and populations.

TABLE 1.1   *(Continued)*

Acronym	URL	Short Description
HGPD–CEPH Database	http://www.cephb.fr/hgdp/main.php	The HGDP–CEPH Diversity Panel Database is designed to receive and store polymorphic marker genotypes, copy number variant (CNVs) calls, and Sanger DNA sequences generated by users of the HGDP–CEPH Diversity Panel.
ClinVar	https://www.ncbi.nlm.nih.gov/clinvar/	ClinVar is a freely accessible, public archive of reports of the relationships among human variations and phenotypes, with supporting evidence.
GTEx	https://www.gtexportal.org/home/	The Genotype-Tissue Expression (GTEx) project aims to provide to the scientific community a resource with which to study human gene expression and regulation and its relationship to genetic variation. This project collects and analyzes multiple human tissues from donors who are also densely genotyped, to assess genetic variation within their genomes.
POPaffiliator	http://cracs.fc.up.pt/~nf/popaffiliator2/	Prediction of an individual affiliation to a major population group based on information from a small set of autosomal STRs.
rSNPBase	http://rsnp.psych.ac.cn/index.do	rSNPBase is a database that provides reliable, comprehensive, and user-friendly regulatory annotations on rSNPs.

with three or four allelic forms. Note that the reference allele is the base represented in the genome reference sequence and is not necessarily the most frequent or the ancestral allele. In order to identify the ancestral allele, a comparison with an outgroup (nonhuman) species is necessary to determine which allele is shared between the two. This may reveal that the ancestral allele is the reference, or the alternative, or, in some cases, a third allele not observed in humans.

Due to the presence of only two alleles, the heterozygosity of one SNP (the expected percentage of heterozygous individuals at that position, or locus) has, in most cases, an upper limit of only 50%. In its final phase, the 1KGP (The 1000 Genomes Project Consortium 2015) has identified 84.5, 3.4 million, and 62,000 SNPs and small indels on the autosomes, X and Y chromosomes, respectively. The majority of variants are rare: approximately 64 million autosomal variants have a frequency of <0.5%, 12 million have a frequency between 0.5% and 5%, and only 8 million have a frequency of >5%. However, these findings refer to the aggregate sample, and it is essential to analyze how this reservoir is apportioned among genomic regions, individuals, and populations around the globe.

When we consider an average individual, he/she carries an alternative allele at 4.9–5.0 million SNP and indel sites. The vast majority of these are found to be shared among individuals, whereas only 11,000–14,000 sites are singletons, on average. Thus, the individuality of the genome is the result of a particular combination of not only particularly rare variants, but also a few really private ones. The prediction is that, upon continued resequencing of additional subjects, the number of very rare or private variants will grow, but with a little increase in the number of variants in a typical genome.

Only approximately 2% of the human genome encodes for polypeptides. The occurrence of SNPs in the coding regions (exons) is particularly informative, as they can affect the protein sequence, properties, and levels of expression. An average genome carries an alternative allele at 20,000–25,000 exonic SNPs, half of which are nonsynonymous (i.e., determine an amino acid change) and half are synonymous. These proportions show an impoverishment in nonsynonymous substitutions (as compared to predictions based on the genetic code), which is interpreted as a result of ongoing removal of deleterious variants by natural selection (purifying selection). In addition to exonic variants, the average genome also carries approximately 1.7–2 million and ~500,000 variants in introns and other regulatory regions, respectively. As to the putative effect of this baggage of variants in the average genome, 150–180 variants are predicted to cause a loss of function in the corresponding protein, and 2000 have been reported associated with multifactorial traits.

Major advances in the description of coding variants derive from exome sequencing studies. In this approach, the coding (and immediately flanking) regions in DNA are isolated from the rest of DNA and sequenced, with the possibility of reaching complete coverage at high depth with an order of magnitude drop in sequencing costs. More than seven million variants have been detected by assembling the results of more than 60,000 exomes (Lek et al., 2016), most of which are rare and not represented in the 1KG data. By virtue of its size, this study has opened new perspectives on the impact of rare variants and the propensity of some positions to undergo mutation.

The occurrence of variants along the 22 autosomes and the sex chromosomes is highly nonrandom. After excluding those regions of the genome (e.g., the pericentromeric regions) in which the detection of variation is difficult due to the highly repetitive DNA sequence, some genomic regions are enriched and others depleted in SNPs (The 1000 Genomes Project Consortium 2010). The HLA region (short arm of chromosome 6) and the subtelomeric regions show high rates of variation, while a 5-Mb gene-dense and highly conserved region around 3p21 shows very low levels of variation. The Y chromosome is particular in having an extremely low level of SNP variation (Malaspina et al., 1990). This is not currently attributed to a different proneness to mutations but rather to the haploidy and the particular evolutionary history of this chromosome (Jobling and Tyler-Smith, 2017).

One particular feature of the distribution of variants across human continental populations is the higher amount of diversity in Africa and in persons of African ancestry. Here, higher numbers of SNPs and singletons per person are observed, and a higher percentage of variants is private to the Continent. This is currently considered one of the strongest genetic evidence in favor of a relatively recent exit of modern humans from Africa to colonize the rest of the world, and it is replicated for other markers (see later in the chapter). The observation that the amount of diversity decreases with increasing distance from Eastern Africa, calculated across landmasses (Li et al., 2008; Ramachandran et al., 2005), fits the serial founder effect model of colonization. In this model, the first groups exiting Africa bore only a subset of the diversity of the Continent; from this point on, successive migrants, who expanded further the inhabited range, replicated this process of subsampling from the respective sources, thus producing populations progressively depleted in diversity. The intervening mutational process has not yet reestablished comparable diversity levels among Continents.

A major achievement in understanding the genome organization has been the discovery of its block structure (Gabriel et al., 2002; Wall and

Pritchard, 2003). Briefly, the occurrence of a particular allele at a variable site may be not independent of the alleles found at the preceding or following variable site along the chromosome (so-called *Linkage Disequilibrium*). A full array of alleles in this condition may persist in the population, as far as it is transmitted unaltered from parents to descendants, until a recombination event occurs within the array. Since the average recombination rate in the human genome is approximately 1.1 cM/Mb, at the scale of kilobases many generations are required until a recombination event occurs. The result, in practice, is that the genome can be considered a mosaic of relatively stable segments: the combinations of alleles (the so-called haplotypes) found in each of these segments across different subjects are far less than those expected by random assortment of alleles. The separation between adjacent segments is the result of historical recombination events, and adjacent segments can be recognized because the alleles in one are independent or nearly independent from those in the other. Here, we notice that the occurrence of recombination events in the genome is all but uniformly distributed, with extreme local rate variation spanning four orders in magnitude, in which 50% of all recombination events take place in less than 10% of the sequence (McVean et al., 2004). Additionally, the occurrence of recombination varies across populations with different ancestry, leading to varying patterns of *Linkage Disequilibrium* (Hinch et al., 2011).

The consequences of these phenomena are far reaching. First, for some analyses, the resequencing results of a diploid genome require the recognition of the segments and the reconstruction of the haplotype in each homolog, a procedure called "phasing" (see, e.g., Table 1.1 in The 1000 Genomes Project Consortium 2015). Second, haplotypes can be usefully taken into consideration in pedigree and GWAS studies (Altshuler et al., 2008), and for reconstructing population histories (Lawson et al., 2012; Loh et al., 2013; Gattepaille and Jakobsson 2012; Conrad et al., 2006). In fact, a given genomic segment displaying different haplotypes can be treated as a multiallele locus, whose heterozygosity can largely exceed 50%. In the two regions of the genome that do not undergo recombination, that is, the mitochondrial DNA and the male-specific portion of the Y chromosome (Skaletsky et al., 2003), *Linkage Disequilibrium* is extreme, and each haplotype corresponds to an independent lineage, transmitted through successive generations (Underhill and Kivisild, 2007).

More than 336 million SNPs were recorded in Single Nucleotide Polymorphism Database (dbSNP) (build 150), representing the total number of sites found to vary (Table 1.1).

1.3 SHORT TANDEM REPEATS (STRs)

Short tandem repeats are a class of abundant repetitive elements comprised of recurring DNA units of 2–6 bases. In a locus, all repeated units may be identical (forming the so-called perfect or uninterrupted repeat), or they may show variation around a common motif. Often, units which vary in their internal sequence or in their length are interspersed in an otherwise perfect stretch, leading to the so called "interrupted repeat."

Allelic variation at STR loci consists in different numbers of repetitions of the units. These loci are highly prone to mutations, due to their susceptibility to slippage events during DNA replication, resulting in high polymorphism and multiple alleles at each of them. By virtue of this property, STRs play an important role in population genetics and are the tool of choice in forensics and paternity testing. In fact, with a low number of loci, one person's genotype can be distinguished from any of the other person.

Classically, STR genotyping is obtained by PCR followed by capillary electrophoresis, to obtain a neat separation of alleles based on their molecular weight. Several loci can be multiplexed, and the PCR product of each of them labeled with one of a large selection of fluorescent dyes, resulting in complex profiles that are highly individual specific.

A complete view of occurrence and properties of STRs across the entire genome is still missing, because only recently methods for recognizing STR loci and reconstructing an individual genotype from next generation sequencing (NGS) reads have become available. In fact, the short read length of some sequencing platforms limits the ability of assembling the true sequence, more so for a diploid heterozygous genotype (Chaisson et al., 2015b). For example, in the most comprehensive study so far (Willems et al., 2014), the comparison between capillary and NGS genotyping revealed a remarkable proportion of instances of "allelic dropout" with the latter method, that is, the miscalling of a heterozygous genotype as homozygous. This effect was more pronounced for long alleles.

New single-molecule sequencing methods are revealing that STR detection has been most likely underestimated, that STRs occur preferentially in the last 5 Mb of each chromosome and this enrichment correlates with recombination rate (Chaisson et al., 2015a; Huddleston and Eichler, 2016). However, these methods have not been applied to population-scale studies, yet.

With the above caveats in mind, a genome-wide view of the occurrence of STRs as emerged from the 1KG data reported 700,000 such loci, 75% of which are di- and tetranucleotide, whereas the remaining loci are tri-, penta-, and hexanucleotide STRs (Willems et al., 2014). In general, the diversity at a STR locus takes the form of a unimodal allelic spectrum, that is, a most common allele and other alleles with progressively decreasing frequencies differing of + or − 1, 2, 3... repeats from that one.

Loci with a dinucleotide motif in noncoding regions of the genome appear the most variable, with 48% displaying polymorphism (30% with more than three alleles with a frequency of >5%) and heterozygosity averaged over all loci of the order of 0.1. These figures decrease across loci as the length of the repeated motif increases. While this observation could be considered the direct consequence of a higher mutation rate at dinucleotide STRs, a finer examination of mutational changes in Y-linked STRs (Willems et al., 2016) arrived at a different conclusion. In this study, tetranucleotide repeat STRs emerged as the most mutable ($\mu = 1.76 \times 10^{-4}$ mutations per generation, mpg), but the mutational change consisted in the addition/subtraction of a single repeat in most cases. Conversely, dinucleotide STRs had a lower μ (7.7×10^{-5} mpg), but more often a change in the number of repeats larger than one.

For all types of motifs, heterozygosity at autosomal STRs tends to increase with increasing length of the most common allele, in agreement with the expectation that a higher number of repeats across all alleles augments the chances of slippage during replication, and thus mutability. In this case, a direct relationship with mutational change is supported by Y-linked STRs (Willems et al., 2016), for which the main determinant of mutation is the length of uninterrupted repeats.

STRs falling in coding regions display a radically different pattern of diversity. Here, the length of the motif is key in determining whether a variation impacts on the reading frame. In fact an increase/decrease in the number of repeats of a coding tri- or hexanucleotide STR may cause the addition/subtraction of amino acid(s) in the corresponding polypeptide, but it does not alter the reading frame of the mRNA. Conversely, if the motif length is not a multiple of three, any change in the number of repeats will cause a disruption of the reading frame, an event very poorly tolerated within coding regions. In agreement with these considerations, the heterozygosity of coding STRs is one order of magnitude lower than noncoding STRs, with a peak only for tri- and hexanucleotide loci.

Studies that included a large number of STR loci have provided a broad view of the structuring of the human population (Rosenberg et al., 2002; Pemberton et al., 2013), anticipating the conclusions supporting the Out of Africa model discussed earlier (Ramachandran et al., 2005). While this list of loci could not be considered unbiased, these same findings were also replicated by the top 10% most variable autosomal loci of the genome-wide series (Willems et al., 2014). All the authors of these findings reported a higher heterozygosity in African than Eurasian populations and an excellent power to cluster populations according to their continental origin. At shorter distances, the power of STRs in detecting structuring declines rapidly, because the large number of alleles inflates the interindividual diversity and obscures the tiny fraction of interpopulation diversity (Algee-Hewitt et al., 2016). Only datasets obtained with a large number of autosomal loci are able to clusterize populations correctly within continents (Pemberton et al., 2013). On the Y chromosome, it is not uncommon that particular alleles at STR loci are tightly linked with some lineages defined by SNPs. Thus, a relatively small number of STR loci is often able to reveal population differentiation also within continents, and even at smaller scales (Roewer et al., 2005).

STRs in each of the haplotypic blocks of the genome should be expected to be in linkage disequilibrium with SNPs nearby. However, this expectation is only partially verified, as the STR–SNP disequilibrium is generally lower than the SNP–SNP disequilibrium, at comparable distances (Willems et al., 2014). This is thought to be the result of the mutational pattern at STRs, which is able to produce alleles equal in state on multiple occasions (and on multiple haplotypic backgrounds). The consequence is that, when an STR is the real causal contributor to a phenotype, its detection in a SNP-based association study is extremely difficult, as there might be many SNP haplotypes associated with the causal STR allele(s).

1.4 STRUCTURAL VARIANTS (SVs)

The SVs are defined as variations of the genome involving $\geq$ 50 bp. It is a heterogeneous class, since it includes deletions, duplications, insertions (mainly Mobile Elements Insertions and Nuclear Mitochondrial Insertions), inversions and translocations. Deletions and duplications (unbalanced variations) are also called copy number variants or CNVs; they can be biallelic (0 or 1 copy of a specific DNA region in the haploid genome for the deletions, one or two copies for the duplications) or multiallelic (presence of a variable number of copies, mCNV).

Until about 15 years ago, it was believed that SVs (especially those involving loss or gain of a stretch of DNA) were confined to individuals affected by genetic disorders. Only after the introduction of new technologies and studies specifically addressed to discover this type of variation (Sebat et al., 2004, Iafrate et al., 2004), it became evident that also "normal" individuals harbor a huge number of SVs. Nowadays, our knowledge on SVs mainly derives from the results of the 1KG Project (Sudmant et al., 2015) and from various studies focused on specific multifactorial pathological conditions for which the involvement of structural variants has been demonstrated or strongly suggested (Weischenfeldt et al., 2013: Perry et al., 2007: Cantsilieris and White, 2013). A catalog of SVs found in "normal" individuals can be found at the DGV site, whereas DECIPHER reports all the disease-causing or disease-associated SVs (Table 1.1).

Despite the considerable progress on our knowledge on SVs, much remains to be elucidated. A strong limitation concerns the bias on the rate of discovery of the different types of SVs when using NGS. In fact, due to technical reasons, CNVs are the most easily discovered SVs and, among CNVs, it is far easier to detect deletions than duplications. Another bias in discovery concerns the size of the SVs. In this respect, both ends of the size spectrum are adversely affected (Sudmant et al., 2015). Moreover, as far as the mCNVs class is concerned, the assessment of the number of copies of each haplotype is hampered by the fact that individuals with the same diploid number of copies (e.g., 6), could have different haplotype combinations (e.g., 3 PLUS 3, vs 4 PLUS 2, vs 5 PLUS 1); this assignment becomes more problematic as the number of copies increases (Handsaker et al., 2015). Nevertheless, despite these and other limitations, some features of SVs can be delineated, especially for biallelic and multiallelic CNVs which, although unbalanced, are the most numerous.

Each individual harbors a mean number of 4405 SVs, corresponding to 18.4 Mb, which is a proportion of genome fourfold higher than that affected by SNPs. SVs are unevenly distributed in the genome, with differences among chromosomes and along chromosomes, with a general enrichment in the pericentromeric and subtelomeric regions, partially due to the richness in segmental duplications of these chromosome regions (Zarrei et al., 2015). Furthermore, hotspots of SV mutations have been identified. Coding genes (introns included), transcription factor binding sites, and evolutionarily highly conserved sequences show a significant SV depletion (especially of deletions), compared to a random background model. Genes more intolerant to mutations exhibit the most pronounced depletion. Moreover, as deletion sizes increase, SVs become rarer. All these features strongly suggest purifying selection acting on SVs (Sudmant et al., 2015).

However, some functional classes of genes are enriched in SVs (particularly in CNVs). Among them, we find genes involved in a variety of functions that mediate the interactions with the environment (Zarrei et al., 2015): genes coding for the olfactory receptors; genes involved in starch and sucrose metabolism, or in xenobiotic, drug, and steroid metabolism; genes of the immune response. More than 1400 SVs (580 of which encompassing coding sequences) show a strong population structure and are thus potential targets to search for adaptive selection or genetic drift (Sudmant et al., 2015).

By using transcriptome data from lymphoblastoid cell lines of 462 individuals, the involvement of SVs, SNPs, and indels in expression quantitative trait loci (eQTL) was tested (Sudmant et al., 2015). SVs are disproportionally enriched for association with eQTL, both as lead markers and as they are in *Linkage Disequilibrium* with a SNP or an indel.

The final phase of the 1KG project (The 1000 Genomes Project Consortium 2015) has identified more than 68,000 SVs, 68% of which are rare (with a Variant Allele Frequency or VAF < 0.2%) and confined to one major continental group, whereas almost all the SVs showing a VAF > 2% are shared across continents. Similarly to the other types of variations, individuals of African ancestry show a higher amount of diversity.

1.5   DISCUSSION

The three classes of DNA variants briefly discussed earlier do not represent the sole sources of interindividual differences. Their abundance in the genome is only one of the reasons why their catalogs are so vast. With the advent of massive sequencing technologies, SNPs, STRs, and SVs have left behind other types of variation that are difficult to characterize with short-read platforms. For example, genes for rRNA are present in numerous copies, tandemly arranged at different genomic locations for 45S RNA (the precursor of 18S, 5.8S, and 28S) and 5S RNA, forming clusters of several hundred of kilobases, hard to quantify with the current sequencing technologies. Yet, electrophoresis-based methods have shown that the size of these blocks is highly variable among individuals and displays high rates of mutation across generations (Stults et al., 2008). These findings were replicated in NGS data from the 1KG project (Parks et al., 2018). In addition, a positive correlation is observed between the sizes (and hence the number of copies) of 45S and 5S clusters, despite they are located on different chromosomes. This interdependency, dubbed "concerted copy number variation," has been interpreted as a mechanism to ensure an equalized availability of material for ribosomal assembly (Gibbons et al., 2015).

Alpha satellite DNA can also be highly polymorphic. For example, on chromosome 17, the repeated arrays can vary of more than 2 Mb

(Aldrup-MacDonald et al., 2016), with different arrangements of the repeated units related to features as relevant as the position of the centromere.

It is then to be remembered that our knowledge of genomic variation is biased in favor of more easily detectable variant types. Moreover, given the widely differences between alleles across different classes (from 1 bp to several Kb), the most numerous variations (SNPs) contribute to the overall interindividual differences with an amount of DNA lower than the other classes of variants. This further increases the difficulties to associate a variation in the genotype with one or more phenotypic feature(s), either pathologic or not. A key goal in understanding the human genome is to discover and interpret all functional elements encoded within its sequence, by one of three main approaches, that is, the "biochemical," "genetic," and "evolutionary" ones (Kellis et al., 2014). However, naturally occurring variation within our species should be expected to have subtle effects as compared to genomic changes that underlie divergence with even closely related species. Massive DNA and RNA sequencing efforts are promising in this context, as they can relate a naturally occurring variant found in a subject, with the levels of mRNA abundance in his/her tissues (GTEx Consortium 2017). Certainly, this is producing a genome-wide view of the landscape of gene expression up to its first step, that is, mRNA. Filling the subsequent step will be challenging, in view of the incomplete correlation between mRNA and the corresponding protein's levels, at least as revealed in mice (Chick et al., 2016).

Finally, it has to be remembered that quantitative genetics theory predicts that, for traits contributed by many loci, the effect of alleles at each of these loci is expected to be small. This prediction has been verified for a vast number of qualitative traits with an underlying liability threshold (Albert and Kruglyak, 2015) and for a vast number of quantitative traits, including the mRNA measurements (GTEx Consortium 2017). In this line, the UK10K project (The UK10K Consortium 2015) was designed to characterize rare and low frequency variation in the UK population and to study its contribution to a broad spectrum of biomedically relevant quantitative traits and diseases, with different predicted genetic architectures.

DECLARATION

All illustrations, photographs, and tables in this chapter are original and have not been published elsewhere. They have been assembled and drawn by Andrea Novelletto and Bianca Maria Ciminelli.

KEYWORDS

- genetic diversity
- polymorphism
- single-nucleotide polymorphisms
- structural variants
- short tandem repeats

REFERENCES

Albert, F. W.; Kruglyak, L. The role of regulatory variation in complex traits and disease. *Nat. Rev. Genet.* **2015**, 16, 197–212.

Aldrup-MacDonald, M. E.; Kuo, M. E.; Sullivan, L. L.; Chew, K.; Sullivan, B. A. Genomic variation within alpha satellite DNA influences centromere location on human chromosomes with metastable epialleles. *Genome Res.* **2016**, 26, 1301–1311.

Algee-Hewitt, B. F. B.; Edge, M. D.; Kim, J.; Li, J. Z.; Rosenberg, N. A. Individual identifiability predicts population identifiability in forensic microsatellite markers. *Curr. Biol.* **2016**, 26, 935–942.

Altshuler, D.; Daly, M. J.; Lander, E. S. Genetic mapping in human disease. *Science* **2008**, 322, 881–888.

Brown, E. A. Genetic explorations of recent human metabolic adaptations: Hypotheses and evidence. *Biol. Rev.* **2012**, 87, 838–855.

Cantsilieris, S.; White, S. J. Correlating multiallelic copy number polymorphisms with disease susceptibility. *Hum. Mutat.* **2013**, 34, 1–13.

Cavalli-Sforza, L. L.; Menozzi, P.; Piazza, A. *The history and geography of human genes*, Princeton, NJ: Princeton University Press, **1994**.

Chaisson, M. J. P.; Huddleston, J.; Dennis, M. Y.; Sudmant, P. H.; Malig, M.; Hormozdiari, F.; Antonacci, F.; Surti, U.; Sandstrom, R.; Boitano, M.; Landolin, J. M ; Stamatoyannopoulos, J. A.; Hunkapiller, M. W.; Korlach, J.; Eichler, E. E. Resolving the complexity of the human genome using single-molecule sequencing. *Nature* **2015**a, 517, 608–611.

Chaisson, M. J. P.; Wilson, R. K.; Eichler, E. E. Genetic variation and the *de novo* assembly of human genomes. *Nat. Rev. Genet.* **2015**b, 16, 627–640.

Chick, J. M.; Munger, S. C.; Simecek, P.; Huttlin, E. L.; Choi, K.; Gatti, D. M.; Raghupathy, N.; Svenson, K. L.; Churchill, G. A.; Gygi, S. P. Defining the consequences of genetic variation on a proteome-wide scale. *Nature* **2016**, 534, 500–505.

Conrad, D. F.; Jakobsson, M.; Coop, G.; Wen, X.; Wall, J. D.; Rosenberg, N. A.; Pritchard, J. K. A worldwide survey of haplotype variation and linkage disequilibrium in the human genome. *Nat. Genet.* **2006**, 38, 1251.

Gabriel, S. B.; Schaffner, S. F.; Nguyen, H.; Moore, J. M.; Roy, J.; Blumenstiel, B.; Higgins, J.; DeFelice, M.; Lochner, A.; Faggart, M.; Liu-Cordero, S. N.; Rotimi, C.; Adeyemo, A.;

Cooper, R.; Ward, R.; Lander, E. S.; Daly, M. J.; Altshuler, D. The structure of haplotype blocks in the human genome. *Science* **2002**, 296, 2225–2229.

Gattepaille, L. M.; Jakobsson, M. Combining markers into haplotypes can improve population structure inference. *Genetics* **2012**, 190, 159.

Gibbons, J. G.; Branco, A. T.; Godinho, S. A.; Yu, S.; Lemos, B. Concerted copy number variation balances ribosomal DNA dosage in human and mouse genomes. *Proc. Natl. Acad. Sci. USA* **2015**, 112, 2485.

GTEx Consortium. Genetic effects on gene expression across human tissues. *Nature* **2017**, 550, 204.

Hancock, A. M.; Witonsky, D. B.; Alkorta-Aranburu, G.; Beall, C. M.; Gebremedhin, A.; Sukernik, R.; Utermann, G.; Pritchard, J. K.; Coop, G.; Di Rienzo, A. Adaptations to climate-mediated selective pressures in humans. *PLoS Genet.* **2011**, 7, e1001375.

Handsaker, R. E.; Van Doren, V.; Berman, J. R.; Genovese, G.; Kashin, S.; Boettger, L. M.; McCarroll, S. A. Large multiallelic copy number variations in humans. *Nat. Genet.* **2015**, 47, 296–303.

Hinch, A. G.; Tandon, A.; Patterson, N.; Song, Y.; Rohland, N.; Palmer, C. D.; Chen, G. K.; Wang, K.; Buxbaum, S. G.; Akylbekova, E. L.; Aldrich, M. C.; Ambrosone, C. B.; Amos, C.; Bandera, E. V.; Berndt, S. I.; Bernstein, L.; Blot, W. J.; Bock, C. H.; Boerwinkle, E.; Cai, Q.; Caporaso, N.; Casey, G.; Adrienne Cupples, L.; Deming, S. L.; Ryan Diver, W.; Divers, J.; Fornage, M.; Gillanders, E. M.; Glessner, J.; Harris, C. C.; Hu, J. J.; Ingles, S. A.; Isaacs, W.; John, E. M.; Linda Kao, W. H.; Keating, B.; Kittles, R. A.; Kolonel, L. N.; Larkin, E.; Le Marchand, L.; McNeill, L. H.; Millikan, R. C.; Murphy, A.; Musani, S.; Neslund-Dudas, C.; Nyante, S.; Papanicolaou, G. J.; Press, M. F.; Psaty, B. M.; Reiner, A. P.; Rich, S. S.; Rodriguez-Gil, J. L.; Rotter, J. I.; Rybicki, B. A.; Schwartz, A. G.; Signorello, L. B.; Spitz, M.; Strom, S. S.; Thun, M. J.; Tucker, M. A.; Wang, Z.; Wiencke, J. K.; Witte, J. S.; Wrensch, M.; Wu, X.; Yamamura, Y.; Zanetti, K. A.; Zheng, W.; Ziegler, R. G.; Zhu, X.; Redline, S.; Hirschhorn, J. N.; Henderson, B. E.; Taylor Jr, H. A.; Price, A. L.; Hakonarson, H.; Chanock, S. J.; Haiman, C. A.; Wilson, J. G.; Reich, D.; Myers, S. R. The landscape of recombination in African Americans. *Nature* **2011**, 476, 170–175.

Huddleston, J.; Eichler, E. E. An incomplete understanding of human genetic variation. *Genetics* **2016**, 202, 1251.

Iafrate, A. J.; Feuk, L.; Rivera, M. N.; Listewnik, M. L.; Donahoe, P. K.; Qi, Y.; Scherer, S. W.; Lee, C. Detection of large-scale variation in the human genome. *Nat. Genet.* **2004**, 36, 949–951.

Itan, Y.; Jones, B. L.; Ingram, C. J.; Swallow, D. M.; Thomas, M. G. A worldwide correlation of lactase persistence phenotype and genotypes. *BMC Evol. Biol.* **2010**, 9, 10–36.

Jobling, M. A.; Tyler-Smith, C. Human Y-chromosome variation in the genome-sequencing era. *Nat. Rev. Genet.* **2017**, 18, 485–497.

Kellis, M.; Wold, B.; Snyder, M. P.; Bernstein, B. E.; Kundaje, A.; Marinov, G. K.; Ward, L. D.; Birney, E.; Crawford, G. E.; Dekker, J.; Dunham, I.; Elnitski, L. L.; Farnham, P. J.; Feingold, E. A.; Gerstein, M.; Giddings, M. C.; Gilbert, D. M.; Gingeras, T. R.; Green, E. D.; Guigo, R.; Hubbard, T.; Kent, J.; Lieb, J. D.; Myers, R. M.; Pazin, M. J.; Ren, B.; Stamatoyannopoulos, J. A.; Weng, Z.; White, K. P.; Hardison, R. C. Defining functional DNA elements in the human genome. *Proc. Natl. Acad. Sci. USA* **2014**, 111, 6131–6138.

Kitts, A.; Phan, L.; Ward, M.; Holmes, J. B. (eds.). *The database of Short Genetic Variation (dbSNP)*, Bethesda, MD: National Center for Biotechnology Information, **2014**.

Lawson, D. J.; Hellenthal, G.; Myers, S.; Falush, D. Inference of population structure using dense haplotype data. *PLoS Genet.* **2012**, 8, e1002453.

Lek, M.; Karczewski, K. J.; Minikel, E. V.; Samocha, K. E.; Banks, E.; Fennell, T.; O'Donnell-Luria, A. H.; Ware, J. S.; Hill, A. J.; Cummings, B. B.; Tukiainen, T.; Birnbaum, D. P.; Kosmicki, J. A.; Duncan, L. E.; Estrada, K.; Zhao, F.; Zou, J.; Pierce-Hoffman, E.; Berghout, J.; Cooper, D. N.; Deflaux, N.; DePristo, M.; Do, R.; Flannick, J.; Fromer, M.; Gauthier, L.; Goldstein, J.; Gupta, N.; Howrigan, D.; Kiezun, A.; Kurki, M. I.; Moonshine, A. L.; Natarajan, P.; Orozco, L.; Peloso, G. M.; Poplin, R.; Rivas, M. A.; Ruano-Rubio, V.; Rose, S. A.; Ruderfer, D. M.; Shakir, K.; Stenson, P. D.; Stevens, C.; Thomas, B. P.; Tiao, G.; Tusie-Luna, M. T.; Weisburd, B.; Won, H.-H.; Yu, D.; Altshuler, D. M.; Ardissino, D.; Boehnke, M.; Danesh, J.; Donnelly, S.; Elosua, R.; Florez, J. C.; Gabriel, S. B.; Getz, G.; Glatt, S. J.; Hultman, C. M.; Kathiresan, S.; Laakso, M.; McCarroll, S.; McCarthy, M. I.; McGovern, D.; McPherson, R.; Neale, B. M.; Palotie, A.; Purcell, S. M.; Saleheen, D.; Scharf, J. M.; Sklar, P.; Sullivan, P. F.; Tuomilehto, J.; Tsuang, M. T.; Watkins, H. C.; Wilson, J. G.; Daly, M. J.; MacArthur, D. G.; Exome Aggregation Consortium Analysis of protein-coding genetic variation in 60,706 humans. *Nature* **2016**, 536, 285–291.

Li, J. Z.; Absher, D. M.; Tang, H.; Southwick, A. M.; Casto, A. M.; Ramachandran, S.; Cann, H. M.; Barsh, G. S.; Feldman, M.; Cavalli-Sforza, L. L.; Myers, R. M. Worldwide human relationships inferred from genome-wide patterns of variation. *Science* **2008**, 319, 1100–1104.

Loh, P.-R.; Lipson, M.; Patterson, N.; Moorjani, P.; Pickrell, J. K.; Reich, D.; Berger, B. Inferring admixture histories of human populations using linkage disequilibrium. *Genetics* **2013**, 193, 1233–1254.

Mackay, T. F. C.; Stone, E. A.; Ayroles, J. F. The genetics of quantitative traits: Challenges and prospects. *Nat. Rev. Genet.* **2009**, 10, 565–577.

Malaspina, P.; Persichetti, F.; Novelletto, A.; Iodice, C.; Terrenato, L.; Wolfe, J.; Ferraro, M.; Prantera, G. The human Y chromosome shows a low level of DNA polymorphism. *Ann. Hum. Genet.* **1990**, 54 (Pt 4), 297–305.

McVean, G. A.; Myers, S. R.; Hunt, S.; Deloukas, P.; Bentley, D. R.; Donnelly, P. The fine-scale structure of recombination rate variation in the human genome. *Science* **2004**, 304, 581–584.

Parks, M. M.; Kurylo, C. M.; Dass, R. A.; Bojmar, L.; Lyden, D.; Vincent, C. T.; Blanchard, S. C. Variant ribosomal RNA alleles are conserved and exhibit tissue-specific expression. *Sci. Adv.* **2018**, 4, eaao0665.

Pemberton, T. J.; DeGiorgio, M.; Rosenberg, N. A. Population structure in a comprehensive genomic data set on human microsatellite variation. *G3: Genes|Genomes|Genetics* **2013**, 3, 891–907.

Perry, G. H. Parasites and human evolution. *Evol. Anthropol.* **2014**, 23, 218–228.

Perry, G. H.; Dominy, N. J.; Claw, K. G.; Lee, A. S.; Fiegler, H.; Redon, R.; Werner, J.; Villanea, F. A.; Mountain, J. L.; Misra, R.; Carter, N. P.; Lee, C.; Stone, A. C. Diet and the evolution of human amylase gene copy number variation. *Nat. Genet.* **2007**, 39, 1256–1260.

Ramachandran, S.; Deshpande, O.; Roseman, C. C.; Rosenberg, N. A.; Feldman, M. W.; Cavalli-Sforza, L. L. Support from the relationship of genetic and geographic distance in human populations for a serial founder effect originating in Africa. *Proc. Natl. Acad. Sci. USA* **2005**, 102, 15942–15947.

Roewer, L.; Croucher, P. J.; Willuweit, S.; Lu, T. T.; Kayser, M.; Lessig, R.; de Knijff, P.; Jobling, M. A.; Tyler-Smith, C.; Krawczak, M. Signature of recent historical events in the European Y-chromosomal STR haplotype distribution. *Hum. Genet.* **2005**, 116, 279–291.

Rosenberg, N. A.; Huang, L.; Jewett, E. M.; Szpiech, Z. A.; Jankovic, I.; Boehnke, M. Genome-wide association studies in diverse populations. *Nat. Rev. Genet.* **2010**, 11, 356–366.

Rosenberg, N. A.; Pritchard, J. K.; Weber, J. L.; Cann, H. M.; Kidd, K. K.; Zhivotovsky, L. A.; Feldman, M. W. Genetic structure of human populations. *Science* **2002**, 298, 2381–2385.

Sankararaman, S.; Mallick, S.; Dannemann, M.; Prufer, K.; Kelso, J.; Paabo, S.; Patterson, N.; Reich, D. The genomic landscape of Neanderthal ancestry in present-day humans. *Nature* **2014**, 507, 354–357.

Sebat, J.; Lakshmi, B.; Troge, J.; Alexander, J.; Young, J.; Lundin, P.; Månér, S.; Massa, H.; Walker, M.; Chi, M.; Navin, N.; Lucito, R.; Healy, J.; Hicks, J.; Ye, K.; Reiner, A.; Gilliam, T. C.; Trask, B.; Patterson, N.; Zetterberg, A.; Wigler, M. Large-scale copy number polymorphism in the human genome. *Science* **2004**, 305, 525–528.

Shendure, J.; Balasubramanian, S.; Church, G. M.; Gilbert, W.; Rogers, J.; Schloss, J. A.; Waterston, R. H. DNA sequencing at 40: Past, present and future. *Nature* **2017**, 550, 345.

Skaletsky, H.; Kuroda-Kawaguchi, T.; Minx, P. J.; Cordum, H. S.; Hillier, L.; Brown, L. G.; Repping, S.; Pyntikova, T.; Ali, J.; Bieri, T.; Chinwalla, A.; Delehaunty, A.; Delehaunty, K.; Du, H.; Fewell, G.; Fulton, L.; Fulton, R.; Graves, T.; Hou, S. F.; Latrielle, P.; Leonard, S.; Mardis, E.; Maupin, R.; McPherson, J.; Miner, T.; Nash, W.; Nguyen, C.; Ozersky, P.; Pepin, K.; Rock, S.; Rohlfing, T.; Scott, K.; Schultz, B.; Strong, C.; Tin-Wollam, A.; Yang, S. P.; Waterston, R. H.; Wilson, R. K.; Rozen, S.; Page, D. C. The male-specific region of the human Y chromosome is a mosaic of discrete sequence classes. *Nature* **2003**, 423, 825–837.

Strachan, T.; Read, A. *Human molecular genetics—4th ed.*, Garland Science, **2011**.

Stults, D. M.; Killen, M. W.; Pierce, H. H.; Pierce, A. J. Genomic architecture and inheritance of human ribosomal RNA gene clusters. *Genome Res.* **2008**, 18, 13–18.

Sudmant, P. H.; Rausch, T.; Gardner, E. J.; Handsaker, R. E.; Abyzov, A.; Huddleston, J.; Zhang, Y.; Ye, K.; Jun, G.; Hsi-Yang Fritz, M.; Konkel, M. K.; Malhotra, A.; Stutz, A. M.; Shi, X.; Paolo Casale, F.; Chen, J.; Hormozdiari, F.; Dayama, G.; Chen, K.; Malig, M.; Chaisson, M. J. P.; Walter, K.; Meiers, S.; Kashin, S.; Garrison, E.; Auton, A.; Lam, H. Y. K.; Jasmine Mu, X.; Alkan, C.; Antaki, D.; Bae, T.; Cerveira, E.; Chines, P.; Chong, Z.; Clarke, L.; Dal, E.; Ding, L.; Emery, S.; Fan, X.; Gujral, M.; Kahveci, F.; Kidd, J. M.; Kong, Y.; Lameijer, E.-W.; McCarthy, S.; Flicek, P.; Gibbs, R. A.; Marth, G.; Mason, C. E.; Menelaou, A.; Muzny, D. M.; Nelson, B. J.; Noor, A.; Parrish, N. F.; Pendleton, M.; Quitadamo, A.; Raeder, B.; Schadt, E. E.; Romanovitch, M.; Schlattl, A.; Sebra, R.; Shabalin, A. A.; Untergasser, A.; Walker, J. A.; Wang, M.; Yu, F.; Zhang, C.; Zhang, J.; Zheng-Bradley, X.; Zhou, W.; Zichner, T.; Sebat, J.; Batzer, M. A.; McCarroll, S. A.; The 1000 Genomes Project Consortium; Mills, R. E.; Gerstein, M. B.; Bashir, A.; Stegle, O.; Devine, S. E.; Lee, C.; Eichler, E. E.; Korbel, J. O. An integrated map of structural variation in 2,504 human genomes. *Nature* **2015**, 526, 75–81.

The 1000 Genomes Project Consortium. A map of human genome variation from population-scale sequencing. *Nature* **2010**, 467, 1061–1073.

The 1000 Genomes Project Consortium. A global reference for human genetic variation. *Nature* **2015**, 526, 68–74.

The UK10K Consortium. The UK10K project identifies rare variants in health and disease. *Nature* **2015**, 526, 82–90.

Underhill, P. A.; Kivisild, T. Use of Y chromosome and mitochondrial DNA population structure in tracing human migrations. *Annu. Rev. Genet.* **2007**, 41, 539–564.

Wall, J. D.; Pritchard, J. K. Haplotype blocks and linkage disequilibrium in the human genome. *Nat. Rev. Genet.* **2003**, 4, 587.

Weischenfeldt, J.; Symmons, O.; Spitz, F.; Korbel, J. O. Phenotypic impact of genomic structural variation: Insights from and for human disease. *Nat. Rev. Genet.* **2013**, 14, 125.

Willems, T.; Gymrek, M.; Highnam, G.; The Genomes Project Consortium; Mittelman, D.; Erlich, Y. The landscape of human STR variation. *Genome Res.* **2014**, 24, 1894–1904.

Willems, T.; Gymrek, M.; Poznik, G. D.; Tyler-Smith, C.; Erlich, Y. Population-scale sequencing data enable precise estimates of Y-STR mutation rates. *Am. J. Hum. Genet.* **2016**, 98, 919–933.

Yi, X.; Liang, Y.; Huerta-Sanchez, E.; Jin, X.; Cuo, Z. X. P.; Pool, J. E.; Xu, X.; Jiang, H.; Vinckenbosch, N.; Korneliussen, T. S.; Zheng, H.; Liu, T.; He, W.; Li, K.; Luo, R.; Nie, X.; Wu, H.; Zhao, M.; Cao, H.; Zou, J.; Shan, Y.; Li, S.; Yang, Q.; Asan; Ni, P.; Tian, G.; Xu, J.; Liu, X.; Jiang, T.; Wu, R.; Zhou, G.; Tang, M.; Qin, J.; Wang, T.; Feng, S.; Li, G.; Huasang; Luosang, J.; Wang, W.; Chen, F.; Wang, Y.; Zheng, X.; Li, Z.; Bianba, Z.; Yang, G.; Wang, X.; Tang, S.; Gao, G.; Chen, Y.; Luo, Z.; Gusang, L.; Cao, Z.; Zhang, Q.; Ouyang, W.; Ren, X.; Liang, H.; Zheng, H.; Huang, Y.; Li, J.; Bolund, L.; Kristiansen, K.; Li, Y.; Zhang, Y.; Zhang, X.; Li, R.; Li, S.; Yang, H.; Nielsen, R.; Wang, J.; Wang, J. Sequencing of 50 human exomes reveals adaptation to high altitude. *Science* **2010**, 329, 75–78.

Zarrei, M.; MacDonald, J. R.; Merico, D.; Scherer, S. W. A copy number variation map of the human genome. *Nat. Rev. Genet.* **2015**, 16, 172–183.

CHAPTER 2

Single-Nucleotide Polymorphisms: An Overview of the Sequence Polymorphisms

EUGENIA D'ATANASIO,[1] FULVIO CRUCIANI[2] and
BENIAMINO TROMBETTA[2*]

[1]*Institute of Molecular Biology and Pathology, National Research Council,
Piazzale A. Moro 5, 00185 Rome, Italy*

[2]*Department of Biology and Biotechnology, Sapienza University of Rome,
Piazzale A. Moro 5, 00185, Rome, Italy*

Corresponding author. E-mail: beniamino.trombetta@uniroma1.it

ABSTRACT

Single nucleotide polymorphisms (SNPs), that is, substitutions or insertions/
deletions of a single nucleotide, are the most common variants in the human
genomes. Because of their low mutation rate, they are mostly biallelic
and evolutionary stable and a higher number of SNPs is required to have
a discrimination capacity similar to microsatellites. Nonetheless, these
markers can have several applications in forensic genetics, for example, as
ancestry informative markers. Due to their importance, in this chapter we will
explore the main molecular mechanisms leading to the onset of new SNPs
(namely, spontaneous mutations, induced mutations, and gene conversion)
and the *de novo* mutation rate in the human genome. We will also consider
two main aspects of the *de novo* mutation rate: (1) the paternal age effect,
that is, the increase of the mutation rate in offspring of elderly fathers and
(2) the presence in the genome of hyper-mutational sites such as the CpG
dinucleotides. Finally, we will explore the possible use of SNPs as analysis
tools, taking as an example the human Y chromosome, which represents an
interesting case because of its haploidy and paternal inheritance pattern.

2.1   INTRODUCTION

All humans are different from each other, and part of these differences has a genetic background due to variations in our DNA. In all living organisms, the genetic material may be subject to permanent changes called mutations, which generate different forms of homologous molecules that contribute to the allelic diversity of a population.

The simplest and smallest scale difference that can be observed between two DNA sequences is the base substitution in which one base is replaced by another one. For example, a G and a T may exist in two homologous sequences at a particular nucleotide position and, in this example, a G-to-T mutation (or vice versa) has occurred in one of the two molecules.

In animals, mutations can be divided into two types based on the tissues where they occur. When the mutation occurs in the germ cells (i.e., the cells that generate gametes), it is called germ line mutation. The germ cells are involved in transmitting genetic material to future generations; thus, such mutation is passed to the offspring. The other type of mutation can occur in any other cell of the body. This type is called somatic mutation and cannot be transmitted to the next generation.

In this context, we are only interested in the germ line mutations (i.e., the random changes of DNA that occur during the formation of gametes). If a mutation occurs in the germ line of one individual, it will be introduced within the population as a new allelic variant, whose destiny (in terms of allelic frequency) will depend on the evolutionary and demographic forces acting on the population. If the new borne allele (called derived allele) will increase in frequency to the detriment of the ancestral allele, it could be possible to observe the occurrence of a new genetic polymorphism, which is defined as a genetic variation in which the less frequent allele is present (within the population) with a frequency of 1% or greater.

When a genetic polymorphism involves a single base (a substitution or a deletion) it is called single-nucleotide polymorphism (SNP, pronounced "snip"). Although the insertions or deletions of a single base can also be defined as SNPs, the single base substitutions are the most common SNPs observed in the human genome. From a chemical point of view, it is possible to classify SNPs into two categories: the substitutions of a pyrimidine (T or C) with another pyrimidine or a purine (A or G) with another purine are defined transitions, whereas the exchange of a purine with a pyrimidine (or vice versa) is called transversion.

By comparing two different human genomes, the great majority of nucleotides are nearly always the same. Occasionally, different variants may be seen at any nucleotide position, and though each of them is rare, SNPs are the most abundant class of genetic variants within the human genome. By comparing two homologous chromosomes within a population, it is possible to observe a single nucleotide difference about every 1000 bp. This is not a strict rule, indeed in duplicated regions of the human genome it is possible to observe clusters of SNPs (defined as groups of two or more SNPs occurring in close proximity and showing the derived alleles on the same chromosome) (Hallast et al., 2005; Trombetta et al., 2016).

Due to the very low mutation rate (about 10^{-8} changes per nucleotide per generation) (Campbell and Eichler, 2013) SNPs can be usually considered as biallelic polymorphisms (with only two alleles - for example an A or a G in a certain position), but few rare polymorphic sites show more complex variation pattern, with SNPs involving three or all the four DNA bases (The 1000 Genomes Project Consortium 2015). Moreover, with a few exceptions, SNPs can also be defined as Unique Event Polymorphisms, implying that in case of genetic variation in a population the identity in state between two sequences can be also considered an identity by descent. It means that the two identical molecules probably originated from a common ancestral molecule through its replication during the evolution of the population. This evolutionary stability also implies that it can be possible to infer the ancestral state of a SNP observed in the human population by analyzing the orthologous region in a closely related species, such as the chimpanzee. For example, if it has been observed a T/G SNP in a human population, the allele corresponding to the base of the chimpanzee will be considered as the ancestral one. So, the presence of the G in chimpanzee indicates that a G-to-T mutation occurred in the human lineage.

All the SNPs identified in the 1000 Genomes Project and in other studies are classified and cataloged in public databases such as the dbSNP database (https://www.ncbi.nlm.nih.gov/projects/SNP/) (Reich et al., 2003; Wheeler et al., 2008). It is a free archive for genetic variation within and across different species. Although the name of the database implies a collection of one class of polymorphisms only (i.e., single nucleotide polymorphisms), it contains a range of small molecular variants: SNPs, short deletion and insertion polymorphisms, short tandem repeats (STRs), etc. To date in regard to the human species (*Homo sapiens*), the build 151 of the dbSNP (available since March 2018) contains about 113 million validated variants, which can be used by scientists to investigate a wide variety of genetically based natural phenomena.

The importance of SNPs in humans is highlighted by the fact that in January 2008 it has been launched a new project which intended to sequence 1000 different genomes from worldwide populations (1KGP—http://www.

internationalgenome.org) in order to establish the most detailed catalogs of human genetic variation (Gibbs et al., 2015; Sudmant et al., 2015).

SNPs have great potential for many applications in forensic genetics for several reasons. First, they are very simple to analyze. Second, they can be easily multiplexed (so it is possible to analyze a lot of loci simultaneously). Third, they can be amplified from DNA fragment less than 50 bp (it means that these markers are especially useful for studies involving degraded DNA - such as ancient DNA), better than STRs that have amplicons usually larger than 100 bp. For example, a recent study showed a better efficacy of the SNP analysis kits than those of STRs to investigate the kinship relationship between ancient samples (Serventi et al., 2018).

On the other hand, because SNPs are usually biallelic, a higher numbers of markers (respect to the number of STRs markers) are needed to have a power of discrimination similar to that obtainable by analyzing microsatellite loci. It has been shown that about 25–45 biallelic loci are needed to obtain similar random match probabilities as in the 13 STRs core loci, with the number of SNPs depending on their allele frequencies in the population (Chakraborty et al., 1999).

Moreover, several studies highlighted that, mainly as consequence of natural selection, the alleles of some autosomal SNPs are population specific, suggesting that it could be possible to predict the geographic origin of the perpetrator of a crime by analyzing only few loci from a biological trace found on the crime scene (Pereira et al., 2017). In this context, giant steps have been taken in the use of the Y-chromosome SNPs that, in combination with the Y-STRs, are yielding interesting results in the identification of the geographic origin of one individual and in the ability to discriminate different individuals within a family (Ralf et al., 2015; van Oven et al., 2013; Wetton et al., 2005; Xue and Tyler-Smith, 2010).

Despite their stability, the use of SNPs to study the genetic diversity among populations may give raise to ascertainment bias. It describes systematic deviations from an expected theoretical result attributable to the sampling processes used to find new SNPs and their population-specific allele frequencies (Lachance and Tishkoff, 2013). Ascertainment bias is a crucial issue in many applications of SNPs. It results from the selection of SNPs from an unrepresentative sample of a population. This selection may lead to study the genetic differences between two populations using loci that are not representative of the spectrum of their allele frequencies. For example, if few individuals are used for SNPs discovery it is possible that not representative SNPs will be used for the genotyping of other populations.

Thus, future genotyping studies using those SNPs will result in a false deficit of rare alleles. Ascertainment bias has the potential to introduce systematic error in the estimate of variation among and within populations (Lachance and Tishkoff, 2013).

Due to the importance of SNPs, understanding the mechanisms by which they arise and estimating the rate of their occurrence are of fundamental importance. The processes which generate a new allelic variant (and the SNPs - after the action of different evolutionary forces) can be grouped into two categories: spontaneous mutations and induced mutations. The former occur spontaneously due to errors in fundamental biological processes (such as DNA replication), whereas the induced mutations are produced when the organism interacts with an external or internal mutagenic agent (i.e., radiation, chemical agents).

All these types of errors may lead to mutation only if they are not correctly repaired before the next round of replication. Thus, the number of mutations (and so the number of SNPs) is the result of a dynamic balance between the number of errors that are introduced and the efficacy of various types of repair (Ségurel et al., 2014).

A third way to introduce new mutations in a population, besides spontaneous and induced, is through gene conversion, a particular molecular repair mechanism strongly active in the maintenance of genome integrity. It is, in fact, the major molecular mechanism used to repair double-strand breaks (DSBs) (Shrivastav et al., 2008; van den Bosch et al., 2002), which represents the most deleterious form of damage to genetic material (O'Driscoll and Jeggo, 2006). As a secondary effect, gene conversion is able to generate clusters of SNPs within duplicated region of the human genome (Trombetta et al., 2010). In this case, it is the repair mechanism itself that generates new mutations physically linked and in a narrow region.

2.1.1 SPONTANEOUS MUTATIONS

Spontaneous mutations mainly occur due to the base misincorporation during the DNA replication, which is the fundamental biological process that produces two identical DNA molecules starting from an ancestral one.

When a human cell divides, all its nuclear DNA must be replicated and included in the two daughter cells. The enzyme responsible for the replication process is the DNA polymerase, which, by exploiting the DNA-pairing laws and the correct binding geometry between the bases, correctly polymerizes the new growing DNA strand. Occasionally, it will occur the incorporation of an incorrect base, possibly due to the presence, within the template strands, of rare tautomeric forms of the bases that have different base pair properties. This polymerization process is subject to a second control. The DNA polymerase is able to re-examine the embedded base and, if it is wrong, the enzyme can excise the wrong base and it will try again to introduce another one. This double checking greatly decreases the probability of mutation but these enzymes still make mistakes in the introduction of bases during the formation of the new strand.

Thus, a higher number of divisions can lead to a higher number of mutations. Indeed, due to the higher number of divisions necessary to form the male gametes (sperms) respect to female gametes (eggs), the *de novo* mutation rate (i.e., the rate for mutations that are present for the first time in one family member as a result of a mutation in a germ cell of one of the parents or in the fertilized egg itself) is higher in males than in females (Kong et al., 2012).

2.1.2   INDUCED MUTATIONS

Mutations in the germ line can also be introduced by external agents or internal chemical changes. There are three main external agents that can induce mutation: ionizing radiations (that produce DSBs in the DNA molecule and that can produce cluster of SNPs after the gene conversion repair process), UV radiation (that may cross-link adjacent pyrimidines and has no role in the evolution of SNPs in a population), and chemical external compounds that can chemically modify the DNA.

The DNA stability can also be compromised by endogenous chemical events such as: depurination (the random loss of an A or a G due to the spontaneous hydrolysis of the base) and deamination (the elimination of a $-NH_2$ group from a cytosine). The latter event is of particular importance in the onset of new polymorphisms as it induces hyper-mutability in some sites of the genome that thus turn out to be more polymorphic than others.

2.2   GENE CONVERSION: THE CASE OF CLUSTERED SNPs IN THE HUMAN GENOME

One remarkable feature of the human genome is the abundance of duplicated elements that can be divided into two classes: (1) small interspersed repetitive elements whose features are to be at high copy number within the genome and (2) large low copy number duplications characterized by a high degree of sequence identity. About 41% of the genome is covered by the elements of the first class, whereas it has been estimated that about 5% of the human genome is composed of segmental duplications (SDs) (i.e., sequences that are duplicated either on the same or different chromosomes, with an identity >90% and a length >1 kb) (Bailey et al., 2001, 2002; She et al., 2004; Zhang et al., 2004). Once initially formed, SDs can promote further genomic rearrangements through nonallelic homologous recombination (HR); thus playing an important role in genome evolution and disease (Armengol et al., 2003; Cheng et al., 2005; Eichler, 2001; Samonte and Eichler, 2002; Stankiewicz et al., 2004). By analyzing public and private human genome sequences it has been observed that duplicated sequences of the human genome such as SD are particularly enriched of SNPs. It has been suggested that the excess of SNPs in these genomic regions may be nothing more than differences between paralogous sequences (paralogous sequence variants, PSVs), which have been misassembled in the draft of the human genome sequence; but recently several studies revealed that in repeated region of the human genome it is possible to observe an excess of clustered SNPs (Chen et al., 2007; Cruciani et al., 2011; Hallast et al., 2005; Trombetta et al., 2014, 2010). Moreover, an excess of clustered SNPs has been also observed within the long terminal repeats elements, a particular class of interspersed repetitive elements (belonging to the first class described earlier) that are found at the either ends of human endogenous retroviruses (Trombetta et al., 2016).

The presence of a group of derived alleles of several SNPs tightly linked on the same chromosome is often due to gene conversion: The main molecular mechanism used to repair DSBs in DNA. DSBs are strong inducers of HR, which will potentially lead to chromosomal aberrations if the template sequence is a paralogous rather than allelic region (Richardson et al., 1998). However, 98% of the DSBs, which are repaired by HR, are resolved by ectopic gene conversion rather than crossing-over (Chen et al., 2007). The repair of DSBs involves gene conversion between homologous chromosomes or sister chromatids, but it could also occur between paralogous regions.

Gene conversion is a standard type of recombination that, unlike crossing-over, involves the nonreciprocal transfer of genetic information from a "donor" sequence to a highly similar "acceptor" (Chen et al., 2007). In mammals, it constitutes the main form of HR and it always starts with a DSB in the acceptor sequence. During this process, the broken region uses the intact homologous strand as a template to repair itself and the main effect is that the acceptor sequence becomes identical to the donor, which remains unchanged. Despite its misleading name, gene conversion does not take place only within genes. Indeed, it can potentially occur in any duplicated region of the genome. However, efficient gene conversion usually requires a sequence similarity of >88%. Gene conversion has important evolutionary consequences. Its main effect is to increase the similarity between the interacting paralogs, making them more closely related to each other than to their orthologous counterparts (Hurles and Jobling, 2001). Moreover, inter-locus gene conversion can also increase the allelic diversity in the acceptor sequence by generating a clusters of SNPs (Nielsen, 2003; Trombetta et al., 2010, 2016). Indeed, when gene conversion involves several PSVs (i.e., single nucleotide differences between the two interacting paralogs), the bases on the donor sequence will change the status of the paralogous bases on the acceptor chromosome. As a consequence, the PSVs will disappear and new SNPs will be introduced in the population (Trombetta and Cruciani, 2017). It has been observed that gene conversion could favor some variants over others (Marais, 2003). A conversion bias is to be expected when one paralog bearing a particular state variant is more prone to DSBs. This process, known as biased gene conversion (bGC), tends to favor the paralog bearing the G (or C) variant as a donor rather than the paralog with the A (or T) variant which will act as acceptor sequence. The result of this process is an increased number of A/G SNPs in duplicated region of the genomes (Hallast et al., 2013). Recently, bGC has been described within the ampliconic region of the avian W chromosome (Backström et al., 2005) and for Y–Y gene conversion occurring between the arms of the P6 palindrome of the human MSY (Hallast et al., 2013).

Often the gene conversion rate is similar (or higher) than the mutation rate (Chen et al., 2007). It implies that it is a strong inducer of SNPs and that attention should be paid in interpreting an identity by state as an identity by descent for the SNPs in duplicate regions of the genome (Adams et al., 2006).

2.3 *DE NOVO* MUTATION (DNM) RATE OF THE HUMAN GENOME: THE ONSET OF NEW SNPs

Germ line DNMs are the main source of the genetic variability at the basis of all the human evolutionary adaptations and heritable diseases (Ségurel et al., 2014).

Because of the importance of the *de novo* mutations, several studies have been focused on the estimation of the *de novo* mutation rate by the analysis of different members of the same family. Due to technical difficulties, most of the first studies about germline mutation rate were restricted to specific genes involved in Mendelian diseases or to defined regions of the human genome (Crow, 2000; Kondrashov, 2003; Neale et al., 2012; Xue et al., 2009).

Over the past decade, the next generation sequencing technologies have allowed the analysis of the whole genome of several individuals at reduced costs and this technological improvement was exploited in several studies to obtain a better estimation of the DNM rate analyzing several trios (i.e., familiar groups composed by father, mother, and one child) or, in some cases, multisibling families (Campbell and Eichler, 2013; Conrad et al., 2011; Goldmann et al., 2016; Kong et al., 2012; Michaelson et al., 2012; Rahbari et al., 2016; Ségurel et al., 2014). All the studies led to comparable estimates of the DNM rate, whose average figure is of 1×10^{-8} mutations/nucleotide/generation, roughly corresponding to 60 DNMs/diploid genome (Campbell and Eichler, 2013).

However, the DNM rate is not uniform along the human genome. For example, CpG sites show a higher mutation rate compared to the rest of the genome, and it has been estimated that they account for about the 19% of the DNMs, even though they only represent 2% of the genome (Hodgkinson and Eyre-Walker, 2011; Ségurel et al., 2014).

Another factor affecting the DNM rate is the parental age, due to an increasing number of DNMs as the number of cell divisions and DNA replication increase. A maternal age effect is well known for the occurrence of novel structural variants and aneuploidy, such as the trisomy 21 (Nagaoka et al., 2012). However, the maternal age effect has been found to be small for DNMs while, on the other hand, the paternal age effect for the insurgence of DNMs was repeatedly confirmed by several studies (Francioli et al., 2014; Goldmann et al., 2016; Kong et al., 2012; Nagaoka et al., 2012; Ségurel et al., 2014; Wong et al., 2016).

2.3.1 GERMLINE MUTATIONS AND THE PATERNAL AGE EFFECT

A higher mutation rate in men than in women was first proposed in 1947 by Haldane in a pioneering work on hemophilia, when the nature of the genetic material was still unknown (Haldane, 1947). This finding has been repeatedly confirmed by studies focused on Mendelian diseases (Ségurel et al., 2014) and by several recent genome-wide studies, which highlighted that the number of DNMs of paternal origin inherited by the offspring increases with the father's age (Goldmann et al., 2016; Goriely and Wilkie, 2012; Kong et al., 2012; Michaelson et al., 2012; Momand et al., 2013; Rahbari et al., 2016; Roach et al., 2010).

The differences between the paternal and maternal DNM rate can be explained considering the difference between the male and female gametogenesis. During the female gametogenesis, called oogenesis, the primary oocytes are produced before the birth of the woman and have experienced a fixed number of cell divisions and genome replications (about 23 from the primordial female germ cell to the female gamete) (Nagaoka et al., 2012). On the contrary, the male gametogenesis, or spermatogenesis, lasts all the man's life and the spermatogenic stem cells undergo continuous genome replications. It has been estimated that the germ line of a 20-year-old man has experienced about 160 genome replications and this number increases about four times to 610 when the man is 40 years old (Wilson Sayres and Makova, 2011).

It has been proposed that, in some specific cases, the increase of DNMs with the father's age could be further enhanced by a selfish spermatogonial selection that occurs when mutated stem cells acquire a growth advantage. This leads in turn to a faster clonal proliferation and to a disproportion of mutated sperms as paternal age increases. This theory seems to be supported by the analysis of some Mendelian disorders due to SNPs that arose in loci involved in the RAS pathway, which also controls the stem cell proliferation (Arnheim and Calabrese, 2016; Campbell and Eichler, 2013; Goriely and Wilkie, 2012; Paul and Robaire, 2013). For example, Apert syndrome and achondroplasia are due to single nucleotide mutations occurring in the fibroblast growth factor receptor 2 and 3 (*FGFR2* and *FGFR3*), respectively. In both cases, a strong paternal age effect has been reported, with the 95%–100% of the reported cases of these rare syndromes that are due to missense gain-of-function DNMs of paternal origin (Campbell and Eichler, 2013; Goriely and Wilkie, 2012).

The increased number of DNMs because of the paternal age effect is thought to be also involved in other congenital anomalies that were found to be more frequent in children of elderly fathers (Bille et al., 2005; Nybo Andersen and Urhoj, 2017; Su et al., 2015; Urhoj et al., 2015; Zhu et al., 2005).

In addition, some studies have been focused on the link between the higher number of DNMs transmitted by elderly fathers and childhood cancers, since this type of tumors are probably due to single nucleotide mutations which may have been inherited from parents in the affected children (Nybo Andersen and Urhoj, 2017). A consistent bulk of observations seems to point toward an increase of the risk of childhood acute lymphoblastic leukemia and retinoblastoma in the children of old fathers (Dockerty et al., 2001; Heck et al., 2012; Larfors et al., 2012; Moll et al., 1996; Sergentanis et al., 2015).

Finally, advanced paternal age has also been linked to neurodevelopmental outcomes in children, with several studies showing an association with schizophrenia and autism spectrum disorders (Malaspinas et al., 2014; Nybo Andersen and Urhoj, 2017).

The paternal age effect has been almost exclusively analyzed in families in which the fathers were not older than 45, even though few studies involving over 55 fathers have been conducted (Francioli et al., 2015; Goldmann et al., 2016; Jónsson et al., 2018; Kong et al., 2012; Rahbari et al., 2016). The observations collected so far seem to fit with a linear model explaining the higher number of paternally inherited DNMs over time, with an estimated increase of 2.0–2.9 per year (Francioli et al., 2015; Kong et al., 2012; Rahbari et al., 2016). However, other data seem to point toward a model in which the paternal DNMs increase exponentially with the father's age (Kong et al., 2012) and this difference has been explained, at least in part, by cases of selfish spermatogonial selection (Campbell and Eichler, 2013).

2.3.2 HYPER-MUTATIONAL SITES IN THE HUMAN GENOME: THE CASE OF THE CpG DINUCLEOTIDES

The mutational model for single nucleotide substitutions provides that the number of possible transversions is twice that of the transitions; therefore, by analyzing the distribution of the SNPs in a population, one would expect to observe more transversions than transitions. On the contrary, in the human genome there is an increased number of transitions, partially due to the high mutation rate at a particular dinucleotide: a C followed by a G (known as CpG site).

CpGs show a mutation rate about 10 times higher than the observed mutation rate at non-CpG sites (Awadalla et al., 2010; Conrad et al., 2011; Hodgkinson and Eyre-Walker, 2011; Kong et al., 2012). The higher mutability reported for these sites is explained considering that cytosine can experience deamination. The deamination of a cytosine produces uracil, which is not one of the four default DNA bases and can be easily recognized and corrected by the mismatch repairing system during the DNA replication. However, cytosine can be methylated (about 75% of CpG in the human shown a –CH_3 group at the 5-carbon of the cytosine ring), as part of the epigenetic genomic regulation, and the 5′-methylecytosine (5′-meC) can experience a spontaneous deamination, yielding a thymine. Since thymine is one of the default DNA bases, the mismatch is often not recognized by the repairing machinery, leading to a C-to-T mutation in the successive step of replication. The final result is that CpG sites are the hot spots of mutations and that the sharing of the derived state of a SNPs in these particular sites may not indicate an identity by descent but simply an identity by state due to the high mutation rates of these sites.

Importantly, demethylation of 5'-meC cannot fully explain the mutational pattern at CpG sites. For example, also the rate of transversions is higher in CpGs compared with the rest of the genome and, on the other hand, the mutation rate at CpGs was found to be about seven times lower in CG-rich portions of the genome. This finding, that seems to be at odds with the higher CpG mutability generally observed, has been partly explained considering two features of the GC-rich sequences: (1) their higher stability and (2) their lower methylation level. The first explanation is based on the fact that deamination requires the separation of the two DNA strands, which occurs less easily in GC-rich sequences because of the strongest strand pairing due to the three hydrogen bonds between C and G (compared to the weaker two hydrogen bonds between A and T) (Ségurel et al., 2014).

Regarding the second feature, the low methylation can explain only in part the lower mutation rate observed in these regions and a negative selection effect has been proposed as a possible explanation for the lower mutation rate observed (Panchin et al., 2016).

Another clue suggesting that methylation is not the only factor affecting CpGs higher mutation rate, came from a recent study investigating how the sequence context affect the mutational pattern (Aggarwala and Voight, 2016). The authors found that two different sequences contexts (GTACGCA and GATCGCA), both with a methylation level higher that 94% in sperms, show a difference in the C-to-T mutation probability at CpGs of about twice. All these data seem to suggest that, although demethylation of 5'-meC and subsequent C-to-T transition can explain much of the high CpG mutation rate, other factors can be important as well, such as the sequence context, which in turns correlates with different biological features and mechanisms (Aggarwala and Voight, 2016; Panchin et al., 2016; Ségurel et al., 2014).

2.4   THE SNPs AS ANALYSIS TOOLS: THE CASE OF THE HUMAN Y CHROMOSOME

The human Y chromosome, with its unique genetic features, is a useful tool for investigating many issues regarding a wide range of fields including forensic science (Jobling et al., 1997), human population genetics (Underhill and Kivisild, 2007), medical genetics (Krausz et al., 2004), and the analysis of the dynamics of fundamental evolutionary mechanisms of the human genome (Bosch et al., 2004; Repping et al., 2006; Rosser et al., 2009; Trombetta et al., 2010).

For more than 20 years, the Y chromosome diversity has been used by geneticists to solve specific forensic cases in which routinely used autosomal SNPs could be uninformative. These cases range from fatherless paternity tests to generation of male-specific profiles in presence of strongly unbalanced male - female mixture (Maiquilla et al., 2011; Roewer, 2009).

To date, these analyses were mainly based on highly variable microsatellite markers (Y-STR), but, with the introduction of NGS technologies, the forensic interest on Y-SNPs has rapidly increased (Xue and Tyler-Smith, 2010).

One of the most important advantages in the forensic use of Y-SNPs with respect to Y-STRs is their potential as ancestry informative markers (AIMs) in suspect-less cases, allowing hypotheses to be formulated on the geographic origin/ethnicity of a DNA trace (Ralf et al., 2015; van Oven et al., 2013; Wetton et al., 2005), with the due cautions (King et al., 2007a, b). To be considered as a useful AIM, a *de novo* identified Y-SNP should be restricted to a certain geographic area and its frequency distribution must be known in a worldwide population sample (D'Atanasio et al., 2018; Trombetta et al., 2015; van Oven et al., 2013).

2.4.1 STRUCTURE AND FEATURES OF THE HUMAN Y CHROMOSOME

The male-specific portion of the human Y chromosome (MSY), along with the mitochondrial DNA (mtDNA), represents a particular region of the human genome, because of its peculiar inheritance pattern. Indeed, most of the human genome is diploid, is passed down from one generation to the next one by both parents and undergoes meiotic crossing-over, which reshuffles the loci between maternal and paternal chromosomes. On the contrary, the MSY escapes this rule: it is haploid and lacks the meiotic recombination with the X chromosome (Jobling et al., 2013). For these reasons, the Y-SNPs are simpler to analyze compared to the autosomal SNPs, making the MSY an excellent tool to analyze the genetic features of the human genome.

The MSY represents the largest portion of the human Y chromosome, covering about 95% of its length, whereas the remaining 5% is represented by two subtelomeric pseudoautosomal regions (PARs) (Skaletsky et al., 2003). The PARs take their name from their inheritance pattern, since they undergo meiotic crossing-over and pass down to the following generation as autosomes. On the contrary, the MSY lacks meiotic recombination and is transmitted unaltered to the offspring. More precisely, the presence of the Y chromosome determines the male sex in humans, so the MSY is transmitted with a male uniparental inheritance pattern, from fathers to sons along the patrilineages (Jobling and Tyler-Smith, 2003, 2017). In this regard, it represents the male counterpart of the mitochondrial DNA, which is inherited along the matrilineages (Torroni et al., 2006; Underhill and Kivisild, 2007). Within the MSY, three classes of sequences can be recognized: the X-transposed region, the X-degenerate region, and the ampliconic region (Skaletsky et al., 2003).

The X-transposed region was formed by a transpositional event from the X chromosome to the Y chromosome in recent times, after the divergence between the human and the chimpanzee lineages. Because of its recent origin, this region shows about 99% of sequence similarity with the X chromosome (Skaletsky et al., 2003). The X-degenerate portion of the MSY represents the remains of the ancient pair of autosomes from which the sex chromosomes evolved (Bachtrog, 2013; Hughes and Rozen, 2012) and shows a sequence similarity with the X chromosome from 60% to 95%, depending on the time when the block of crossing-over occurred (Bachtrog, 2013; Skaletsky et al., 2003). Finally, the ampliconic region is characterized by eight palindromic structures, whose arms show a sequence identity of > 99%, maintained by gene conversion events (Trombetta et al., 2017).

The main source of variability of the MSY is the sequential accumulation of mutations, mainly SNPs. The Y-SNPs can be considered stable variants, because they usually arise with a low rate (Balanovsky, 2017; Helgason et al., 2015; Xue et al., 2009), and they are not reshuffled by the meiotic crossing-over, being passed down to the next generation as a unique block. So, if two Y chromosomes share the same SNPs, they probably descend from the same ancestor chromosome, where the variants firstly arose. Following this line of reasoning, it is possible to group together the Y chromosomes on the basis of the shared SNPs: each group of Y chromosomes can be considered a monophyletic entity, since all its members descend from the same common ancestor, and it is defined as a haplogroup (Jobling et al., 2013).

The haplogroups can be in turn organized in an unambiguous phylogenetic tree (Underhill and Kivisild, 2007). The main elements of a phylogenetic tree are the branches (or lineages or clades), corresponding to haplogroups, and the nodes, representing the points where two or more lineages diverge. Assuming a negligible effect of selection, we can assume that the rate of onset of new SNPs is constant over time and along a phylogeny. So, it is possible to use the variability accumulated along two or more clades as a measure of the Time of Their Most Recent Common Ancestor (TMRCA) (Jobling et al., 2013), since the two figures as directly related according to the following equation, where v is a measure of the accumulated variability along a lineage, t is the TMRCA, and μ is the mutation rate:

$$v = \mu \times t$$

This approach is known as the molecular clock hypothesis and has been widely used to estimate the TMRCA of the Y chromosome haplogroups to make inferences about the past human evolution (Batini and Jobling, 2017).

2.4.2 Y-SNPs MUTATION RATES

To obtain accurate TMRCA estimates, an accurate estimate of the mutation rate (μ) must be used. Over time, several studies have been focused on the estimate of the MSY mutation rate and several approaches have been used (Wang et al., 2014).

The first mutation rate estimates relied on the sequence comparison between Y chromosome of human and chimpanzee (Kuroki et al., 2006; Thomson et al., 2000). Counting the number of single-nucleotide substitutions (SNSs) between human and chimpanzee in a sequence of length l (expressed as the number of analyzed bases) and knowing the split time T between their evolutionary lineages, the mutation rate was calculated according to the following formula:

μ = (Number of SNSs between human and chimpanzee MSY)/2Tl.

In this context, it is worth noting that the single nucleotide differences between different species cannot be defined as SNPs, since, as explained earlier, the term "polymorphism" means that there are at least two alleles, with the less common observed with a frequency higher than 1%, within the same population. This is not the case for the interspecies SNSs, because each state of the variant site may have been fixed in each species. This estimate method needs at least three assumptions: (1) the parameter T is precisely known; (2) it is possible to perform a precise sequence alignment between different portions of the human and chimpanzee MSY despite the structural differences shown by this genomic region in the two species (Hughes and Page, 2015); (3) the evolution rate was the same in the human and chimpanzee lineages. However, none of three assumptions have not been definitively verified (Wang et al., 2014).

Another way to estimate the human Y mutation rate is to derive it from the human autosomal mutation rate, taking into account the strict patrilineal inheritance of the MSY (Mendez et al., 2013; Scozzari et al., 2014). The advantage of this approach is that the autosomal mutation rate was repeatedly confirmed and is based on a high number or reliable SNPs (Kong et al., 2012). However, this calculation assumes that the mutational process is the same in the autosomes and the Y chromosomes, without considering the specific features of the MSY.

Because of the issues linked in the use of a Y mutation rate calculated from interspecies comparisons or derived from the autosomal one, intraspecies Y-specific estimation methods have been preferred over the last years. These methods can be grouped in three main categories (Balanovsky, 2017): pedigree-based estimates, estimates based on calibration on known historical events, and estimates based on calibration on radiocarbon dated ancient human remains.

The first pedigree-based estimate of the Y chromosome mutation rate was 1.0×10^{-9} mutation/nucleotide/year and was based on the analysis of two Chinese individuals belonging to the same pedigree and separated by 13 generations (Xue et al., 2009). Taking advantage of the technological improvement due to NGS (Jobling and Tyler-Smith, 2017), a recent study recalculated the MSY mutation rate analyzing the whole-genome sequences of 753 Icelandic males organized in 274 patrilineages, for a total of 2449 meiosis considered (Helgason et al., 2015). The obtained rate was 0.83×10^{-9} mutation/nucleotide/year (0.88×10^{-9} mutation/nucleotide/year for only the X-degenerate portion), consistently with the previous estimate.

Differently from the former approach, the estimates calibrated on historical events or ancient remains are based on the variability accumulated in the Y phylogeny rather than on the number of new mutational events in a pedigree and the obtained mutation rate is defined "evolutionary mutation rate."

The calibration based on historical event relies on the assumption that a specific and well-known fact is causally related with the origin/expansion of a specific Y haplogroup. For example, linking a Sardinian specific Y subhaplogroup with the Neolithic colonization of this island, this approach was used to calibrate the Y phylogeny including more than 1000 Sardinian males, yielding a mutation rate of 0.65×10^{-9} mutation/nucleotide/year (Francalacci et al., 2013). However, the same approach led to a faster mutation rate (0.82×10^{-9} mutation/nucleotide/year) when applied to a phylogeny of 69 males, where the calibration point was the origin of the Q-L54/M3 haplogroup (Poznik et al., 2013). The coalescence age of this haplogroup is thought to be linked to the peopling of the Americas, which is usually dated to 15,000 years ago.

Finally, the calibration on ancient remains is performed including the Y chromosome data of at least one fossil in the phylogeny composed of modern Y sequences. The branch representing the ancient Y chromosome will be shorter than the modern ones, because that lineage have stopped accumulating new mutations since the moment of the death of the ancient specimen. So, the ancient lineage can be considered a sort of snapshot of the Y variability at the time when the ancient man lived (and died). Estimating the mean difference in the number of SNPs between ancient and modern samples, and knowing the radiocarbon date of the ancient specimen, it is possible to calibrate the whole Y phylogeny and to estimate the mutation rate (Balanovsky, 2017). Several studies used this approach, using one or more Y chromosomes from ancient males as calibration points and all the estimated mutation rates were comparable, about 0.75×10^{-9} mutation/nucleotide/year (D'Atanasio et al., 2018; Fu et al., 2014; Karmin et al., 2015; Trombetta et al., 2015).

All the three Y-specific approaches to estimate the MSY mutation rate have pros and cons. The main advantage of the pedigree-based methods is the direct estimate of the mutation rate, without the possible errors linked to the assumptions made in the calibration approaches. However, it does not take into account the loss of SNPs over time due to the effects of selection, yielding a faster mutation rate. When the pedigree mutation rate is used to estimate deep nodes of the Y phylogeny, this can lead to an under-estimation of their coalescence ages. For example, the coalescence age of an ancient node of the Y phylogeny (node A0'T) has been dated to about 170 thousand years ago with a rate calibrated on ancient remains (D'Atanasio et al., 2018), but a pedigree-based rate yielded a younger time estimate, of about 120 kilo-years ago (Hallast et al., 2015).

The calibration based on historical events has two main limits. First, it assumes a causal link between a Y haplogroup and a historical event, but the existence of this correlation and its exact date are often uncertain and matter of debate (Balanovsky, 2017). Second, the mutation rate estimate is usually based on the variability accumulated in only one haplogroup, that can have experienced different evolutionary processes compared with the rest of the Y phylogeny (Wang et al., 2014). For example, it has been observed a statistically significant reduction in the number of SNPs along the basal A0 lineage and the possible explanations can be population-specific differences in the mutation rate and/or differences in the selective pressure (Scozzari et al., 2014). The possible bias linked to this aspect can be solved using two or more calibration points, possibly linked to different haplogroups in the same phylogeny, to estimate a more reliable mutation rate (Wang et al., 2014).

The calibration with ancient remains relies on less assumptions and uses as temporal reference points the radiocarbon dates of the ancient remains, which are highly precise and reliable. Some issues linked to this method are due to the degradation and contamination of the ancient DNA, which can be addressed thanks to the technological improvement of the next generation sequencing techniques (Marciniak and Perry, 2017).

2.4.3   THE USE OF THE Y-SNPs: THE Y CHROMOSOME PHYLOGENETIC TREE

In the MSY, sequential accumulation of mutational events is the only source of intrapopulation genetic diversity (Rozen et al., 2003; Skaletsky et al., 2003). This process creates monophyletic entities, known as "haplogroups," which show a strong geographic differentiation due to molecular divergence during the dispersal of mankind over the continents(Jobling and Tyler-Smith, 2003). The phylogeographic approach keeps into account the phylogenetic relations among haplogroups and their ethnogeographic distribution. Thus, taking into account the Y-SNPs distribution around the world and the evolutionary relationships among different SNPs it is possible to understand some demographic processes behind the origin of *Homo sapiens* and the dispersal of human populations (Chiaroni et al., 2009).

Haplogroups are stable entities, as they are defined by markers (usually SNPs) with a low mutation rate; they can thus be arranged in an unambiguous maximum parsimony phylogenetic tree. The most recent high-resolution tree to encompass all haplogroups contains 20 main clades, indicated with letters from A to T (Karafet et al., 2008). Each clade is subdivided into subclades. The nomenclature of the branches (and therefore of the various clades) is alphanumeric, in which the first letter, corresponding to the main haplogroup (from A to T), is followed by a number indicating the subhaplogroup and then by another letter. The alternation of numbers and letters in the name of the clade gives us the necessary information to map a specific sample within the phylogenetic tree of the Y chromosome. By using this nomenclature, it is possible to classify every Y chromosome existing in the world (Karmin et al., 2015).

As new lineages are discovered and larger amounts of sequence are surveyed, the structure of the MSY phylogenetic tree is perpetually adjusted to accommodate the new findings. For example, in recent years, the deepest portion of the phylogeny was remarkably susceptible to such changes. The deepest split, separating haplogroup A from the rest of the phylogeny (Karafet et al., 2008), was challenged by the discovery of a completely different structure (Cruciani et al., 2011), which showed the polyphyletic nature of the lineages formerly grouped into haplogroup A. As a result, such linages were no more grouped together in a single clade, and haplogroup A1b (recently renamed as A0) was identified as the deepest-rooting branch. An even more recent work (Mendez et al., 2013) discovered a very deep, rare lineage, named A00, whose split from the rest of the phylogeny long predates that of A1b. Such radical changes in structure directly lead to adjustments of time estimates and geographic inferences associated with the phylogenetic tree; these subjects will be discussed in detail in the following sections.

2.4.4 DISTRIBUTION OF THE Y-CHROMOSOME HAPLOGROUPS

The geographic distribution of haplogroups, seen in the light of the phylogenetic relations linking them, provides clues on the dispersal of human population over the world. In a similar fashion, the distribution of the deepest branches can be informative on the evolutionary events that involved the oldest representatives of our species.

The deepest-rooting branches of the Y phylogeny, namely A00, A1b, A1a, A2, A3, and B, are found, with some exceptions, only in the African continent, though they only represent a small fraction of the overall genetic variation in the continent (Batini et al., 2011; Chiaroni et al., 2009; Cruciani et al., 2002, 2011; Jobling et al., 2013; King et al., 2007a, b; Mendez et al., 2013; Wood et al., 2005). A00 and A1b have only been reported, at very low frequencies, in small populations in central Africa (Cruciani et al., 2011; Mendez et al., 2013). A1a has been found at low frequencies too, having been reported in less than 30 individuals coming from a wide area spanning from Morocco to Senegal to Niger (with the exception of three Afro-Americans and an individual from Cape Verde) (Cruciani et al., 2002; Gonçalves et al., 2003; King et al., 2007a, b; Rosa et al., 2007; Vallone and Butler, 2004; Wood et al., 2005).

The presence of the deepest branches of the phylogeny within the African continent has been interpreted as an African origin of human male genetic variability. The man who gave origin of all the human male diversity (allegorically called "Adam" of the Y chromosome) lived in Africa. Obviously, this does not mean that he was the only man alive at the time, but that all lines of descent of the other males have been lost over time.

A2 and A3 clades are sister clades stemming from a short branch (Batini et al., 2011; Scozzari et al., 2012). A2 is mostly found in Khoisan populations from Southern Africa; a specific A2 branch has recently been observed in Central Africa pygmies (Batini et al., 2011). A3 shows a dual distribution with A3a being found in Eastern Africa only, and its sister clade A3b displaying a clear differentiation between South Africa and Central-Eastern Africa.

Haplogroup B is mainly confined to sub-Saharan Africa (Butler, 2003; Consortium, 2002; Cruciani et al., 2002; Gomes et al., 2010; Karafet et al., 2008; Semino et al., 2002; Underhill et al., 2000, 2001; Vallone and Butler, 2004) and is divided in two main branches; the first, B1, has been so far observed Cameroon, Mali, and Burkina Faso; the other, B2, has a wider distribution, being found in Eastern, Central, and Southern Africa, with its subhaplogroups reaching frequencies as high as 70% in some ethnic groups (Berniell-Lee et al., 2009; Knight et al., 2003; Tishkoff et al., 2007; Wood et al., 2005).

Proceeding further down the tree after haplogroup B, we found the split between macrohaplogroups DE and CT.

Haplogroup DE is characterized by the derived state of the only polymorphic Alu insertion in the MSY known to date (YAP, Y Alu Polymorphism). Haplogroup D is mainly found in Central and South-East Asia (Karafet et al., 2001), whereas haplogroup E is the most common haplogroup in Africa, but it is also found in Europe and Middle East. Within the African continent, different E subhaplogroups display a strong differential localization and peak at frequencies as high as 80% in some regions or populations (Battaglia et al., 2009; Beleza et al., 2005; Scozzari et al., 1999; Semino et al., 2004, 2002; Underhill et al., 2000; Wood et al., 2005; Cruciani et al., 2007, 2002, 2004; Gomes et al., 2010; Henn et al., 2008; Knight et al., 2003; Luis et al., 2004; Rosa et al., 2007).

Haplogroup CT is split into haplogroup C, found at high frequency in New Guinea and Australia (Underhill et al., 2001) and at lower frequency in Southern and Eastern Asia (Zhong et al., 2010), and macrohaplogroup F, which is widely distributed over the world, although it is rarely found in sub-Saharan Africa. This macrohaplogroup contains several branches, namely G, H, IJ, and macrohaplogroup KT. Haplogroup G is mainly found in the Mediterranean basin and the Caucasian region, whereas H is mostly present in India (Sengupta et al., 2006). Haplogroup I is distinctive of Europe (Battaglia et al., 2009; Rootsi et al., 2004), whereas J is more widely distributed and is found in Europe, Middle East, India, Central Asia, and Northern

Africa (Chiaroni et al., 2010; Di Giacomo et al., 2004; Hammer et al., 2000; Underhill et al., 2001).

K lineages are present in India (K1), Oceania and Indonesia (K2 to K4) (Consortium, 2002; Karafet et al., 2008; Underhill et al., 2001). Other main haplogroups within K are also found in India (L), Indonesia (M, S), and Oceania (O, S), but also in Northern Eurasia (N), Central Asia (O, T), Africa and Middle East (T) (Capelli et al., 2001; Jobling and Tyler-Smith, 2003; Karafet et al., 2001, 2008; Kayser et al., 2006; King et al., 2007a, b; Mona et al., 2007; Rootsi et al., 2007; Sanchez et al., 2005; Underhill et al., 2001). Haplogroup Q is peculiar of the American continent (Karafet et al., 2008), whereas haplogroup R is one of the most important contributors to the European MSY diversity (Balaresque et al., 2010; Myres et al., 2011; Underhill et al., 2010) but is also found at very high frequency in Central-Western Africa (Cruciani et al., 2010).

KEYWORDS

- **single-nucleotide polymorphisms**
- ***de novo* mutation rate**
- **human Y chromosome**
- **Y-SNPs mutation rate**
- **gene conversion**
- **clusters of SNPs**

REFERENCES

Adams, S. M.; et al.; The Case of the Unreliable SNP: Recurrent Back-Mutation of Y-Chromosomal Marker P25 through Gene Conversion. *Forensic Sci. Int.* **2006**, *159* (1), 14–20.

Aggarwala, V.; and Voight, B. F.; An Expanded Sequence Context Model Broadly Explains Variability in Polymorphism Levels across the Human Genome. *Nat. Genet.* **2016**, *48* (4), 349–355.

Armengol, L.; et al.; Enrichment of Segmental Duplications in Regions of Breaks of Synteny between the Human and Mouse Genomes Suggest Their Involvement in Evolutionary Rearrangements. *Hum. Mol. Genet.* **2003**, *12* (17), 2201–2208.

Arnheim, N.; and Calabrese, P.; Germline Stem Cell Competition, Mutation Hot Spots, Genetic Disorders, and Older Fathers. *Annu. Rev. Genomics Hum. Genet.* **2016**, *17* (1), 219–243.

Awadalla, P.; et al.; Direct Measure of the De Novo Mutation Rate in Autism and Schizophrenia Cohorts. *Am. J. Hum. Genet.* **2010**, *87* (3), 316–324.

Bachtrog, D.; Y-Chromosome Evolution: Emerging Insights into Processes of Y-Chromosome Degeneration. *Nat. Rev. Genet.* **2013**, *14* (2), 113–124.

Backström, N.; et al.; Gene Conversion Drives the Evolution of HINTW, an Ampliconic Gene on the Female-Specific Avian W Chromosome. *Mol. Biol. Evol.* **2005**, *22* (10), 1992–1999.

Bailey, J. A.; et al.; Segmental Duplications: Organization and Impact within the Current Human Genome Project Assembly. *Genome Res.* **2001**, *11* (6), 1005–1017.

Bailey, J. A.; et al.; Recent Segmental Duplications in the Human Genome. *Science (80-.).* **2002**, *297* (5583), 1003–1007.

Balanovsky, O.; Toward a Consensus on SNP and STR Mutation Rates on the Human Y-Chromosome. *Hum. Genet.* **2017**, *136* (5), 575–590.

Balaresque, P.; et al.; A Predominantly Neolithic Origin for European Paternal Lineages. *PLoS Biol.* **2010**, *8* (1), e1000285.

Batini, C.; et al.; Signatures of the Preagricultural Peopling Processes in Sub-Saharan Africa as Revealed by the Phylogeography of Early Y Chromosome Lineages. *Mol. Biol. Evol.* **2011**, *28* (9), 2603–2613.

Batini, C.; and Jobling, M. A.; Detecting Past Male-Mediated Expansions Using the Y Chromosome. *Hum. Genet.* **2017**, *136* (5), 1–11.

Battaglia, V.; et al.; Y-Chromosomal Evidence of the Cultural Diffusion of Agriculture in Southeast Europe. *Eur. J. Hum. Genet.* **2009**, *17* (6), 820–830.

Beleza, S.; et al.; The Genetic Legacy of Western Bantu Migrations. *Hum. Genet.* **2005**, *117* (4), 366–375.

Berniell-Lee, G.; et al.; Genetic and Demographic Implications of the Bantu Expansion: Insights from Human Paternal Lineages. *Mol. Biol. Evol.* **2009**, *26* (7), 1581–1589.

Bille, C.; et al.; Parent's Age and the Risk of Oral Clefts. *Epidemiology* **2005**, *16* (3), 311–316.

Bosch, E.; et al.; Dynamics of a Human Interparalog Gene Conversion Hotspot. *Genome Res.* **2004**, *14* (5), 835–844.

van den Bosch, M.; et al.; DNA Double-Strand Break Repair by Homologous Recombination. *Biol. Chem.* **2002**, *383* (6), 873–892.

Butler, J. M.; Recent Developments in Y-Short Tandem Repeat and Y-Single Nucleotide Polymorphism Analysis. *Forensic Sci. Rev.* **2003**, *15* (2), 91–111.

Campbell, C. D.; and Eichler, E. E.; Properties and Rates of Germline Mutations in Humans. *Trends Genet.* **2013**, *29* (10), 575–584.

Capelli, C.; et al.; A Predominantly Indigenous Paternal Heritage for the Austronesian-Speaking Peoples of Insular Southeast Asia and Oceania. *Am. J. Hum. Genet.* **2001**, *68* (2), 432–443.

Chakraborty, R.; et al.; The Utility of Short Tandem Repeat Loci beyond Human Identification: Implications for Development of New DNA Typing Systems. *Electrophoresis* **1999**, *20* (8), 1682–1696.

Chen, J.-M.; et al.; Gene Conversion: Mechanisms, Evolution and Human Disease. *Nat. Rev. Genet.* **2007**, *8* (10), 762–775.

Cheng, Z.; et al.; A Genome-Wide Comparison of Recent Chimpanzee and Human Segmental Duplications. *Nature* **2005**, *437* (7055), 88–93.

Chiaroni, J.; et al.; Y Chromosome Diversity, Human Expansion, Drift, and Cultural Evolution. *Proc. Natl. Acad. Sci.* **2009**, *106* (48), 20174–20179.

Chiaroni, J.; et al.; The Emergence of Y-Chromosome Haplogroup J1e among Arabic-Speaking Populations. *Eur. J. Hum. Genet.* **2010**, *18* (3), 348–353

Conrad, D. F.; et al.; Variation in Genome-Wide Mutation Rates within and between Human Families. *Nat. Genet.* **2011**, *43* (7), 712–714.

Consortium, T. Y. C.; A Nomenclature System for the Tree of Human Y-Chromosomal Binary Haplogroups. *Genome Res.* **2002**, *12* (2), 339–348.

Crow, J. F.; The Origins, Patterns and Implications of Human Spontaneous Mutation. *Nat. Rev. Genet.* **2000**, *1* (1), 40–47.

Cruciani, F.; et al.; Tracing Past Human Male Movements in Northern/Eastern Africa and Western Eurasia: New Clues from Y-Chromosomal Haplogroups E-M78 and J-M12. *Mol. Biol. Evol.* **2007**, *24* (6), 1300–1311.

Cruciani, F.; et al.; A Back Migration from Asia to Sub-Saharan Africa Is Supported by High-Resolution Analysis of Human Y-Chromosome Haplotypes. *Am. J. Hum. Genet.* **2002**, *70* (5), 1197–1214.

Cruciani, F.; et al.; Phylogeographic Analysis of Haplogroup E3b (E-M215) Y Chromosomes Reveals Multiple Migratory Events Within and Out of Africa. *Am. J. Hum. Genet.* **2004**, *74* (5), 1014–1022.

Cruciani, F.; et al.; Human Y Chromosome Haplogroup R-V88: A Paternal Genetic Record of Early Mid Holocene Trans-Saharan Connections and the Spread of Chadic Languages. *Eur. J. Hum. Genet.* **2010**, *18* (7), 800–807.

Cruciani, F.; et al.; A Revised Root for the Human Y Chromosomal Phylogenetic Tree: The Origin of Patrilineal Diversity in Africa. *Am. J. Hum. Genet.* **2011**, *88* (6), 814–818.

D'Atanasio, E.; et al.; The Peopling of the Last Green Sahara Revealed by High-Coverage Resequencing of Trans-Saharan Patrilineages. *Genome Biol.* **2018**, *19* (1), 20.

Dockerty, J. D.; et al.; Case-Control Study of Parental Age, Parity and Socioeconomic Level in Relation to Childhood Cancers. *Int. J. Epidemiol.* **2001**, *30* (6), 1428–1437.

Eichler, E. E.; Recent Duplication, Domain Accretion and the Dynamic Mutation of the Human Genome. *Trends Genet.* **2001**, *17* (11), 661–669.

Francalacci, P.; et al.; Low-Pass DNA Sequencing of 1200 Sardinians Reconstructs European Y-Chromosome Phylogeny. *Science (80-.)* **2013**, *341* (6145), 565–569.

Francioli, L. C.; et al.; Whole-Genome Sequence Variation, Population Structure and Demographic History of the Dutch Population. *Nat. Genet.* **2014**, *46* (8), 818–825.

Francioli, L. C.; et al.; Genome-Wide Patterns and Properties of De Novo Mutations in Humans. *Nat. Genet.* **2015**, *47* (7), 822–826.

Fu, Q.; et al.; Genome Sequence of a 45,000-Year-Old Modern Human from Western Siberia. *Nature* **2014**, *514* (7253), 445–449.

Di Giacomo, F.; et al.; Y Chromosomal Haplogroup J as a Signature of the Post-Neolithic Colonization of Europe. *Hum. Genet.* **2004**, *115* (5), 357–371.

Gibbs, R. A.; et al.; A Global Reference for Human Genetic Variation. *Nature* **2015**, *526* (7571), 68–74.

Goldmann, J. M.; et al.; Parent-of-Origin-Specific Signatures of De Novo Mutations. *Nat. Genet.* **2016**, *48* (8), 935–939.

Gomes, V.; et al.; Digging Deeper into East African Human Y Chromosome Lineages. *Hum. Genet.* **2010**, *127* (5), 603–613.

Gonçalves, R.; et al.; Y-Chromosome Lineages in Cabo Verde Islands Witness the Diverse Geographic Origin of Its First Male Settlers. *Hum. Genet.* **2003**, *113* (6), 467–472.

Goriely, A.; and Wilkie, A. O. M. O. M.; Paternal Age Effect Mutations and Selfish Spermatogonial Selection: Causes and Consequences for Human Disease. *Am. J. Hum. Genet.* **2012**, *90* (2), 175–200.

Haldane, J. B. S.; The Mutation Rate of the Gene for Haemophilia, and Its Segregation Ratios in Males and Females. *Ann. Eugen.* **1947**, *13* (4), 262–271.

Hallast, P.; et al.; Recombination Dynamics of a Human Y-Chromosomal Palindrome: Rapid GC-Biased Gene Conversion, Multi-Kilobase Conversion Tracts, and Rare Inversions. *PLoS Genet.* **2013**, *9* (7), e1003666.

Hallast, P.; et al.; Segmental Duplications and Gene Conversion: Human Luteinizing Hormone/ Chorionic Gonadotropin Beta Gene Cluster. *Genome Res.* **2005**, *15* (11), 1535–1546.

Hallast, P.; et al.; The Y-Chromosome Tree Bursts into Leaf: 13,000 High-Confidence SNPs Covering the Majority of Known Clades. *Mol. Biol. Evol.* **2015**, *32* (3), 661–673.

Hammer, M. F.; et al.; Jewish and Middle Eastern Non-Jewish Populations Share a Common Pool of Y-Chromosome Biallelic Haplotypes. *Proc. Natl. Acad. Sci.* **2000**, *97* (12), 6769–6774.

Heck, J. E.; et al.; Perinatal Characteristics and Retinoblastoma. *Cancer Causes Control* **2012**, *23* (9), 1567–1575.

Helgason, A.; et al.; The Y-Chromosome Point Mutation Rate in Humans. *Nat. Genet.* **2015**, *47* (5), 453–457.

Henn, B. M.; et al.; Y-Chromosomal Evidence of a Pastoralist Migration through Tanzania to Southern Africa. *Proc. Natl. Acad. Sci.* **2008**, *105* (31), 10693–10698.

Hodgkinson, A.; and Eyre-Walker, A.; *Variation in the Mutation Rate across Mammalian Genomes. Nat. Rev. Genet.* **2011**, *12*, 756–766.

Hughes, J. F.; and Rozen, S.; Genomics and Genetics of Human and Primate Y Chromosomes. *Annu. Rev. Genom. Hum. Genet.* **2012**, *13* (1), 83–108.

Hughes, J. F.; and Page, D. C.; The Biology and Evolution of Mammalian Y Chromosomes. *Annu. Rev. Genet.* **2015**, *49* (1), 507–527.

Hurles, M. E.; and Jobling, M. A.; Haploid Chromosomes in Molecular Ecology: Lessons from the Human Y. *Mol. Ecol.* **2001**, *10* (7), 1599–1613.

Jobling, M. A.; and Tyler-Smith, C.; The Human Y Chromosome: An Evolutionary Marker Comes of Age. *Nat. Rev. Genet.* **2003**, *4* (8), 598–612.

Jobling, M. A.; and Tyler-Smith, C.; Human Y-Chromosome Variation in the Genome-Sequencing Era. *Nat. Rev. Genet.* **2017**, *18* (8), 485–497.

Jobling, M. A.; et al.; The Y Chromosome in Forensic Analysis and Paternity Testing. *Int. J. Legal Med.* **1997**, *110* (3), 118–124.

Jobling, M. A.; et al.; *Human Evolutionary Genetics*, Second ed.; Garland Science, 2013.

Jónsson, H.; et al.; Multiple Transmissions of De Novo Mutations in Families. *Nat. Genet.* **2018**, *50* (12), 1674–1680.

Karafet, T. M.; et al.; New Binary Polymorphisms Reshape and Increase Resolution of the Human Y Chromosomal Haplogroup Tree. *Genome Res.* **2008**, *18* (5), 830–838.

Karafet, T.; et al.; Paternal Population History of East Asia: Sources, Patterns, and Microevolutionary Processes. *Am. J. Hum. Genet.* **2001**, *69* (3), 615–628.

Karmin, M.; et al.; A Recent Bottleneck of Y Chromosome Diversity Coincides with a Global Change in Culture. *Genome Res.* **2015**, *25* (4), 459–466.

Kayser, M.; et al.; Melanesian and Asian Origins of Polynesians: MtDNA and Y Chromosome Gradients across the Pacific. *Mol. Biol. Evol.* **2006**, *23* (11), 2234–2244.

King, T. E.; et al.; Thomas Jefferson's Y Chromosome Belongs to a Rare European Lineage. *Am. J. Phys. Anthropol.* **2007a**, *132* (4), 584–589.

King, T. E.; et al.; Africans in Yorkshire? The Deepest-Rooting Clade of the Y Phylogeny within an English Genealogy. *Eur. J. Hum. Genet.* **2007b**, *15* (3), 238–293.

Knight, A.; et al.; African Y Chromosome and MtDNA Divergence Provides Insight into the History of Click Languages. *Curr. Biol.* **2003**, *13* (6), 464–473.

Kondrashov, A. S.; Direct Estimates of Human per Nucleotide Mutation Rates at 20 Loci Causing Mendelian Diseases. *Hum. Mutat.* **2003**, *21* (1), 12–27.

Kong, A.; et al.; Rate of De Novo Mutations and the Importance of Father's Age to Disease Risk. *Nature* **2012**, *488* (7412), 471–475.

Krausz, C.; et al.; Y Chromosome Polymorphisms in Medicine. *Ann. Med.* **2004**, *36* (8), 573–583.

Kuroki, Y.; et al.; Comparative Analysis of Chimpanzee and Human Y Chromosomes Unveils Complex Evolutionary Pathway. *Nat. Genet.* **2006**, *38* (2), 158–167.

Lachance, J.; and Tishkoff, S. A.; SNP Ascertainment Bias in Population Genetic Analyses: Why It Is Important, and How to Correct It. *BioEssays* **2013**, *35* (9), 780–786.

Larfors, G.; et al.; Parental Age, Family Size, and Offspring's Risk of Childhood and Adult Acute Leukemia. *Cancer Epidemiol. Biomarkers Prev.* **2012**, *21* (7), 1185–1190.

Luis, J. R.; et al.; The Levant versus the Horn of Africa: Evidence for Bidirectional Corridors of Human Migrations. *Am. J. Hum. Genet.* **2004**, *74* (3), 532–544.

Maiquilla, S. M. B.; et al.; Y-STR DNA Analysis of 154 Female Child Sexual Assault Cases in the Philippines. *Int. J. Legal Med.* **2011**, *125* (6), 817–824.

Malaspinas, A.-S.; et al.; Two Ancient Human Genomes Reveal Polynesian Ancestry among the Indigenous Botocudos of Brazil. *Curr. Biol.* **2014**, *24* (21), R1035–R1037.

Marais, G.; Biased Gene Conversion: Implications for Genome and Sex Evolution. *Trends Genet.* **2003**, *19* (6), 330–338.

Marciniak, S.; and Perry, G. H.; Harnessing Ancient Genomes to Study the History of Human Adaptation. *Nat. Rev. Genet.* **2017**, *18* (11), 659–674.

Mendez, F. L.; et al.; An African American Paternal Lineage Adds an Extremely Ancient Root to the Human Y Chromosome Phylogenetic Tree. *Am. J. Hum. Genet.* **2013**, *92* (3), 454–459.

Michaelson, J. J.; et al.; Whole-Genome Sequencing in Autism Identifies Hot Spots for De Novo Germline Mutation. *Cell* **2012**, *151* (7), 1431–1442.

Moll, A. C.; et al.; High Parental Age Is Associated with Sporadic Hereditary Retinoblastoma: The Dutch Retinoblastoma Register 1862–1994. *Hum. Genet.* **1996**, *98* (1), 109–112.

Momand, J. R.; et al.; The Paternal Age Effect: A Multifaceted Phenomenon. *Biol. Reprod.* **2013**, *88* (4), 108.

Mona, S.; et al.; Patterns of Y-Chromosome Diversity Intersect with the Trans-New Guinea Hypothesis. *Mol. Biol. Evol.* **2007**, *24* (11), 2546–2555.

Myres, N. M.; et al.; A Major Y-Chromosome Haplogroup R1b Holocene Era Founder Effect in Central and Western Europe. *Eur. J. Hum. Genet.* **2011**, *19* (1), 95–101.

Nagaoka, S. I.; et al.; Human Aneuploidy: Mechanisms and New Insights into an Age-Old Problem. *Nat. Rev. Genet.* **2012**, *13* (7), 493–504.

Neale, B. M.; et al.; Patterns and Rates of Exonic De Novo Mutations in Autism Spectrum Disorders. *Nature* **2012**, *485* (7397), 242–245.

Nielsen, K. M.; Gene Conversion as a Source of Nucleotide Diversity in Plasmodium Falciparum. *Mol. Biol. Evol.* **2003**, *20* (5), 726–734.

Nybo Andersen, A. M.; and Urhoj, S. K.; Is Advanced Paternal Age a Health Risk for the Offspring? *Fertil. Steril.* **2017**, *107* (2), 312–318.

O'Driscoll, M.; and Jeggo, P. A.; The Role of Double-Strand Break Repair—Insights from Human Genetics. *Nat. Rev. Genet.* **2006**, *7* (1), 45–54.

van Oven, M.; et al.; Multiplex Genotyping Assays for Fine-Resolution Subtyping of the Major Human Y-Chromosome Haplogroups E, G, I, J, and R in Anthropological, Genealogical, and Forensic Investigations. *Electrophoresis* **2013**, *34* (20–21), 3029–3038.

Panchin, A. Y.; et al.; Preservation of Methylated CpG Dinucleotides in Human CpG Islands. *Biol. Direct* **2016**, *11* (1), 11.

Paul, C.; and Robaire, B.; Ageing of the Male Germ Line. *Nat. Rev. Urol.* **2013**, *10* (4), 227–234.

Pereira, V.; et al.; Evaluation of the Precision ID Ancestry Panel for Crime Case Work: A SNP Typing Assay Developed for Typing of 165 Ancestral Informative Markers. *Forensic Sci. Int. Genet.* **2017**, *28*, 138–145.

Poznik, G. D.; et al.; Sequencing Y Chromosomes Resolves Discrepancy in Time to Common Ancestor of Males versus Females. *Science* **2013**, *341* (6145), 562–565.

Rahbari, R.; et al.; Timing, Rates and Spectra of Human Germline Mutation. *Nat. Genet.* **2016**, *48* (2), 126–133.

Ralf, A.; et al.; Simultaneous Analysis of Hundreds of Y-Chromosomal SNPs for High-Resolution Paternal Lineage Classification Using Targeted Semiconductor Sequencing. *Hum. Mutat.* **2015**, *36* (1), 151–159.

Reich, D. E.; et al.; Quality and Completeness of SNP Databases. *Nat. Genet.* **2003**, *33* (4), 457–458.

Repping, S.; et al.; High Mutation Rates Have Driven Extensive Structural Polymorphism among Human Y Chromosomes. *Nat. Genet.* **2006**, *38* (4), 463–467.

Richardson, C.; et al.; Double-Strand Break Repair by Interchromosomal Recombination: Suppression of Chromosomal Translocations. *Genes Dev.* **1998**, *12* (24), 3831–3842.

Roach, J. C.; et al.; Analysis of Genetic Inheritance in a Family Quartet by Whole-Genome Sequencing. *Science* **2010**, *328* (5978), 636–639.

Roewer, L.; Y Chromosome STR Typing in Crime Casework. *Forensic Sci. Med. Pathol.* **2009**, *5* (2), 77–84.

Rootsi, S.; et al.; Phylogeography of Y-Chromosome Haplogroup I Reveals Distinct Domains of Prehistoric Gene Flow in Europe. *Am. J. Hum. Genet.* **2004**, *75* (1), 128–137.

Rootsi, S.; et al.; A Counter-Clockwise Northern Route of the Y-Chromosome Haplogroup N from Southeast Asia towards Europe. *Eur. J. Hum. Genet.* **2007**, *15* (2), 204–211.

Rosa, A.; et al.; Y-Chromosomal Diversity in the Population of Guinea-Bissau: A Multiethnic Perspective. *BMC Evol. Biol.* **2007**, *7* (1), 124.

Rosser, Z. H.; et al.; Gene Conversion between the X Chromosome and the Male-Specific Region of the Y Chromosome at a Translocation Hotspot. *Am. J. Hum. Genet.* **2009**, *85* (1), 130–134.

Rozen, S.; et al.; Abundant Gene Conversion between Arms of Palindromes in Human and Ape Y Chromosomes. *Nature* **2003**, *423* (6942), 873–876.

Samonte, R. V.; and Eichler, E. E.; Segmental Duplications and the Evolution of the Primate Genome. *Nat. Rev. Genet.* **2002**, *3* (1), 65–72.

Sanchez, J. J.; et al.; High Frequencies of Y Chromosome Lineages Characterized by E3b1, DYS19-11, DYS392-12 in Somali Males. *Eur. J. Hum. Genet.* **2005**, *13* (7), 856–866.

Scozzari, R.; et al.; Combined Use of Biallelic and Microsatellite Y-Chromosome Polymorphisms to Infer Affinities among African Populations. *Am. J. Hum. Genet.* **1999**, *65* (3), 829–846.

Scozzari, R.; et al.; Molecular Dissection of the Basal Clades in the Human Y Chromosome Phylogenetic Tree. *PLoS One* **2012**, *7* (11), e49170.

Scozzari, R.; et al.; An Unbiased Resource of Novel SNP Markers Provides a New Chronology for the Human Y Chromosome and Reveals a Deep Phylogenetic Structure in Africa. *Genome Res.* **2014**, *24* (3), 535–544.

Ségurel, L.; et al.; Determinants of Mutation Rate Variation in the Human Germline. *Annu. Rev. Genomics Hum. Genet.* **2014**, *15* (1), 47–70.

Semino, O.; et al.; Ethiopians and Khoisan Share the Deepest Clades of the Human Y-Chromosome Phylogeny. *Am. J. Hum. Genet.* **2002**, *70* (1), 265–268.

Semino, O.; et al.; Origin, Diffusion, and Differentiation of Y-Chromosome Haplogroups E and J: Inferences on the Neolithization of Europe and Later Migratory Events in the Mediterranean Area. *Am. J. Hum. Genet.* **2004**, *74* (5), 1023–1034.

Sengupta, S.; et al.; Polarity and Temporality of High-Resolution Y-Chromosome Distributions in India Identify Both Indigenous and Exogenous Expansions and Reveal Minor Genetic Influence of Central Asian Pastoralists. *Am. J. Hum. Genet.* **2006**, *78* (2), 202–221.

Sergentanis, T. N.; et al.; Risk for Childhood Leukemia Associated with Maternal and Paternal Age. *Eur. J. Epidemiol.* **2015**, *30* (12), 1229–1261.

Serventi, P.; et al.; Iron Age Italic Population Genetics: The Piceni from Novilara (8th-7th Century BC). *Ann. Hum. Biol.* **2018**, *45* (1), 34–43.

She, X.; et al.; Shotgun Sequence Assembly and Recent Segmental Duplications within the Human Genome. *Nature* **2004**, *431* (7011), 927–930.

Shrivastav, M.; et al.; Regulation of DNA Double-Strand Break Repair Pathway Choice. *Cell Res.* **2008**, *18* (1), 134–147.

Skaletsky, H.; et al.; The Male-Specific Region of the Human Y Chromosome Is a Mosaic of Discrete Sequence Classes. *Nature* **2003**, *423* (6942), 825–837.

Stankiewicz, P.; et al.; Serial Segmental Duplications during Primate Evolution Result in Complex Human Genome Architecture. *Genome Res.* **2004**, *14* (11), 2209–2220.

Su, X. J.; et al.; Paternal Age and Offspring Congenital Heart Defects: A National Cohort Study. *PLoS One* **2015**, *10* (3), e0121030.

Sudmant, P. H.; et al.; Global Diversity, Population Stratification, and Selection of Human Copy-Number Variation. *Science.* **2015**, *349* (6253), aab3761.

The 1000 Genomes Project Consortium; A global reference for human genetic variation. *Nature.* 2015, *526* (7571), 68–74.

Thomson, R.; et al.; Recent Common Ancestry of Human Y Chromosomes: Evidence from DNA Sequence Data. *Proc. Natl. Acad. Sci.* **2000**, *97* (13), 7360–7365.

Tishkoff, S. A.; et al.; History of Click-Speaking Populations of Africa Inferred from MtDNA and Y Chromosome Genetic Variation. *Mol. Biol. Evol.* **2007**, *24* (10), 2180–2195.

Torroni, A.; et al.; Harvesting the Fruit of the Human MtDNA Tree. *Trends Genet.* **2006**, *22* (6), 339–345.

Trombetta, B.; and Cruciani, F.; Y Chromosome Palindromes and Gene Conversion. *Hum. Genet.* **2017**, *136* (5), 1–15.

Trombetta, B.; et al.; Footprints of X-to-Y Gene Conversion in Recent Human Evolution. *Mol. Biol. Evol.* **2010**, *27* (3), 714–725.

Trombetta, B.; et al.; Inter- and Intraspecies Phylogenetic Analyses Reveal Extensive X-Y Gene Conversion in the Evolution of Gametologous Sequences of Human Sex Chromosomes. *Mol. Biol. Evol.* **2014**, *31* (8), 2108–2123.

Trombetta, B.; et al.; Phylogeographic Refinement and Large Scale Genotyping of Human Y Chromosome Haplogroup E Provide New Insights into the Dispersal of Early Pastoralists in the African Continent. *Genome Biol. Evol.* **2015**, *7* (7), 1940–1950.

Trombetta, B.; et al.; Evidence of Extensive Non-Allelic Gene Conversion among LTR Elements in the Human Genome. *Sci. Rep.* **2016**, *6*, 28710.

Trombetta, B.; et al.; Patterns of Inter-Chromosomal Gene Conversion on the Male-Specific Region of the Human Y Chromosome. *Front. Genet.* **2017**, *8* (May), 1–7.

Underhill, P. A.; and Kivisild, T.; Use of Y Chromosome and Mitochondrial DNA Population Structure in Tracing Human Migrations. *Annu. Rev. Genet.* **2007**, *41* (1), 539–564.

Underhill, P. A.; et al.; Y Chromosome Sequence Variation and the History of Human Populations. *Nat Genet.* **2000**, *26* (3), 358–361.

Underhill, P. A.; et al.; The Phylogeography of Y Chromosome Binary Haplotypes and the Origins of Modern Human Populations. *Ann. Hum. Genet.* **2001**, *65* (1), 43–62.

Underhill, P. A.; et al.; Separating the Post-Glacial Coancestry of European and Asian Y Chromosomes within Haplogroup R1a. *Eur. J. Hum. Genet.* **2010**, *18* (4), 479–484.

Urhoj, S. K.; et al.; Advanced Paternal Age and Risk of Musculoskeletal Congenital Anomalies in Offspring. *Birth Defects Res. Part B Dev. Reprod. Toxicol.* **2015**, *104* (6), 273–280.

Vallone, P. M.; and Butler, J. M.; Y-SNP Typing of U.S. African American and Caucasian Samples Using Allele-Specific Hybridization and Primer Extension. *J. Forensic Sci.* **2004**, *49* (4), 723–732.

Wang, C.-C. C.; et al.; Evaluating the Y Chromosomal Timescale in Human Demographic and Lineage Dating. *Investig. Genet.* **2014**, *5* (1), 1–7.

Wetton, J. H.; et al.; Inferring the Population of Origin of DNA Evidence within the UK by Allele-Specific Hybridization of Y-SNPs. *Forensic Sci. Int.* **2005**, *152* (1), 45–53.

Wheeler, D. L.; et al.; Database Resources of the National Center for Biotechnology Information. *Nucleic Acids Res.* **2008**, *36* (Database issue), D13–D21.

Wilson Sayres, M. A.; and Makova, K. D.; Genome Analyses Substantiate Male Mutation Bias in Many Species. *BioEssays* **2011**, *33* (12), 938–945.

Wong, W. S. W.; et al.; New Observations on Maternal Age Effect on Germline De Novo Mutations. *Nat. Commun.* **2016**, *7* (1), 10486.

Wood, E. T.; et al.; Contrasting Patterns of Y Chromosome and MtDNA Variation in Africa: Evidence for Sex-Biased Demographic Processes. *Eur. J. Hum. Genet.* **2005**, *13* (7), 867–876.

Xue, Y.; and Tyler-Smith, C.; The Hare and the Tortoise: One Small Step for Four SNPs, One Giant Leap for SNP-Kind. *Forensic Sci. Int. Genet.* **2010**, *4* (2), 59–61.

Xue, Y.; et al.; Human Y Chromosome Base-Substitution Mutation Rate Measured by Direct Sequencing in a Deep-Rooting Pedigree. *Curr. Biol.* **2009**, *19* (17), 1453–1457.

Zhang, L.; et al.; Patterns of Segmental Duplication in the Human Genome. *Mol. Biol. Evol.* **2004**, *22* (1), 135–141.

Zhu, J. L.; et al.; Paternal Age and Congenital Malformations. *Hum. Reprod.* **2005**, *20* (11), 3173–3177.

PART II
Forensic Genetic Markers

CHAPTER 3

Forensic Identity Markers: An Overview of Forensic Autosomal STRs and SNPs

DEBORA VERGANI

Dipartimento di Scienze biochimiche, sperimentali e cliniche "Mario Serio," Università degli Studi di Firenze, Viale Morgagni 50, 50134 Florence, Italy. E-mail: debora.vergani91@gmail.com

ABSTRACT

A genetic marker is defined as a DNA sequence with known physical locations on chromosomes. Good genetic markers largely used in forensic for human identification purposes are short tandem repeats (STRs) also called microsatellites polymorphisms that are characterized by high heterozygosity and high power of discrimination and that are easily amplified by polymerase chain reaction (PCR) technique. Before PCR advent other forensic identity markers were employed, from the AB0 system antigens, to serum proteins polymorphisms to DNA technique fingerprinting but, for their critical issues related with degradation and amount of biological material required for highly discriminating results, they were replaced. In addition to STRs, other markers of interest are single nucleotide polymorphisms (SNPs), considered stable genetic markers for lineage-based analyses because of the lower hyper-variability that emerge to be used by the forensic community, especially with NGS technologies advent. NGS technologies improve the information about the composition of STR locus increasing the statistical power of the STR investigation and essentially reduce the necessary number of loci needed to be typed to solve a case. They also increase the multiplexing capability for SNP loci to be analyzed in one reaction. Moreover, the main advantage of NGS compared to conventional methods is the simultaneous use of many genetic markers with high resolution of genetic data for complex biological sample in which mixed stain derived from different contributors. High-throughput sequencing of a large number of targets (including length and sequence polymorphisms) and the high read depth per base further allow sensitive detection and quantitative resolution also of minor variants in mixtures.

3.1   THE STORY OF FORENSIC IDENTITY MARKERS

"Any action of an individual, and obviously, the violent actions of a crime, cannot occur without leaving a trace," writes the French criminologist, Edmond Locard in 1934 in his book *La police et les methodes scientifiques* (Locard, 1934). This has become the fundamental principle recognized in forensic science. Locard's principle and the idea that "every contact leaves a trace" is the starting point for forensic scientists' studies.

Clearly, forensic studies and the concept of identity are inherently linked. Indeed, the main aim of investigating authorities is to establish the identity of those individuals responsible for committing crimes, and this goal is increasingly achieved with the aid of science.

Human forensic identity testing can trace its modern origins to the late 19th century when the British science writer Francis Galton proposed, for the first time, digital fingerprint analysis as a method for human identification in criminal cases. Galton's own studies of the various fingerprint patterns on the surfaces of the distal phalanges spread rapidly to police and investigative agencies around the world (Stigler, 1995).

During the first decades of the 20th century, two scientists, Karl Landsteiner and Paul Uhlenhuth, identified the presence of specific carbohydrate sugars on the surface of red blood cell membranes, N-acetylgalactosamine and D-galactose that respectively constitute the A antigen and the B antigen. Both these sugars are built upon a H antigen that is synthesized by an enzyme that adds a fucose residue on the glycolipid chain's end in erythrocyte membrane. The terminal fucose residue is the precursor for the addition of antigen A and antigen B monosaccharide. If the H antigen is left unmodified, the resulting blood group is 0 because neither the A nor the B antigen can attach to the red blood cell's surface. According with the antigen that is expressed on the surface of red blood cells, individuals will naturally develop antibodies in the serum against the AB0 antigens they do not have. For example, individuals with blood group A will have anti-B antibodies, and individuals with blood group 0 will have both anti-A and anti-B. The specific combination of these components, antigens and antibodies, allows the discrimination of distinct blood groups: A, B, AB, and 0. The AB0 blood group is controlled by a single gene *AB0* located on the long arm of chromosome 9 that encodes for glycosyltransferase, an enzyme that modifies the carbohydrate content of the red blood cell antigens. AB0 allele inheritance obeys Mendelian principles, and so each individual has two AB0 blood type alleles, one from the mother and one from the father. Since there are three different alleles, there are a total of six different genotypes at the human AB0 genetic locus: AA, A0, BB, B0, AB, and 00.

Before the discovery of the AB0 blood system, blood transfusions were a cause of injury and death related to massive agglutination. In fact, when antibodies and antigens of the same type come together, the phenomenon of agglutination takes place. The central role of this discovery became clear not only for blood transfusions, but the human blood groups were quickly recognized as useful genetic markers for the study of human population genetics and for their forensic utility in paternity disputes and criminal investigations. A pioneer in this work was Leone Lattes, a forensic doctor and blood expert, who developed the method for detecting the AB0 antibodies in blood, the so-called Lattes test (Giusti, 1982).

Subsequently, a variety of methods were developed for the AB0 system forensic testing based on antigens' type, which are more stable in dried bloodstream. The most commonly used technique is the absorption elution test that consists of exposing a portion of the stain bearing the blood for a sufficient time to absorb the homologous antibody, eventually allowing agglutination that can be viewed macroscopically. In the 1930s, scientists discovered that other body fluids like semen, vaginal secretion, and saliva can also contain the AB0 blood group substances, and people with this genetically controlled characteristic are called "secretors." People who do not have the gene, and thus do not have the blood group substances in their fluids, are called "nonsecretors." Provider of secretor status indicator in blood is called the Lewis antigen system and it inherited independently from the AB0 group. The technique used for typing AB0 antigens in body fluids is the adsorption inhibition test, in which an antiserum containing antibody is added and mixed with the specimen. If the blood group antigen corresponding to the antibody is present, a bond occurs. Afterward, adding the control test cells, no antibody will remain to agglutinate them because the agglutination is inhibited by previous binding of the antibody to the antigen in the specimen.

Other blood group systems besides AB0 were discovered in the 20th century like the Rh, MNS, Kell, Duffy, and Kidd systems that are typed in addition to AB0 antigens, with basically the same technique. By the 1940s, with the development of new techniques such as electrophoresis, it became possible to perform the separation of molecules according to their electric charge and size on an inert medium made of paper, cellulose acetate, or agarose gel. Studying with the help of this new method, the scientist found that many of the blood proteins showed several different genetically determined forms. These are called serum proteins polymorphims and are studied in forensic field: Gg system (heavy chain IgG), Km system (light chain IgG), haptoglobin system (Hp), transferrin (Tf), Pi system (alfa 1 antitripsin), erythrocyte enzymes (acidic erythrocyte phosphatase, adenylate kinase, phosphoglucomutase, etc.). The serological techniques were a powerful tool but limited in many forensic cases by the amount of biological material that was required to provide highly discriminating results. However, this method offered poor results, especially in the typing of blood stains, because proteins are also quickly prone to degradation on exposure to the environment (Jobling et al., 2004). For this reason, the characterization of protein polymorphisms has been progressively abandoned and replaced with new molecular techniques. In 1985, Alec Jeffreys, professor and geneticist at the University of Leicester in the United Kingdom (UK), pioneered DNA-based identity testing discovering the DNA technique fingerprinting by the characterization of repeated sequences over and over next to each other in DNA. Because the number of repetitions could differ from an individual to another, these highly polymorphic repeated sequences, known as variable number of tandem repeats (VNTRs), were used to perform human identity tests. Jeffreys introduced the technique called restriction fragment length polymorphism (RFLP) that used restriction enzymes that cut the region of DNA surrounding the VNTRs, originating a pattern of fragments with different lengths separated by gel electrophoresis used to compare the suspect's sample and the one originated from the stain. The huge power of discrimination of RFLP goes at the expense of the requirement of a great amount and better quality of starting DNA. In fact RFLP testing requires DNA with an average fragment size of about 20–25 kb. Breakage of DNA into smaller fragments caused by degradation, associated with environmental factor exposure, can limit the usefulness of DNA typing leading to false interpretation of data (Nakamura et al., 1987). However, the impact of this discovery on personal identification in criminal investigations and forensic paternity tests has been fundamental and remains one of the best known applications of human molecular genetics.

The decisive turning point in forensic genetics has been determined from the introduction of the polymerase chain reaction (PCR) technique, developed by Kary Mullis and members of the Human Genetics group at the Cetus Corporation starting from the 1990s onward, that allows to a specific portion of DNA of interest to be copied with high fidelity, increasing its amount, thanks to an amplification reaction. This enzymatic process consists of different cycles, and in each cycles the two DNA template strands are firstly denatured by heat, then cooled to an appropriate temperature to allow the annealing of oligonucleotide primers that act as reaction trigger, and the temperature is finally raised to the optimal condition allowing the enzyme DNA polymerase (extracted from a bacterium named *Thermus aquaticus*) to extend the primers and produce a copy of each DNA template strand (Erlich, 1989). DNA samples prepared using PCR can be analyzed in different ways ensuring less variation per locus than RFLP loci. The first system to become available for forensic analysis of PCR amplified DNA was called HLA DQα that considers the DQ gene cluster region on chromosome 6 (Blake et al., 1992). Variations in this region are detected using specially designed molecular probes complementary to particular subregions within this locus, and the results are seen as series of dots on a paperlike strip that represents the hybridization between probes and DNA sample. In forensic analysis, the comparison between the pattern of the dots is studied for identity purposes (Kawasaki et al., 1993). An expansion of the technique used in HLA DQA1 analysis was the poly-marker AmpliType PM + DQA1 system that combines the analysis of the DQA1 locus with the multiplexing, so the PCR amplification, of five more different loci at the same time, increasing the power of discrimination. A disadvantage of this method remains the difficult results' interpretation of mixtures of DNA samples. Another further PCR system briefly used until the 1990s was the amplified fragment length and, precisely, the D1S80 system that has the name of the locus that is amplified and typed. This locus is characterized by a size order of magnitude smaller than the fragment normally analyzed in RFLP typing and the variation resides in the length itself. D1S80 loci, each of which contains two alleles common among many people, are detected as discrete alleles after PCR amplification and can be compared directly to a standard rule made up of most alleles found in the population, called the allelic ladder. This analysis allows us to combine the effectiveness of PCR to amplify limited quantity and quality DNA with the greater variation of length-based polymorphism and represents a meaningful improvement for the subsequent development of the STR system.

3.2 DNA GENETIC MARKERS

The human nuclear genome consists of about 3300 Mb of DNA, conventionally divided into genic and extra genic regions. By the sequencing of the human genome, it has emerged that 1.5% of the DNA is composed of protein coding regions, whereas the remaining 98.5% is represented by noncoding sequences (Gregory, 2005). Overall, most of the human genetic material (more than 99.5%) does not vary between individuals, but only a very small fraction of our genome, less than 0.5%, contributes to total interindividual variability. This minimum percentage, however, consists of millions of polymorphic positions, and it is, therefore, sufficient to make each individual unique (the 1000 Genomes Project Consortium, 2015). More than 50% of the extra genic regions are composed of repetitive DNA, divided into dispersed sequences and repeated sequences in tandem, whereas the other half is composed of unique DNA sequence (monomorphic). Depending on the average size of the individual repeating units and the total amount of DNA occupied, the repeated sequences in tandem can be subdivided into subclasses: satellite, minisatellite or VNTRs and microsatellite or short tandem repeats (STRs) (Lander et al., 2001). In the satellite DNA, the blocks vary from 100 Kb to 1 Mb and are formed by the repetition of units of about 170 bp. A part of this satellite DNA is located near the centromeres, important functional regions during the cell replication phase. Thus, a well-known example of satellite human DNA is alfoid DNA, which forms part of the centromere. The minisatellite DNA has units ranging from 8 to 100 bp, which are repeated from 5 to more than 1000 times (Brown, 2007). They are useful as genetic markers and have copies number on average from a few repetitions, less than 10 to more than 30 (Duitama et al., 2014). VNTRs were the first polymorphisms used in DNA profiling in forensic casework, even if their use was limited by the type of sample analyzed, because a large amount of high molecular weight DNA was required and because of the problematic interpretation. For these reasons their use in forensic genetics has been replaced by STRs.

3.2.1   SHORT TANDEM REPEATS (STRs)

Microsatellites polymorphisms (STRs) consist of DNA regions with repeat units that are 2 to 7 bp in length. STRs are named according to the number of times a basic sequence is repeated and with their length. They also vary in the rigor with which they conform to an incremental repeated pattern. The main STRs classification, based on the repeated pattern, divides microsatellites into several categories: simple repeats that contain units of identical length and sequence, compound repeats that comprise two or more adjacent simple repeats, and complex repeats that may contain several repeat blocks of variable unit length or variable intervening sequences. There are also complex hypervariable repeats that differ in both size and sequence, but this category is not commonly used in forensics because of difficulties with allele nomenclature and reproducibility.

Perfect STR satellites have the repetition made up of units that are completely identical to each other, but if the repetitions do not have the same length of the single unit or the units are not always identical to each other, they are composite microsatellites. For example, in the locus D12S391, "AGAT" repetitions are followed by "AGAC" repetitions. In some other cases, there is not a complete number of repeated units in all the locus' alleles, so they are broken STR satellites and represent the microallelic variants. One of the most complete examples of a microvariant is the allele 9.3 in the locus TH01, which contains nine repetitions of the tetranucleotide 5'-AATG-3' and an incomplete repetition made of three nucleotides in which a single adenine is missing compared to the repetition unit (Puers et al., 1993). The microsatellite mutation rate tends to vary according to the number of repetitions length and the frequency of the expansion events, and it seems to be independent from the overall length of the repetitions; whereas if the allele has a higher repeat number, the rate of reduction events is higher (Brinkmann et al., 1998; Xu et al., 2000). This property explains why alleles with a low length are equally distributed in the genome, while the large ones (>50 repeat) are very rare. The mutation rate of microsatellites was estimated by a direct analysis of a father–mother–child trio (Brinkmann et al., 1998) and by an analysis of broad pedigrees in which the living descendants are separated by several genera-tions (Heyer et al., 1997). The characteristics of the mutation processes have also been studied in patients with colon cancer, which have a high microsatel-lite instability (Di Rienzo et al., 1994). Estimates for STRs mutation rates are around 10^{-3} to 10^{-4} events/locus/generation and most of the mutations (> 85%) involve an increase or decrease of only one repeated unit. The loci with repeated units composed of two nucleotides turn out to be much more variable than the tri- and tetranucleotides (Chakraborty et al., 1997). This last feature is fundamental in choosing the tetranucleotide STRs loci as good genetic markers for personal identification (Edwards et al., 1991).

3.2.1.1 CHARACTERISTICS AND NOMENCLATURE OF STRs FOR PERSONAL IDENTIFICATION

A genetic marker is defined as a DNA sequence with known physical locations on chromosomes. They are variation points with Mendelian characteristics that can be used to follow the chromosomal segment inheritance through a family tree or population. Thus, they can be used to identify individuals or species. The hypervariability of autosomal STRs allows their use as markers in human genetics, especially in cases where it is useful to detect an extreme level of distinction between individuals. STRs are considered good genetic markers for human identification purposes and they have some important advantages over other marker systems: They are present in huge numbers; they are evenly distributed throughout the genome (Payseur et al., 2011); they have a low mutation rate; and they can be easily analyzed by PCR, producing small amplicons (100–500 bp). The repeated unit succession represents the "repeated region" of the microsatellite and the number of repetitions, which varies from one gene copy to another, constitutes the polymorphism itself. The determination of an individual's genotype in a specific locus consists of the determination of the number of repetitions in each of the allelic copies (Gill et al., 2000).

The main criteria that make microsatellites ideal in the field of forensic genetics are the following (Butler, 2012):

1. Widely separated chromosomal positions to avoid the joint transmission of alleles due to genetic linkage and real independence even at the population level;

2. High heterozygosity, determined by the number of different alleles and their frequency, which are characteristics that influence the power of discrimination;

3. Amplification in short PCR products with flanking sequences that are bona fide single copy, ensuring a high specificity of the primers near the repeated region; a limited length of the repetitive stretch to be amplified maximizes the probabilities of success in the allelic recognition since, in proportion, the difference between alleles is more conspicuous;

4. The different alleles have to be well separable by electrophoresis or differ for a large number of bases; the loci with tetranucleotide repeats are among the most used STRs for human identification, because of their high frequency in the genome and their molecular structure, which make them easily usable even in the presence of degraded DNA;

5. Reproducibility of the results in multiplex reactions;

6. Reduced phenomena of stuttering; the use of repeated units of 4 bp makes it possible to obtain more stable amplicons and to minimize amplification artifacts, improving the reliability of the analysis of mixed traces or microtraces (Edwards et al., 1991);

7. Low mutation rate especially for the purposes of paternity examination.

To ensure reproducibility and comparison of data between different laboratories, a universal nomenclature system has been developed to indicate specific repetitive regions of DNA. From 1993 to 1997, the International Society of Forensic Genetics (ISFG) has drew up useful guidelines for the designation of alleles and for the unambiguous nomenclature of all markers, defining the choice of the strand and motifs and the allele designation.

Relatively to the choice of the strand STRs that map within genes, but also for STRs located in an intron, coding strands should be used. If the STRs map into a gene, it is assigned the name of the gene in which they are localized. For example, in the STR TH01 locus, located within the human gene Tiroxina hydroxylase, the suffix 01 indicates that the repeated region is located within the intron 1 of the gene. Sometimes, the prefix HUM is included at the beginning of the name to indicate that it comes from the human genome. Thus, the locus TH01 can be correctly referred also to HUMTH01. Meanwhile, for STRs falling into intergenic regions, there is a modular nomenclature. For example, in the abbreviation D16S539, "D" indicates DNA, "16" the chromosome on which the locus STR is located, "S" the fact that the locus is in single copy in the genome, and "539" is a progressive identification code that indicates the 539th locus described on chromosome 16 (Butler, 2005). For the repeated sequences without any connection to encoding protein's genes, the sequence originally described in the literature of the first public database should become the official reference for the nomenclature. If the allelic nomenclature has already been established in the forensic field, but it is not in agreement with the aforementioned guidelines, the nomenclature should be maintained to avoid unnecessary confusion.

Regarding the choice of the motif and allele designation, the repetitive unit sequence should be determined by taking into consideration the first nucleotide at the 5' end that can define a repeated motif. For example, the sequence 5'-GG TCA TGG-3 could be interpreted as 3 TCA or 3 CAT. In any case, only the first (3 TCA) is correct because it determines the first possible repeating unit. The alleles that contain incomplete repetitions, called microvariants, should contain the number of complete repetitions and, separated by a decimal point, the number of base pairs in the incomplete repetition.

STRs used in forensics are localized on both autosomal and sex chromosomes X and Y. Because of their unique transmission properties, markers on sex chromosomes can be very useful in kinship analysis and can complement the autosomal STRs marker analysis. A more detailed explanation about the Y-STRs and X-STRs and their usefulness in forensic will be dealt within the following chapters (see Chapters 4 and 5 of this book).

3.2.1.2   DEVELOPMENT OF STR KITS FOR PERSONAL IDENTIFICATION

For identification purposes in forensic genetics, it is important to shortly analyze highly informative DNA markers that can discriminate samples between each other, and it is necessary to exploit the advantages of the PCR technique that not only allow the production of multiple copies of a DNA region, but also to do it simultaneously with multiple target sequences. This process of co-amplification, named "multiplex PCR" requires the simple addition to the mixture reaction of a number of primers' pairs, according with the number of STRs to amplify, which must, however, be compatible in term of *annealing* temperatures. So the biggest obstacle in setting up multiple PCR is, however, represented by the total number of the loci that have to be simultaneously analyzed. For this reason, a good primer design is fundamental to ensure an adequate separation of the amplicons that are generated and to allow the correct examination of all the loci without overlapping phenomena. Almost all modern commercial kits for STRs typing have obviated this inconvenience, thanks to the use of primers labeled with fluorochromes. This allowed to simultaneously amplify microsatellites of overlapping dimensions using different dyes separated by suitable optical filters. The microsatellites used today by the forensic community were initially characterized and developed by Edwards and Caskey at Baylor College of Medicine, who in 1991 published the first article on fluorescence detection of STR markers and patented their work, which was then licensed to Promega Corporation and Thermo-Fisher (Butler, 2009). The "first-generation multiplex" was one of the first STR multiplexes to be developed, and it is a quadruplex that comprised four loci: TH01, FES/FPS, vWA, and F13A1 (Kimpton et al., 1994). It then followed a second-generation multiplex, made up of six polymorphic STRs: TH01, vWA, FGA, D8S1179, D18S51, and D21S11 and a gender identification marker Amelogenin (Kimpton, 1996).

In 1996, the FBI Laboratory sponsored a large project for the determination of a group of STRs to be used in the establishment of the national DNA database, better known as Combined DNA Index System (CODIS). The project, which involved 22 laboratories specialized in DNA genotyping and the evaluation of 17 STRs loci, ended in November 1997 with the choice of 13 loci, listed below: CSF1P0, FGA, TH01, TPOX, VWA, D3S1358, D5S818, D7S820, D8S1179, D13S317, D16S539, D18S51, and D21S11 (Budowle et al., 1998). A genotype obtained by typing the 13 microsatellites of CODIS makes it possible to identify the subject in an unequivocal way. Using the classification scheme previously described, the 13 CODIS loci can be divided into four categories:

1. Simple repetitions consisting of a repetitive unit: TPOX, CSF1P0, D5S818, D13S317, D16S539;
2. Simple repetitions with nonconsensus alleles: TH01, D18S51, D7S820;
3. Repetitions composed with nonconsensus alleles: VWA, FGA, D3S 1358, D8S1179;
4. Complex repetitions: D21S11.

In 1999, the European Standard Set (ESS) of STR loci were selected, many of which were in common with the STR loci used in the United States. In 2005, several new European STR loci were recommended for inclusion in future European STR typing kits and in 2009, the European Network of Forensic Science Institutes voted the extension of the ESS, recommended to enable DNA data exchange across Europe. The loci described earlier can be easily typed using the numerous kits developed by specialized companies that allow the co-amplification of multiple STRs (included CODIS microsatellites). Two primary vendors were Promega Corporation (Madison, Wisconsin) and Thermo Fisher (Oyster Point, California). In Europe, companies such as Serac (Bad Homburg, Germany), Biotype (Dresden, Germany), and QIAGEN (Hilden, Germany) have begun offering commercial STR kits. Table 3.1 presents a list of the commercially available STRs multiplex kits developed by Promega, Thermo-Fisher, and QIAGEN.

All these STRs kits allow in a single reaction the amplification of the 13 CODIS systems, along with the sexual marker for Amelogenin and additional STR loci specific for each kit. Among the most innovative kits available on the market, there is the AmpFlSTR® MiniFiler™ kit (Thermo Fisher), which increases the probability of obtaining profiles from particularly degraded samples and the amplification results in the reduced size of the amplicons. These smallest PCR products are, in fact, obtained through the use of redesigned primers able to pair near the STR repeated region, producing miniSTRs. An artificial mixture of the most STRs alleles present in the population, containing alleles sequenced and named according to recommendations listed above, should be used as a reference for the allelic designation of unknown samples. These mixtures are named allelic ladders and are prepared using multiple individuals in a population that have alleles representative of the variability of a given STR. Generally, forensic genetic laboratories use commercially available ladders, supplied with co-amplification kits. Other improvements such as new buffer formulations, new DNA polymerases, additives to the PCR reaction, substitution of high-stability nucleic acid analogs along the primers to improve annealing stability, and energy-transfer dye labeled primers to improve PCR product sensitivity were introduced into next-generation STRs kits like:

TABLE 3.1 Overview of Commercially Available STRs Multiplex Kits Developed by Promega, Thermo Fisher, and QIAGEN.

Kit Name	Release Year
Thermo Fisher	
AmpFlSTR Blue (no longer available)	1996
AmpFlSTR Green I (no longer available)	1997
AmpFlSTR Profiler	1997
AmpFlSTR Profiler Plus	1997
AmpFlSTR COfiler	1998
AmpFlSTR SGM Plus	1999
AmpFlSTR Identifiler	2001
AmpFlSTR Profiler Plus ID (extra unlabeled D8-R primer)	2001
AmpFlSTR SEfiler (no longer available)	2002
AmpFlSTR MiniFiler	2007
AmpFlSTR SEfiler Plus (improved buffer)	2007
AmpFlSTR Sinofiler	2008
AmpFlSTR Identifiler Direct (same primers, improved reagents)	2009
AmpFlSTR Identifiler Plus (same primers, improved reagents)	2010
AmpFlSTR NGM	2010
AmpFlSTR NGM Select	2010
Promega	
CTTv	1997
FFFL	1997
GammaSTR	1997
PowerPlex 1.1, PowerPlex 1.2	1997, 1998
PowerPlex 2.1 (for Hitachi FMBIO users)	1999
PowerPlex 16	2000
PowerPlex 16 BIO (for Hitachi FMBIO users)	2001
PowerPlex ES	2002
PowerPlex 16 HS (same primers, improved reagents)	2009
PowerPlex ESX 16 & ESX 17	2009
PowerPlex 18D	2011
QIAGEN	
Investigator ESSplex	2010
Investigator Decaplex SE	2010
Investigator Triplex AFS QS	2010
Investigator Triplex DSF	2010
Investigator IDplex	2010
Investigator HDplex	2010
Investigator Hexaplex ESS	2010
Investigator Nonaplex ESS	2010
Investigator ESSplex SE	2010

- Globalfiler STRs kit (Thermo Fisher Scientific, Waltham, MA, USA) that combines the 13 original CODIS loci with 7 nonoverlapping loci from the expanded ESS, as well as the highly discriminating SE33 locus, two Y-based loci and the sex determining maker, Amelogenin. The full complement of loci in the GlobalFiler™ Kit are: D13S317, D7S820, D5S818, CSF1PO, D1S1656, D12S391, D2S441, D10S1248, D18S51, FGA, D21S11, D8S1179, vWA, D16S539, TH01, D3S1358, AMEL, D2S1338, D19S433, DYS391, TPOX, D22S1045, SE33, and a Y-specific insertion/deletion locus (Y-indel);
- PowerPlex Fusion 6C System (Promega) that allows the amplification and detection by fluorescence of the 20 autosomal loci in the expanded CODIS core loci (CSF1PO, D3S1358, D5S818, D7S820, D8S1179, D13S317, D16S539, D18S51, D21S11, FGA, TH01, TPOX, vWA, D1S1656, D2S441, D2S1338, D10S1248, D12S391, D19S433, and D22S1045), as well as Amelogenin for gender determination. The loci Penta D, Penta E, and SE33 are also included, and three exclusive Y chromosome alleles (DYS391, DYS576 and DYS570), allowing allelic attribution in a total of 27 loci;
- Investigator ESSplex SE QS (QIAGEN) that amplifies 16 STRs, including SE33, and Amelogenin. The reaction mix is supplemented with two quality sensors that consist of a short fragment and a long fragment, sensitive to inhibitors in the amplified samples.

3.2.1.3   STRs ANALYSIS AND GENOTYPING

Following PCR amplification, the overall length of the STRs amplicons is measured to determine the number of repeats present in each allele of the DNA profile. This length measurement is made via a size-based separation involving capillary electrophoresis (CE). Each STR amplicon has been fluorescently labeled during PCR, since either the forward or reverse locus specific primer contains a fluorescent dye. Thus, by recording the dye color and by the migration time of each DNA fragment, the size for each STR allele may be determined following its separation from other STRs alleles in comparison with internal size standard (Butler, 2007).

The electrophoresis data just allows the display of the alleles as spikes in an electropherogram. The information contained in the various peaks must be converted into a common language to allow comparison of data between several laboratories. From this conversion, the genotype, or genetic profile, is obtained and it is formed, for each locus, by one allele in case of homozygosis, and by two alleles in case of heterozygosis.

A commonly used instrument for STR allele separation and sizing is the ABI 3500xL Genetic Analyzer produced by Thermo Fisher Scientific, which also developed sophisticated software for genotype assignment of DNA samples. The main functions of these data collection software are generally to check the conditions of electrophoretic runs, to check which wavelengths emitted by the fluorochromes must be collected inside of the CCD camera through virtual filters, and to allow the creation of a list of samples that have to be submitted to electrophoresis with the relative run setup (order and sample injection conditions, electrophoretic run conditions, virtual filter to use). At the end of the electrophoretic run, a file called raw data is produced for each sample and a Cartesian graph that correlates the relative fluorescence units on the *y*-axis with the number of data points on the *x*-axis. The GeneScan and Genotyper or GeneMapper programs are then needed for the conversion of the raw data into a genetic profile for the analysis of the STRs. In particular, the GeneScan Analysis software:

1. recognizes the peaks by height threshold value and also determines the height and area of the various peaks;
2. separates the emission spectra of the fluorochromes based on the matrix;
3. assigns the sizes to the fragments based on comparison with the internal standard peaks.

The Genotyper software then converts the peaks, to which the size has been assigned, in alleles by comparison with the ladder peaks. At the end of this process the electropherogram is shown on different lines, one for each color, containing the various loci from the shortest to the longest, with related alleles. In November 2003, Thermo Fisher Scientific developed and marked the software GeneMapperID that combines together the functions of GeneScan and Genotyper with new features, including the Process Component-Based Quality Values system, which automatically assigns quality values on the process of size determination and allelic call made by the software. This feature facilitates the identification of problems during the preparation and analysis phases. The results can then be printed or exported to an electronic sheet for further analysis or directly included in a database.

The interpretation and reporting of DNA typing results for human identification purposes requires professional judgment and expertise. It is a complex process that draws upon empirical data and the overall training and experience of the scientist involved. Additionally, laboratories that analyze DNA samples for forensic casework purposes are required by the Quality Assurance Standards for Forensic DNA Testing Laboratories to establish and follow documented procedures for the interpretation of DNA typing results and reporting (SWGDAM, 2017). A correct interpretation of the STR analysis data is done according to the SWGDAM Interpretation Guidelines for Autosomal STR Typing by Forensic DNA Testing Laboratories, approved in 2017.

3.2.2 SINGLE-NUCLEOTIDE POLYMORPHISMS (SNPs)

Other markers of interest that are emerging to the forensic community are the SNPs single-base variations as substitutions, insertions, or deletions that occur at single positions and that are highly abundant in the human genome (around 1 in every 1000 bases). They represent the most common class of human polymorphisms. SNPs variation can occur in the coding regions of genes, altering function or structure of the encoded proteins, or in noncoding regions without detectable impact on the phenotype of an individual. These noncoding SNPs are suitable for forensic studies and useful as markers due to some characteristics (Gill, 2001):

1. They have lower mutation rates than STR so are stable genetic markers for lineage-based analyses, such as inheritance cases, missing person cases, and situations where no direct reference sample may be available;
2. They can be analyzed from short amplicons, less than 100 bp in size, allowing successful amplification of degraded samples;
3. They can be multiplexed and the sample processing and data analysis can be more fully automated because a size-based separation is not needed;
4. They are particularly suitable for analysis using high-throughput technologies, which have become increasingly important for the successful implementation of large criminal DNA databases and to perform the large-population studies for allele frequencies estimation.

According with their use, SNP markers may be classified into four general categories: Identity SNPs, lineage SNPs, ancestry informative SNPs, and phenotype informative SNPs (Budowle et al., 2008).

Individual identification or identity-testing SNPs provides genetic information to differentiate people collectively given very low probabilities of two individuals having the same multilocus genotype. The best SNPs for identity testing are those that have the highest heterozygosity and the low fixation index (F_{ST}), a measure of population differentiation, to reach high levels of discrimination power. Lineage-informative SNPs generally reside on the mtDNA genome and on the Y chromosome, but they have limited power of discrimination, so sets of tightly linked markers have also been identified on the autosomes with the function as multiallelic markers to identify relatives with higher probabilities than simple biallelic SNPs. These linked SNPs can move as a haplotype block through generational transmission, providing more allelic states than single loci. As such, they can be helpful for kinship analyses (Ge et al., 2010). The most likely forensic use of lineage SNPs is for missing persons cases or mass disaster identifications.

Ancestry informative SNPs are markers distributed throughout the human genome that occur at very different frequencies in different world populations and that can reveal ancestral origin by indirect method, assessing phenotype according to the phenotypic expression of certain features. For example, skin pigmentation is lighter in Northern Europeans than in any other population, thus with proper databases defining regional and various global reference of ancestral populations with skin pigmentation measurements, light skin color of a genetically defined Northern European donor of an evidence sample can be predicted from a precise genomic ancestry estimate. Due to much lower mutation rate, SNPs are more likely fixed in a population than STRs and collectively give a high probability of an individual's ancestry being from one part of the world. SNPs are thus usually the better predictors of ethnicity (Lao et al., 2006).

Phenotype-informative SNPs are markers that able to provide with high probability the phenotypic traits of an individual (skin color, hair color and eye color, among others) to identify, for example, the perpetrator of a crime. They also may be of value in anthropological studies for the facial reconstruction of unknown human remains (Bouakaze et al., 2009). Prediction of externally visible characteristics (EVCs) can provide forensic intelligence about the physical features; however, this direct method requires an assessment of the genetic variation that strongly affects a specific phenotype as well as the development of databases to relate these variants to the specific traits (Frudakis, 2008). The first human gene shown to be associated with normal pigment variation was the melanocortin 1 receptor (MC1R) gene. Thus numerous SNPs in this gene have been linked to red hair and fair skin (Branicki et al., 2007).

3.2.2.1 SNPs ANALYSIS TECHNIQUE

Over the past years, thanks to the rapid and continuous evolution, a large number of different SNPs typing technologies have been developed. Different aspects such as the sensitivity, the reproducibility, the accuracy, the capability of multiplexing, and the level of throughput should be considered to determine the most suitable technology for forensic purposes. The choice of the technique to be used is based on allelic discrimination reaction and detection platforms. According to the molecular mechanism, SNP genotyping assays can be divided in four groups: allele specific hybridization, primer extension, oligonucleotide ligation, and invasive cleavage. Products of the allelic discrimination reactions can be detected with one or more method (like fluorescence, luminescence, mass measurement, and so forth), and the same detection method can analyze products obtained with different reactions or assay formats (Sobrino et al., 2005). A comprehensive review on SNP genotyping techniques is provided by Sobrino et al. that include high resolution melting analysis, TaqMan hybridization probes, invader technology, hybridization microarrays, massively parallel sequencing (MPS) and the SNaPshot minisequencing method. One of the most commonly applied technique to forensic DNA analysis, thanks to its sensitivity and high multiplexing capability with the added advantage of not requiring additional equipment to that already utilized in forensic laboratories, was SNaPshot. SNaPshot or minisequencing is a genotyping method, developed in 1990, which belongs to the group of primer extension techniques and is used mainly for diagnosis of genetic disorders and genotyping proteins (Sokolov, 1990). The protocol of this technique consists in the generation of target amplicons containing the SNPs of interest through multiplex PCR starting from the DNA template. Subsequently, purification reaction of PCR product is performed by adding exonuclease I and shrimp alkaline phosphatase to degrade unbound primers and unincorporated dNTPs, which would interfere with the subsequent primer extension reaction. The 3' end of the oligonucleotide SNaPshot primer, immediately adjacent to the SNP of interest, is extended by Taq DNA polymerase which incorporates a fluorescently labeled dideoxyribonucleotide triphosphate complementary to the base on the opposite strand at the SNP position. Purified products are spatially separated with automated capillary electrophoresis sequencer (ABI 3500xL Genetic Analyzer) that detects fluorescence at timed intervals to record the electrophoretic mobility of the fragment and its fluorescent signal's wavelength. The separation of PCR amplification reaction from the subsequent SNP detection reaction leads to much improved performance especially when analyzing highly degraded DNA due to the small size of the PCR amplicons. This technology also allows considerable multiplexing capacity for the simultaneous individualization of multiple primers extended in parallel in a combined extension reaction. The multiplexing capability in SNP genotyping is feasible for forensic requirements even if it requires lot of work to optimize the design and the concentration of the primers for PCR and minisequencing reaction of each set of SNPs. Fondevila et al. (2017) compiled a technical review for adoption of single-base extension (SBE) tests for forensic SNP genotyping detailing a set of guidelines for optimizing SNaPshot assay designs and for making the most reliable SNP profile interpretations.

Recently the interest in SNP typing has become focused on sequence-based NGS technologies that are gaining traction as a more extensive form of forensic SNP testing. Small SNaPshot-based assays will continue to contribute to forensic casework while NGS matures and becomes simpler to run as a routine genotyping approach. NGS provides much more data per assay than CE-based tests and SNaPshot assays, which amplify a smaller proportion of markers compared to the PCR scales possible with NGS (Fondevila et al., 2017). Forensic SNaPshot assays are classified into four categories based on their application (Mehta et al., 2017): IISNP assays (identity-informative SNP), LISNP assays (lineage-informative SNP), AISNP assays (ancestral-informative SNP), and PISNP assays (phenotype-informative SNP). IISNP assays are divided in blood grouping assay, which analyze SNPs representing the antigen and amino acid changes associated with each blood group, and other (nonblood group) human identification SNP assays. One of the earliest human identification assays was SNPforID 52-plex assay, incorporating a set of two multiplexes (a 23-plex and a 29-plex), which provided a combined power of exclusion greater than 99.999% (Sanchez et al., 2006). More recently, a 55-plex IISNP assay (54 highly informative SNPs and an Amelo-genin sex marker) has been developed (Wang et al., 2016), which expanded the precedent 44 plex (Børsting et al., 2009) and reoptimized the concentra-tions of PCR primers and SBE primers, as well as the reaction volumes and conditions, in order to increase the effectiveness of the system and enhance the robustness of the method.

LISNP assays include Y chromosome and mitochondrial DNA markers. A major Y chromosome haplogroup typing kit consisting of 29 Y-LISNPs and then, more recently, a 28 Y-SNP SBE multiplex assay enabling the discrimination of major Y chromosome haplogroups worldwide have been developed, even if this assay can provide an assessment of the continental biogeographical male lineage only and requires additional SNPs for detailed phylogenetic classification. For mtDNA haplogroups, a 12-SNP multiplex assay was developed defining the broad for different population (Nelson et al., 2007); more recently, a 36-mtSNP multiplex system has been employed to efficiently infer maternal ancestry at the continental level, with the possibility to differentiate 43 different haplotypes (van Oven et al., 2011).

AISNPs are designed to provide biogeographical ancestry information about the donor of a DNA sample and are designed with ideal characteristics such as low heterozygosity and high fixation index (F^{ST}). The SNPforID 34-plex SNaPshot assay is a well-established ancestry-informative assay, differentiating between Europeans, Asians, and Africans (Phillips et al., 2007). There are also tools such as Eurasiaplex (Phillips et al., 2013) and EurEas_Gplex (Daca-Roszak et al., 2016) that can further assist in offering higher-resolution differentiation of Europeans and Asians (East Asians), whereas Pacifiplex could play a critical role in differentiating Oceanian populations (such as Australian Aboriginals and Papua New Guinea) from global populations (Santos et al., 2016), which is useful for the analysis of samples in the Asia-Pacific region.

PISNP assays include two SNaPshot-based phenotypic assays that have been validated for the European population, the IrisPlex, which is a blue and brown eye color classification system comprised of six highly predictive eye color SNPs and HIrisPlex, which is a 24-plex assay (23 SNPs and 1 INDEL) capable of predicting eye and hair color collectively and includes the six IrisPlex SNPs. Moreover an 8-plex SNaPshot was developed to predict eye and skin color that had three SNPs in common with the IrisPlex (Hart et al., 2013). Other EVCs of potential forensic value with associated SNPs such as male pattern baldness, hair texture, facial characteristics, fingerprint patterns, and age estimation may be incorporated in future SNaPshot assays.

3.2.3 STRs AND SNPs IN NEXT GENERATION SEQUENCING (NGS) ERA

DNA from biological forensic samples can be highly fragmented and present in limited quantity. When DNA is highly fragmented, conventional PCR-based STR analysis may fail as primer binding sites, may not be present on a single template molecule. As already mentioned, SNPs can serve as an alternative type of genetic marker for analysis of degraded samples because the targeted variation is a single base. However, conventional PCR-based SNP analysis methods still require intact primer binding sites for target amplification. Recently, the advent of first NGS technologies quickly changed and involved also forensic genetic laboratories offering new possibilities in the resolution of forensic genetic case work. Because of the extreme importance of STRs in large national database constituted by profiles from criminal offenders, NGS applications focused on the sequencing of STR loci. Compared to fragment length analysis by PCR-CE that provides information only about the number of repetitions that compose the STR locus, sequencing also reveals the variations in the repetition sequence of the STR locus and in the flanking regions, allowing to detect not only previously unknown STR alleles but also mainly complex and compound STRs (Dalsgaard et al., 2013). Complex and compound STRs consist of different subrepeats and, if the individual subrepeats are polymorphic, the number of possible alleles will be much higher than they are in simple repeats. More identifiable alleles imply more statistical power of the STR investigation and essentially reduce the necessary number of loci that need to be typed to solve a case to a certain level. The possibility to distinguish between individuals with identical allele lengths as far as the characterization of mutation events could be essential in forensic or kinship analysis (Børsting et al., 2015). It may also be easier to resolve DNA mixtures in crime case investigations when alleles that appear identical in CE-analyses may be further characterized by NGS.

Discovery of many new STR and SNP–STR alleles with the same sizes makes the old PCR-CE based nomenclature for STR alleles inadequate. A new transparent description of STR sequences is much in demand and the ISFG has initiated a working group for finding a common definition for naming sequenced STR alleles (Børsting et al., 2015). Despite this new improvement in STRs, most NGS studies focused on SNPs increasing the multiplexing capability and allowing to a higher number of SNP loci to be analyzed in one reaction. The two companies Verogen and Thermo Fisher Scientific developed marker panels and specific platforms for forensic genetics: MiSeqFGx™ Forensic Genomics System and the HID-Ion Personal Genome. These platforms are coupled with the commercially available panels for human identification, the ForenSeq™ DNA Signature Prep kit (Verogen) that sequence in one reaction 173 SNP markers with additional 59 STR markers, and the HID-Ion AmpliSeq™ Identity Panel (Thermo Fisher Scientific) that sequence 124 SNP markers simultaneously. These two panels have in common 83 SNP markers that spread across the 22 autosomes, have high heterozygosity and low fixation index (Fst), and have relatively small amplicon sizes, thus increasing the likelihood of successful DNA profiling of degraded DNA (Apaga et al., 2017).

Therefore, the main advantage of NGS compared to conventional methods, is the simultaneous use of a large number of genetic markers with high resolution of genetic data. Most of the PCR-CE assays may be combined into a single NGS assay to develop a capture for the relevant loci. More information may be obtained from unique samples in a single experiment by analyzing combinations of large batteries of markers. An MPS offers also new solution for mixed stain derived from different contributors that are common biological evidence samples in forensic practice. These complex biological samples present challenges in interpreting the results, especially for those imbalanced genomic mixtures. In fact PCR-CE in STR typing does not work successfully if the proportion of the DNA quantities of the two contributors is more extreme than 1:10 (Triggs et al., 2004). Thus the high throughput sequencing of a large number of targets (including length and sequence polymorphisms) and the high read depth per base further allow sensitive detection and quantitative resolution of minor variants in mixtures.

Although traditional forensic genetics has been oriented toward using human DNA in criminal investigation and civil court cases, currently forensic genetics is progressively incorporating the analysis of nonhuman genetic material to a greater extent. The analysis of this material, which includes other animal species, plants, or microorganisms are now broadly used, providing ancillary evidence in criminalistics cases, such as animal attacks, trafficking of species, bioterrorism and biocrimes, as well as identification of fraudulent food composition, among many others. This topic will be better detailed in Chapter 13.

3.2.3.1 INSERTION–DELETION POLYMORPHISMS

Indel (Insertion–Deletion Polymorphism) is the insertion or deletion of a segment of DNA ranging from one nucleotide to hundreds of nucleotides in length that is derived from a single mutation event. Their low mutation frequency makes them suitable in forensics. Such polymorphisms may be examined using as small amplicon size as SNP (about 100 bp) but could be analyzed by techniques used for routine STR analysis, thus combining advantages of both STRs and SNPs. INDEL typing procedures include selection of marker, design of specific primers, and amplification with a simple fluorescent PCR followed by capillary electrophoresis (Fondevila et al., 2012). Actually there are two multiplexed INDEL typing assays available for forensic identification, namely QIAGEN Investigator DIPplex® kit of 30 INDELs and a 38-INDEL multiplex assay (LaRue et al., 2012).

INDEL typing was proved to be useful in population studies as well as the studies of genetic diseases, but it is suitable on forensic and parentage testings, as well as for highly degraded DNA and highly decomposed remains or skeletonized.

KEYWORDS

- **genetic markers**
- **personal identification**
- **STRs**
- **SNPs**
- **INDEL**

REFERENCES

Apaga, D. et al.; Comparison of two massively parallel sequencing platforms using 83 single nucleotide polymorphisms for human identification. *Sci. Rep.* **2017**; *7 (1)*, 398.

Blake, E.; et al.; Polymerase chain reaction (PCR) amplification and human leukocyte antigen (HLA)-DQ alpha oligonucleotide typing on biological evidence samples: Casework experience. *J. Forensic Sci.* **1992**, *37 (3)*, 700–726.

Børsting, C.; et al.; Validation of a single nucleotide polymorphism (SNP) typing assay with 49 SNPs for forensic genetic testing in a laboratory accredited according to the ISO 17025 standard. *Forensic Sci. Int. Genet.* **2009**, *4 (1)*, 34–42.

Børsting, C.; et al.; Next generation sequencing and its applications in forensic genetics. *Forensic Sci. Int. Genet.* **2015**, *18*, 78–89.

Bouakaze, C.; et al.; Pigment phenotype and biogeographical ancestry from ancient skeletal remains: Inferences from multiplexed autosomal SNP analysis. *Int. J. Legal Med.* **2009**, *123 (4)*, 315–325.

Branicki, W.; et al.; Determination of phenotype associated SNPs in the MC1R gene. *J. Forensic Sci.* **2007**, *52 (2)*, 349–354.

Brinkmann, B.; et.al.; Mutation rate in human microsatellites: Influence of the structure and length of the tandem repeat. *Am. J. Hum. Genet.* **1998**, *62*, 1408–1415.

Brown, T.; *Genomes 3, 3rd ed.* **2007**. New York: Garland Science.

Budowle, B.; et.al.; CODIS and PCR-based short tandem repeat loci: Law enforcement tools. *Promega Corporation (ed) Genetic Identity Conference Proceedings of the Second European Symposium on Human Identification.* **1998**, Madison, WI, 73–88.

Budowle, B.; et al.; Forensically relevant SNP classes. *BioTechniques* **2008**, *44*, 603–610.

Butler, J.; *Forensic DNA Typing: Biology, Technology, and Genetics of STR Markers, 2nd ed.* **2005**, New York: Elsevier Academic Press.

Butler, J.; Short tandem repeat typing technologies used in human identity testing. *BioTechniques* **2007**, 43 (4), ii–v. doi:10.2144/000112582.

Butler, J.; *Fundamentals of Forensic DNA Typing*. **2009**, Academic Press/Elsevier.

Butler, J.; *Advanced Topics in Forensic DNA Typing: Methodology*. **2012**, Waltham, MA: Elsevier/Academic Press.

Chakraborty, R.; et. al.; Relative mutation rates at di-,tri-, and tetranucleotide microsatellite loci. *Proc. Natl. Acad. Sci. USA*. **1997**, *94*, 1041–1046.

1000 Genomes Project Consortium; A global reference of human genomic variation. *Nature* **2015**, *526*, 68–74.

Daca-Roszak, P.; et al.; EurEAs_Gplex—A new SNaPshot assay for continental population discrimination and gender identification. *Forensic Sci. Int. Genet.* **2016**, *20*, 89–100.

Dalsgaard, S.; et al.; Characterization of mutations and sequence variations in complex STR loci by second generation sequencing. *Forensic Sci. Genet. Suppl.* **2013**, *4*, e218–e219.

Di Rienzo, A.; Mutational processes of simple-sequence repeat loci in human population. *Proc. Natl. Acad. Sci. USA* **1994**, *91*, 3166–3170.

Duitama, J.; et al.; Large-scale analysis of tandem repeat variability in the human genome. *Nucleic Acids Res.* **2014**, *42*, 5728–5741.

Edwards, A.; et al.; DNA typing and genetic mapping with trimeric and tetrameric tandem repeats. *Am. J. Hum. Genet.* **1991**, *49*, 746–756.

Erlich, H. E.; *PCR Technology: Principles and Applications for DNA Amplification*. **1989**, New York: Stockton Press.

Fondevila, M.; et al.; Forensic performance of two insertion–deletion marker assays. *Int. J. Legal Med.* **2012**, *126(5)*, 725–737.

Fondevila, M.; et al.; Forensic SNP genotyping with SNaPshot: Technical considerations for the development and optimization of multiplexed SNP assays. *Forensic Sci. Rev.* **2017**, *29(1)*, 57–76.

Frudakis, T.; *Molecular Photofitting: Predicting Ancestry and Phenotype from DNA*. **2008**, Amsterdam, the Netherlands: Academic Press (Elsevier).

Ge, J.; et al.; Haplotype block: a new type of forensic DNA markers. *Int. J. Legal Med.* **2010**, *124 (5)*, 353–361.

Gill, P.; et al.; An investigation of the rigor of interpretation rules for STRs derived from less than 100 pg of DNA. *Forensic Sci. Int.* **2000**, *112*, 17–40.

Gill, P.; An assessment of the utility of single nucleotide polymorphisms. *Int. J. Legal Med.* **2001**, *114*, 204–210.

Giusti, G.; Leone Lattes: Italy's pioneer in forensic serology. *Am. J. Forensic Med. Pathol.* **1982**, *3*(1), 79–81.

Gregory, R.; Synergy between sequence and size in large-scale genomics. *Nat. Rev. Genet.* **2005**, *6*, 699–708.

Hart, K.; et al.; Improved eye- and skin-color prediction based on 8 SNPs. *Croat. Med. J.* **2013**, *54 (3)*, 248–256.

Heyer, E.; et.al; Estimating Y chromosome specific microsatellite mutation frequencies using deep rooting pedigrees. *Hum. Mol. Genet.* **1997**, *6*, 799–803.

Jobling, M.; et al.; Encoded evidence: DNA in forensic analysis. *Nat. Rev. Genet.* **2004**, *5(10)*, 739–751.

Kawasaki, E.; et al.; Genetic analysis using polymerase chain reaction-amplified DNA and immobilized oligonucleotide probes: Reverse dot-blot typing. *Methods Enzymol.* **1993**, *218*, 369–381.

Kimpton, C. P.; et al.; Evaluation of an automated DNA profiling system employing multiplex amplification of four tetrameric STR loci. *Int. J. Legal Med.* **1994**, *106*, 302–311.

Kimpton, C. P.; et al.; Validation of highly discriminating multiplex short tandem repeat amplification systems for individual identification. *Electrophoresis.* **1996**, *17 (8)*, 1283–1293.

Lander, E. et al.; Initial sequencing and analysis of the human genome. *Nature.* **2001**, *409*, 860–921.

Lao, O.; et al.; Proportioning whole-genome single-nucleotide-polymorphism diversity for the identification of geographic population structure and genetic ancestry. *Am. J. Hum. Genet.* **2006**, *78 (4)*, 680–690.

LaRue B.L.; et al.; A validation study of the Qiagen Investigator DIPplex® kit; an INDEL-based assay for human identification. *Int. J. Legal Med.* **2012**, *126* (4), 533–540.

Locard, E; *La police et les méthodes scientifiques.* **1934**, Paris: Editions Riede.

Mehta, B.; et al.; Forensically relevant SNaPshot® assays for human DNA SNP analysis: A review. *Int. J. Legal. Med.* **2017**, *131(1)*, 21–37.

Nakamura, Y.; et al.; Variable number of tandem repeat (VNTR) markers for human gene mapping. *Science* **1987**, *237*, 1616–1622.

Nelson, T. et al.; Development of a multiplex single base extension assay for mitochondrial DNA haplogroup typing. *Croat. Med. J.* **2007**, *48 (4)*, 460–472.

Payseur, B.; et al.; A genomic portrait of human microsarellite variation. *Mol. Bio. Evol.* **2011**, *28 (1)*, 303–312.

Phillips, C.; et al.; Inferring ancestral origin using a single multiplex assay of ancestry-informative marker SNPs. *Forensic Sci. Int. Genet.* **2007**, *1 (3–4)*, 273–280.

Phillips, C.; et al.; Eurasiaplex: A forensic SNP assay for differentiating European and South Asian ancestries. *Forensic Sci. Int. Genet.* **2013**, *7 (3)*, 359–366.

Puers, C.; et al.; Identification of repeat sequence heterogeneity at the polymorphic short tandem repeat locus HUMTH01 [AATG]n and reassignment of alleles in population analysis by using a locus-specific allelic ladder. *Am. J. Hum. Genet.* **1993**, *53*, 953–958.

Sanchez, J.; et al.; A multiplex assay with 52 single nucleotide polymorphisms for human identification. *Electrophoresis* **2006**, *27 (9)*, 1713–1724.

Santos, C.; et al.; Pacifiplex: An ancestry-informative SNP panel centred on Australia and the Pacific region. *Forensic Sci. Int. Genet.* **2016**, *20*, 71–80.

Sobrino, B.; et al.; SNPs in forensic genetics: A review on SNP typing methodologies. *Forensic Sci. Int.* **2005**, *154 (2–3)*, 181–194.

Sokolov, B. Primer extension technique for the detection of single nucleotide in genomic DNA. *Nucleic Acids Res.* **1990**, *18 (12)*, 3671.

Stigler, S; Galton and identification by fingerprints. *Genetics.* **1995**; *140 (3)*, 857–860.

SWGDAM.; *Interpretation Guidelines for Autosomal STR Typing by Forensic DNA Testing Laboratories.* **2017**.

Triggs, C.; et al.; *Forensic DNA Evidence Interpretation.* **2004**, Boca Raton, FL: CRC Press.

van Oven, M.; et al.; Multiplex genotyping system for efficient inference of matrilineal genetic ancestry. *Investig. Genet.* **2011**, *2*, 1–14.

Wang, Q.; et al.; Expansion of a SNaPshot assay to a 55-SNP multiplex: Assay enhancements, validation, and power in forensic science. *Electrophoresis* **2016**, *37 (10)*, 1310–1317.

Xu, X.; et al.; The direction of microsatellite mutations is dependent upon allele length. *Nat. Genet.* **2000**, *24*, 396–399.

CHAPTER 4

The Y-Chromosomal STRs in Forensic Genetics: Y Chromosome STRs

DEBORA VERGANI

Dipartimento di Scienze Biochimiche, Sperimentali e Cliniche "Mario Serio," Università degli Studi di Firenze, viale Morgagni 50, 50134 Firenze, Italy. E-mail: debora.vergani91@gmail.com

ABSTRACT

In males, one X and one Y chromosomes are present compared with females who have only two X chromosomes. The presence of the sex-determining region Y (*SRY*) gene determines the human sex and is one of the main features, but not only, from the forensic point of view. The sex-determining function of the Y chromosome also directs the uniparental inheritance within paternal lineages, which is remarkable. In forensic genetics, polymorphic loci, which are in linkage disequilibrium and scattered over the entire nonrecombining part of the Y chromosome, are analyzed, especially the rapidly mutating Y-STRs loci (short tandem repeats). Y-STRs are polymorphisms with higher mutation frequency and higher heterozygosity than Y-SNPs (single nucleotide polymorphism). Several Y-STR specific kits are being improved by different companies and online databases with the collection of Y-STR haplotype information were published. The importance of Y-STR haplotyping finds application for paternal lineage identification, to build phylogenetic trees and in special cases of missing persons and disaster victim identification involving men, but also in crime scene investigations to exclude male suspects from involvement in crime, in particular, in the case of male–male or male–female DNA mixtures. The Y chromosome can provide information about the geographic region from which a person's paternal ancestors originate, so it is also useful for bio-geographic ancestry.

4.1   THE Y CHROMOSOME

Mammalian sex chromosomes, X and Y, form two of the 23 pairs of human chromosomes in each cell. The Y chromosome is one of the smallest chromosomes in the genome and spans more than 59 million building blocks of DNA (base pairs), representing almost 2% of the total DNA in cells. The first era in the history of human Y chromosome research started in the opening decades of the 20th century, when proponents of Mendel's concept of the gene observed three modes of inheritance in our species: autosomal recessive, autosomal dominant, and X-linked recessive. Contemporaneously, other scholars sought to identify traits that exhibited Y-linked, father to son, transmission. Meanwhile, light microscopic studies of human cells provided strong physical evidence of the existence of a male-specific chromosome (Painter, 1921). The second era was dominated by the view that the Y chromosome was a genetic wasteland, based on the debunking of earlier studies and a dearth of new evidence for genes. In the 1960s, Ohno proposed that the mammalian X and Y chromosomes had evolved from an ordinary pair of autosomes (Ohno, 1967). Ohno speculated that the X chromosome had retained the ancestral autosome's gene content, whereas the Y chromosome had lost all but perhaps the one gene involved in sex determination. Thus, there emerged the understanding of the human Y chromosome as a profoundly degenerate X chromosome. The hallmark of the recent decades is related to the application of recombinant DNA and genomic technologies to the Y chromosome, culminating in molecular-based conclusions about its genes. The Y chromosome is present in males, who have one X and one Y chromosome, while females have two X chromosomes. Cytogenetically, the human Y is an acrocentric chromosome composed of two pseudoautosomal regions (PARs), the euchromatic region, and heterochromatic region.

The PARs are localized at the terminal part of the short-arm Yp (PAR1) and at the terminal part of the long-arm Yq (PAR2). The main PAR is PAR1 and extends for 2.6 Mb at the terminal ends of both the X and Y short arms.

The euchromatic region is distal to PAR1 and consists of the short-arm paracentromeric region (about 8 Mb), the centromere, and the long-arm paracentromeric region (about 14.5 Mb). This euchromatic portion can also be divided into three other classes: X-transposed, X-degenerate, and ampliconic. The X-transposed sequences are 99% identical to DNA sequences in Xq21, a band in the midst of the long arm of the human X chromosome. The X-transposed sequences are named so because their presence in the human Y is the result of a massive X-to-Y transposition that occurred about 3–4 million years ago (Page et al., 1984). Subsequently, an inversion within the Y short arm cleaved the X-transposed block into two noncontiguous segments (Schwartz, 1998). The X-transposed sequences do not participate in X–Y crossing over during male meiosis and exhibit the lowest density of genes as only two genes have homologs in Xq21 among the three sequence classes in the Y euchromatin. Furthermore, the X-transposed sequences have the highest density of interspersed repeat elements, in particular, long interspersed nuclear element 1 (LINE1). The X-degenerate segments are dotted with single-copy gene, or pseudogene, homologs of 27 different X-linked genes. These single-copy genes and pseudogenes display between 60% and 96% nucleotide sequence identity to their X-linked homologues, and they seem to be surviving relics of ancient autosomes from which the X and Y chromosomes co-evolved. The third class of euchromatic sequences, the ampliconic segments, is composed largely of sequences that exhibit marked similarity, as much as 99.9% identity, to other sequences in the Y chromosome, and they are amplicons (Skaletsky, 2003). Amplicon sequences exhibit the lowest density of LINE1 and interspersed repeating elements and the highest density of coding and noncoding genes. Finally, the heterochromatic region comprises distal Yq corresponding to Yq12, and it is a genetically inert region, rich in highly repeated sequences (Colaco et al., 2018).

Genomic studies revealed that the PARs are the only parts of the Y chromosome in which there is exchange of genetic material between X and Y chromosomes during male meiosis. In addition, the region flanked on both sides by the PARs, comprising 95% of the Y chromosome length, is called the nonrecombining region on the Y chromosome (NRY). It is characterized by the absence of X–Y crossing over (Rozen, 2003). The number of genes localized on the Y chromosome is limited with respect to the other chromosomes and is present both in the PAR and the NRY. Genes that are distributed in PARs are present on both sex chromosomes, are essential for normal development, and are inherited in the same manner as autosomal genes. Many genes are unique in the Y chromosome and are distributed in the NRY region, where they can be divided into two categories. The first category comprises those genes that are ubiquitously expressed and exhibit housekeeping cell functions. The second category includes genes expressed specifically in the testis, that exist in multiple copies on the NRY, and that encode proteins with more specialized functions (Quintana-Murci et al., 2001). All of these genes are responsible for several phenotypes, and most of these are male-specific. Because only males have the Y chromosome, its most characteristic features remain its implication in human sex determination and in male germ cell development and maintenance. The most interesting gene, also from the forensic point of view, is sex-determining region Y (SRY), also called testis determining factor (TDF) that is located on the short arm of the Y chromosome, close to the pseudoautosomal boundary. This intronless gene encodes a transcription factor, a protein of 201 amino acids that is a member of the high mobility group box family of DNA-binding proteins, suggesting that this protein regulates gene expression. In fact, many other genes interact with SRY protein, such as Wilm's tumor gene, Steroidogenic Factor 1, and SOX-9. SRY has been shown to be essential for the regulation of the cascade of testis determination, for initiating testis development, and in the differentiation of the indifferent, bipotential, gonad into the testicular pathway. Because of its distinctive role in sex determination, the Y chromosome has long attracted special attention from geneticists, evolutionary biologists, and even the lay public. It is known that the Y chromosome consists of regions of DNA that show quite distinctive genetic behavior and genomic characteristics (Huntington, 2003).

4.2   THE Y-CHROMOSOMAL MARKERS

Scattered over the entire nonrecombining part of the human Y chromosome, specifically in the heterochromatic region, lots of polymorphic loci have been identified. These polymorphisms on the Y chromosome can be classified as follows:

- biallelic markers with a low mutation rate representing unique (or near-unique) mutation events in human evolution, such as single base-pair substitutions [single nucleotide polymorphisms (SNPs)] (Undehill et al., 1997), ALU insertion/deletion polymorphisms (Hammer, 1994), or a LINE insertion (Santos et al., 2000);
- moderately fast evolving microsatellites or simple tandem repeats (STRs) (Kayser et al., 2000);
- fast evolving loci, such as the minisatellite locus MSY1 (Jobling et al., 1998).

Y-STRs have a mutation rate $\sim$1 in 10^3, so they change more rapidly compared to Y-SNPs that have a mutation rate $\sim$1 in 10^9. Thus, the Y-STRs find larger use in forensic application.

A peculiarity of different loci allele variants in the Y chromosome is that they are in linkage disequilibrium. This means that, differently from other autosomal variants, several loci are in a nonrandom association with each other. Hence, a haplotype is the combination of allelic variants of a set of polymorphic markers with loci in linkage disequilibrium, physically located on the same chromosome. These alleles are associated in haplotypes due to the lack of recombination phenomena that allow them to be inherited in uniparental mode from paternal lineage in the case of Y chromosome. In the Y chromosome, a haplotype consists of the sum of the variability of microsatellite polymorphisms (STRs). A set of haplotypes form a haplogroup that is defined by the sharing of specific slow evolution mutations for biallelic markers (SNPs) (Butler, 2011).

4.3   THE ROLE OF Y-CHROMOSOME MARKERS IN FORENSIC BIOLOGY

The sex-determining function of the Y chromosome and the uniparental inheritance of the non-pseudoautosomal portion as haplotypes within paternal lineages are important features of the Y chromosomes. In principle, it is possible to reconstruct the history of paternal lineages and build phylogenetic trees by comparing modern Ys. Using DNA polymorphisms (Jobling et al., 1995), autosomal DNA profiling is preferred, since it provides a higher power of discrimination, and Y chromosome DNA analysis has different important applications in forensic biology. Y-STR haplotyping, applied in crime scene investigations, can exclude male suspects from involvement in crime, in particular, in the case of male/male DNA mixture or male/female DNA mixture. The majority of the cases in which identification of male-specific DNA is essential are sexual assault cases where admixed samples contain low concentrations of male DNA masked by extremely high levels of female DNA. Y-STR analysis allows for the targeted amplification of male DNA, producing only a genetic profile for the male donor(s) in a sample. This also has proven advantages in cases where mixed-gender DNA cannot be segregated by differential extraction. Y-STR profiles resulting in exclusions are perhaps more helpful to an investigation, as a match can only indicate that the individual and their paternal relatives could have contributed to the biological stain. Increasing the discrimination power of the Y-STR amplification system used for analysis increases the exclusionary power and the accuracy of profile matches. Y-STR haplotype analysis is employed in paternal lineage identification, paternity disputes of male offspring, and other types of paternal kinship testing, including historical cases, as well as in special cases of missing persons and disaster victim identification involving men (Manfred, 2017). The Y chromosome can also provide information about the geographic region from which a person's paternal ancestors originate, so forensic DNA testing is also useful for bio-geographic ancestry (Kayser, 2015) and for tracing historical human migration patterns (Jobling et al., 1995).

The feature of the Y chromosome that gives it an advantage in forensic testing, maleness, is also its biggest limitation in identification because this part of the Y chromosome lacks the meiotic phenomenon of crossing over and recombination, which is the same as mitochondrial DNA and is passed down from father to son unchanged except by the gradual accumulation of mutations (Jobling et al, 1997). One of the main limitations is due to the identity between Y-STR profiles in paternal lineage that does not allow distinguishing among brothers or even distant paternal relatives. Thus, considering the random match probability, inclusions with Y chromosome testing are not as meaningful as autosomal STR matches (de Knijff, 2003).

4.3.1   Y-STR MARKERS

The increase in the number of Y-STR loci to use in human identity allowed in 1997 to establish a set of nine Y-short tandem repeat loci, commonly referred to as the "minimal haplotype loci" set, which still forms the core of all Y-STR kits in current forensic use. These loci are comprised of DYS19, DYS385a and b, DYS389I and II, DYS390, DYS391, DYS392, and DYS393. The rapid growth in the discovery of new Y-STR markers is a direct result of the availability of DNA sequence information from the Human Genome Project and improved bioinformatics tools for searching DNA sequence databases. Most Y-chromosome data have been generated with these loci. In early 2003, the US Scientific Working Group on DNA Analysis Methods (SWGDAM) selected a core set of markers that included the nine markers in the minimal haplotype plus DYS438 and DYS439. New markers were added to databases as their value is demonstrated, and they became part of commercially available kits (Butler, 2003).

4.3.2   Y-STR KIT AND DATABASES

Several Y-STR specific kits are being developed and improved by different companies to provide successful amplification of Y-STR alleles (as shown in Table 4.1), and currently, the most used among these kits for forensic purposes are: Yfiler Plus PCR Amplification Kit (Thermo Fisher Scientific,

Waltham, MA, USA) that simultaneously targets 27 markers, and PowerPlex Y23 System (Promega, Madison, WI, USA) that targets 23 markers on the Y chromosome.

TABLE 4.1 Overview of Commercially Available Y-STR Kits

Kit Name	Release Year
ReliaGene Technologies	
Y-PLEX 6	2001
Y-PLEX 5	2002
Y-PLEX 12	2003
Serac	
genRES DYSplex-1	2002
genRES DYSplex-2	2002
Promega	
PowerPlex Y	2003
PowerPlex Y23	2012
Biotype	
MenPlex Argus Y-MH	2004
Applied Biosystem - Thermo Fisher Scientific	
Yfiler	2004

The PowerPlex Y23 System is a five-dye multiplex system that combines the 17 Y-STR loci currently included in Y-STR kits (DYS19, DYS385a/b, DYS389I/II, DYS390, DYS391, DYS392, DYS393, DYS437, DYS438, DYS439, DYS448, DYS456, DYS458, DYS635, and Y-GATA-H4) with six new highly discriminating Y-STR loci (DYS481, DYS533, DYS549, DYS570, DYS576, and DYS643). The six additional loci included in the PowerPlex Y23 System are characterized by high mutation rates that contribute to more allelic diversity and, therefore, to a better ability to distinguish individuals (Thompson et al., 2012).

The Yfiler Plus multiplex consists of 27 loci in a six-dye configuration, which includes the Yfiler loci (DYS19, DYS385a/b, DYS389I/II, DYS390, DYS391, DYS392, DYS393, DYS437, DYS438, DYS439, DYS448, DYS456, DYS458, DYS635 (Y GATA C4), and Y GATA H4) in addition to ten new loci. The ten new loci consist of three highly polymorphic loci (DYS460, DYS481, and DYS533) and seven well-characterized, rapidly mutating (RM) loci (DYF387S1a/b, DYS449, DYS518, DYS570, DYS576, and DYS627). Yfiler Plus is a dual-application kit designed for efficient amplification of extracted DNA casework samples as well as direct amplification of blood and buccal reference samples on various substrates (Gopinath et al., 2016).

Improvements in newly developed kits have led to a more successful amplification of Y-STR alleles as compared to older kits. Consequently, this improvement provided a higher discriminative capacity, even in samples with a low quantity of Y chromosome DNA and a high female:male DNA ratio (Ferreira-Silva et al., 2018).

Over the past few years, in addition to the description of new Y chromosome STR polymorphisms, there has been a large amount of population and sequencing data published in online databases that collect Y-STR haplotype information coming from anonymous volunteer contributors. One of the most important databases, created by Lutz Roewer and colleagues at Humbolt University in Berlin, is the Y-Chromosome STR Haplotype Reference Database (YHRD) (https://yhrd.org/). This is the result of the worldwide activity of geneticists mainly working in the field of forensics. It is the largest online source for Y chromosome-encoded haplotypes; it is based on a compulsive quality control system and has been available online since 2000 (Roewer, 2003; Willuweit et al., 2007). YHRD latest release R62 provides more than 21,000 haplotypes, of which 1400 typed also with SNPs.

Another important project is US Y-STR Database, funded by the National Institute of Justice and managed by the National Center for Forensic Science in conjunction with the University of Central Florida, which currently includes a total of 32,972 haplotypes with 11 loci.

4.3.3   Y-STR ANALYSIS AND INTERPRETATION

Y-STR analysis follows a similar analytical workflow used for autosomal STRs. However, the interpretation of the Y-STRs results must be done considering one specific feature of Y-STR loci: their haploid nature. Generally, a single Y-STR locus produces one amplicon, and issues related to stochastic effects due to too few template molecules in the PCR are less than the ones for autosomal loci. Nevertheless, it is possible to observe multiple signals that could be related to the presence of more contributors in the tested sample or with a copy number variant (CNV) that involved that specific locus. In fact, many regions of Y chromosome are characterized by the CNV (duplications and deletions), and it is important to consider this to avoid premature conclusions and errors of interpretation (Butler et al., 2005).

There are three possible interpretations resulting from a comparison between Y-STR haplotypes obtained from two different DNA samples:

- exclusion, when Y-STR profiles are different and could not belong to the same source;
- inconclusive when the data are not sufficient to be interpreted;
- inclusion as the Y-STR haplotype results are the same.

When the evidence and reference sample exhibits the same Y-STR haplotype, they may have originated from either a common individual source from any male within the same paternal lineage or unrelated individuals. Barring mutation, all male relatives within the same paternal lineage have the same Y-STR profile, but unrelated individuals may also exhibit the same Y-STR haplotype. As mentioned above, because of the nonrecombining features of the Y-STR loci, the statistical approach for estimating the rarity of a Y DNA profile differs from that applied to autosomal DNA markers (Budowle et al., 2005). Among the approaches for evaluation of coincidental match rarity, the counting method is included (Budowle et al., 2003). Each haplotype is treated as an allele, and according to this method, the profile of a Y-STR haplotype, generated from an evidence sample, is searched against a reference database of unrelated individuals, to determine the number of times the haplotype was observed in that database. The frequency of the haplotype in the database is then estimated by dividing the count by the number of haplotypes that are present in the reference database(s). A confidence interval is then placed on the proportion of count/total profiles in a database. Confidence intervals may be used to reflect the reliability of a statistical estimate and to offer assurance that all data obtained with a procedure should include the true value of the data with a given level of confidence. This confidence interval generally is 95% and can be used to adjust possible effects of population substructure that are more substantial for Y loci compared with those observed for the autosomal STR loci, because Y-STR loci are not shuffled during meiosis and because of the smaller effective population size that contributes to population-specific distribution, genetic drift, and geographic differentiation.

The counting method with the upper bound of 95% is considered as the normal approach with features that make it desirable for forensic application. First, it is conservative because of the assumption of quite complete linkage disequilibrium. All the loci are treated as physically linked, even if the rate of mutation could destabilize the linkage effect with not all the Y-STR loci in linkage disequilibrium; second, Y-STR profiles are not as individualizing as are an equal number of autosomal STR loci, so it is still unlikely to draw two unrelated people at random with the same minimal haplotype, but loci with higher mutation rates may also enhance the ability to distinguish relatives in the same paternal lineage (Ballantyne et al., 2012). Problems related to the normal confidence interval appear in situations of a small sample size and with a rare haplotype. In this situation, it is better to apply the Clopper–Pearson formula (Clopper et al., 1934; Buckleton et al., 2011). This provides a more conservative value, as described in the *Interpretation Guidelines for Y-Chromosome STR Typing by Forensic DNA Laboratories* in 2014, provided by the SWGDAM as a revision of the previous guidelines issued in 2009. This guidance is provided for forensic casework analyses and, in particular, for the identification and application of thresholds for allele detection and interpretation, describing appropriate statistical approaches to the interpretation of Y-STR haplotypes including guidance on mixture interpretation.

Guidelines regarding the interpretation of mixtures are described in *SWGDAM Interpretation Guidelines for Autosomal STR Typing by Forensic DNA Testing Laboratories,* approved in 2010 (SWGDAM, 2010). Furthermore, the ability to combine data from the autosomes and the Y chromosome is particularly important in cases where the signal from the male autosomal markers is largely obscured by the overwhelming amount of a female victim's DNA. To combining match probabilities for autosomal and Y-STR typing results, it is necessary to compute joint match probabilities by multiplying the Y haplotype frequency with the appropriately corrected autosomal frequency. In addition to correcting for autosomal frequency differences between groups, a further correction may be required. Since two individuals sharing the same Y haplotype are likely to be more recently related than two randomly chosen individuals, the autosomal frequencies have to be adjusted by a correction used to account for population substructure (Walsh et al., 2008).

4.3.4   Y-STR MARKER MUTATION RATE

Around 95% of the Y chromosome does not recombine with the X chromosome. Thus, the only source of genetic variation on the Y chromosome between men is the occurrence of mutations on the NRY during meiosis. The fast mutating Y-STRs are polymorphisms that have high mutation frequency and high heterozygosity; thus, they are used to obtain a unique Y haplotype. Several studies have examined mutation rates among the commonly used Y-STR loci focusing on the minimal haplotype loci. In fact, a more precise knowledge of mutation rate variability between (inter) and within (intra) Y-STR loci is important to further improve most recent common ancestor estimations for applications such as forensic familial searching or genealogy research. The mutation rates for Y-STRs are in the same range as autosomal STRs and, specifically, one to four per thousand generational events (0.1%–0.4%). However, a number of criticisms have been raised, in particular concerning the susceptibility of STRs to homoplasy events.

According to the stepwise mutation model of STRs, when two consecutive mutations happen at the same locus, the latter will elide the former in half of the cases, and consequently, identical (or very similar) Y-STR haplotypes may not be the result of a recent shared paternal ancestor. In this condition, homoplasy haplotypes would, therefore, mask the phylogenetic relationships between individuals (Ballantyne et al., 2010). Ballantyne et al. studied 186 Y-STRs through genotyping 2000 father–son couples and making it possible to identify 13 rapidly mutating (RM) Y-STRs with a median mutation rate of 1.97×10^{-2}. Due to the discovery, RM Y-STR's average mutation rate increased by a factor of 10 compared to the conventional Y-STRs, and this makes it more likely for mutations to occur in the meiosis separating the patrilineal relatives and allowing forensic DNA analysis to individualize relatives. In particular, these markers were reported to discriminate between fathers and sons in nearly 50% of cases, brothers in 60%, and cousins in 75%, thus contributing to solving cases of homoplasy.

KEYWORDS

- **Y-STRs**
- **SRY**
- **linkage disequilibrium**
- **paternal kinship testing**

REFERENCES

Ballantyne, K.; et al.; Mutability of Y-chromosomal microsatellites: Rates, characteristics, molecular bases, and forensic implications. *Am. J. Hum. Genet.* **2010**, *87(3)*, 341–353.

Ballantyne, K.; et al.; A new future of forensic Y-chromosome analysis: Rapidly mutating Y-STRs for differentiating male relatives and paternal lineages. *Forensic Sci. Int. Genet.* **2012**, *6*(2), 208–218.

Buckleton, J., et al.; The interpretation of lineage markers in forensic DNA testing. *Forensic Sci. Int. Genet.* **2011** 5(2), 78–83.

Budowle, B.; et al.; Utility of Y-chromosome short tandem repeat haplotypes in forensic applications. *Forensic Sci. Rev.* **2003**, *15*(2), 153–164.

Budowle, B.; et al.; *Molecular Diagnostic Applications in Forensic Science.* **2005**, Amsterdam, The Netherlands, Elsevier.

Butler, J.; Recent developments in Y-short tandem repeat and Y-single nucleotide polymorphism analysis. *Forensic Sci. Rev.* **2003**, *15*, 91.

Butler, J.; *Advanced Topics in Forensic DNA Typing: Methodology.* **2011**, Academic Press.

Butler, J.; et al.; Chromosomal duplications along the Y-chromosome and their potential impact on Y-STR interpretation. *J. Forensic Sci.* **2005**, *50*, 853–859.

Clopper, C.; et al.; The use of confidence or fiducial limits illustrated in the case of the binomial. *Biometrika*, **1934**, *26*(4), 404–413.

Colaco, S.; et al.; Genetics of the human Y chromosome and its association with male infertility. *Reproductive Biol. Endocrinol.* **2018**, *16*(1), 14.

de Knijff, P.; *Son, Give Up Your Gun: Presenting Y-STR Results in Court.* **2003**, Promega Corporation.

Ferreira-Silva, B.; et al.; A comparison among three multiplex Y-STR profiling kits for sexual assault cases. *J. Forensic Sci.* **2018**, *63*(6), 1836–1840

Gopinath, S.; et al.; Developmental validation of the Yfiler® Plus PCR Amplification Kit: An enhanced Y-STR multiplex for casework and database applications. *Forensic Sci. Int. Gen.* **2016**, *24*, 164–175.

Hammer, M.; A recent insertion of an alu element on the Y chromosome is a useful marker for human population studies. *Mol. Biol. Evol.*, **1994**, *5*(11), 749–761.

Huntington, F. W.; Tales of the Y chromosome. *Nature.* **2003**, *423*, 810–813.

Jobling, M.; et al.; Fathers and sons: The Y-chromosome and human evolution. *Trends Genet.* **1995**, 11, 449–456.

Jobling, M.; et al.; Hypervariable digital DNA codes for human paternal lineages: MVR-PCR at the Y-specific minisatellite, MSY1 (DYF155S1). *Hum. Mol. Genet.* **1998**, *7*(4), 643–653.

Jobling, M.; The Y-chromosome in forensic analysis and paternity testing. *Int. J. Legal. Med.* **1997**, *110*, 118–124.

Kayser, M.; Forensic DNA phenotyping: Predicting human appearance from crime scene material for investigative purposes. *Forensic Sci. Int. Genet.* **2015**, *18*, 33–48.

Kayser, M.; et al.; Characteristics and frequency of germline mutations at microsatellite loci from the human Y chromosome, as revealed by direct observation in father/son pairs. *Am. J. Hum. Genet.* **2000**, 66(5), 1580–1588.

Manfred, K.; Forensic use of Y-chromosome DNA: A general overview. *Hum. Genet.* **2017**, *136*, 621–635.

Ohno, S.; *Sex Chromosomes and Sex-Linked Genes.* **1967**, Berlin, Germany, Springer.

Page, D.; et al.; Occurrence of a transposition from the X chromosome long arm to the Y-chromosome short arm during human evolution. *Nature.* **1984**, *311*, 119–123.

Painter, T.; The Y-chromosome in mammals. *Science.* **1921**, *53*, 503–504.

Quintana-Murci, L.; The human Y chromosome: The biological role of a "functional wasteland." *J. Biomed. Biotechnol.* **2001**, *1*(1), 18–24.

Roewer, L.; The Y-Short Tandem Repeat Haplotype Reference Database (YHRD) and male population stratification in Europe: Impact on forensic genetics. *Forensic Sci. Rev.* **2003**, *15*(2), 165–172.

Rozen, S.; Abundant gene conversion between arms of palindromes in human and ape Y. *Nature.* **2003**, *423*, 873–876.

Santos, F.; A polymorphic L1 retroposon insertion in the centromere of the human Y chromosome. *Hum. Mol. Genet.* **2000**, *9*(3), 421–430.

Schwartz, A.; Reconstructing hominid Y evolution: X-homologous block, created by X-Y transposition, was disrupted by Yp inversion through LINE-LINE recombination. *Hum. Mol. Genet.* **1998**, *7*, 1–11.

Skaletsky H.; The male-specific region of the human Y chromosome is a mosaic of discrete sequence classes. *Nature.* **2003**, *423* (6942), 825–837.

SWGDAM; *Interpretation Guidelines for Y-Chromosome STR Typing.* **2014**

SWGDAM; *Interpretation Guidelines for Autosomal STR Typing by Forensic DNA Testing Laboratories.* **2010**

Thompson, J.; et al.; *The PowerPlex® Y23 System: A New Y-STR Multiplex for Casework and Database Applications.* **2012**, Promega Corporation.

Undehill, P.; et al.; Detection of numerous Y chromosome biallelic polymorphisms by denaturing high-performance liquid chromatography. *Genome Res.* **1997**, *7*(10), 996–1005.

Walsh, B.; et al.; Joint match probabilities for Y chromosomal and autosomal markers. *Forensic Sci. Int.* **2008** *174* (2–3), 234–38.

Willuweit, S.; et al.; Y Chromosome Haplotype Reference Database (YHRD): Update. *Forensic Sci. Int. Genet.* **2007** *1*(2), 83–87.

CHAPTER 5

The X-Chromosomal STRs in Forensic Genetics: X Chromosome STRs

VÂNIA PEREIRA[1] and LEONOR GUSMÃO[2*]

[1]Section of Forensic Genetics, Department of Forensic Medicine, Faculty of Health and Medical Sciences, University of Copenhagen, Frederik V's Vej, 11, DK-2100 Copenhagen, Denmark

[2]DNA Diagnostic Laboratory, State University of Rio de Janeiro, Pavilhão Haroldo Lisboa da Cunha, São Francisco Xavier, 524-Maracanã, 20550-900 Rio de Janeiro, Brazil

*Corresponding author. E-mail: leonorbgusmao@gmail.com

ABSTRACT

Because of the unique transmission properties, markers located in the X chromosome are an important tool in the field of forensic genetics, more specifically in kinship analysis. In the majority of the casework presented in forensics, the autosomal markers are the most informative and most widely used, since they present the highest power of discrimination among individuals within a population. However, situations arise where markers located in other regions of the genome can be more informative and should be used instead to complement autosomal information. This is the case of mtDNA, for example, that has a prominent role in the analysis of ancient or degraded samples, due to the high number of copies present in each cell. In contrast, the Y-chromosome-specific markers are more suitable than autosomal to recover male genetic profiles in mixtures with high amounts of female DNA. The X-chromosome-specific markers represent the best choice in kinship cases where the information provided by autosomal markers alone is not sufficient. The presence of only one X chromosome in males that does not suffer recombination during meiosis and that is transmitted to all female descendants as a haplotype has proven to be of great importance in cases where autosomal markers have no power of exclusion, namely to investigate paternal half-sisters or paternal grandmother/granddaughter relationships. While X-chromosomal markers present obvious advantages in some forensic scenarios, a certain degree of complexity arises in the statistical interpretation of genetic evidence from linked markers. The present chapter will briefly introduce the X chromosome as an important tool in forensic genetics and will present the main characteristics of this type of markers when applied to kinship analysis.

5.1   THE X CHROMOSOME

The X and Y chromosomes are the sex chromosomes in the human karyotype. The two sex chromosomes originated from an ancestral autosomal pair around 300 million years ago (Ohno, 1967). Throughout time, the two chromosomes suffered structural changes that culminated in two very different chromosomes that differ both in size and structure (Charlesworth et al., 2005; Graves, 2006). While the Y chromosome is one of the smallest chromosomes in humans, the X chromosome is one of the biggest with around 155 million base pairs. The Y chromosome has lost most of its genomic material and does not suffer recombination in 95% of its extension (Skaletsky et al., 2003). The X chromosome represents around 5% of the total human genetic information and still retains traces of its autosomal past suffering recombination along its entire length during female gametogenesis. Homology between the two chromosomes is still present in the telomeric pseudoautosomal regions (PAR 1 and PAR 2).

5.2   CHARACTERISTICS OF THE X CHROMOSOME

Because of the presence of two very distinct sex chromosomes, the number of X chromosomes present in each cell varies between males and females. Males have one Y chromosome transmitted by the father, and one X chromosome that they inherit from their mothers. Females, on the other hand, have two X chromosomes inherited from each parent (see Figure 5.1). The paternal X chromosome they receive does not suffer recombination (except in the pseudo-autosomal regions) and is transmitted directly from the father to the daughters. Sisters have, therefore, the same X chromosome inherited from their father (safe mutation). The maternal X chromosome contains recombined genetic information from the two X chromosomes present in the mother.

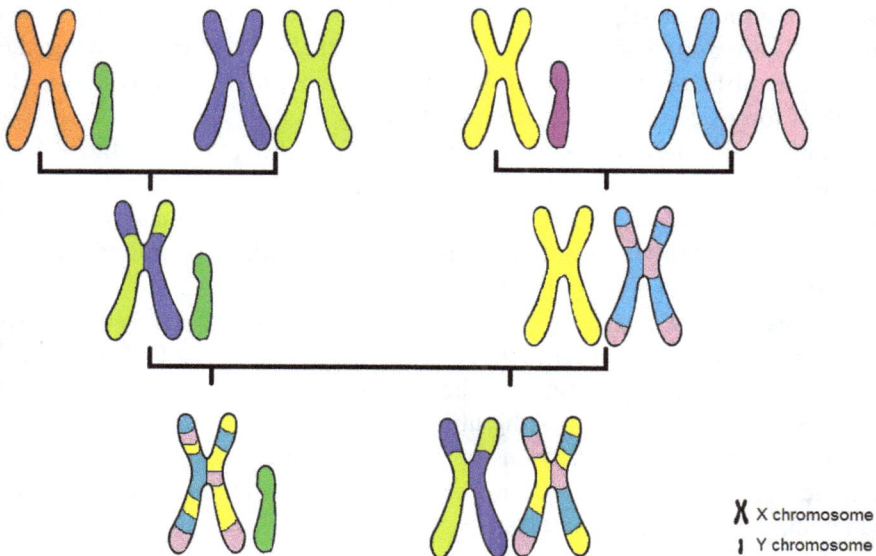

FIGURE 5.1   Genetic transmission of X and Y chromosomes.

This chromosomal number imbalance between genders has made the X chromosome an interesting subject for genetic studies, especially in the clinical field. Many genetic conditions have already been described as being related to mutations in specific genes on the X chromosome (Ross et al., 2005). Hemophilia is a classic example of an X-chromosome-associated disease, among others. These diseases are typically observed and detected in males that carry the X chromosome that has the causative mutation. In females, the symptoms of the disease can go undetected, as long as the other X chromosome copy is fully functional and does not have the causative mutation.

Owing to its particular mode of inheritance, the interest in the study of the X-chromosomal markers as tools for forensic and population genetic studies has been growing in the last decades (Szibor et al., 2003; Schaffner, 2004; Szibor, 2007; Tillmar et al., 2017).

5.3   THE X-CHROMOSOMAL MARKERS IN FORENSIC GENETICS

The high degree of variation that exists in the human genome allows discriminating individuals within and between populations, and therefore, genetic markers become the main identification tool in the forensic field.

Depending on their sequence variation and genome location, different types of DNA polymorphisms are available and can be selected allowing the genetic identification of individuals and biological relationships in a wide range of forensic scenarios under investigation.

Markers located in the X-chromosome-specific region (which does not recombine with the Y chromosome during male meiosis) can be used to solve kinship cases where Y-chromosomal and mtDNA markers are not informative, and the information from autosomal markers is limited (e.g., to investigate paternal half-sisters' relationship).

Forensic genetics casework is mainly related to three areas: analysis of trace samples, individual identification, and establishment of biological relationships (paternity testing or other kinship).

This section demonstrates the utility of the X-chromosomal markers in the forensic context, in situations where the information provided by other genetic markers is not as informative, and where X chromosome analysis can complement autosomal data.

5.3.1 INDIVIDUAL IDENTIFICATION AND THE ANALYSIS OF TRACE SAMPLES

Owing to the high power of discrimination (PD) and easiness of typing, autosomal markers [more specifically, short tandem repeats (STRs)] are the first choice in the analysis of trace samples in forensic routine casework. For equally polymorphic markers, X-chromosomal and autosomal loci will have the same power to discriminate females, but the PD will be lower in males for X-chromosomal loci that only have one allele per locus.

Quite often, the trace samples collected at a crime scene or from a victim are in fact a mixture from one or several donors, and the victim's DNA. Depending on the context, the sex of the individuals involved, and the nature of the trace, X-chromosomal markers can be more informative than the autosomes.

If female traces are to be search in a female background (female epithelial cells under a woman's fingernails, for instance), the information obtained by the analysis of X chromosome yields the same results as autosome analysis, with no gain in PD. When male traces ought to be searched on male background, the use of X chromosome markers is not advisable at all. In this case, the PD value for X markers will be lower, since only one X chromosome (and one allele at each locus) can be analyzed.

In samples that contain DNA from female and male individuals, the applicability of the X-chromosomal markers varies. If a male profile is to be searched on a female background, the use of the X chromosome is not advisable. Since males carry one X chromosome, the probability of the male profile being "hidden" within the female profile is high.

The situation where X-analysis can be an advantage is when a female trace needs to be identified in a male background. In this case, the PD for the X markers will be higher than for the autosomes. The markers selected for forensic purposes are so diverse that the probability of having all the female alleles included in the male profile is very low.

Besides the described applications, X chromosome analysis can also be useful in old and degraded samples, when autosomal information may be absent, or when family relationships must be established based on few genetic markers (e.g., disaster victim identification).

5.3.2 PATERNITY CASES AND OTHER KINSHIP TESTING

As for the trace samples, the bulk of kinship casework is routine paternity cases involving trios (child, mother, and putative father). Mostly, these cases can be easily solved with autosomal markers. Analysis of X-chromosomal markers can be particularly advantageous in situations where genealogical and pedigree reconstruction is needed (as long as the X-chromosomal lineages are not interrupted by father–son relationships) (see Figure 5.2) and, even more so, in situations where the putative father is not immediately available, and his closest relatives must be analyzed instead (see Figure 5.2).

X-chromosomal markers can also be more informative than autosomes when resolving relationships that involve two sisters or paternal half-sisters (see Figure 5.2a and b), since they will certainly share one pair of identical by descent (IBD) X-alleles, being equally likely that they share one or no pair of IBD autosomal alleles. The same happens in paternity investigations where only the putative paternal grandmother is available for genotyping (see Figure 5.2c). Since males will inherit their X chromosome from the mother, the putative father's haplotype (that he then will pass to his daughter) can be inferred from the paternal grandmother. Thus, when the alleged father is not available for testing, X-specific markers should be prioritized whenever his mother (or one daughter) is accessible for typing, since they will have a higher informative power than equally polymorphic markers on autosomes. X-chromosomal markers are also more informative than autosomes in father–daughter duos, since there is only one allele that can be transmitted from the father to the daughter. Therefore, they can be useful for supplementing autosomal information from partial profiles obtained due to a poor quality of the DNA (Tillmar et al., 2017) or in cases showing few incompatibilities between the alleged father and the daughter (Gomes et al., 2012).

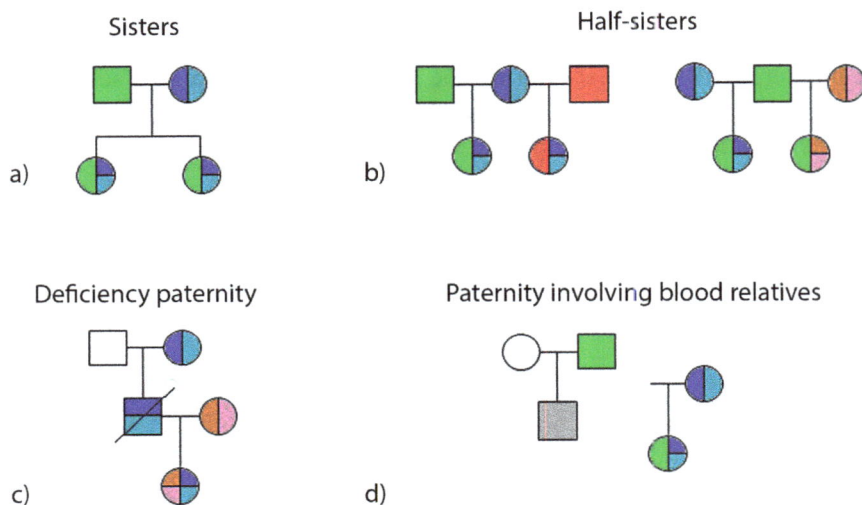

FIGURE 5.2 Examples where the analysis of the X chromosome is more informative than the autosomal data. Paternity can be more easily established using the X-chromosomal markers, since full sisters or paternal step-sisters share the X chromosome transmitted by the father (a and b). X-chromosomal markers are also an advantage in deficiency paternity investigations, where the putative father is not available for testing. In this situation, the putative paternal grandmother can be analyzed instead. If the individuals are related, the putative father's haplotype (that he then will pass to his daughter) can be inferred from the paternal grandmother (c). Since the X chromosome is not shared between male relatives, the analysis of X-chromosomal markers can be used to ascertain paternity when the two alleged fathers are father and son (d).

Since the X chromosome is not transmitted from fathers to sons, when trying to establish kinship between men, the analysis of X-chromosomal markers is not useful. However, on a paternity testing where the two alleged fathers are father and son, the analysis of the X chromosome can be more helpful to establish paternity than the autosomes, since the two males will not share X chromosome alleles identical by descent (see Figure 5.2d).

The application of X-chromosomal information in population and forensic genetics is relatively recent compared to the well-established autosomal protocols. Nevertheless, the examples described demonstrate the potential applications of X-chromosomal markers in complex cases of kinship investigation.

5.4 THE X-CHROMOSOMAL MARKERS IN POPULATION GENETICS

Forensic genetics is largely based on population genetic studies. The presentation of the weight of forensic genetic evidence in court is done by likelihood ratios (LRs) that statistically compare the likelihood of a certain scenario under two mutually exclusive hypotheses, with the random population serving as reference.

As recombination throughout the X chromosome only occurs in females, the genetic information contained in this chromosome is disproportionately influenced by female demography. The study of X chromosomes and autosomes in a population can reveal genetic patterns that are different between males and females. Usually, when addressing these differences in demography, the choice relies on the comparison of the information provided by the haploid markers (mitochondrial DNA and Y chromosome that provide information on female or male mediated histories, respectively). The advantage of using the X-chromosomal information is that it contains information from both genders. Owing to recombination, the X chromosome is composed of a block-like pattern with different chromosomal regions being informative of distinct genetic histories, unlike uniparental markers that are transmitted as a single locus and where all the markers share the same genealogic history.

The copy number imbalance among males and females also leads to differences in the recombination and mutation rates between the X chromosome and the autosomes. Due to these characteristics, and also due to younger age, the diversity on the X chromosome is, in general, lower when compared to autosomes.

From a population genetics point of view, evolutionary forces such as selection and genetic drift are more pronounced and maintained for longer in the X chromosome (Schaffner, 2014). The same is observed for linkage disequilibrium (LD) patterns. LD is the nonrandom association of alleles in a population, at two or more loci (not necessarily linked). LD can be created when two populations with very different allele frequencies exchange genetic information. For a given amount of time, the alleles of the parental populations will be associated in a nonrandom manner. Only after some generations, LD will be broken, and these effects will gradually fade. Several factors are responsible for breaking the extent of LD in a chromosome, such

as the physical distance between the markers, and recombination and mutation rates. Given that recombination only occurs in females, for markers at
the same genetic distance, more time will be necessary to break down LD in
the X chromosome compared to autosomes. As a result, LD is greater when
compared to the autosomes, and the size of regions with a single genetic
history is larger, making it a better and more accurate tool to detect patterns
of LD in populations.

In forensic analysis, when computing likelihoods (and LRs), it is necessary to account for LD by using haplotype instead of allele frequencies
(Tillmar et al., 2017; Kling et al., 2015a). For X-chromosomal markers, the
presence of LD in a population can be tested in male samples, which allows
the direct access to their haplotypes. In the presence of LD, some haplotypes
will be present in a population more frequently than expected by chance, due
to a nonrandom association between alleles at different loci.

The LD structure of one population cannot be extrapolated to others, since,
in addition to the physical distance between markers, the aforementioned
factors related to the population history, as well as population sub-structure,
will impact the degree of LD.

In the last decade, there has been an increase in the publication of data
concerning X-STRs, but further studies are still needed on allele frequency
distributions, mutation rates, and LD, in order to continue to establish reference population databases.

Figure 5.3 displays a geographic overview of published population data
(1999–2016), which shows the lack of data for certain geographic regions,
especially outside Europe, and the imbalance between the numbers of publications by country.

5.5   GENETIC MARKERS ON THE X CHROMOSOME

Motivated by the need of solving complex kinship cases, which are frequently
encountered in the identification of missing persons or victims from mass
disasters, different types of markers have been described along the X chromosome, including single-nucleotide polymorphisms (SNPs) (Zarrabeitia et
al., 2007; Tomas et al., 2008; Li et al., 2010; Oki et al., 2012), insertion/dele-
tions (indels) (Freitas et al., 2010; Pereira et al., 2012; Fan et al., 2015) and
STRs (Gusmão et al., 2009; Diegoli and Coble, 2011; Edelmann et al., 2012;
Prieto-Fernández et al., 2016). Figure 5.4 presents an illustrative description
of some of the X-SNPs and X-indels that have been published.

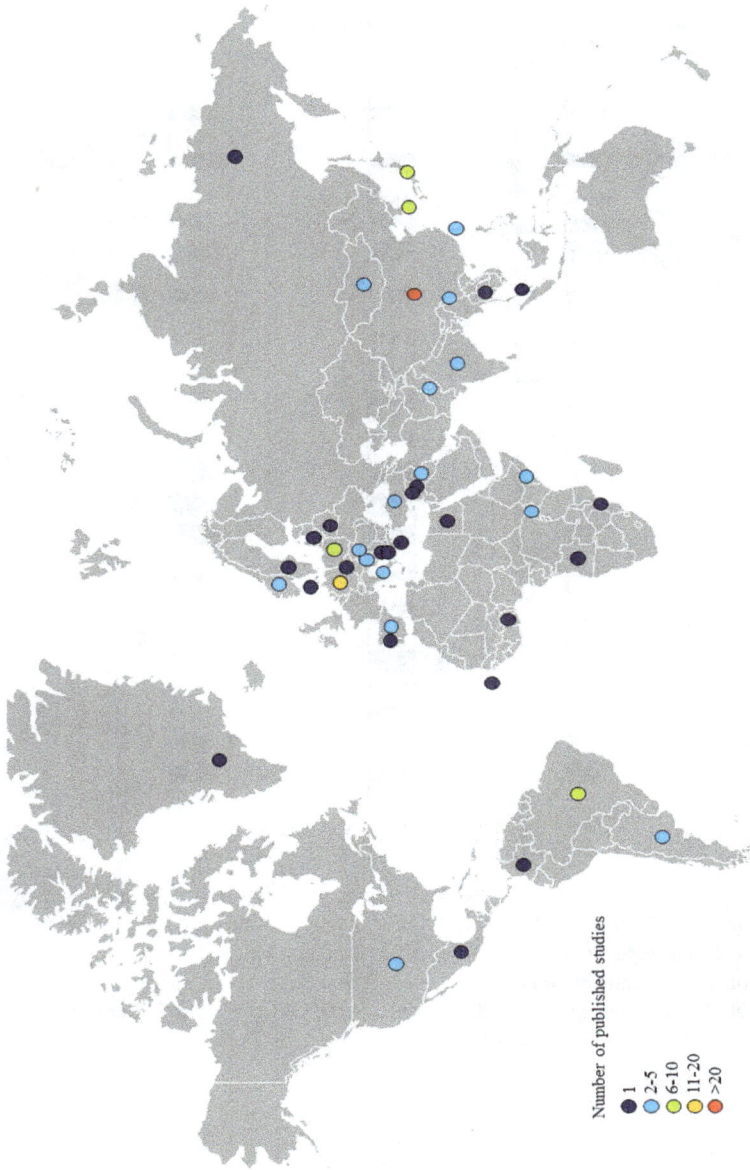

FIGURE 5.3 Geographical overview of population data published for the X chromosome

The STRs are the type of genetic markers most widely used in forensics, since their multiallelic state and high diversity allow obtaining high levels of discrimination with a reduced number of loci. For this reason, the remaining sections of this chapter will focus on X-chromosomal STRs.

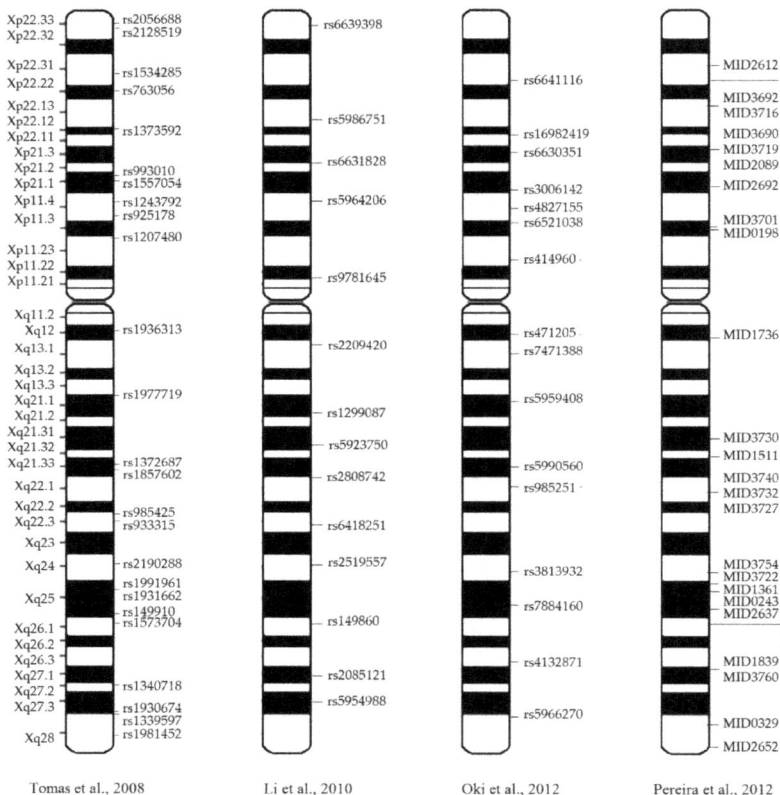

FIGURE 5.4 Example of some of the SNPs (rs [locus accession reference assigned by the National Centre for Biotechnology Information (NCBI) website https://www.ncbi.nlm.nih.gov/], numbers) and indels (MID [locus adentifier assigned by the Marshfield Diallelic Insertion/Deletion Polymorphisms database] numbers) that have been described for the X chromosome (data from Tomas et al., 2008; Li et al., 2010; Oki et al., 2012; Pereira et al., 2012). Chromosomal locations are merely indicative.

5.5.1 X-CHROMOSOMAL STRs

STRs are DNA sequences composed of tandem repetitions (2–6 bp) that are present in different numbers in individuals.

STRs can also be categorized into simple, compound, or complex, according to their structure. The complexity of the motif and its size has repercussions on the mutation rates and the number of different alleles.

STRs have become the marker of election in forensic genetics because of their high diversity (between individuals and between populations) and easiness of genotyping.

It is estimated that STRs represent around 3% of the total human genome variation and occur every 10,000 nucleotides/bases. Although scattered throughout the genome, the majority of STRs are located in noncoding regions. These markers are selectively neutral and highly polymorphic (with average mutations rates of around 2.1×10^{-3}).

A large number of STR loci have been described for autosomes and the Y chromosome (in humans, and other mammals). Selected markers have been included in commercially available kits that have been used by forensic laboratories and facilitated the development of standardized databases that became valuable tools for national and international intelligence agencies.

5.5.2 X-STR MULTIPLEX

Although autosomal and Y-STR analyses have been standard in forensic casework, only very recently has science focused on the potential of X-chromosomal STRs.

Several human X-chromosome STR multiplexes have been described. A multiplex consisting of 10 markers (X Decaplex) was developed in 2008 as a result of a collaborative work carried out by the Spanish and Portuguese Speaking Working Group of the International Society for Forensic Genetics (ISFG) (Gusmão et al., 2009). The first commercially available kit soon followed, containing eight X-STRs (Argus X-8), plus amelogenin for gender determination. Later, this multiplex was expanded by including four additional X-STRs (Argus X-12).

More recently, a multiplex containing 17 X-STRs has been introduced (Prieto-Fernández et al., 2016) aiming to increase the resolution power and forensic applicability for the X chromosome. This multiplex combines markers from the two previous multiplexes plus six additional markers. The work demonstrated that the new set of 17 X-STRs can be a good alternative to the current X-STR multiplexes. Table 5.1 presents the STR markers including in these multiplexes in more detail.

In the past few years, forensic genetic laboratories have been exploring STR and SNP sequencing using massively parallel sequencing (MPS) platforms (Seo et al., 2013; Dalsgaard et al., 2014; Rockenbauer et al., 2014; Van Neste et al., 2014; Warshauer et al., 2015). Commercial companies are also making the transition from the common capillary electrophoresis methods to MPS. Several kits have been launched in the market containing the most common STRs used by the forensic genetic community. In 2012–2013, Thermo Fisher Scientific released the Precision ID GlobalFiler NGS STR Panel, which contains 33 markers, including 21 autosomal STR CODIS loci, three male-specific markers, and amelogenin for gender determination. A few years later in 2015, Illumina® released the ForenSeq™ DNA Signature Prep Kit. The kit contains 29 autosomal STRs, 9 X-STRs, 24 Y-STRs, 86 autosomal human identification SNPs, 56 autosomal ancestry informative SNPs, and 22 autosomal SNPs associated with phenotypic traits.

TABLE 5.1 Overview of STR Markers Present in Some of the Multiplexes Described for the X Chromosome. BUILD 37 hg19

Marker	Physical Location (bps)	Argus X-8	Decaplex	Argus X-12	17 X-STRs
DXS6807	4 743 347				x
DXS10148	9 238 978			x	
DXS10135	9 306 342	X		x	
DXS8378	9 370 150	X	X	x	x
DXS9902	15 323 462		X		x
DXS7132	64 655 268	X	X	x	x
DXS10079	66 715 903			x	x
DXS10074	66 977 187	X		x	
DXS10075	66 998 226				x
DXS6800	78 680 324				x
DXS6803	86 431 165				x
DXS9898	87 796 419		X		x
DXS6801	92 510 985				x
DXS6809	94 938 089		X		x
DXS6789	95 449 242		X		x
DXS6799	97 378 874				x
DXS7133	109 041 339		X		x
GATA172D05	113 174 984		X		x
DXS10103	133 418 989			x	
HPRTB	133 615 405	X		x	
DXS10101	133 654 515	X		x	
GATA31E08	140 234 252		X		x

TABLE 5.1 *(Continued)*

Marker	Physical Location (bps)	Argus X-8	Decaplex	Argus X-12	17 X-STRs
DXS10146	149 584 306			X	
DXS10134	149 650 120	X		X	
DXS7423	149 710 903	X	X	X	X

MPS is gradually making its way in forensics, and although its application in the forensic field sounds promising, there are still some challenges that need to be addressed.

5.5.3 MUTATION IN X-CHROMOSOMAL STRs

It is a general consensus that STRs are originated by random mutations (Levinson and Gutman 1987; Schlotterer 2000), and that the loss or gain of repeat units is due to DNA replication slippage (Ellegren 2000; Schlotterer 2000).

Since the repetitive motive does not expand indefinitely, the currently accepted mutation model for STRs integrates mutational forces acting in opposite directions. Besides replication slippage, studies have shown that the frequency of point mutations increases with an increase in the length of the STR. The point mutations split the initial motif into smaller stretches, and this has been perceived as an evolutionary mechanism to control the average size of the fragment (Ellegren, 2004). The process of replication slippage can also be artificially introduced during polymerase chain reaction (PCR) amplification. This process creates PCR products-*stutter*-that have different number of repeats than the true allele. These artifacts can complicate STR analyses in samples with low-template/low-quality DNA or mixtures, as they can be confounded as part of the profile and influence the interpretation of results.

The application of thresholds in the analysis parameters can help overcome this issue and discriminate between a true allele or an artifact.

For forensic genetic purposes, the STRs typically included in commercial kits have a four-base-pair motif. Motifs with more nucleotides are usually less common, and motifs with two and three base pairs are less stable and tend to produce more stutter in the amplification.

In forensic casework, in order to address if the incompatibilities between two profiles are due to mutation, it is necessary to have accurate information about the mutation rate of each marker. Not many studies have addressed this

TABLE 5.2 Compilation of X-STR Mutation Rates Described in the Literature

Marker	Number of Mutations	Number of Meioses	Pooled Mutation Rate ($\times10^{-3}$)	95% CI ($\times10^{-3}$)
DXS8377	10	1702	5.88	2.8–10.8
DXS10135	13	2663	4.88	2.6–8.3
DXS10148	9	1943	4.63	2.1–8.8
DXS10075	3	984	3.05	0.63–8.9
DXS10079	8	2638	3.03	1.3–6.0
DXS10134	7	2372	2.95	1.2–6.1
DXS7132	12	5310	2.26	1.2–3.9
DXS10074	9	3359	2.68	1.2–5.1
DXS6803	2	1015	1.97	0.24–7.1
DXS6809	4	2133	1.88	0.51–4.8
DXS10146	4	1603	2.50	0.7–6.4
DXS10103	5	1655	3.02	1.0–7.0
HPRTB	6	4530	1.32	0.49–2.9
DXS7424	2	1805	1.11	0.13–4.0
DXS8378	4	3882	1.03	0.28–2.6
GATA31E08	1	1127	0.89	0.02–4.9
DXS6789	3	3478	0.86	0.18–2.5
DXS7423	2	3515	0.57	0.07–2.1
DXS9898	1	1936	0.52	0.01–2.9
DXS10101	3	2318	1.29	0.3–3.8
DXS101	1	2534	0.39	0.01–2.2
DXS10011	0	50	0	0–71.1
DXS10147	0	54	0	0–66.0
DXS6810	0	100	0	0–36.2
DXS6793	0	100	0	0–36.2
DXS6797	0	168	0	0–21.7
DXS9902	0	458	0	0–8.0
DXS6807	0	598	0	0–6.2
GATA172D05	0	876	0	0–4.2
DXS9895	0	917	0	0–4.0
GATA165B12	0	958	0	0–3.8
DXS6801	0	1084	0	0–3.4
DXS7133	0	1459	0	0–2.5
DXS6800	0	1694	0	0–2.2
DXS981	0	2099	0	0–1.8

issue, although an increase in published population data has been observed. In 2014, Diegoli and collaborators published mutation data for 15 X-STRs, together with a revision of literature (Diegoli et al., 2014). Table 5.2 presents the most updated information regarding the mutation rates per marker, for the most commonly used X-STRs.

Note: mutation rates were calculated based on the following references: Athanasiadou et al. (2003), Becker et al. (2008), Castaneda et al. (2012), Diegoli et al. (2014), Edelmann et al. (2001), Edelmann et al. (2002), García et al. (2017), Glesmann et al. (2009), Hering et al. (2001), Huang et al. (2003), Hundertmark et al. (2008), Liu et al. (2008), Liu et al. (2012), Nadeem et al. (2009), Nishi et al. (2013), Nothnagel et al. (2012), Pepinski et al. (2005, 2006, 2007), Poetsch et al. (2005, 2009), Shin et al. (2004), Szibor et al. (2000, 2003), Tabbada et al. (2005), Tang et al. (2006), Tariq et al. (2008), Tetzlaff et al. (2012), Tomas et al. (2012), Turrina et al. (2004, 2007), Wiegand et al. (2003), Zalan et al. (2007), Zarrabeitia et al. (2002a, 2002b).

5.6 BIOSTATISTICAL EVALUATION OF X-STRs IN KINSHIP ANALYSIS

In forensic genetics, the weight of the evidence is usually evaluated based on LR principles (Morling et al., 2003; Gill et al., 2006; Gjertson et al., 2007). Therefore, in the statistical evaluation of kinships, it is necessary to calculate the probability of the observed phenotypic constellations of the tested individuals, assuming two mutually exclusive hypotheses. Centered on this principle, the DNA commission of the ISFG has recently formulated recommendations for the biostatistical evaluations of kinships, based on X-STRs genetic profiles (Tillmar et al., 2017).

For an X-chromosomal marker, the genotypic probabilities can be easily calculated for pairs of individuals assuming different pedigrees, but differently than for autosomal markers, the formulas will depend on the sex of the individuals involved (Toni et al., 2007; Pinto et al., 2011). This is, however, more complex on the evaluation of evidence based on several X-chromosomal markers (Krawczak, 2007), since both linkage between loci and LD among alleles at different loci will have an impact on the final LR (Tillmar et al., 2011; Kling et al., 2015a; Kling, 2018).

In the presence of LD, the conditional probabilities calculated for each locus cannot be multiplied, and LRs must be calculated based on haplotype frequencies. Although LD can also affect unlinked markers (e.g., in the presence of intrapopulation substructure), linked markers are expected to retain LD for longer periods. Moreover, as noted above, LD tends to be lower for autosomal than for X-chromosomal loci that only recombine in female germline.

In contrast to LD that varies among populations and along generations, linkage concerns the physical association between loci that do not segregate independently within a family. Although linkage will not be relevant in the simplest cases of paternity or maternity duos investigations, in other kinship problems, it can be necessary to account for linkage when computing the LR.

Two markers are said to be linked if more than 50% of the gametes are expected to have the same segment as the parental chromosome, which is related to the genetic distance between them.

A relatively large number of STRs are required to obtain high exclusion probabilities and LRs. Because of the limited size of the X chromosome (188.22 cM, according to the deCODE map, on https://www.ncbi.nlm.nih. gov), some markers will be necessarily in linkage, and the recombination rates between them must be calculated. Figure 5.5 depicts the genetic position for some X-STRs that are frequently used in forensic analysis.

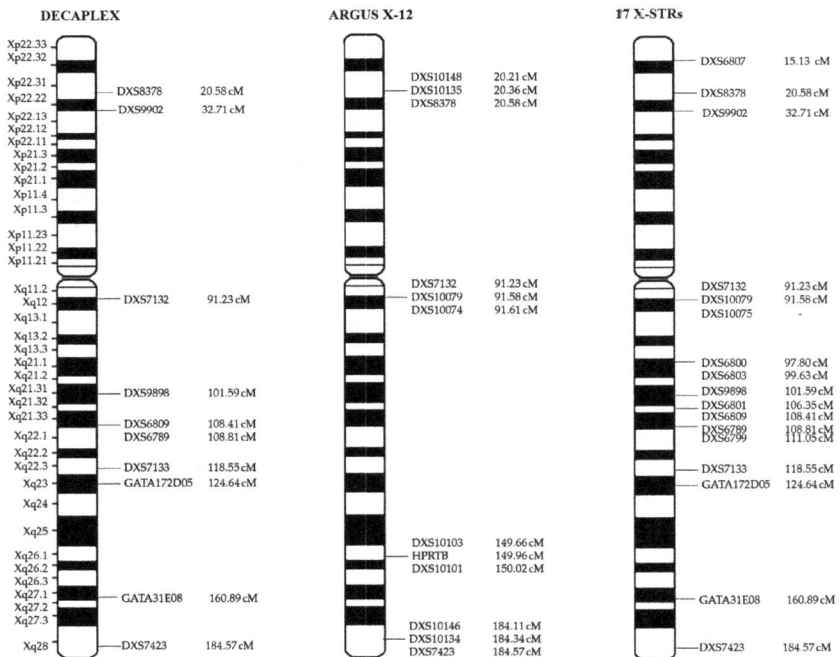

FIGURE 5.5   Genetic position of the most common X-STRs that have been described for the X chromosome. Chromosomal locations are merely indicative.

Recombination rates between X-STR loci can be estimated by segregation analysis in multigeneration families (Nothnagel et al., 2012; Diegoli et al., 2016). In the absence of segregation data, recombination rates may also be inferred from genetic distances that are given in centimorgans (cM). For very close markers, 1 cM will roughly correspond to approximately 1% of recombination. However, when the genetic distance increases, this rule is no longer valid, and there are several mapping functions designed to convert genetic distances to recombination rates [e.g., Haldane's (Haldane, 1919) and Kosambi's (Kosambi, 1944)]. Using Haldane's mapping function, a genetic distance of 50 cM will correspond to a recombination rate of approximately 32%, and recombination rates around 50% are only obtained for genetic distances larger than 200 cM (Tillmar et al., 2017).

Because of the greater complexity of the statistical methods that simultaneously account for linkage and LD among loci, there are fewer available software packages for X-chromosomal applications compared to the autosomal counterpart.

The FamLinkX is a free software (http://famlink.se/fx_index.html) that provides functions in likelihood calculation for family relationships/pedigrees using X-chromosomal genetic marker data, and it simultaneously accounts for linkage, LD, and mutations (Kling et al., 2015a; Kling et al., 2015b).

Because of the relevance of X markers for solving complex kinship cases and in the identification of missing persons, it is expected that in parallel to the developments on methodologies that allow the simultaneous genotyping of large sets of X-chromosomal markers, other software will become available in a near future. According to the recommendations of DNA commission of the ISFG (Tillmar et al., 2017), any software used to calculate LRs based on X-chromosomal markers in kinship analysis "should be able to accommodate linkage, LD, and mutations" and "should follow the recommendations from the DNA Commission of the ISFG on the validation of software programs (Coble et al., 2016)."

KEYWORDS

- **X-STRs**
- **linkage**
- **linkage disequilibrium**
- **paternity testing**
- **kinship analysis**
- **forensics genetics**

REFERENCES

Athanasiadou, D.; et al.; Development of a quadruplex PCR system for the genetic analysis of X-chromosomal STR loci. *Int. Congr. Ser.* **2003**, *1239*, 311–314.

Becker, D.; et al.; Population genetic evaluation of eight X-chromosomal short tandem repeat loci using Mentype Argus X-8 PCR amplification kit. *Forensic Sci. Int. Genet.* **2008**, *2*(1), 69–74.

Castaneda, M.; et al.; Haplotypic blocks of X-linked STRs for forensic cases: Study of recombination and mutation rates. *J. Forensic Sci.* **2012**, *57*(1), 192–195.

Charlesworth, D.; Charlesworth B.; and Marais G.; Steps in the evolution of heteromorphic sex chromosomes. *Heredity* **2005**, *95*(2), 118–128.

Coble, M. D.; et al.; DNA Commission of the International Society for Forensic Genetics: Recommendations on the validation of software programs performing biostatistical calculations for forensic genetics applications. *Forensic Sci. Int. Genet.* **2016**, *25*, 191–197.

Dalsgaard, S.; et al.; Non-uniform phenotyping of D12S391 resolved by second generation sequencing. *Forensic Sci. Int. Genet.* **2014**, *8*(1), 195–199.

Diegoli, T.M.; and Coble, M.D.; Development and characterization of two mini-X chromosomal short tandem repeat multiplexes. *Forensic Sci. Int. Genet.* **2011**, *5*(5), 415–421.

Diegoli, T.M.; et al.; Mutation rates of 15 X chromosomal short tandem repeat markers. *Int. J. Legal Med.* **2014**, *128*(4), 579–587.

Diegoli, T.M.; et al.; Genetic mapping of 15 human X chromosomal forensic short tandem repeat (STR) loci by means of multi-core parallelization. *Forensic Sci. Int. Genet.* **2016**, *25*, 39–44.

Edelmann, J.; and Szibor, R.; DXS101: A highly polymorphic X-linked STR. *Int. J. Legal Med.* **2001**, *114*(4–5), 301–304.

Edelmann, J.; et al.; Validation of the STR DXS7424 and the linkage situation on the X-chromosome. *Forensic Sci. Int.* **2002**, *125*(2–3), 217–222.

Edelmann, J.; et al.; X-chromosomal haplotype frequencies of four linkage groups using the Investigator Argus X-12Kit. *Forensic Sci. Int. Genet.* **2012**, *6*(1), e24–e34.

Ellegren, H; Microsatellite mutations in the germline: Implications for evolutionary inference. *Trends Genet.* **2000**, *16*(12), 551–558.

Ellegren, H.; Microsatellites: Simple sequences with complex evolution. *Nat. Rev. Genet.*, **2004**, *5*(6), 435–445.

Fan, G.; et al.; Use of multi-InDels as novel markers to analyze 13 X-chromosome haplotype loci for forensic purposes. *Electrophoresis.* **2015**, *36*(23), 2931–2938.

Freitas, N.S.; et al.; X-linked insertion/deletion polymorphisms: Forensic applications of a 33-markers panel. *Int. J. Legal Med.* **2010**, *124*(6), 589–593.

García, M. G.; et al.; Mutation rate of 12 X-STRs from investigator Argus X-12 kit in Argentine population. *Forensic Sci. Int. Genet. Suppl. Ser.* **2017**, *6*, e562–e564.

Gill, P.; et al.; DNA Commission of the International Society of Forensic Genetics: Recommendations on the interpretation of mixtures. *Forensic Sci. Int.* **2006**; *160*(2–3), 90–101.

Gjertson, D. W.; et al.; ISFG: Recommendations on biostatistics in paternity testing. *Forensic Sci. Int. Genet.* **2007**; *1*(3–4), 223–231.

Glesmann, L.A.; et al.; Mutation rate of 7 X-STRs of common use in population genetics. *J. Basic Appl. Genet.* **2009**, *20*(2), 37–41.

Gomes, C.; et al.; Comparative evaluation of alternative batteries of genetic markers to complement autosomal STRs in kinship investigations: autosomal indels vs. X-chromosome STRs. *Int. J. Legal Med.* **2012**, *126*(6), 917–921.

Graves, J; Sex chromosome specialization and degeneration in mammals. *Cell.* **2006**, *124*(5), 901–914.

Gusmão, L.; et al.; A GEP-ISFG collaborative study on the optimization of an X-STR decaplex: Data on 15 Iberian and Latin American populations. *Int. J. Legal Med.* **2009**, *123*(3), 227–234.

Haldane, J. B. S.; The combination of linkage values and the calculation of distances between the loci of linked factors. *J. Genet.* **1919**, *8*, 299–309.

Hering, S.; Kuhlisch, E.; and Szibor R.; Development of the X-linked tetrameric microsatellite marker HumDXS6789 for forensic purposes. *Forensic Sci. Int.* **2001**, *119*(1), 42–46.

Huang D; et al.; Development of the X-linked tetrameric microsatellite markers HumDXS6803 and HumDXS9895 for forensic purpose. *Forensic Sci. Int.* **2003**, *133*(3), 246–249.

Hundertmark, T.; et al.; The STR cluster DXS10148-DXS8378-DXS10135 provides a powerful tool for X-chromosomal haplotyping at Xp22. *Int. J. Legal Med.* **2008**, *122*(6), 489–492.

Kling, D.; Curiosities of X chromosomal markers and haplotypes. *Int. J. Legal Med.* **2018**, *132*(2), 361–371.

Kling, D.; et al.; A general model for likelihood computations of genetic marker data accounting for linkage, linkage disequilibrium, and mutations. *Int. J. Legal Med.* **2015a**, *129*(5), 943–954.

Kling, D.; et al.; FamLinkX: Implementation of a general model for likelihood computations for X-chromosomal marker data. *Forensic Sci. Int. Genet.* **2015b**, *17*, 1–7.

Kosambi, D. D.; The estimation of map distance from recombination values. *Ann. Eugen.* **1944**, *12*, 172–175.

Krawczak, M.; Kinship testing with X-chromosomal markers: Mathematical and statistical issues. *Forensic Sci. Int. Genet.* **2007**, *1*(2), 111–114.

Levinson, G.; and Gutman, G. A.; Slipped-strand mispairing: A major mechanism for DNA sequence evolution. *Mol. Biol. Evol.* **1987**, *4*(3), 203–221.

Li, L.; et al.; Analysis of 14 highly informative SNP markers on X chromosome by TaqMan SNP genotyping assay. *Forensic Sci. Int. Genet.* **2010**, *4*(5), e145-e148.

Liu Q. L.; et al.; Development of a five ChX STRs loci typing system. *Int. J. Legal Med.* **2008**, *122*(3), 261–265.

Liu, Q.L.; et al.; Development of multiplex PCR system with 15 X-STR loci and genetic analysis in three nationality populations from China. *Electrophoresis.* **2012**, *33*(8), 1299–1305.

Morling, N.; et al.; Paternity Testing Commission of the International Society of Forensic Genetics: Recommendations on genetic investigations in paternity cases. *Forensic Sci. Int.* 2003; *129*(1), 148–157.

Nadeem, A.; et al.; Development of pentaplex PCR and genetic analysis of X chromosomal STRs in Punjabi population of Pakistan. *Mol. Biol. Rep.* **2009**, *36*(7), 1671–1675.

Nishi, T.; et al.; Application of a novel multiplex polymerase chain reaction system for 12 X-chromosomal short tandem repeats to a Japanese population study. *Leg. Med. (Tokyo).* **2013**, *15*(1), 43–46.

Nothnagel, M.; et al.; Collaborative genetic mapping of 12 forensic short tandem repeat (STR) loci on the human X chromosome. *Forensic Sci. Int. Genet.* **2012**, *6*, 778–784.

Ohno, S.; *Sex Chromosome and Sex Linked Genes.* **1967**, New York: Springer-Verlag.

Oki, T.; et al.; Development of multiplex assay with 16 SNPs on X chromosome for degraded samples. *Leg. Med. (Tokyo).* 2012, *14*(1), 11–16.

Pepinski, W.; et al.; Polymorphism of four X-chromosomal STRs in a Polish population sample. *Forensic Sci. Int.* **2005**, *151*(1), 93–95.

Pepinski, W.; et al.; Polymorphism of four X-chromosomal STRs in a religious minority of Old Believers residing in northeastern Poland. *Int. Congr. Ser.* **2006**, *1288*, 307–309.

Pepinski, W.; et al.; X-chromosomal polymorphism data for the ethnic minority of Polish Tatars and the religious minority of Old Believers residing in northeastern Poland. *Forensic Sci. Int. Genet.* **2007**, *1*(2), 212–214.

Pereira R.; et al.; A method for the analysis of 32 X chromosome insertion deletion polymorphisms in a single PCR. *Int. J. Legal Med.* **2012**, *126*(1), 97–105.

Pico A.; et al.; Genetic profile characterization and segregation analysis of 10 X-STRs in a sample from Santander, Colombia. *Int. J. Legal Med.* **2008**, *122*(4), 347–351.

Pinto, N.; et al.; X-chromosome markers in kinship testing: A generalisation of the IBD approach identifying situations where their contribution is crucial. *Forensic Sci. Int. Genet.* **2011**, *5*(1), 27–32.

Poetsch, M.; et al.; Development of two pentaplex systems with X-chromosomal STR loci and their allele frequencies in a northeast German population. *Forensic Sci. Int.* **2005**, *155*(1), 71–76.

Poetsch, M.; et al.; Allele frequencies of 11 X-chromosomal loci in a population sample from Ghana. *Int. J. Legal Med.* **2009**, *123*(1), 81–83.

Prieto-Fernández E.; et al.; Development of a new highly efficient 17 X-STR multiplex for forensic purposes. *Electrophoresis.* **2016**, *37*(12), 1651–1658.

Rockenbauer, E.; et al.; Characterization of mutations and sequence variants in the D21S11 locus by next generation sequencing. *Forensic Sci. Int. Genet.* **2014**, *8*(1), 68–72.

Ross, M. T.; The DNA sequence of the human X chromosome. *Nature* **2005**, *434*(7031), 325–337.

Schaffner, S. F.; The X chromosome in population genetics. *Nat Rev Genet.* **2004**, *5*(1), 43–51.

Schlotterer, C.; Evolutionary dynamics of microsatellite DNA. *Chromosoma.* **2000**, *109*(6), 365–71.

Seo, S. B.; et al.; Single nucleotide polymorphism typing with massively parallel sequencing for human identification. *Int. J. Legal Med.*, **2013**, *127*, 1079–1086.

Shin, K. J.; et al.; Five highly informative X-chromosomal STRs in Koreans. *Int. J. Legal Med.* **2004**, *118*(1), 37–40.

Skaletsky, H.; et al.; The male-specific region of the human Y chromosome is a mosaic of discrete sequence classes. *Nature.* **2003**, *423*(6942), 825–837.

Szibor R.; et al.; Population data on the X chromosome short tandem repeat locus HumHPRTB in two regions of Germany. *J. Forensic Sci.* **2000**, *45*(1), 231–233.

Szibor, R.; et al.; Use of X-linked markers for forensic purposes. *Int. J. Legal Med.* **2003**, *117*(2), 67–74.

Szibor, R.; X-chromosomal markers: past, present and future. *Forensic Sci. Int. Genet.* **2007**, *1*(2), 93–99.

Tabbada, K.A.; et al.; Development of a pentaplex X-chromosomal short tandem repeat typing system and population genetic studies. *Forensic Sci. Int.* **2005**, *154*(2–3), 173–180.

Tang, W.M.; and To, K.Y.; Four X-chromosomal STRs and their allele frequencies in a Chinese population. *Forensic Sci. Int.* **2006**, *162*(1–3), 64–65.

Tariq, M.A.; et al.; Allele frequency distribution of 13 X-chromosomal STR loci in Pakistani population. *Int. J. Legal Med.* **2008**, *122*(6), 525–528.

Tetzlaff, S.; Wegener, R.; and Lindner, I.; Population genetic investigation of eight X-chromosomal short tandem repeat loci from a northeast German sample. *Forensic Sci. Int. Genet.* **2012**, *6*(6), e155-e156.

Tillmar, A. O.; et al.; Using X-chromosomal markers in relationship testing: calculation of likelihood ratios taking both linkage and linkage disequilibrium into account. *Forensic Sci. Int. Genet.* **2011**, *5*(5), 506–511.

Tillmar, A. O.; et al.; DNA Commission of the International Society for Forensic Genetics (ISFG): Guidelines on the use of X-STRs in kinship analysis._*Forensic Sci. Int. Genet.* **2017**, *29*, 269–275.

Tomas C.; et al.; X-chromosome SNP analyses in 11 human Mediterranean populations show a high overall genetic homogeneity except in North-west Africans (Moroccans)._*BMC Evol. Biol.* **2008**, *29*(8), 75.

Tomas, C.; Pereira, V.; and Morling, N.; Analysis of 12 X-STRs in Greenlanders, Danes and Somalis using Argus X-12. *Int. J. Legal Med.* **2012**, *126*(1), 121–128.

Toni, C.; Domenici, R.; and Presciuttini, S.; Genotype probabilities of pairs of individuals for X-chromosome markers. *Transfusion.* **2007** *47(7)*, 1276–1280.

Turrina, S.; and De Leo, D.; Population genetic comparisons of three X-chromosomal STRs (DXS7132, DXS7133 and GATA172D05) in North and South Italy. *Int. Congr. Ser.* **2004**, *1261*, 302–304.

Turrina, S.; et al.; Development and forensic validation of a new multiplex PCR assay with 12 X-chromosomal short tandem repeats. *Forensic Sci. Int. Genet.* **2007**, *1*(2), 201–204.

Van Neste, C.; et al.; My-Forensic-Loci-queries (MyFLq) framework for analysis of forensic STR data generated by massive parallel sequencing. *Forensic Sci. Int.* **2014**, *9*(1), 1–8.

Warshauer, D. H.; et al.; Massively parallel sequencing of forensically relevant single nucleotide polymorphisms using TruSeq forensic amplicon. *Int. J. Legal Med.*, **2015**, *129*(1), 31–36.

Wiegand, P.; et al.; Population genetic comparisons of three X-chromosomal STRs. *Int. J. Legal Med.* **2003**, *117*(1), 62–65.

Zalan, A.; et al.; Hungarian population data of four X-linked markers: DXS8378, DXS7132, HPRTB, and DXS7423. *Int. J. Legal Med.* **2007**, *121*(1), 74–77.

Zarrabeitia, M. T.; et al.; Sequence structure and population data of two X-linked markers: DXS7423 and DXS8377. *Int. J. Legal Med.* **2002a**, *116*(6), 368–371.

Zarrabeitia, M. T.; et al.; A new pentaplex system to study short tandem repeat markers of forensic interest on X chromosome. *Forensic Sci. Int.* **2002b**, *129*(2), 85–89.

Zarrabeitia, M. T.; et al.; Forensic efficiency of microsatellites and single nucleotide polymorphisms on the X chromosome. *Int. J. Legal Med.* **2007**, *121*(6), 433–437.

CHAPTER 6

Application of Mitochondrial DNA as a Tool in the Forensic Field: Update and New Perspectives in mtDNA Analysis

MANUEL CRESPILLO MÁRQUEZ[1*], PEDRO A. BARRIO CABALLERO[2], and CAROLINA NÚÑEZ DOMINGO[1]

[1]Instituto Nacional de Toxicología y Ciencias Forense, Carrer de la Mercè 1, 08071 Barcelona, Spain

[2]Instituto Nacional de Toxicología y Ciencias Forense, José Echegaray 4, 28232 Madrid, Spain

*Corresponding author. E-mail: manuel.crespillo@justicia.es

ABSTRACT

The analysis of mitochondrial DNA (mtDNA) is a useful tool in the forensic field as a complementary technique to forensic nuclear DNA thanks to the high sensitivity it provides in those cases in which the integrity or quantity of DNA recovered compromises the study of other forensic genetic markers. Nowadays, mtDNA analysis has been accepted by the majority of courts around the world. However, mtDNA analysis is a type of analysis less used in forensic laboratories than nuclear DNA analysis for several reasons: greater interpretative difficulty, the absence of commercial kits, lower power of discrimination, and increased analytical complexity. This chapter provides an overview of mtDNA analysis, its characteristics, nomenclature, and a methodological overview of how it is typically analyzed in forensic genetics laboratories. In this sense, with the new technologies of massively parallel sequencing (MPS), the platforms used in the forensic field are introduced, as well as the bioinformatics tools for sequences analysis/edition. In addition, a special reference is made to the data interpretation, a key point in forensic laboratories for the statistical evaluation of a match. All the international recommendations existing so far are reviewed.

6.1 INTRODUCTION

The analysis of the polymorphism of the mitochondrial DNA (mtDNA) molecule for genetic identification purposes is a tool of unquestionable usefulness in resolving of forensic cases (Gill et al., 1994; Holland et al., 1993, Holland and Parsons, 1999). However, the use of short tandem repeats (STR) markers for genetic individualization purposes is currently considered the "gold standard" in the field of forensic genetics.

The analysis of mtDNA provides two great advantages over the analysis of autosomal STR markers: first, the high number of copies of mtDNA molecules per cell compared to the two copies of nuclear DNA (Robin, 1988; Bogenhagen, 1980), resulting in higher sensitivity, which is of particular interest in those situations in which the integrity or the quantity of DNA recovered from the specimens subjected to analysis may compromise the study of STR markers; second, the type of inheritance, exclusively maternal, which makes it possible to establish relationship between maternal relatives separated by several generations (Gill et al., 1994; Holland et al., 1993, Holland and Parsons, 1999). This feature is especially useful in cases of cadaver identification, in which there are no direct relatives available. However, despite the advantages described, the absence of recombinant molecules gives it a discrimination power inferior to that offered by nuclear STR markers, thus limiting the individualization usefulness of the mtDNA molecule.

Despite the possibilities that mtDNA analysis offers as a complementary tool in the analysis of autosomal STRs, at the moment, it is not a widely used method in forensic laboratories. There are several reasons that explain this fact: the limited discriminatory power, the greater sensitivity to accidental contamination processes, and higher level of complexity in the analysis and, occasionally, in the interpretation of the results. All these issues require a higher skill level by the staff that performs this type of analysis. Finally, the manufacturers have not openly committed themselves to the development and validation of commercial kits, which involves a time-consuming process for the laboratories and, consequently, with long or protracted execution times.

Currently, the analysis of mtDNA, like the rest of the methods used in the forensic genetics field, has a high degree of standardization, to which different scientific standardization groups have contributed by issuing recommendations and guidelines on their interpretation and use (Carracedo et al., 2000; Parson et al., 2014), as well as the introduction of open-access world population databases that contain high-quality data, such as European DNA Profiling Group Mitochondrial DNA Population Database (EMPOP) (Parson et al., 2007a, 2007b), and the organization of collaborative exercises

(Tully et al., 2004; Salas et al., 2005b; Crespillo et al., 2006; Prieto et al., 2013) by different scientific societies and institutions [i.e., German DNA Profiling Group, European DNA Profiling Group, and Spanish and Portuguese Speaking Working Group of the International Society for Forensic Genetics (GHEP-ISFG)]. Finally, the use of mtDNA analysis in other scientific disciplines, such as anthropology, evolutionary, and population genetics, has provided forensic genetics with a better knowledge of the phylogenetic distribution of mtDNA, as well as significant improvements in the methods and interpretation.

The future introduction of new analytical techniques [i.e., massively parallel sequencing (MPS)] into the field of forensic genetics promises to be a solution for some of the current limitations of mtDNA analysis, by offering a better discriminatory power in the analysis, as well as the possibility of analyzing mixtures of biological fluids, or a greater sensitivity in the detection and identification of heteroplasmy, and the introduction and implementation of new panels, which allow a greater standardization (Woerner et al., 2018; Strobl et al., 2018).

6.2 THE mtDNA MOLECULE

The mitochondria are double-membrane cytoplasm organelles that are present in eukaryotic cells of the superior organisms that use oxygen as an energy source. The mitochondria are responsible for crucial metabolic processes, such as the production of ATP by oxidative phosphorylation. In general, the cells involved in a greater energy output will possess a higher amount of mitochondria.

The mitochondria contain their own genetic material. The number of copies per cell varies between 200 and 2700, depending on the type of tissue (Robin and Wong, 1988). The length of the mitochondrial genome is typically 16,569 pairs, but this number of bases can vary slightly depending on the presence or absence of insertions/deletions (Indels) and the length of determined homopolymeric tracts present in some regions of the mitochondrial genome. For example, there is a dinucleotide repeat, ACACACACAC or $(AC)_5$ that allows some polymorphism between $(AC)_3$ and $(AC)_7$ (Bodenteich et al., 1992; Szibor et al., 1997).

The mtDNA molecule is made up of a double strand, one of them rich in purine bases, which is known as the heavy strand (H), with the complementary strand rich in pyrimidine bases, and called the light strand (L). Most of the mtDNA codes and contains information for 22 different mitochondrial tRNAs, 2 rRNAs (subunits 12S and 16S), and 13 mitochondrial proteins located in the internal membrane. All these take part in the oxidative phosphorylation and respiratory chain processes (Attardi, 1987; Borst, 1972; Borst and Grivell, 1981). The genetic code of mtDNA has some variations as regard nuclear DNA (Barrell et al., 1979; Knight et al.. 2001).

The mutation rate of mtDNA is at least 10 times higher than that occurring in nuclear DNA (Brown et al., 1979; Wallace et al., 1987). There are several causes for this fact: the susceptibility of mtDNA to oxidative damage produced by the free radicals generated during the oxidative phosphorylation process (Nedbal and Flynn, 1998; Williams and Hurst, 2002); the absence of histones that reduces the protective effect that these confer to DNA; and, finally, the mtDNA repair mechanisms that are less efficient than those present in nuclear DNA (Yakes and Van Houten, 1997; Croteau et al., 1999).

The mtDNA does not contain introns, and with the exception of some noncoding nucleotides among some genes, the only noncoding region is known as the displacement loop or D-loop. It is a region of 1.2 kb (1121 bp) located between the pro-tRNA and phe-tRNA genes that contain the promoters for the transcription of the L and H strands and the replication origin of the H-chain. This region accumulates most of the polymorphism of the molecule, and its noncoding character means that certain mutations may be observed without having the damaging effects that other locations of the genome could have.

Traditionally, the forensic laboratories have analyzed the regions that contain more polymorphism within the control region (CR), classically described as hypervariable segment I (HVS-I) and hypervariable segment II (HVS-II). HVS-I extends from position 16024 to 16365, and HVS-II extends from position 73 to 340. There are nucleotide positions within the D-loop that are more prone to mutate. These positions have been defined as hotspots and include the following positions in HVS-I: 16093, 16129, 16153, 16189, 16192, 16293, 16337, and 16309. For HVS-II, the following positions have been described: 72, 153, 189, 207, and 279 (Calloway et al., 2000; Stoneking, 2000). Lutz et al. (2000) have described a third hypervariable region located between nucleotides 438 and 574, called HVS-III, with less polymorphism than the previous ones. Occasionally, the HVS-III region is of great use for increasing the discrimination between individuals with an identical sequence for the HVS-I and HVS-II regions. However, the ISFG, in its latest recommendations for the use of mtDNA, includes the interest in analyzing the entire CR, mainly with two objectives: to increase the discriminatory power of the analysis, and to study the positions with high phylogenetic interest (Parson et al., 2014).

The forensic interest in the analysis of mtDNA resides in two properties. The first one is its high number of copies per cell (200–2700) (Robin and Wong, 1988; Bogenhagen et al., 1980), which enables specimens to be analyzed, in which the quantity and quality of the DNA obtained do not make the analysis using autosomal STRs feasible. The other is that mtDNA is exclusively inherited by the maternal line (Giles et al., 1980) and does not suffer from recombination. This means that all individuals related via the maternal line will share the same mtDNA, making it a tool of indisputable use in order to make comparisons of family members who are not directly related but share a common maternal ancestry. The maternal heredity of mtDNA is due to two circumstances: one of which is due to the important difference in the number of mtDNA molecules between the ovule and the spermatozoid (Chen et al., 1995; Manfredi et al., 1997; Diez-Sanchez et al., 2003), and the other is due to the existence of a recognition mechanism that should eliminate the mtDNA molecules from the spermatozoa that could enter the ovule (Manfredi et al., 1997; Sutovsky et al., 2000).

Not all the population of mtDNA molecules has an identical sequence in individuals, as there are small differences between them. This phenomenon is defined as heteroplasmy. The presence of certain differences in the mtDNA molecule among individuals of the same maternal lineage is explained by the phenomenon called bottleneck, which occurs during human oogenesis (Hawswirth et al., 1984; Hawswirth and Laipis, 1982).

The mtDNA molecules are replicated independently from each other, although the replication is linked to the mitosis and meiosis cell division processes. Thus, in one individual, we may find several mitochondrial variables dividing and segregating independently. During the production of the primary oocytes, a limited group of mtDNA molecules are transferred to these oocytes; in such a way, due to simple randomization, each oocyte may have different proportions of mtDNA variables that are subsequently developed into mature ovules. This could explain the finding of different homoplasmy and heteroplasmy states between generations of the same maternal lineage or even between tissues of the same individual. This circumstance occasionally has important implications in the forensic field when interpreting the results of an mtDNA analysis (Butler, 2012).

It is currently thought that all individuals are heteroplasmic at some level, very likely at a level of intensity much lower than the detection limits currently permitted in mtDNA sequence analysis (Comas et al., 1985; Alonso et al., 2002). Likewise, tissues more prone to the appearance of heteroplasmy than others have been described, as in the case of the hair (Salas et al., 2001), where it appears that the histogenesis of the hair itself is the cause of this tendency to heteroplasmy (Lynch et al., 2001). In contrast, as regard the mutation type, heteroplasmy can be classified into two large groups, by sequence and by length, as will be discussed later.

6.3 REFERENCE SEQUENCE, ALIGNMENT, AND NOTATION

The first human mtDNA sequence was obtained in 1981 from an individual of European descent (Anderson et al., 1981). This 16,569 bp sequence has been known since then as the Cambridge reference sequence (CRS). In order to report mtDNA haplotypes, in both forensic and population genetics applications, the CRS served as reference for the scientific community. However, years later, the CRS was resequenced, and some positions were corrected establishing the revised Cambridge reference sequence (rCRS) (Andrews et al., 1999). Then, the rCRS became the reference relative to which mtDNA haplotypes were reported.

More recently, an alternative to the rCRS has been proposed, a hypothetical "reconstructed sapiens reference sequence" (Behar et al., 2012). Although this approach entails positive features with regard to haplogroup determination and the identification of mtDNA derived states, the change to this notation method would mean a high risk of introducing error among other issues (Salas et al., 2012; Bandelt et al., 2014). Thus, from the ISFG, the recommendation remains to use the rCRS, at least for the time being (Parson et al., 2014).

One of the main challenges when dealing with mtDNA interpretation is converting DNA sequence data into a standard nomenclature for database inclusion and searching. If a uniform notation system does not exist, laboratories would designate DNA sequences in different ways, which could mean that a database search would not provide accurate results. In view of this, guidelines to help in this issue have been published by the Scientific Working Group on DNA Analysis Methods (SWGDAM) and the ISFG.

When an mtDNA sequence is aligned to the rCRS, mutational events relative to this reference are reported as the haplotype. All nomenclature recommendations are compatible with International Union of Pure and Applied Chemistry (IUPAC) codes.

Transitions and transversions are reported with the position number and the nucleotide differing from the reference sequence (see Figure 6.1). If an unresolved ambiguity is observed at any site, that is, all four nucleotides are present at a single position, the base number for the site is listed followed by an "N" (Carracedo et al., 2000). Insertions are reported as first noting the site immediately 5′ to the insertion followed by a decimal point and a number depending on the number of nucleotides that are inserted (Carracedo et al., 2000) (see Figure 6.1). Deletions will be indicated by the missing site followed by "DEL," "del," or "–" (Parson et al., 2014) (see Figure 6.1). When a mixture of deleted/undeleted and inserted/noninserted bases appears, lowercase letters instead of capital letters after the nucleotide position will be used (see Bandelt et al., 2007).

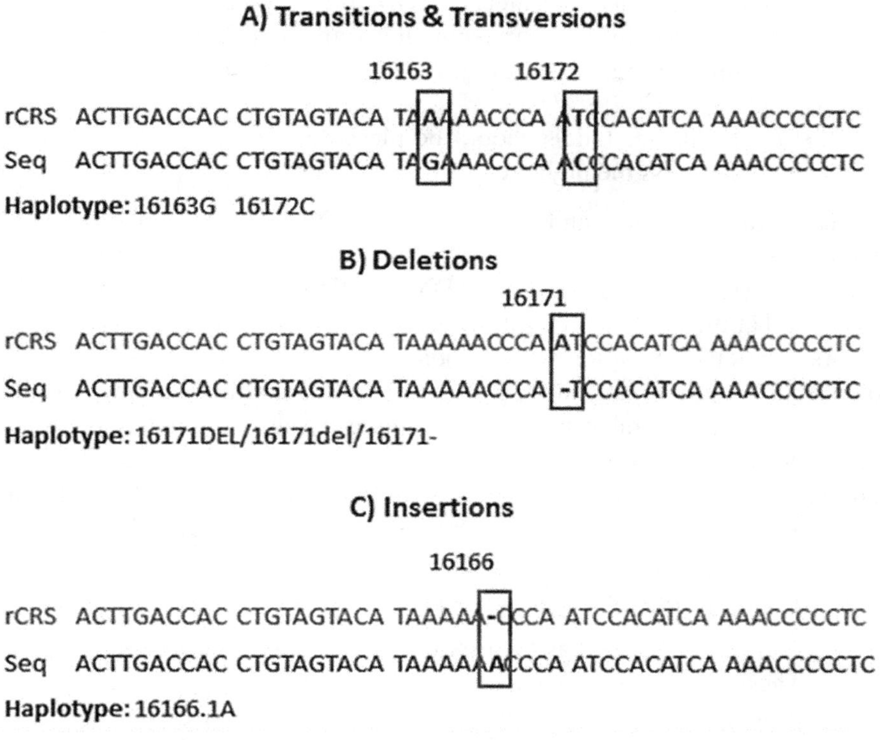

A) Transitions & Transversions

```
           16163          16172
rCRS  ACTTGACCAC CTGTAGTACA TAAAAACCCA ATCCACATCA AAACCCCCTC
Seq   ACTTGACCAC CTGTAGTACA TAGAAACCCA ACCCACATCA AAACCCCCTC
Haplotype: 16163G  16172C
```

B) Deletions

```
                      16171
rCRS  ACTTGACCAC CTGTAGTACA TAAAAACCCA ATCCACATCA AAACCCCCTC
Seq   ACTTGACCAC CTGTAGTACA TAAAAACCCA -TCCACATCA AAACCCCCTC
Haplotype: 16171DEL/16171del/16171-
```

C) Insertions

```
                   16166
rCRS  ACTTGACCAC CTGTAGTACA TAAAAA-CCCA ATCCACATCA AAACCCCCTC
Seq   ACTTGACCAC CTGTAGTACA TAAAAAACCCA ATCCACATCA AAACCCCCTC
Haplotype: 16166.1A
```

FIGURE 6.1 Three different mtDNA nomenclature situations after the alignment of a sequence (Seq) with the rCRS: (A) transitions and transversions, (B) deletions, and (C) insertions.

The alignment of an mtDNA sequence to the rCRS could result in multiple alignments, mainly in regions displaying length variation. Hence, the international recommendation claims that the alignment and notation should be performed in agreement with the mitochondrial phylogeny considering the established patterns of mutations (Bandelt and Parson 2008; Parson et al., 2014). The phylogenetic alignment follows three rules (from Bandelt and Parson 2008).

1. *Phylogenetic rule:* Sequences should be aligned with regard to the current knowledge of the phylogeny. In the case of multiple equally plausible solutions, one should strive for maximum (weighted) parsimony. Variants flanking long C tracts, however, are subject to extra conventions in view of extensive length heteroplasmy (LHP).

2. *C-tract conventions:* The long C tracts of HVS-I and HVS-II should always be scored with 16189C and 310C, respectively, so that phylogenetically subsequent interruptions by novel C to T changes are encoded by the corresponding transition. Length variation of the short A tract preceding 16184 should be notated in terms of transversions.

3. *Indel scoring:* Indels should be placed 3' with respect to the light strand unless the phylogeny suggests otherwise.

There are examples and tools to assist with this notation of mtDNA sequences available at the SWGDAM Interpretation Guidelines for Mitochondrial DNA Analysis by Forensic DNA Testing Laboratories (SWGDAM, 2013) and at the EMPOP site (https://empop.online).

As previously mentioned, heteroplasmy is the presence of more than one mtDNA type in an individual (Comas, 1985). This phenomenon may be observed in several ways: (a) in a single tissue, individuals may have different mtDNA molecules; (b) in different tissues, individuals may have different mtDNA types; and (c) individuals may present heteroplasmy in one tissue but not in another tissue. There are two types of heteroplasmy, point heteroplasmy (PHP) and LHP, which differ in their frequency and cause (Parson et al., 2014; Butler, 2012).

• *PHP:* It is detected as the mixture of two bases in the same position. These nucleotide mixtures should be reported using the nomenclature provided by the IUPAC in capital letters such as A/G=R and C/T=Y (e.g., see Figure 6.2).

• *LHP:* It is detected as the mixture of two mtDNA molecules with different length, and it is typically detected by the presence of overlapping peaks in the sequence electropherogram. LHP often occurs around the homopolimeric C-tracts in HVS-I (positions 16184–16193) and HVS-2 (positions 303–310) (e.g., see Figure 6.3). In such cases, it is often difficult to unambiguously establish the exact number of cytosine residues present. For that reason, insertions and deletions in those tracts are ignored in direct forensic comparisons and database searches (Parson et al., 2014).

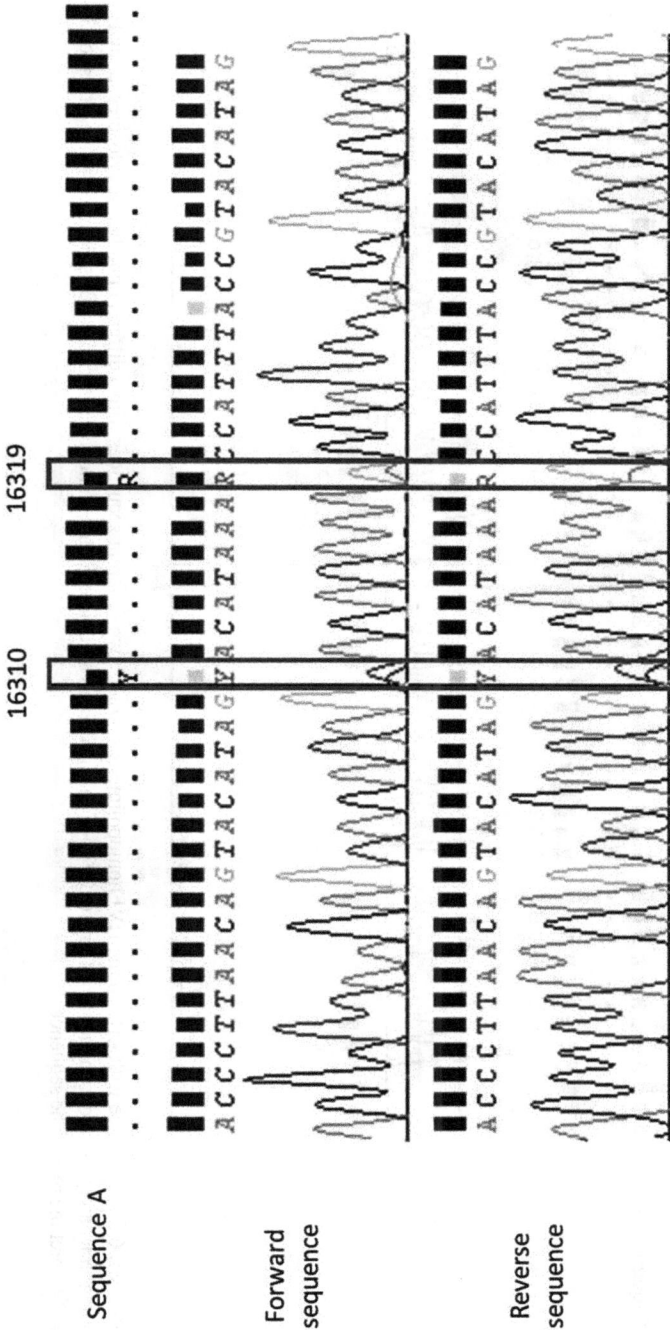

FIGURE 6.2 Sequence with two PHP positions. Position 16310 consists of a mixture of nucleotides C/T (16310Y), while in position 16319, a nucleotide mixture of A and G is detected (16319R).

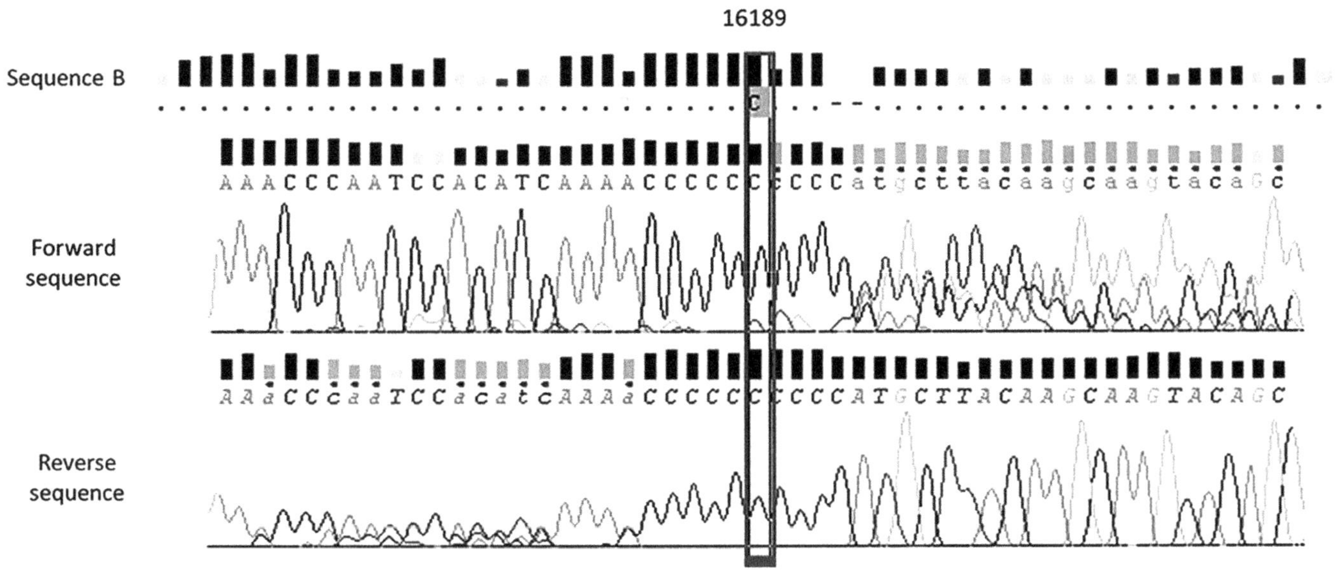

FIGURE 6.3 Sequence with LHP in the HVI homopolimeric C-tract. Two different sequences with a different number of cytosines in the HVI poli-C tract are present due to the transition 16189T→C that generates an uninterrupted homopolymeric tract. This situation makes it impossible to interpret the rest of the sequence.

Forensic laboratories must establish their own interpretation and reporting guidelines regarding point and LHP.

6.4 METHODOLOGY

6.4.1 IMPORTANCE OF THE WORK AREA SEPARATION

Every forensic laboratory requires separate facilities for pre-polymerase chain reaction (PCR) (sample preparation, DNA extraction, quantification, and PCR amplification setup) and post-PCR (product purification and capillary electrophoresis or MPS) to avoid PCR product contamination. Sample preparation requires ventilated hoods with UV lamps to be used after each case manipulation, and this process is evidently best performed in a separate laboratory from other pre-PCR steps. Besides, proper hoods, with biofilter and UV lamps, should be used for DNA extraction and PCR setup. However, special attention must be paid to the separation of areas when analyzing evidence and reference samples. Whenever possible, there must be a physical separation or at least a temporal separation, preferably after evidence samples analysis is completed, to avoid any potential contamination (Butler, 2012). In the case of mtDNA analysis, these considerations are even more important because of its molecular characteristics. The high number of copies per cell makes mtDNA more sensitive to contamination than nuclear DNA. Besides, in those cases in which DNA is degraded, it is more probable to detect mtDNA contamination.

6.4.2 DNA ISOLATION: PARTICULAR CONSIDERATIONS ABOUT mtDNA

Besides preparation and conditioning of samples, DNA extraction will be one of the most important steps in forensic analysis, in particular in the case of mtDNA analysis, due to the molecular characteristics of this kind of DNA, as we have commented. Therefore, extraction of the mtDNA needs to be performed in a very clean laboratory environment. The mtDNA analysis typically involves samples where little DNA is present to begin with. Teeth, hair, and bones (e.g., femur) are samples often used for mtDNA analysis in forensic cases (Butler, 2012). Thus, the mtDNA must be carefully extracted from these samples and often purified away from PCR inhibitors that can be coextracted (Barrio, 2013).

Currently, there are some novel techniques to separate and analyze mtDNA in samples containing DNA from two individuals (Zander et al., 2017). The authors adapted and combined previously developed methods of haplotype-specific extraction, and they were able to subsequently identify the DNA of the two individuals by sequencing.

6.4.3   ESTIMATING mtDNA QUANTITY (mtDNA QUANTIFICATION)

The vast majority of forensic laboratories carry out the quantification of DNA obtained after extraction of nuclear regions by reverse transcription PCR, and Quantifiler Trio® (Thermo Fisher Inc., CA, USA) (Liu, 2014) is the last widely used commercial kit. This kit gives us very useful information about degradation and inhibition. However, we do not obtain real information about mtDNA quantity. A classical approach is post-PCR valuation through agarose gel or automated electrophoresis, such as 2100 Bioanalyzer (Agilent Technologies Inc., CA, USA) (Fernández and Alonso, 2012).

However, mtDNA sequence analysis, as a PCR-based method, requires a minimal amount of template DNA for successful and efficient amplification. The mtDNA quantification ensures that the optimal quantity of template DNA is added to the amplification reaction. Real-time quantitative PCR (qPCR) is a reliable, highly specific, and sensitive method to quantify DNA. Several mtDNA qPCR assays for forensic purpose have been published: mtDNA (Meissner et al., 2000; von Wurmb-Schwark et al., 2002), and nuclear and mtDNA (Andréasson et al., 2002; Alonso et al., 2004; Niederstätter et al., 2007). A last publication (Sprouse et al., 2014) shows an analysis of multiple targets simultaneously, the primary mtDNA target of interest, and an internal positive control to assess possible inhibition. By incorporating a dual real-time nuclear and mtDNA quantitation assay into our workflow, we would be able to reduce our reamplifications when examining casework samples (Niederstätter et al., 2007) and, therefore, reducing time and cost.

6.4.4   IMPORTANCE OF NEGATIVE AND POSITIVE CONTROL USE

Controls are samples processed in parallel with evidentiary samples through each step of the process, and they serve to monitor performance. We will include two types of negative controls: extraction and amplification blanks. Both controls will be performed until the final sequencing analysis to monitor contamination (SWGDAM, 2013). Since mtDNA analysis is a very sensitive technique, the presence of low-level contamination is not uncommon (Isenberg, 2004), and with the more sensitive new MPS techniques, we will observe a higher incidence of it. In any case, if contamination is observed within blanks, results from the unknown sample being run in parallel do not always have to be disregarded. There are some analytical rules that are conservative and reliable, such as the 10:1 rule, where any contamination seen in blanks during post-PCR analysis must be less than 1/10th the amount of the sample being processed (Wilson et al., 1995).

In contrast, a positive control is a sample of known mtDNA sequence that serves to demonstrate that amplification and sequencing reaction components are working properly (Butler, 2012). This positive control is typically an extracted DNA sample that is processed through the steps of amplification, sequencing, and data analysis. For example, AmpFLSTR® Control DNA 007 (Thermo Fisher Inc., CA, USA) could be used as a positive control. However, it could be possible to use samples from interlaboratory exercises or Certified Reference Materials for mtDNA Sequence Analysis (SRM 2392-I and SRM 2392 of the US National Institute of Standards and Technology).

This fact introduces the importance of the laboratory participating in interlaboratory exercises, in particular those in which mtDNA analysis is carried out. Our laboratory participates annually in the proficiency test of the GHEP-ISFG.

6.4.5 CLASSICAL METHODS OF AMPLIFICATION AND SEQUENCING

DNA sequencing of mtDNA is usually performed with the following steps: (1) PCR amplification of the entire CR or a portion of it, depending on the degradation degree of the extracted DNA; (2) removal of remaining deoxyribonucleotide triphosphates (dNTPs) and primers from PCR; (3) performance of DNA sequencing reaction to incorporate fluorescent dideoxyribonucleotide triphosphates (ddNTPs); (4) removal of unincorporated fluorescent dye terminators; (5) separation through a capillary electrophoresis instrument; and (6) sequence analysis of each reaction performed and interpretation.

6.4.5.1 PCR AMPLIFICATION

The HVS-I and HVS-II regions are usually analyzed, and in exceptional cases, when a plus discrimination is needed, the HVS-III region is analyzed.

The PCR is usually performed in 25 µL of final volume of amplification (up to 3 µL of sample template and 22 µL of reaction mixture). The reaction mixture contains 200 µM of each dNTP, 5 U Taq Gold DNA Polymerase (Applied Biosystem Inc., CA, USA), 1 X PCR Buffer (10 mM Tris–HCl, pH 8.3, 50 mM KCl, 1.5 mM $MgCl_2$, and 0.001% gelatin), and 0.2 µM of each primer forward and reverse (see Table 6.1). The PCR amplification is carried out with the following conditions: one cycle of 95 °C for 11 min, then 36 cycles of 95 °C for 10 s, 60 °C for 20 s, and 72 °C for 30 s, and ending 72 °C for 10 min (Wilson et al., 1995). PCR products and negative controls were checked in agarosa gel and visualized with GelRed™ (Biotium, CA, USA) staining. It is possible to perform this assessment through an automated electrophoresis with Bioanalyzer (Agilent Technologies Inc., CA, USA). When inhibition is detected, different strategies could be applied: to add BSA, to add excess Taq, and/or to amplify at double volume. Protocols for highly degraded DNA specimens even call for 42 cycles (Gabriel et al., 2001).

TABLE 6.1 Amplification and Sequencing Primers for mtDNA Control Region: HVS-I, HVS-II, and HVS-III Portions

Region	Lab Code	Primer Name	Primer Sequence
HVS-I	A1	L 15997	5'-CAC CAT TAG CAC CCA AAG CT-3'
	B1	H 16395	5'-CAC GGA GGA TGG TGG TCA AG-3'
	A4	L 16209	5'-CCC CAT GCT TAC AAG CAA GT-3'
	B4	H 16164	5'-TTT GAT GTG GAT TGG GTT T-3'
HVS-II	C1	L 00048	5'-CTC ACG GGA GCT CTC CAT GC-3'
	D1	H 00408	5'-CTG TTA AAA GTG CAT ACC GCC A-3'
HVS-III	E1	L 00361	5'-ACA AAG AAC CCT AAC ACC AGC-3'
	F1	H 00580	5'-TTG AGG AGG TAA GCT ACA TAA-3'

Legend: L (light strand), H (heavy strand).

In relation to the primers used, for the two main hypervariable regions within the CR, HVS-I (16024–16365) and HVS-II (72–340) regions, the primers proposed by Wilson et al. (1995) are usually used. In addition, regarding the third hypervariable region, HVS-III (438–574), for resolving indistinguishable HVS-I/HVS-II samples, we use a modification of the primers proposed by Lutz et al. (2000) (see Table 6.1). This region has one of the most informative mtDNA loci with length variations, a $(CA)_n$ dinucleotide repeat, located between positions 514 and 523 (Szibor et al., 1997).

In highly degraded remains, amplification of entire HVS regions is frequently unattainable due to the high degree of DNA fragmentation. For this reason, some laboratories have adapted their amplification and sequencing strategies of mtDNA to the degradation state of crime scene samples (Gabriel et al., 2001; Berger and Parson, 2009).

6.4.5.2 PCR PRODUCT PURIFICATION

The PCR products are purified to remove excess of primers and unincorporated dNTPs with a treatment with ExoSAP-IT (USB Affymetrix Inc., OH, USA) (Dugan et al., 2002): 25 µL of PCR product was incubated with 5 µL for 15 min at 37 °C followed by 15 min at 80 °C for enzyme inactivation. However, it is also possible through spin filtration, for example, with Microcon® 100 filter (Merck KGaA, Darmstadt, Germany)

6.4.5.3 SEQUENCING REACTION

For mtDNA sequencing, the classic Sanger method has been widely used, first described over 40 years ago (Sanger et al., 1977). The process involves the polymerase incorporation of ddNTPs as chain terminators followed by a separation step capable of single-nucleotide resolution. ddNTPs (ddTTP, ddCTP, ddATP, and ddGTP) are colored with four different fluorescent dyes. Each DNA strand is sequenced in separate reactions with a single primer. In forensic laboratories, both the forward and reverse PCR primers are used for this process.

In our laboratory, sequencing reaction is performed in 20 µL of final volume (up to 3 µL of the purified PCR product and 17 µL of reaction mixture). The reaction mixture contains 8 µL of BigDye Terminator v3.1 Cycle Sequencing Kit (Applied Biosystems, CA, USA), 0.32 µL of the corresponding primer (10 µM), and ultrapure water up to 17 µL. As PCR amplification, sequencing reaction is carried out with the following conditions: one cycle of 96 °C for 1 min and then 25 cycles of 96 °C for 10 s, 50 °C for 5 s, and 60 °C for 4 min.

After sequencing reaction, the products must be purified to remove unincorporated dye terminators; otherwise, they interfere in the base calling, especially at the beginning of the sequence. This purification could be done through Centri-Sep™ Spin Columns (Thermo Fisher, CA, USA) or Microcon® (Merck KGaA, Darmstadt, Germany). However, there are other purification methods, for example, DyeEx 2.0 (QIAGEN, Hilden, Germany), BigDye XTerminator® Purification kit (Thermo Fisher, CA, USA), or precipitation methods (ethanol–EDTA precipitation or ethanol–EDTA–sodium acetate precipitation). There are other combined methods of digestion with Shrimp Alkaline Phosphatase (SAP, GE Healthcare, UK) and precipitation.

Then, sequencing reaction products have to be diluted in formamide, denatured for 3 min in thermal block at 95 °C, and immediately cooled to avoid renaturation. At that time, the samples are ready to be separate through a capillary electrophoresis instrument. There are a great variety of platforms for DNA sequencing. The classical vertical gel sequencer (e.g., ABI 377, Applied Biosystem Inc., CA, USA) was reliable for mtDNA sequencing, but they were quickly replaced by capillary electrophoresis equipment, with one (e.g., ABI 310) or more capillaries (e.g., ABI 3130, four capillaries). One of the last models of Applied Biosystem, ABI 3500 (eight capillaries; ABI 3500xl, 24 capillaries) with 50-cm capillary length, is also good equipment for mtDNA sequencing.

Both the length of the capillary and the polymer used give the ability to sequence. At least, we need a 36-cm-long capillary, and a POP-6 polymer (performance optimized polymers) is necessary, which gives us a resolution of 1 bp. Although POP-4 is used for STR typing (less viscous and lower resolution polymer), it is possible to use it in mtDNA sequencing if we use a 47-cm-long capillary and with appropriate time and temperature (38–52 min at 50 °C).

6.4.6   NEW METHODS: MASSIVELY PARALLEL SEQUENCING

Since the introduction of the first next-generation sequencing (NGS) sequencer in 2004, 454 GS FLX System (Roche, CT, USA) (Margulis et al., 2005), there has been an important revolution. Mikkelsen et al. (2009) first sequenced full mtDNA for forensic use through pyrosequencing NGS. Currently, there is a wide variety of MPS equipment with different chemistries, but MiSeqFGx System (Illumina, CA, USA) and Ion S5 System (Thermo Fisher Inc., CA, USA) are being validated for their forensic use (DNASEQEX, 2019). The *Illumina* MPS technology is based on sequencing by synthesis (SBS) in solid phase and the detection of fluorescently labeled dNTPs into a DNA template strand during sequential cycles of DNA synthesis (Mardis, 2013). In addition, the *Thermo Fisher* MPS technology (Ion Torrent®) is also based on SBS in chip, but on the detection of potential changes (as a consequence of the pH changes) with the incorporation of each dNTP (Mardis, 2013).

The equipment, reagents, and data evaluation software required for this approach are quite expensive; however, the MPS technology is rapidly developing, and prices are expected to fall. Another important limitation is that the MPS process is time consuming and complex. However, there are some solutions, such as Ion Chef System (Thermo Fisher Inc., CA, USA) that automatically performs every phase of the process. All these aspects lead us to think that MPS technology may eventually supplement if not displace Sanger methodologies.

In the case of forensic mtDNA analysis, the potential of MPS technology is very large. Apart from the high number of samples that can be analyzed at the same time, not only we can analyze the hypervariable regions of CR, but also it is possible to analyze the whole genome with quite good resolution (Parson et al., 2013; King et al., 2014a; Peck et al., 2016; Churchill et al., 2017; Woerner et al., 2018; Strobl et al., 2018). In addition, new sequencing platforms are emerging, in which a previous amplification/enrichment is not required (Zascavage et al., 2019).

6.4.6.1 mtDNA MPS ANALYTICAL PHASES

MPS of mtDNA is usually performed with the following steps, with small differences between different technologies: (1) PCR amplification of the targets regions (to complete CR or whole mtDNA genome); (2) library preparation and normalization; (3) template preparation (in the case of Ion Torrent® technology); (4) MPS sequencing; and (5) data analysis.

1. *Target enrichment:* The CR or the whole mtDNA molecule is usually amplified with two overlapping primers pools with different numbers of primers to cover the regions of interest (e.g., Fendt et al., 2009). Amplicons are purified using different kits, for example, QIAquick PCR Purification Kit (QIAGEN, Hilden, Germany). It is possible to make a quality-controlled/quantified, for example, using Bioanalyzer (Agilent Technologies Inc., CA, USA) or Qubit dsDNA BR Quantification Kit (Thermo Fisher Inc., CA, USA). Next, 0.2 ng/mL normalized products are pooled, and 1.0 ng of DNA was used for library preparation. In the case of *Thermo Fisher*, the primers pools are included in its commercial kits: Precision ID mtDNA CR and Whole Genome Panels. *Illumina* (in particular, the genetic forensic division *Verogen*) is preparing a new mtDNA panel (ForenSeq™ mtDNA), which is expected to be commercialized throughout 2019.

2. *Library preparation and normalization:* Regarding *Illumina*, for now, libraries is prepared using the Nextera XT DNA Sample Preparation Kit according to its protocol: "tagment" Genomic DNA (DNA is simultaneously fragmented and tagged with adapters); amplify libraries; clean up libraries [in this step, the libraries could be quantified, for example, through Qubit (Thermo Fisher Inc., CA, USA)]; normalize libraries (cluster optimization), for sequencing to 12 pM; and pool libraries.

   In the case of *Thermo Fisher*, the library construction involves the following three steps: partially digest amplicons, ligation of the adapters to amplicons, and purification. Then, it is recommended to quantify the generated library through qPCR with the Ion Library TaqMan® Quantitation Kit (Thermo Fisher Inc., CA, USA). Once quantified, it should be diluted to 30 pM, according to the manufacturer's recommendations, and it should be pooled. In both cases, the ligation of adapters ("genetic barcode") will allow the unambiguous identification of the samples.

3. *Template preparation* (Thermo Fisher Inc., CA, USA)*:* In the case of the *Thermo Fisher* process, it will also be necessary to carry out the template preparation. The main point of this step is the emulsion PCR, which is a clonal amplification: DNA is localized to Ion Sphere particles (ISPs). Then, the ISPs are enriched, preferably by automated equipment, for example, through Ion Chef (Thermo Fisher Inc., CA, USA).

4. *MPS sequencing and (5) data analysis.* Obviously, the MPS sequencing is the main phase of the whole process. As we have commented previously, the *Illumina* MPS sequencing is based on fluorescently labeled dNTPs detection using the MiSeq platform in an automated way for ~39 h. The mtDNA sequence output data will be processed with on-board software (BaseSpace® mtDNA Variant Processor), which generates output files. These will be analyzed through BaseSpace® mtDNA Variant Analyzer v1.0, obtaining mtDNA variants and being able to compare different samples. In the near future, it is expected that its ForenSeq™ Universal Analysis Software for STR/single-nucleotide polymorphism (SNP) analysis will be updated, and a new mtDNA analysis module will be implemented.

The *Thermo Fisher* MPS sequencing is based on the detection of potential changes using PGM/Ion S5 platform for up to 4 h. In this case, the mtDNA sequences output data will be processed using Torrent Variant

Caller (TVC) software plugin that runs on Torrent Server Suite™ (TSS). The TVC plugin calls SNPs, multinucleotide polymorphisms, insertions, and deletions in a sample across a reference or within a targeted subset of that reference. Currently, the latest update of its Converge™ v2.1 software is able to perform the analysis of mtDNA sequences, both of the CR and the whole mitogenome. This software imports the file generated by the HID Genotyper Plugin v2.1 in the TSS.

6.4.7 BIOINFORMATICS TOOLS FOR SEQUENCES ANALYSIS/EDITION

In the classical methodology of mtDNA analysis in forensic laboratories, the different sequences obtained with direct and reverse primers are aligned on the sequenced region of interest, and the consensus sequence is compared with the revised mtDNA reference sequence (rCRS) (Andrews et al., 1999). Each nucleotide position is interrogated, and variations from the reference are annotated by base difference (e.g., 263G). Although the process is automatically done through different software, the visual inspection of the entire length of the sequence must be done to review the data, especially at the beginning and ends of the sequence. Special attention should be paid to identifying PHP not detected by the software. This revision process must be carried out by two independent analysts (Crespillo, 2012).

Classically, the mtDNA sequence data obtained through the Sanger method had been analyzed and edited using SeqScape® software (Thermo Fisher Inc., CA, USA). This software was designed specifically to address the needs of analyzing and identifying sequence variations accurately and reliably, with less manual data manipulation and shorter turnaround time for the complete analysis.

There are other simpler software with less functionalities, which also allow the analysis and editing of mtDNA sequences: Sequence Scanner (Thermo Fisher Inc., CA, USA), Sequencher (Gene Codes Co., MI, USA), or Chro-masPro (Technelysium Pty Ltd, Australia), in some cases with free versions. However, currently, with the implementation of new MPS technologies, new software has emerged: GeneMarker® HTS or NextGENe® (SoftGenetics, PA, USA) (Holland et al., 2017). With respect to MPS technologies, as we have said, each platform has got its on-board software: BaseSpace® mtDNA Variant Processor (Illumina, CA, USA) and TVC (Thermo Fisher Inc., CA, USA). These software convert raw data to Binary Alignment Map and Variant Call Format (VCF). The output of the variant caller is presented in tabular format, as a list of differences to the rCRS without a graphical display of the aligned reads. At this time, graphical displays could only be visualized with separate tools for alignment and assembly viewing, such as IGV package (Integrative Genomics Viewer) (Robinson et al., 2011), Genome Analysis Toolkit (McKenna et al., 2010), and a wide variety of software, most of which are open-access and open-source. In the mtDNA module of Converge™ v2.1 (Thermo Fisher Inc., CA, USA), the visualization is much more graphic and intuitive, allowing the connection with EMPOP to confirm the variants detected.

In contrast, the existence of tools that allow the evaluation of the mtDNA results, detection of contaminations, etc., is very interesting. Thus, we can use some software, such as eCOMPAGT (Weissensteiner et al., 2010), which was designed to enable error-free postlaboratory data handling of human mtDNA profiles. It allows importing data from SeqScape and Sequencher, and the mtDNA information is stored in eCOMPAGT and can be modified, or the data can be exported for specific applications (EMPOP, mtDNAmanager, FASTA, etc.). Other interesting tool is HaploGrep (Kloss-Brandstätter et al., 2011), which was initially created to provide a fully automated way to determine the haplogroup of mtDNA profiles, based on PhyloTree. Now, the last version, HaploGrep2 (Weissensteiner et al., 2016a), offers several advanced features: a generic rule-based system for immediate quality control (QC) that allows detecting artificial recombinants and missing variants as well as annotating rare and phantom mutations. In the MPS field, this initiative has got the mtDNA-Server (Weissensteiner et al., 2016b), a scalable web server for the analysis of mtDNA studies of any size with a special focus on usability as well as reliable identification and quantification of heteroplasmic variants. There are other simpler software that allow evaluating haplotypes and convert VCF files into a standardized forensic format haplotype, mitoSAVE (King et al., 2014b).

6.5   DATA INTERPRETATION

6.5.1   QUALITY ASSURANCE

A major issue regarding mtDNA typing is the contamination risk. Due to the sensitivity of detection of mtDNA analysis, even low levels of exogenous DNA may be observed. For that reason, as has been commented in previous paragraphs, contamination should be monitored, and special practices should be followed in order to reduce it to the minimum (Carracedo et al., 2000) and to guarantee high-quality results. In this way, special measures have to be taken in the laboratory facilities (see Section 6.4.1). In addition, we will have to monitor the contamination through the use of controls/blanks in the whole analytical process (from extraction to sequencing analysis) (see Section 6.4.4.). If those controls reveal contamination, they must be evaluated to ensure that results for the sample(s) are legitimately from the samples and not the consequence of exogenous contamination. If the situation is the latter and contamination is present above the acceptance parameters established in the laboratory, the data cannot be used for interpretative purposes (SWGDAM, 2003). Another issue when dealing with mtDNA sequencing and documentation is the potential sources of error involved. Indeed, the various kinds of errors have been classified in five major categories (Bandelt et al., 2001; Salas et al., 2005a, 2005b):

- Base shift (Type I): one or several positions are wrongly noted by an alignment, reading shift or a column shift during the preparation of a table.
- Reference bias (Type II): overlooking nucleotide variants relative to the rCRS.
- Phantom mutations (Type III): uncommon mutations generated in the sequencing process itself.
- Base misscoring (Type IV): repeating the rCRS base instead of the variant base in a "dot" table, mistyping transversions as transitions, scoring a base as deleted, disregarding Indel events or mixing up the letters C and G.
- Artefactual recombination (Type V): obtaining a compound haplotype derived from different samples. The fact that most laboratories analyzed separately the different CR segments without overlap is a major reason to generate this kind of error. Other causes can be contamination or the human error while transferring data into a database or table.

Some authors (Bandelt et al., 2001; Salas et al., 2005a) have report recommendations in order to avoid and detect these errors.

The knowledge acquired until now about the mtDNA phylogeny is a powerful tool to uncover discrepancies. When haplotypes are contextualized within the mtDNA phylogeny, unusual or unobserved variants may occur. In this situation, raw data should be double checked (Crespillo, 2012) in order to confirm those rare variants since they could be potential artifacts instead of true ones. The EMPOP tool "NETWORK," based on quasi-median network analysis, was designed for this purpose and has been successfully employed as a QC (Zimmermann et al., 2014).

Haplogroup determination is an additional verification tool of the mtDNA dataset quality (Salas et al., 2005a). Phylotree is a comprehensive phylogenetic tree of global human mtDNA variation (van Oven and Kayser, 2009), where haplogroup-defining mutations are listed and serve as the basis for mtDNAhaplogrouping, manually or through different software tools developed to perform this work: HaploGrep2 (Kloss-Brandstätter et al., 2011; Weissensteiner et al., 2016a), EMMA (Röck et al., 2013), MitoTool (Fan and Yao, 2011, 2013), HmtDB (Rubino et al., 2012; Clima et al., 2017), mtDNAoffice (Soares et al., 2012), and mtDNAmanager (Lee et al., 2008).

When haplogrouping of a given mtDNA sequence is performed, for example, with HaploGrep2, expected and unused polymorphisms are listed for further evaluation. If an expected mutation for haplgroup classification is not found or if, on the contrary, private/unusual mutations are observed, data review must be performed, since errors may have been introduced. In this manner, artificial recombinants, phantom mutations (Weissensteiner et al., 2016a), and documentation errors can be easily recognized and resolve.

EMMA, implemented in EMPOP, is another automated tool to perform haplogroup assignment, which uses both Phylotree virtual haplotypes and a set of 14,990 real haplotypes (Röck et al., 2013). The advantage of using real haplotypes for haplogroup determination is that some private mutations that are not diagnostic motifs can be taken into consideration. Thus, haplogroup assignments could be more accurate and less raw.

6.5.2   INTERPRETING mtDNA RESULTS

6.5.2.1   "MATCH" AND "NO MATCH" CRITERIA

Once mtDNA sequences are appropriately edited (for guidelines of establishing the quality of mtDNA sequences and editing data, see Crespillo, 2012), sequences for the unknown (U) and known (K) samples are aligned and compared. Three possible results are derived from this comparison: exclusion, inconclusive, or failure to exclude (SWGDAM, 2013):

- **Exclusion:** If samples differ at two or more nucleotide positions (excluding LHP), they can be excluded as belonging to the same source or maternal lineage (see Figure 6.4). To reach these conclusion aspects such as tissue specificity (segregation of mutations occurs at different rates in different tissues [Calloway et al., 2000]) and mutation rates (several positions constitute hotspots for mutation [Stoneking, 2000; Calloway et al., 2000; Brandstätter and Parson, 2003]) must be considered in order to ascertain that positions are unequivocally different.

- **Inconclusive:** Samples differ at a single position only (whether or not they share a common length variant between positions 302 and 310) or differ only by not sharing a common length variant between positions 302 and 310 (all other positions are coincident) (see Figure 6.4). These situations are classified as inconclusive since they can be due to the aforementioned aspects (see Crespillo, 2012), that is, discrete differences can be observed between different tissues of the same individual and/or individuals from the same maternal lineage.

- **Failure to exclude:** If samples have the same sequence, they cannot be excluded as belonging to the same source or maternal lineage (see Figure 6.5). Even if samples share some heteroplasmic position, it will represent additional strength of the evidence, and one cannot exclude samples to belong to the same source or maternal lineage.

A) Exclusion

	16150	16160	16170	16180	16190
rCRS	ACTTGACCAC	CTGTAGTACA	TAAAAACCCA	ATCCACATCA	AAACCCCCTC
U	ACTTAACCAC	TTGTAGTACA	TAAAAACCCA	ATCCACATCA	AAACCCCCTC
K	ACTTGACCAC	CTGTAGTACA	TAAAAACCCA	ACCCACATCA	AAACCCCCTC

Sample U	Sample K
16145A	16172C

B) Inconclusive

	16150	16160	16170	16180	16190
rCRS	ACTTGACCAC	CTGTAGTACA	TAAAAACCCA	ATCCACATCA	AAACCCCCTC
U	ACTTAACCAC	TTGTAGTACA	TAAAAACCTA	ATCCACATCA	ACACCCCCTC
K	ACTTGACCAC	CTGTAGTACA	TAAAAACCTA	ACCCACATCA	AAACCCCCTC

Sample U		Sample K
16169T	16182C	16169T

FIGURE 6.4 Interpretation of mtDNA results. (A) *Exclusion:* samples U and K differ at two nucleotide positions (16145A and 16172C). (B) *Inconclusive:* samples U and K differ at only one nucleotide position (16182C).

C) Failure to exclude

	16150	16160	16170	16180	16190
rCRS	ACTTGACCAC	CTGTAGTACA	TAAAAACCCA	ATCCACATCA	AAACCCCTC
U	ACTTAACCAC	TTGTAGTACA	TAAAAACCTA	ATCCACATCA	ACCCCCCTC
K	ACTTGACCAC	CTGTAGTACA	TAAAAACCTA	ACCCACATCA	ACCCCCCTC

Sample U	Sample K
16169T 16182C 16183C	16169T 16182C 16183C

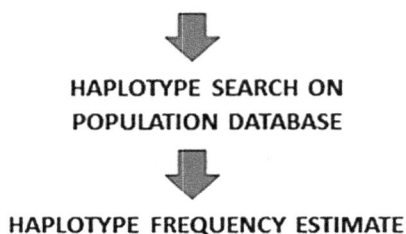

⬇

**HAPLOTYPE SEARCH ON
POPULATION DATABASE**

⬇

HAPLOTYPE FREQUENCY ESTIMATE

FIGURE 6.5   Interpretation of mtDNA results (continued). (C) *Failure to exclude:* samples U and K have the same sequence (16169T 16182C 16183C). Then, this haplotype should be searched in a population database in order to provide a statistical weight to the coincidence.

6.5.2.2   *STATISTICAL EVALUATION OF THE MATCH*

The mtDNA profiles of an unknown and a known sample that cannot be excluded as coming from the same source should be searched in a population database in order to provide a statistical weight to the coincidence. In this context, the question we would like to answer is how much rare is the mtDNA haplotype of the unknown sample, to establish the weight of belonging to a certain individual (or the same maternal lineage) and not to a random individual of the population.

mtDNA is entirely inherited from our mother without recombination, so nucleotide positions must be considered as a single-locus haplotype. The current practice to convey the rarity of a mtDNA haplotype is the so-called counting method, where the number of times a haplotype of interest is observed is divided by the total number of haplotypes in the database used (Butler, 2015) (see Table 6.2). This approach depends on the size of the database, that is, the larger the number of unrelated individuals in the database (haplotypes), the better will be the statistics for a random match frequency estimate.

TABLE 6.2 Summary Statistics for mtDNA Haplotype Frequency Estimates and Confidence Intervals

Calculation of mtDNA Haplotype Frequency Estimates and Confidence Intervals

Frequency Estimates	Counting method:

$$p = \frac{X}{N}$$

X = number of times an haplotype is observed in a database; N = haplotypes in the database

Considering not all haplotypes are represented in the database[1]:

$$p = \frac{x+1}{n+1}$$

$$p = \frac{x+2}{n+2}$$

x = number of times an haplotype is observed in a database; n = haplotypes in the database

Confidence Intervals A 95% upper bound confidence interval can be placed on the haplotype's frequency using[2]:

$$p + 1.96 \sqrt{\frac{(p)(1-p)}{N}}$$

p = haplotype frequency

If the profile has not been observed in the database[2]:

$$p = 1 - \alpha^{1/N}$$

where α is the confidence coefficient (0.05 for a 95% confidence interval)

The Clopper–Pearson formula can be used for a more conservative confidence intervals when very low counts are observed[3]:

$$\sum_{k=0}^{x} \binom{N}{k} p_0^k (1-p_0)^{N-k} = 0.05$$

[1]Balding and Nichols, 1994; [2]Holland and Parsons, 1999; [3]Clooper and Pearson, 1934.

A drawback of this method is that the failure to observe a haplotype in a database could be a consequence of a small size or a poor sampling of the database. In order to include a correction for this fact, alternative probabilistic approaches have been given.

Estimates for probabilistic approaches have been proposed by adding the haplotype of the unknown and reference sample to the database once or twice, the latter under the hypothesis that the profiles of the unknown and reference sample may have come from two different individuals (see Table 6.2) (Balding and Nichols, 1994; Egeland and Salas, 2008).

Holland and Parsons (1999) suggested the use of confidence intervals to estimate the upper and lower bounds of a frequency calculation (see Table 6.2). A more conservative approach that has been widely used for mtDNA (Holland and Parsons, 1999; Tully et al., 2001) is based on the upper bound of a 95% confidence limit calculated by Clopper and Pearson (1934). This formula provides a more conservative value when very low counts are observed and is recommended in the SWGDAM (2013) guidelines. Further discussions on the estimation of rare or unseen mtDNA haplotype frequencies have been given by Egeland et al. (2004) and Brenner (2010). Finally, reporting in court the likelihood ratio (LR) expressed as LR=$1/p$, where p is the frequency of the haplotype, is a common practice among forensic laboratories.

In any case, international recommendations claim that laboratories must be able to justify the choice of database(s) and statistical approach used (Parson et al., 2014).

Another issue to consider while searching a haplotype in a database is the occurrence of population substructure. Because it is recognized that population substructure exists for mtDNA haplotypes, the choice of database(s) used for reporting results should be carefully considered within the context of the case since frequencies of mtDNA types can differ significantly at a local level (Parson et al., 2014). In this sense, although statistical approaches accounting for subpopulation effects do exist (see Butler, 2015), a consensus for an appropriate recommendation on this respect has not yet been reached (SWGDAM, 2013).

6.5.2.3   mtDNA POPULATION DATABASES

The choice of the population database for mtDNA haplotype search is a fundamental step, especially in a forensic context (Salas et al., 2007). Over the past, a great effort has been made in order to gather mtDNA sequences from worldwide populations, and many population genetic studies have been published. However, some of this freely available population genetic literature may not have passed appropriate forensic standardization (Salas et al., 2007), leading to awaken several concerns about their use for reliable estimates of haplotype frequencies. Later on, the use of strict QC measures, including phylogenetic analysis, has served to significantly improve mtDNA data quality (Parson and Dür, 2007).

The EMPOP (https://empop.online/) has become a reference mtDNA database, since it applies phylogenetic analysis of the mtDNA data for QC purposes (Parson, 2004; Parson and Dür, 2007) as well as implements a string-based sequence search algorithm for mtDNA database queries that ensures the appropriate search of a haplotype regardless of its alignment (Röck et al., 2011) and that was recently updated and improved (Huber et al., 2018). Nowadays, EMPOP (release 12) contains 42,839 quality-controlled mtDNA haplotypes with at least HVS-I variation (16024–16365) from worldwide populations (https://empop.online/empop_stats); thereof, 41,385 cover HVS-I and HVS-II (16024–16365 and 73–340); 33,447 cover the CR (16024-576); and 1366 cover the entire mitogenome (ALL). It is recommended for haplotype frequency assessments by the SWGDAM mtDNA interpretation guidelines (2013) and the updated ISFG guidelines for mtDNA analysis (Parson et al., 2014). It is expected that soon there will be new updates in EMPOP for its complete integration with the new MPS technologies (DNA. bases, 2019).

The SWGDAM also harbors a population database, the SWGDAM mtDNA population database available only to CODIS users (Monson et al., 2002), which is an appropriate database for assessing the relative frequency of mtDNA haplotypes within the US (SWGDAM, 2013). This database was created in collaboration with the Armed Forces DNA Identification Laboratory, EMPOP, and the FBI Laboratory.

6.6 CONCLUDING REMARKS

The utility of mtDNA in the forensic field has been amply demonstrated. Although the use of autosomal STRs is more decisive, due to the high discriminatory power that is reached with them, in some cases, their application is not possible. In several situations, forensic casework entails dealing with samples containing few amounts or degraded DNA; therefore, in such cases, the analysis of mtDNA could be the only possibility due to its molecular characteristics. However, its analysis is quite complex and requires a highly standardized methodology as well as a high level of specialization and training in order to ensure the quality of its analysis and the interpretation of the results.

Methodologically, the evolution of mtDNA analysis has been huge. The new Sanger sequenchers have increased their sensitivity, with the limitations that implies. Now, we are able to detect low-level contaminations, which were previously hidden in the background noise. With the new MPS technologies, this power increases even more. Fortunately, we have more and better informatics tools that allow a better evaluation of our results (eCOMPAGT, HaploGrep2, etc.).

In contrast, although the analysis of the mtDNA whole genome is very interesting because it allows us increasing mtDNA power of discrimination, it poses new challenges at the bioethical level (Budowle et al., 2005). We will be able to identify genetic mutations associated with diseases that we were not able to identify with the analysis of the CR only. This disease information does not have any interest at the forensic level. In addition, there are some countries legislations, such as Spanish one, which explicitly would not allow such analysis.

Finally, although the entire mtDNA analytical process will be relevant for obtaining reliable results in the field of forensic genetics, the interpretation of data will be crucial for obtaining correct conclusions and subsequent communication to our final recipient, the Court. Today, we have numerous bioinformatics tools that allow us to ensure the authenticity of the results before their final interpretation.

KEYWORDS

- **mtDNA**
- **forensic genetics**
- **heteroplasmy**
- **mutation**
- **sequencing**
- **MPS**
- **bioinformatics tools**
- **EMPOP**
- **data interpretation**

REFERENCES

Alonso, A.; et al.; Results of the 1999–2000 collaborative exercise and proficiency testing program on mitochondrial DNA of the GEP-ISFG: An inter-laboratory study of the observed variability in the heteroplasmy level of hair from the same donor. *Forensic Sci Int.* **2002**, *125*(1), 1–7.

Alonso, A.; et al.; Real-time PCR designs to estimate nuclear and mitochondrial DNA copy number in forensic and ancient DNA studies. *Forensic Sci Int.* **2004**, *139*(2–3), 141–9.

Anderson, S.; et al.; Sequence and organization of the human mitochondrial genome. *Nature.* **1981**, *290*(5806), 457–65.

Andréasson, H.; Gyllensten, U.; and Allen, M.; Real-time DNA quantification of nuclear and mitochondrial DNA in forensic analysis. *Biotechniques.* **2002**, *33*(2), 402–4, 407–11.

Andrews, R.M.; et al.; Reanalysis and revision of the Cambridge reference sequence for human mitochondrial DNA. *Nat Genet.* **1999**, *23*(2), 147.

Attardi, G.; The elucidation of the human mitochondrial genome: A historical perspective. *Bioessays.* **1987**, *5*, 34–9.

Balding, D.J.; and Nichols, R.A.; DNA profile match probability calculation: How to allow for population stratification, relatedness, database selection and single bands. *Forensic Sci Int.* **1994**, *64*(2–3), 125–40.

Bandelt, H.J.; and Dür, A.; Translating DNA data tables into quasi-median networks for parsimony analysis and error detection. *Mol Phylogenet Evol.* **2007**, *42*(1), 256–71.

Bandelt, H.J.; and Parson, W.; Consistent treatment of length variants in the human mtDNA control region: A reappraisal. *Int J Legal Med.* **2008**, *122*(1), 11–21.

Bandelt, H.J.; et al.; Detecting errors in mtDNA data by phylogenetic analysis. *Int J Legal Med.* **2001**, *115*(2), 64–9.

Bandelt, H.J.; et al.; The case for the continuing use of the revised Cambridge Reference Sequence (rCRS) and the standardization of notation in human mitochondrial DNA studies. *J Hum Genet.* **2014**, *59*(2), 66–77.

Barrell, B.; et al.; A different genetic code in human mitochondria. *Nature.* **1979**, *282*,189–94.

Barrio, P.A.; Revisión de Métodos de Extracción de ADN a partir de Restos Óseos en el Laboratorio Forense. *Rev Esp Med Legal.* **2013**, *39*, 54–62.

Behar, D.M.; et al.; A "Copernican" reassessment of the human mitochondrial DNA tree from its root. *Am J Hum Genet.* **2012**, *90*(4), 675–84.

Berger, C.; and Parson, W.; Mini-midi-mito: adapting the amplification and sequencing strategy of mtDNA to the degradation state of crime scene samples. *Forensic Sci Int Genet.* **2009**, *3*(3), 149–53.

Bodenteich, A.; et al.; Dinucleotide repeat in the human mitochondrial D-loop. *Hum Mol Genet.* **1992**, *1*(2), 140.

Bogenhagen, D.; and Clayton, D.A.; The number of mitochondrial deoxyribonucleic acid genomes in mouse L and HeLa cells: Quantitative isolation of mitochondrial deoxyribonucleic acid. *J Biol Chem.* **1980**, *136*(3), 507–13.

Borst, P.; Mitochondrial nucleic acids. *Ann Rev Biochem.* **1972**, *41*, 333.

Borst, P.; and Grivell, L.A.; Small is beautiful. Portrait of a mitochondrial genome. *Nature.* **1981**, *290*, 443–4.

Brandstätter, A.; and Parson, W.; Mitochondrial DNA heteroplasmy or artefacts—A matter of the amplification strategy? *Int J Legal Med.* **2003**, *117*(3), 180–4.

Brenner, C.H.; Fundamental problem of forensic mathematics—The evidential value of a rare haplotype. *Forensic Sci Int Genet.* **2010**, *4*(5), 281–91.

Brown, W.M.; et al.; Rapid evolution of animal mitochondrial DNA. *Proc Acad Natl Sci USA.* **1979**, *76*, 1967–71.

Budowle, B.; et al.; Forensic analysis of the mitochondrial coding region and association to disease. *Int J Legal Med.* **2005**, *119*(5), 314–5.

Butler, J.M. Mitochondrial DNA analysis. In *Advanced Topics in Forensic DNA Typing: Methodology*; Academic Press: New York, **2012**.

Butler, J.M.; Lineage marker statistics. In *Advanced Topics in Forensic DNA Typing: Interpretation*; Academic Press: San Diego, CA, USA, **2015**.

Calloway, C.D.; et al.; The frequency of heteroplasmy in the HVII region of mtDNA differs across tissue types and increases with age. *Am J Hum Genet.* **2000**, *66*(4),1384–97.

Carracedo, A.; et al.; DNA Commission of the International Society for Forensic Genetics: Guidelines for mitochondrial DNA typing. *Forensic Sci Int.* **2000**, *110*(2), 79–85.

Chen, X.; et al.; Rearranged mitochondrial genomes are present in human oocytes. *Am J Hum Genet.* **1995**, *57*, 239–47.

Churchill, J.D.; et al.; Working towards implementation of whole genome mitochondrial DNA sequencing into routine casework. *Forensic Sci Int Genet Suppl Ser.* **2017**, *6*, e388–9.

Clima, R.; et al.; HmtDB 2016: Data update, a better performing query system and human mitochondrial DNA haplogroup predictor. *Nucleic Acids Res.* **2017**, *45*(D1), D698–706.

Clopper, C.J.; and Pearson, E.S.; The use of confidence or fiducial limits illustrated in the case of the binomial. *Biometrika*, **1934**, *26*, 404–13.

Comas, D.; et al.; Heteroplasmy in the control region of human mitochondrial DNA. *Genes Res.* **1985**, *5*, 89–90.

Crespillo, M. Interpretation guidelines of mtDNA control region sequence electropherograms in forensic genetics. In *DNA Electrophoresis Protocols for Forensic Genetics*; Alonso, A., Ed.; Humana Press: New York, **2012**.

Crespillo, M.; et al.; Results of the 2003–2004 GEP-ISFG collaborative study on mitochondrial DNA: Focus on the mtDNA profile of a mixed semen-saliva stain. *Forensic Sci Int.* **2006**, *160*(2–3), 157–67.

Croteau, D.L.; et al.; Mitochondrial DNA repair pathways. *Mutat Res.* **1999**, *434*(3), 137–48.

Diez-Sanchez, C.; et al.; Mitochondrial DNA content of human spermatozoa. *Biol Reprod.* **2003**, *68*, 180–85.

DNA.bases, Empowering forensic genetic DNA databases for the interpretation of next generation sequencing profiles. [Online]. Available: https://www.researchgate.net/project/Empowering-forensic-genetic-DNA-databases-for-the-interpretation-of-next-generation-sequencing-profiles-DNAbases (accessed March 09, 2019).

DNASEQEX, DNA-STR Massive Sequencing & International Information Exchange. [Online]. Available: https://dnadatabank.forensischinstituut.nl/binaries/dnaseqex-letter- 160531_tcm127–629975_tcm37–209493.pdf (https://www.researchgate.net/project/DNASEQEX) (accessed March 09, 2019).

Dugan, K.A.; et al.; An improved method for post-PCR purification for mtDNA sequence analysis. *J Forensic Sci.* **2002**, *47*(4), 811–8.

Egeland, T.; and Salas, A.; Estimating haplotype frequency and coverage of databases. *PLoS One.* **2008**, *3*(12), e3988.

Egeland, T.; et al.; Inferring the most likely geographical origin of mtDNA sequence profiles. *Ann Hum Genet.* **2004**, *68*(Pt5), 461–71.

Fan, L.; and Yao, Y.G.; MitoTool: A web server for the analysis and retrieval of human mitochondrial DNA sequence variations. *Mitochondrion.* **2011**, *11*(2):351–6.

Fan, L.; and Yao, Y.G.; An update to MitoTool: Using a new scoring system for faster mtDNA haplogroup determination. *Mitochondrion.* **2013**, *13*(4), 360–3.

Fendt, L.; et al.; Sequencing strategy for the whole mitochondrial genome resulting in high quality sequences. *BMC Genomics.* **2009**, *10*, 139–50.

Fernández, C.; and Alonso, A. Microchip capillary electrophoresis protocol to evaluate quality and quantity of mtDNA amplified fragments for DNA sequencing in forensic genetics.

In *DNA Electrophoresis Protocols for Forensic Genetics*; Alonso, A., Ed.; Humana Press: New York, **2012**.

Gabriel, M.N.; et al.; Improved MtDNA sequence analysis of forensic remains using a "mini-primer set" amplification strategy. *J Forensic Sci.* **2001**, *46*(2), 247–53.

Giles, R.E.; et al.; Maternal inheritance of human mitochondrial DNA. *Proc Nat Acad Sci USA.* **1980**, *77*, 6715–9.

Gill, P.; et al.; Identification of the remains of the Romanov family by DNA analysis. *Nat Genet.* **1994**, *6*(2), 130–5.

Hawswirth, W.W.; and Laipis, P.J.; Mitochondrial DNA polymorphism a maternal lineage of Holstein Cows. *Proc Natl Acad Sci USA.* **1982**, *79*, 4686–90.

Hawswirth, W.W.; et al.; Heteogenous mitochondrial DNA D-loop sequences in bovine tissue. *Cell.* **1984**, *37*, 1001–7.

Holland, M.M.; and Parsons, T.; Mitochondrial DNA sequence analysis—Validation and use for forensic casework. *Forensic Sci Rev.* **1999**, *11*(1), 21–50.

Holland, M.M.; et al.; Mitochondrial DNA sequence analysis of human skeletal remains: Identification of remains from the Vietnam War. *J Forensic Sci.* **1993**, *38*(3), 542–45.

Holland, M.M.; Pack, E.D.; and McElhoe, J.A.; Evaluation of GeneMarker® HTS for improved alignment of mtDNA MPS data, haplotype determination, and heteroplasmy assessment. *Forensic Sci Int Genet.* **2017**, *28*, 90–98.

Huber, N.; Parson, W.; Dür, A.; Next generation database search algorithm for forensic mitogenome analyses. *Forensic Sci Int Genet.* **2018**, *37*, 204–14.

Huel, R.; et al.; DNA extraction from aged skeletal samples for STR typing by capillary electrophoresis. In *DNA Electrophoresis Protocols for Forensic Genetics*; Alonso, A., Ed.; Humana Press: New York, **2012**.

Isenberg, A. R. Forensic mitochondrial DNA analysis. In *Forensic Science Handbook*; Saferstein, R.; Ed.; Pearson/Prentice-Hall: Upper Saddle River, NJ, USA, **2014**; Vol. II; pp. 297–327.

King, J.L.; et al.; High-quality and high-throughput massively parallel sequencing of the human mitochondrial genome using the Illumina MiSeq. *Forensic Sci Int Genet.* **2014a**, *12*, 128–35.

King, J.L.; Sajantila, A.; and Budowle, B.; mitoSAVE: Mitochondrial sequence analysis of variants in Excel. *Forensic Sci Int Genet.* **2014b**, *12*, 122–5.

Kloss-Brandstätter, A.; et al.; HaploGrep: A fast and reliable algorithm for automatic classification of mitochondrial DNA haplogroups. *Hum Mutat.* **2011**, *32*(1), 25–32.

Knight, R.; et al.; How mitochondria redefine the code. *J Mol Evol.* **2001**, *53*, 299–13.

Lee, H.Y.; et al.; mtDNAmanager: A Web-based tool for the management and quality analysis of mitochondrial DNA control-region sequences. *BMC Bioinformatics.* **2008**, *9*, 483.

Liu, J.Y.; Direct qPCR quantification using the Quantifiler® Trio DNA quantification kit. *Forensic Sci Int Genet.* **2014**, *13*, 10–9.

Lutz, S.; et al.; Is it possible to differentiate mtDNA by means of HVIII in samples that cannot be distinguished by sequencing the HVI and HVII regions? *Forensic Sci Int.* **2000**, *113*(1–3), 97–101.

Lynch, C.A.; et al.; Human hair histogenesis for the mitochondrial DNA forensic scientists. *J Forensic Sci.* **2001**, *46*, 844–53.

Manfredi, G.; et al.; The fate of human sperm-derived mtDNA in somatic cells. *Am J Hum Genet.* **1997**, *61*, 953–60.

Mardis, E.R.; Next-generation sequencing platforms. *Annu Rev Anal Chem (Palo Alto Calif).* **2013**, 6, 287–303.

Margulies, M.; et al.; Genome sequencing in microfabricated high-density picolitre reactors. *Nature*. **2005**, *437*(7057), 376–80.

McKenna, A.; et al.; The Genome Analysis Toolkit: A MapReduce framework for analyzing next-generation DNA sequencing data. *Genome Res*. **2010**, *20*(9), 1297–303.

Meissner, C.; et al.; Quantification of mitochondrial DNA in human blood cells using an automated detection system. *Forensic Sci Int*. **2000**, *113*(1–3), 109–12.

Mikkelsen, M.; et al.; Application of full mitochondrial genome sequencing using 454 GS FLX pyrosequencing. *Forensic Sci Int Genet*. **2009**, *2*(1), 518–519.

Monson, K.L.; et al.; The mtDNA population database: An integrated software and database resource for forensic comparison. *Forensic Sci Commun*. **2002**, *4* (2).

Nedbal, M.; and Flynn, J.; Do the combined effects of the asymmetric process of replication and DNA damage from oxygen radicals produce a mutation-rate signature in the mitochondrial genome? *Mol Biol Evol*. **1998**, *15*, 219–23.

Niederstätter, H.; et al.; A modular real-time PCR concept for determining the quantity and quality of human nuclear and mitochondrial DNA. *Forensic Sci Int Genet*. **2007**, *1*(1), 29–34.

Parson, W.; and Bandelt, H.J.; Extended guidelines for mtDNA typing of population data in forensic science. *Forensic Sci. Int. Genet*. **2007**, *1*(1), 13–9.

Parson, W.; and Dür, A.; EMPOP—A forensic mtDNA database. *Forensic Sci Int Genet*. **2007**, *1*(2), 88–92.

Parson, W.; et al.; The EDNAP mitochondrial DNA population database (EMPOP) collaborative exercises: Organisation, results and perspectives. *Forensic Sci Int*. **2004**, *139* (2–3), 215–26.

Parson, W.; et al.; Evaluation of next generation mtGenome sequencing using the Ion Torrent Personal Genome Machine (PGM). *Forensic Sci Int Genet*. **2013**, *7*(5), 543–9.

Parson, W.; et al.; DNA Commission of the International Society for Forensic Genetics. DNA Commission of the International Society for Forensic Genetics: Revised and extended guidelines for mitochondrial DNA typing. *Forensic Sci Int Genet*. **2014**, *13*, 134–42.

Peck, M.A.; et al.; Concordance and reproducibility of a next generation mtGenome sequencing method for high-quality samples using the Illumina MiSeq. *Forensic Sci Int Genet*. **2016**, *24*, 103–111.

Prieto, L.; et al.; GHEP-ISFG proficiency test 2011: Paper challenge on evaluation of mitochondrial DNA results. *Forensic Sci Int Genet*. **2013**, *7*, 10–15.

Robin, E.D.; and Wong, R.; Mitochondrial DNA molecules and virtual number of mitochondria per cell in mammalian cells. *J Cell Physiol*. **1988**, *136*(3), 507–13.

Robinson, J.T.; et al.; Integrative genomics viewer. *Nat Biotechnol*. **2011**, *29*(1), 24–6.

Röck, A.W.; et al.; SAM: String-based sequence search algorithm for mitochondrial DNA database queries. *Forensic Sci Int Genet*. **2011**, *5*(2), 126–32.

Röck, A.W.; et al.; Concept for estimating mitochondrial DNA haplogroups using a maximum likelihood approach (EMMA). *Forensic Sci Int Genet*. **2013**, *7(6)*, 601–9.

Rubino, F.; et al.; HmtDB, a genomic resource for mitochondrion-based human variability studies. *Nucleic Acids Res*. **2012**, *40*(Database issue), D1150–9.

Salas, A.; et al.; A cautionary note on switching mitochondrial DNA reference sequences in forensic genetics. *Forensic Sci Int Genet*. **2012**, *6*(6), e182–4.

Salas, A.; et al.; A practical guide to mitochondrial DNA error prevention in clinical, forensic, and population genetics. *Biochem Biophys Res Commun*. **2005a**, *335*(3), 891–9.

Salas, A.; et al.; Heteroplasmy in mtDNA and the weight of evidence in forensic mtDNA analysis: A case report. *Int J Legal Med*. **2001**, *114*(3), 186–90.

Salas, A.; et al.; Mitochondrial, error prophylaxis: Assessing the causes of errors in the GEP'02–03 proficiency testing trial. *Forensic Sci Int.* **2005b**, *148*, 191–98.

Salas, A.; et al.; Phylogeographic investigations: The role of trees in forensic genetics. *Forensic Sci Int.***2007**, *168*(1), 1–13.

Sanger, F.; Nicklen, S.; and Coulson, A.R.; DNA sequencing with chain-terminating inhibitors. *Proc Natl Acad Sci USA.* **1977**, *74*(12), 5463–7.

Soares, I.; Amorim, A.; and Goios, A.; mtDNA office: A software to assign human mtDNA macro haplogroups through automated analysis of the protein coding region. *Mitochondrion.* **2012**, *12*(6), 666–8.

Sprouse, M.L.; et al.; Internal validation of human mitochondrial DNA quantification using realtime PCR. *J Forensic Sci.* **2014**, *59*(4), 1049–56.

Stoneking, M.; Hypervariable sites in the mtDNA control region are mutational hotspots. *Am J Hum Genet.* **2000**, *67*(4), 1029–32.

Strobl, C.; et al.; Evaluation of the precision ID whole MtDNA genome panel for forensic analyses. *Forensic Sci Int Genet.* **2018**, *35*, 21–5.

Sutovsky, P.; et al.; Ubiquitinated sperm mitochondria, selective proteolysis, and the regulation of mitochondrial inheritance in mammalian embryos. *Biol Reprod.* **2000**, 63:582–90.

SWGDAM. Interpretation Guidelines for Mitochondrial DNA Analysis by Forensic DNA Testing Laboratories (approved Jul 18, 2013). [Online]. Available: https://www.swgdam. org/publications (accessed Mach 09, 2019)

Szibor, R.; et al.; Mitochondrial D-loop 3'(CA)n repeat polymorphism: optimization of analysis and population data. *Electrophoresis.* **1997**, *18*, 2857–60.

Tully, G.; et al.; Considerations by the European DNA profiling (EDNAP) group on the working practices, nomenclature and interpretation of mitochondrial DNA profiles. *Forensic Sci Int.* **2001**, *124*, 83–91.

Tully, G.; et al.; Results of a collaborative study of the EDNAP group regarding mitochondrial DNA heteroplasmy and segregation in hair shafts. *Forensic Sci Int.* **2004**, *140*, 1–11.

van Oven, M.; and Kayser M.; Updated comprehensive phylogenetic tree of global human mitochondrial DNA variation. *Hum Mutat.* **2009**, *30*(2), E386–94.

von Wurmb-Schwark, N.; et al.; Quantification of human mitochondrial DNA in a real time PCR. *Forensic Sci Int.* **2002**, *126*(1), 34–9.

Wallace, D.; et al.; Sequence analysis of cDNAs for the human and bovine ATP synthase b subunit: Mitochondrial DNA genes sustain seventeen times more mutations. *Curr Genet.* **1987**, *12*, 81–90.

Weissensteiner, H.; et al.; eCOMPAGT integrates mtDNA: Import, validation and export of mitochondrial DNA profiles for population genetics, tumour dynamics and genotype-phenotype association studies. *BMC Bioinformatics.* **2010**, *11*, 122.

Weissensteiner, H.; et al.; HaploGrep 2: Mitochondrial haplogroup classification in the era of high-throughput sequencing. *Nucleic Acids Res.* **2016a**, *44*(W1), W58–63.

Weissensteiner, H.; et al.; mtDNA-Server: Next-generation sequencing data analysis of human mitochondrial DNA in the cloud. *Nucleic Acids Res.* **2016b**, *44*(W1), W64–9.

Williams, E.; and Hurst, L.; Is the synonymous substitution rate in mammals gene-specific? *Mol Biol Evol.* **2002**, 19, 1395–98.

Wilson, M.R.; et al.; Validation of mitochondrial DNA sequencing for forensic casework analysis. *Int J Legal Med.* **1995**, *108*(2), 68–74.

Woerner, A.E.; et al.; Evaluation of the precision ID mtDNA whole genome panel on two massively parallel sequencing systems. *Forensic Sci Int Genet.* **2018**, *36*, :213–24.

Yakes, M.F.; and Van Houten, B.; Mitochondrial DNA damage is more extensive and persist longer than nuclear DNA damage in human cells following oxidative stress. *Proc Natl Acad Sci USA*. **1997**, *94*, 514–19.

Zander, J.; et al.; New application for haplotype-specific extraction: Separation of mitochondrial DNA mixtures. *Forensic Sci Int Genet.* **2017**, *29*, 242–9.

Zascavage, R.R.; Thorson, K. Planz, J.V.; Nanopore sequencing: An enrichment-free alternative to mitochondrial DNA sequencing. *Electrophoresis*. **2019**, *40(2)*, 272–80.

Zimmermann, B.; et al.; Improved visibility of character conflicts in quasi-median networks with the EMPOP NETWORK software. *Croat Med J*. **2014**, *55*(2), 115–20.

PART III
Novelties in Forensic Genetics

CHAPTER 7

Sequencing Technology in Forensic Science: Next-Generation Sequencing

RUNA DANIEL[1*] and SALLYANN HARBISON[2]

[1]*Office of the Chief Forensic Scientist, Victoria Police Forensic Services Centre, Macleod, VIC 3085, Australia*

[2]*Institute of Environmental Science and Research Ltd., Private Bag 92021, Auckland 1142, New Zealand*

Corresponding author. E-mail: Runa.Daniel@police.vic.gov.au

ABSTRACT

The advancement in DNA sequencing technologies and its application to forensic analysis has enabled an expansion of forensic capabilities. This chapter reviews the evolution of first-generation sequencing to second- and third-generation technologies, chemistries, platforms, and forensic considerations.

7.1 FIRST-GENERATION SEQUENCING

The characterization of the three-dimensional structure of DNA in 1953 (Watson and Crick, 1953) was followed by two decades of research to develop methodology to determine the sequence composition and the order of nucleotides in DNA fragments. Although protein sequencing methods were developed in the early 1950s (Sanger and Tuppy, 1951) and RNA was sequenced in the mid-1960s (Holley et al., 1965), these methods were not readily applicable to DNA. Compared to proteins, DNA molecules are longer and are made of fewer distinguishable units, that is, four nucleotides compared to 20 amino acid residues, which complicated their separation. RNA sequencing (RNA-Seq) was not complicated by a complementary strand, and

RNase enzymes known to cleave RNA chains at specific sites were in use (Ari and Arikan, 2016; Heather and Chain, 2016).

Assisted by the ability to purify and produce vast quantities of bacteriophages with DNA genomes creating an ideal abundant template, Wu and Kaiser (1968) obtained the first DNA sequence. This was achieved by sequencing the 3′ ends of Enterobacteria phage λ using DNA polymerase to copy DNA using radioactive nucleotides (Wu and Kaiser, 1968). Although restricted to short DNA fragments, the principle of adding single radiolabeled nucleotides and measuring incorporation, as well as the generalized use of specific oligonucleotides to prime the DNA polymerase, could be used to determine the order of nucleotides anywhere within the sequence, not only at the 3′ end. Greater resolution power was achieved using polyacrylamide gel electrophoresis to sequence fragments replacing the 2D separation (often consisting of electrophoresis and chromatography) previously used to separate fragments (Heather and Chain, 2016). This separation method was used by two influential techniques. Sanger and Coulson (1975) introduced a rapid approach to sequence DNA known as the *plus and minus method* (Sanger and Coulson, 1975), and a fragmentation technique was introduced by Maxam and Gilbert in 1977 (Maxam and Gilbert, 1977).

The plus and minus method required a primer for synthesis using DNA polymerase to incorporate radiolabeled oligonucleotides. A "plus" reaction only contained a single nucleotide type, for example, only an "A"; therefore, all strand extensions ended in that specific base. A "minus" reaction contained three nucleotides resulting in sequences up to the position before the missing nucleotide. The position of each nucleotide in the DNA strand was inferred (excluding homopolymeric regions) by comparing the products of the reactions, which were electrophoresed on polyacrylamide gels. This method was used to sequence the first DNA genome by determining the sequence of the entire genome of bacteriophage phi X174 of approximately 5375 nucleotides (Sanger et al., 1977a).

In contrast, the fragmentation technique did not utilize DNA polymerase but instead required 32P labeling of the 3′ end of the fragment and subjecting the DNA to partial degradation, breaking terminally labeled DNA molecules at a specific base. The lengths of the labeled fragments identified the position of that base allowing the sequence to be inferred (Maxam and Gilbert, 1977). The Maxam and Gilbert technique was the first method to be widely adopted, as the plus and minus method was considered to be time consuming, and it could not be used to determine the internal positions of sequences. The Maxam and Gilbert method may be considered the first "first-generation sequencing" method.

About this time, Sanger and colleagues began to consider the use of chemical analogs of deoxynucleotide triphosphates (dNTPs), dideoxynucleotide triphosphates (ddNTPs). Kornberg et al. (1974) had demonstrated that ddTTP was a substrate for DNA polymerase, but its lack of a 3′ hydroxyl group prevented it from forming a bond with the 5′ phosphate of the next dNTP, and no further nucleotides could be incorporated (Kornberg, 1974). Utilizing the chain-terminating inhibitor properties of ddNTPs, Sanger and colleagues developed a sequencing method which changed the progress of DNA sequencing technology. In 1977, the Sanger "chain-termination" or dideoxy technique was published (Sanger et al., 1977b). Also known as Sanger sequencing, this method was the beginning of the revolution of the field of genomics.

Sanger sequencing reactions employed radiolabeled ddNTPs (added at lower concentrations) mixed with dNTPs resulting in random termination of the DNA strand extension when a dideoxy base is incorporated. This process generates all possible fragment lengths of the target sequence. Four reactions each containing an individual ddNTP were performed. After separation by polyacrylamide gel electrophoresis, the products of each reaction were visualized by autoradiography with the terminal base of each fragment radiolabeled. This dideoxy chain termination method, due to its accuracy, robustness, and ease of use, became the most widely used sequencing method (Heather and Chain, 2016; Sanger et al., 1977b; van Dijk et al., 2014a).

In the three decades that followed, the Sanger method was gradually improved achieving sequence lengths of up to approximately 1–1.2 kilobase (kb) with per base "raw" accuracies as high as 99.999% (Shendure and Ji, 2008). Limitations in the length of DNA that could be sequenced were overcome by the development of Shotgun sequencing (Anderson, 1981). Shotgun sequencing involves fragmenting DNA, either mechanically or enzymatically, into smaller fragments. These fragments are cloned into sequencing vectors and sequenced individually. Multiple overlapping sequenced strands of the target are generated by performing several rounds of fragmentation and sequencing. The sequence of the DNA fragment is obtained by aligning and reassembling the multiple fragments *in silico* based on partial sequence overlaps (Zhang et al., 2011). Aligning overlapping sequences forms the basis of future high throughput DNA sequencing technologies.

A number of technological advances also contributed to improvements in the Sanger method. The development of the polymerase chain reaction (Mullis and Faloona, 1987; Mullis et al., 1986; Saiki et al., 1985) enabled the generation of numerous copies of specific DNA targets providing a means of obtaining high concentrations of DNA template for sequencing. Subsequent to improvements to fluorescent dyes, fluorescently labeled chain terminators replaced the use of radioactively labeled nucleotides (Rosenblum et al., 1997; Smith et al., 1986), and thermostable polymerases specifically designed for sequencing were utilized (Reeve and Fuller, 1995).

A growing need for greater sequencing output led to laboratory automation and process parallelization. In 1986, LeRoy Hood from the Californian Institute of Technology developed the first semiautomated DNA Sequencing machine (Smith et al., 1986). Marketed by Applied Biosystems (USA), the ABI Model 370A closely followed by the Model 373A model (Halloran et al., 1993), automated the detection of DNA bases using Sanger sequencing, and became a key instrument in mapping and sequencing genetic material. The ABI range of sequencers resulted in the establishment of high-throughput sequencing laboratories (van Dijk et al., 2014a). The ABI Prism 377, a polyacrylamide gel-based instrument, was an early choice in forensic analysis to increase the throughput of short tandem repeat (STR) detection (Frazier et al., 1996).

Separation of sequencing products using polyacrylamide gels was replaced by capillary electrophoresis utilizing novel polymer chemistry. The ABI Prism 310, released in 1996, was a single capillary instrument designed for a wide range of sequencing and fragment analysis approaches (Barba et al., 2014). This improved fragment resolution allowed the reaction to occur in one vessel instead of four (Heather and Chain, 2016). Two years later, the ABI Prism 3700 with 96 capillaries was released, truly automating DNA sequencing.

The notion of sequencing the entire human genome was proposed between 1984 and 1986, and in late 1990s, the publicly funded Human Genome Project (HGP) was launched (Lander et al., 2001). The objective was to determine the entire euchromatic genome in 15 years at an estimated cost of 3 billion US$ (Hutchison, 2007). In 1998, Celera Genomics, founded by Applera Corporation and Craig Venter, in direct competition with the HGP, entered the race to sequence the human genome applying Venter's method of whole genome shotgun sequencing. Celera and the HGP both published the first draft of the human genome in 2001 (Lander et al., 2001; Venter et al., 2001). Following the release of the completed human genome sequence in 2004 (Consortium 2004), the National Human Genome Research Institute initiated a program to achieve a $1000 human genome in 10 years (Reuter et al., 2015). This initiative was aimed at the development and commercialization of next-generation sequencing technologies to achieve the goal of high-throughput, automated, whole genome sequencing (Schloss 2008).

Sanger sequencing has been the gold standard for the analysis of mito-chondrial genome for forensic purposes since the determination of the human mitochondrial sequence in 1981 (Anderson et al., 1981). Early work involved sequencing of mtDNA from single hair (Higuchi et al., 1988). Sample sequences are aligned to the revised Cambridge reference sequence (rCRS), and the sequence information recorded is generally limited to the differences between the sample sequence and this sequence. Sanger sequencing has provided an understanding of heteroplasmy in mtDNA, and extensive guide-lines have been established to allow robust and reliable mtDNA profiling (Carracedo et al., 2000; Parson et al., 2014; SWGDAM 2013). Although mtDNA sequencing in forensic analysis has focused on the analysis of the control region, next-generation sequencing is a cost-effective, faster alterna-tive with greater resolution of DNA mixtures including heteroplasmic vari-ants also enabling whole mtDNA genome sequencing (Woerner et al., 2018).

7.2 SECOND-GENERATION SEQUENCING

The defining characteristic of Sanger sequencing is that each reaction sequences a single, predefined target (approximately 1 kb). The DNA frag-ments are labeled and applied to a sequencer to be separated by electropho-resis where the fragments are detected. In contrast, in second-generation sequencing, thousands to millions of sequencing reactions occur at the same time with sequencing and detection occurring simultaneously. Second-gener-ation sequencing is collectively referred to as next generation sequencing (NGS) or massively parallel sequencing.

In NGS, fragmented DNA is captured on a solid surface such that a single, target molecule occupies one of the million or billions of spatially identifiable locations or features on the surface. Examples of such surfaces include the flow cells used by Illumina sequencers or the semiconductor chips used by the Ion Torrent sequencers. In NGS, sequencing of multiple targets is performed cyclically and in parallel, or simultaneously, in a single run. This led to the massive parallelization which enabled the significant increase in throughput per reaction, compared to Sanger sequencing, and decrease in cost. In addition, compared to Sanger, the NGS technologies do not require bacterial cloning of DNA fragments. The preparation of DNA fragments for sequencing, known as library preparation, occurs in a cell-free system, and the sequencing output is detected directly without the need for electrophoresis. Compared to the read lengths of 1000–1200 bps achieved by Sanger sequencing, NGS generates relatively short fragments of between

35 and 500 bps depending on the specific technology used. The relatively short reads of NGS presented challenges for genome assembly and required development of novel alignment algorithms (Moorthie et al., 2011; van Dijk et al., 2014a).

The increased sensitivity of NGS allows detection and identification of variants present in low numbers of cells, including mosaic variation. Sanger sequencing was limited to the discovery of substitutions and small insertions and deletions (indels). Based on the application, the sensitivity of NGS to detect variants can be adjusted by increasing the depth of coverage. Coverage is the number of times a specific nucleotide is sequenced. High depth of coverage is used to generate accurate data and detect low-level human variation. Higher accuracy can be achieved with low depth of coverage when using appropriate quality scores. Not limited to requiring prior knowledge of the DNA sequence, NGS can be used for *de novo* sequencing or in a targeted NGS approach, where individual genes or regions of interest can be sequenced (Behjati and Tarpey, 2013).

The selection of a suitable sequencing methodology is largely dependent on the application. Factors such as the size (or expected size) of the genome to be studied and the complexity of the genome (guanine-cytosine [GC] content, repetitive sequences, etc.) are considered. Sequencing platforms are commonly compared on performance metrics such as sequencing depth, coverage, read length, errors, and accuracy. Longer read lengths may be required for *de novo* sequencing, while shorter read lengths may be appropriate for targeted amplicon sequencing. Factors such as cost per base, cost per run, sample preparation time and cost, instrument run time, and sequencing error rates are more challenging to compare given the vast differences in chemistries and sample preparation workflows of the NGS platforms (Barba et al., 2014; Levy and Myers, 2016).

Depth of coverage, coverage, and sequencing depth refer to the number of times a base is sequenced. Therefore, a depth of 20× indicates that a base has been sequenced 20 times. Depth can be affected by the complexity of the genome (including high or low GC content) and is not uniform due to repetitive elements, nonuniform targeting, and variable GC content, which affects amplification and sequencing efficiency. Depth may vary depending on the accuracy of the platform, variant detection method, the template sequence, and the required sensitivity or specificity. Therefore, it may be necessary to increase the overall coverage depending on the application (Moorcraft et al., 2015, 2011).

Sanger sequencing has an extremely low error rate of 10^{-4}–10^{-5} for single calls; however, the limit of detection of low-level variants such as mosaic and somatic mutation is approximately 20% (with respect to minor allele representation). NGS has enabled sequencing of individual genomes and detection of rare variants across populations. In contrast to Sanger sequencing, detection of low-level variants using NGS is 0.1%–1%; however, it is accompanied by higher raw error rates of 10^{-2}–10^{-3} depending on read length. The desired accuracy can be achieved by increasing read depth (consensus accuracy) (Moorthie et al., 2011; Stasik et al., 2018).

In addition to amplification errors, random and systematic errors are associated with all NGS methods. Errors can include insertion and deletion of bases as well as incorrectly assigned bases (miscalls). Base call errors are known to occur more frequently at the end of a sequence read. Systematic errors are many individual base call errors from separate sequence reads occurring at the same genomic location (Meacham et al., 2011). Different sequencing technologies are prone to different systematic errors, for example, sequencing homopolymeric regions can be challenging using pyrosequencing or Ion Torrent sequencing due to intermediate fluorescence signal intensities or detection of voltage changes from the incorporation of multiple same nucleotides (Moorthie et al., 2011). Substitution errors are more common in some platforms such as Illumina and SOLiD (Yang et al., 2013). Robasky et al. (2014) highlight the sources of experimental error in NGS and the role of replicates in error mitigation (Robasky et al., 2014).

Raw accuracy of the sequencing process and the base calling quality are important factors in NGS. Quality scoring is the process of assigning a score to each base call that indicates the degree of confidence of the call. This is known as the Phred score. Phred scores are logarithmically related to base calling error probabilities. A Phred score of 10 (Q10) refers to a 1 in 10 chance of an incorrect call, that is, a 10% probability of a miscall. Q20 equates to an error of 1 in 100, Q30 equates to an error of 1 in 1000, and so on. Factors that affect the quality score are signal intensity and background noise in the reaction or generated by the instrument (Ewing and Green, 1998; Ewing et al., 1998; Moorthie et al., 2011).

7.2.1 NGS SAMPLE PREPARATION

7.2.1.1 SAMPLE PREPARATION

DNA is extracted and quantified following standard forensic methods (Butler, 2011). Library and template preparation processes are specific to the NGS platform and application used. Generally, the recommended DNA input amount is 1 ng for NGS-based assays developed specifically for forensic analysis, such as the ForenSeq™ Signature DNA Prep Kit (Verogen) and the human identification (HID) Ion AmpliSeq™ panels (Thermo Fisher Scientific). However, full DNA sequence profiles can be obtained with lower template input amounts and is dependent on the number of samples analyzed and the application (Jager et al., 2017). Full profiles can also be achieved with lower template amounts by increasing the polymerase chain reaction (PCR) amplification cycle numbers (Al-Asfi et al., 2018). Section 7.2.3 describes Ion Torrent PGM/S5 and Illumina MiSeq FGx sequencing.

7.2.1.2   LIBRARY PREPARATION

A library is a collection of DNA fragments which contain the genomic regions of interest to be sequenced. Each library represents an individual sample. DNA library fragments consist of the target DNA with adapters and barcodes (in some workflows) attached to the ends. Adapters are specific oligonucleotide sequences which enable hybridization of the library fragments to a solid surface and provide a priming location for amplification and/or sequencing primers. Barcodes, or indices, are unique identifier (oligonucleotide) sequences which are used to label library fragments within a sample, analogous to a sample ID. Barcoding allows multiple samples to be combined and sequenced simultaneously in a high-throughput, cost-effective manner. At the end of the sequencing process, bioinformatic software is used to group sequenced fragments from the same sample together for analysis (see Section 7.4).

An important factor in library preparation is to create DNA fragments of optimal lengths, which can be sequenced. The overall library fragment length is determined by the DNA target region and the length of the adapters (which is constant, i.e., does not change) and barcodes/indices. The optimal library fragment length depends on the sequencing platform and application, for example, the optimal insert size is impacted by cluster generation in bridge amplification and the clonal amplification method in Illumina sequencing (Head et al., 2014).

Broadly, in targeted sequencing methods, three general approaches are used for library preparation; PCR-based methods, circularization methods, and the hybridization capture approach. In PCR-based methods, generating a target DNA fragment is achieved using primers specific to the flanking regions of the target DNA. In circularization methods, optimal fragment length is achieved by circularization of large panels of target molecules in a single reaction using specially designed probes containing universal sequences.

The target sequences can be amplified using the universal sequences. In the hybridization capture approach, optimal length is achieved by fragmenting the DNA either mechanically (e.g., by sonication) or enzymatically. This may not be required for degraded DNA. DNA capture probes are then used to hybridize to the fragments of interest (whole fragmented genomic DNA) to enable enrichment of the target DNA (Moorcraft et al., 2015, 2011). Hybridization-based DNA capture has been used to sequence whole mitochondrial genomes from highly degraded human skeletal remains (ranging from 10 to 2500 years old) for HID for which standard nuclear PCR methods were unsuccessful (Templeton et al., 2013).

Targeted amplicon sequencing is limited due to its requirement for prior knowledge of the sequences flanking the target DNA. However, numerous regions can be targeted simultaneously by utilizing primer sets for each region of interest in a multiplex amplification. Currently, most NGS-based forensic applications use targeted amplicon sequencing of specific, forensically relevant loci (Ambers et al., 2016; Hollard et al., 2017). The circularization method can be used to overcome the limitations of multiplexing in PCR-based methods. Hybridization capture is not limited by the requirement to know the exact sequence of the flanking region specific DNA sequences, however, it is a less specific approach and is highly dependent on the design of the probes (Moorthie et al., 2011).

Once the DNA fragment is generated, the fragment ends are repaired, and adapters and barcodes/indices are attached either by ligation or by amplification. The final step is normalization. The normalization step aims to achieve uniform sequencing coverage between the libraries. However, the normalization does not account for the potentially uneven distribution of amplicons resulting from PCR bias in the initial PCR amplification. Normalization typically involves quantitating and diluting barcoded libraries to equimolar concentrations and pooling libraries in equal volumes to achieve even sequencing of DNA fragments. Normalization can also be achieved using beads with the total yield of libraries determined by the maximum binding capacity of the bead.

A number of important considerations for library preparation are the amount and quality of starting material, the genomic region being sequenced as well as the sequencing application. For example, libraries generated from genomes with high or low GC content may be susceptible to amplification bias. Consideration of specific polymerases for PCR amplification, thermocycling, conditions, and buffers can be used to address these issues. For more information on library preparation considerations and biases, see (Head et al., 2014), (van Dijk et al., 2014a), and (van Dijk et al., 2014b).

7.2.1.3   TEMPLATE PREPARATION

Template preparation, also referred to as clonal amplification, is a process of generating numerous copies of the library fragments. Clonal amplification of isolated targets is a requirement of most NGS systems in order to generate sufficient signal for detection during the sequencing process. Generally, the library fragments are clonally amplified *in situ* on a solid substrate (surface), and many thousands of identical DNA targets are generated in clusters using a PCR method specific to the platform.

Roche and Life Technologies (Thermo Fisher Scientific) sequencers employ emulsion PCR (emPCR). emPCR involves amplification of DNA fragments on oligonucleotide-coated beads which are suspended in a water-in-oil emulsion (Dressman et al., 2003). The oligonucleotides on the surface of the beads are complementary to the adapter sequences ligated to the library fragments. This enables binding of the library fragment to the bead, that is, a solid surface. PCR amplification results in each bead coated with millions of copies of the DNA fragment.

Illumina sequencers employ bridge PCR where library fragments bind to complementary oligonucleotides which coat the surface of a glass flow cell. The library fragments have two different adapters attached to their ends that enable the formation of a bridge by the attachment of the fragment at both ends. Millions of copies of the library fragments are generated through bridge PCR which generates clusters on the surface of the flow cell.

Once library fragments are clonally amplified, the fragments are sequenced. The sequencing platforms differ in the chemistries and detection systems. Generally, the sequencing process involves the addition of nucleotides, signal detection upon nucleotide incorporation, and the removal/washing of the reagents. This process is repeated in a cyclical fashion until the DNA template is sequenced.

7.2.2   NGS PLATFORMS

The first NGS technology was the pyrosequencing-based method by 454 Life Sciences released in 2005. Between 2005 and 2010, a number of NGS technologies rapidly emerged with vastly different sequencing chemistries and detection methods. Low-, medium-, and high-throughput platforms enabled sequencing outputs of 200,000 reads to 100 million reads with varying read lengths of 35–1200 bps (van Dijk et al., 2014a). For diagrams illustrating NGS chemistries, see (Garrido-Cardenas et al., 2017; Kchouk et al., 2017; Metzker 2010; Shendure and Ji, 2008).

7.2.2.1 ROCHE 454/LIFE SCIENCES PYROSEQUENCING - SEQUENCING BY SYNTHESIS

The detection of pyrophosphate in DNA sequencing was first described by Hyman in 1988 (Hyman, 1988). Pyrosequencing relies on the detection of light when pyrophosphate is released following the incorporation of a complementary dNTP. The released pyrophosphate provides energy for luciferase to oxidize luciferin, generating light. Nucleotides are sequentially added and removed from the reaction, and light is only produced when a nucleotide is incorporated. For an early review, see (Ronaghi, 2001). Two pyrosequencing strategies can be employed. Pyrosequencing in a solid phase (Nyren, 1987; Nyren et al., 1993) where the DNA is to be sequenced is immobilized on a solid support and requires washes between reactions. Pyrosequencing in a liquid phase relies on the activity of an enzyme (apyrase) to degrade nucleotides between each step (Ronaghi et al., 1998).

The 454 Life Sciences Genome Sequencer FLX instrument (Roche) was the first high-throughput microfluidic-based instrument, based on principles described in 2005 (Margulies et al., 2005). This method was the first to utilize emPCR on DNA-coated beads for library preparation to obtain sufficient copies of identical sequences for reliable light detection. Barcoding was employed to pool individual samples together enabling sequencing of up to 96 samples in microtiter plate format. Both the 454 instrument and the benchtop version, the GS Junior, were evaluated for forensic applications with the long read lengths (400–1200 bp) seen as advantageous, including sequencing of STRs (Fordyce et al., 2011; Gelardi et al., 2014), hypervariable segment I of the mtDNA control region (Holland et al., 2011), and the16S rRNA genes of bacterial communities found on various handled surfaces and the skin of volunteers (Fierer et al., 2010). However, its application was limited due to an error rate of approximately 1% and signal detection compromised by homopolymeric stretches (Heather and Chain, 2016).

Although the 454 platform is no longer commercially available, pyrosequencing is still utilized in forensic DNA analysis predominantly for the detection of DNA methylation (epigenetics). The PyroMark® technology by Qiagen enables the sequencing of DNA and quantitation of epigenetic and other genetic variants (Qiagen). Pyromark® sequences single stranded biotinylated PCR products using DNA polymerase, ATP sulfurylase, luciferase, and apyrase, and the substrates adenosine 5' phosphosulfate and luciferin. In a defined order, dNTPs are added sequentially and incorporation of a complementary dNTP is accompanied by the release of pyrophosphate (PPi) in an amount proportional to the number of nucleotides incorporated. The detection of PPi occurs through a biochemical enzyme cascade which results in the production of light that is detected in the sequencing instrument. Examples of the use of PyroMark® technology include the validation of epigenetic markers for the identification of blood, semen, and saliva (Silva et al., 2016) and the estimation of human chronological age in blood samples (Zbieć-Piekarska et al., 2015).

7.2.2.2   APPLIED BIOSYSTEMS SOLiD - SEQUENCING BY LIGATION

The SOLiD® (Sequencing by Oligonucleotide Ligation and Detection) technique, developed by the Church group in 2005 (Shendure et al., 2005) and released commercially in 2007, utilizes a unique sequencing process catalyzed by DNA ligase and is based on the multiplex polony sequencing technology (Mardis, 2008). SOLiD®'s sequencing-by-ligation approach employs emPCR, similar to 454, with small magnetic beads coated in complementary oligonucleotides to amplify the DNA fragment for sequencing in parallel (Anderson and Schrijver, 2010). The beads are immobilized to a solid surface, that is, a glass slide.

In the SOLiD® technique, sequencing is driven by a DNA ligase rather than a polymerase (Shendure and Ji, 2008). A universal sequencing primer hybridizes to the SOLiD®-specific adapter sequence preceding the DNA template attached to the beads. Each sequencing cycle involves fluorescently labeled 8-mer oligonucleotide probes in which the first two nucleotides of the probe represent each of the 16 dinucleotide combinations (e.g., TT, GT, TC, GG, etc.) and the remaining six nucleotides of the probe are degenerate (Anderson and Schrijver, 2010). Each probe, labeled with one of four fluorescent labels, competes for ligation to the sequencing primer. Upon ligation, the fluorescence captured corresponds to the probe which ligated. The oligonucleotide probe is then cleaved between nucleotide positions 5 and 6 removing the fluorescent label. The 5' phosphate is regenerated to enable seven subsequent cycles of the ligation reaction. The newly synthesized strand is denatured from the template to reset the system (Shendure and Ji, 2008). A second round of sequencing is initiated with a new sequencing primer, which is offset by one nucleotide relative to the initial sequencing primer ($n - 1$), annealed to the template (Anderson and Schrijver, 2010).

The primer offsetting scheme allows a universal sequencing primer that is offset by one base from the adapter-fragment junction to hybridize to DNA templates in the cycling reactions which permits the entire fragment to be sequenced. Each ligation step is followed by fluorescence detection and another round of ligation (Zhang et al., 2011). In addition, the 2-base encoding is an error-correction mechanism, in which two bases, rather than a single base, are correlated with the label, and therefore, each base is interrogated twice and miscalls can be readily identified (Shendure and Ji, 2008). SOLiD® sequencing generates read lengths up to 50 bps with a base accuracy of 99.94%. Although the SOLiD® instrument is capable of generating 4 Gb of sequencing data, this was achievable after a five- to six-day run (Anderson and Schrijver, 2010).

The Polonator G. 007 was developed in collaboration with Dover and the Church group that developed SOLiD® (Shendure et al., 2005). The Polonator G. 007, based on sequencing by ligation, employs a bead-based emPCR to amplify DNA fragments in parallel. Unlike SOLiD®, which uses dual-base coding, the Polonator G. 007 decodes the bases by using a single-base probe in nonanucleotides (nonamers) (Liu et al., 2012). The Polonator G.007 was intentionally developed as a low-cost, high-performance, open-architecture system with freely downloadable, open-source software and protocols to increase competition in the sequencing market and make genomics more affordable.

7.2.2.3   HELICOS HELISCOPE™—SEQUENCING BY SYNTHESIS

HeliScope™ single molecule sequencing was developed by Quake's group in 2003 (Braslavsky et al., 2003) and licensed by Helicos Biosciences in 2007. This methodology is unique in that, unlike other sequencing methods that require clonal amplification, HeliScope™ does not require amplified DNA templates. Instead, single DNA molecules are interrogated via sequencing by synthesis. Therefore, due to its unique ability to sequence single-DNA molecules without amplification, the HeliScope™ is considered to be the first single molecule sequencing technology, defined as Single Molecule Real Time (SMRT) DNA sequencing (Zhang et al., 2011).

Template libraries are prepared by randomly fragmenting genomic DNA to generate fragments of 100–200 bps and by the addition of multiple adenosines to the 3′ end of the fragment (poly A tailing). These fragments are hybridized to poly-T oligonucleotides covalently linked to the surface of the flow cell. This forms a disordered array of single-molecule sequencing

(SMS) templates. The terminal adenosine on the library fragments is fluorescently labeled enabling identification of the position of each template molecule on the array. However, this fluorescent label is removed prior to sequencing. The sequencing relies on cyclic interrogation, where the DNA templates are exposed to DNA polymerase and one of four fluorescently labeled nucleotides at each cycle resulting in template-dependent extension of the DNA templates. Similar to 454 pyrosequencing, the sequencing is asynchronous as not all templates will incorporate a nucleotide at each round of sequencing. At the end of each sequencing cycle, the fluorescence signal is detected across the array by a highly sensitive fluorescence detection system, then, the fluorescent labeled is chemically cleaved and released which allows the next cycle of extension and imaging (Anderson and Schrijver 2010; Shendure et al., 2005).

HeliScope™ initially yielded an average read length of 25 bps or greater after hundreds of rounds of sequencing (in a seven day run) and produced more than 20 Gb of data (Harris et al., 2008). The overall accuracy is high (>99.99%) when utilizing a two-pass strategy, where the template molecules (with adapters at both ends) are sequenced, copied, and then sequenced in the opposite orientation (Shendure and Ji, 2008). As this technique does not require amplification, it has reduced errors which arise from PCR artefacts. However, similar to the 454, errors arise from sequencing of homopolymer regions from multiple nucleotide incorporations (Anderson and Schrijver, 2010). The predominant error types are deletions (2%–7% error rate with one pass; 0.2%–1% with two passes) possibly due to incorporation of unlabeled nucleotides or detection errors. Substitution error rates are lower (0.01%–1% with one pass; approaching 0.001% with two passes) (Shendure and Ji, 2008).

7.2.3 NGS IN FORENSICS

Forensic DNA analysis has utilized capillary electrophoresis to visualize and analyze data generated from STRs for over 20 years. Forensic STR kits have evolved to include over 20 STR markers multiplexed in a single reaction with sufficient sensitivity and reproducibility for routine application to casework using capillary electrophoresis (CE) (Ensenberger et al., 2014; Srivastava et al., 2019). In addition, CE has been used to analyze single-nucleotide polymorphisms (SNPs) for forensic identity and intelligence testing (Phillips et al., 2009; Sanchez et al., 2006a; Walsh et al., 2013).

Although robust and reliable, DNA analysis using CE is based on fragment length. It is limited by the availability of fluorophores to distinguish PCR products from multiple STRs with amplicons which must also vary in size in order to be differentiated. In contrast, NGS reveals the underlying sequence variation of the amplicon and size separation of amplicons is not required. Using NGS, multiple marker types are analyzed simultaneously including STRs (autosomal, Y and X), SNPs, and microhaplotype markers reducing the depletion of valuable, often scant, evidential material which occurs from multiple analyses.

The application of NGS to forensic DNA analysis enables an expansion of forensic DNA capabilities. Early studies applied pyrosequencing to quantify mtDNA mixtures (Andreasson et al., 2006) and SOLiD for the detection of pathogens in biocrime (Cummings et al., 2010). Research, development, and validation efforts have since focused on a number of forensic applications, including predicting the biological origin of stains using mRNA (Dorum et al., 2018), mixture resolution (Bennett et al., 2019; Young et al., 2019), age estimation (Aliferi et al., 2018), ancestry prediction (Eduardoff et al., 2016), whole mtDNA genome analysis (Strobl et al., 2018), alternative DNA markers (Oldoni et al., 2019; van der Gaag et al., 2018), microbial forensics (Schmedes et al., 2016), traditional medicines (Coghlan et al., 2012), and wildlife crime (Ogden 2011).

To date, the forensic community has predominantly adopted Ion Torrent™ semiconductor sequencing technology (Thermo Fisher Scientific) or MiSeq FGx™ (Verogen) platforms for targeted amplicon sequencing.

7.2.3.1 ION TORRENT™ SEQUENCING TECHNOLOGY - SEQUENCING BY SYNTHESIS

Jonathan Rothberg (also the founder of 454 Life Sciences) and colleagues (Rothberg et al., 2006) invented the specific complementary metal–oxide semiconductor (CMOS) chip massively parallel sequencing device in 2006 (Merriman and Rothberg, 2012). In 2007, Ion Torrent™ was founded and subsequently developed semiconductor chip-based DNA sequencing technology. This development overcame the limitations of the requirement for imaging technology and specialized nucleotides in DNA sequencing. In 2010, Ion Torrent™ was acquired by Life Technologies (now Thermo Fisher Scientific), and the first instrument was released, the Ion Personal Genome Machine™ (PGM) (Thermo Fisher Scientific). The PGM was the first commercial sequencing machine that did not require fluorescence or camera scanning, resulting in higher speed, lower cost, smaller instrument size, and portability (Liu et al., 2012).

Unlike pyrosequencing, Ion Torrent™ semiconductor sequencing technology measures pH changes resulting from the release of a hydrogen ion (H+), or a proton, from the 3' OH incorporation site on the synthesized stand (Merriman and Rothberg, 2012). This introduced two unique features to DNA sequencing. First, a simple sequencing chemistry based on the detection of pH changes during DNA sequencing using native, unlabeled nucleotides, therefore, the DNA sequence is not determined using fluorescence, optics, or light. Second, the sequencing occurs in the millions of wells on the CMOS sensor array chip with the sensor surface at the bottom of each well on the chip. CMOS processes, widely used in constructing integrated circuits, also allow for scaling of the device to higher densities and larger arrays (Rothberg et al., 2011).

Each well on the Ion chip serves as an individual pH meter which is achieved by an ion-sensitive field effect transistor (ISFET) below each well detecting pH changes resulting from H+ release. The change is recorded as a voltage change by the ion-sensor layer indicating nucleotide incorporation. Therefore, this technology overcomes the limitations associated with optical-based sequencing platforms and the requirement for labeled nucleotides imaging technology which allows for faster sequencing (Reuter et al., 2015; Rothberg et al., 2011).

7.2.3.1.1   *Manual and Automated Library and Template Preparation*

Ion Torrent sequencing has options for manual and automated library and template preparation. The Ion One Touch™ 2 system automates multiple manual template preparation steps and enables parallel processing of multiple samples. However, this requires manual library preparation and loading onto the Ion chip. The system consists of two modules: the Ion One Touch™ 2 instrument that performs template preparation and the Ion OneTouch Enrichment System that performs template enrichment. In 2014, the Ion Chef™ system was released enabling automated library and template preparation as well as chip loading minimizing operator variability and increasing productivity. The Ion Chef functions include thermal cycling, liquid transfer, centrifugation, bead enrichment, and chip loading (Thermo Fisher Scientific).

7.2.3.1.2   Library Preparation

Most Ion Torrent NGS-based forensic applications use PCR-based targeted sequencing of specific, forensically relevant markers. These applications generally use Ion AmpliSeq™ technology for library construction targeting specific human genes or genomic regions (Thermo Fisher Scientific).

Forensic DNA markers are PCR amplified using an Ion AmpliSeq™ primer pool (see Figure 7.1A). The primer sequences of the PCR amplicon are partially digested using FuPa reagent (Thermo Fisher Scientific) to create blunt ends. Adapters are ligated randomly to the blunt ends of the forward or reverse PCR amplicon fragments. The P1 adapter (41 base pairs (bps) in length) assists in the binding of the library fragment to the solid surface on which sequencing occurs. The A adapter (30 bps) or the X barcode adapter (43 bps) creates a nonbarcoded or barcoded library. The X barcode adapter consists of same 30 nucleotides as the A adapter, an additional 10 nucleotides are the unique barcode identifier sequences used to label each individual library and three nucleotides, which are the barcode adapters. The Ion Xpress™ Barcode Adapters Kit (Thermo Fisher Scientific) can be used to barcode up to 96 samples, while the IonCode™ Barcode adapters can be used to barcode up to 384 samples. However, barcoding is limited to 32 samples for forensic applications using the Ion Chef™ for automated library preparation.

7.2.3.1.3   Normalization

In addition to achieving uniform sequencing coverage between the libraries, normalization assists in achieving optimal template preparation of Ion Sphere Particles (ISPs) to avoid low-quality sequencing reads or mixed signal during sequencing generated by polyclonal ISPs. In manual library preparation, a TaqMan®-based assay, the Ion Library TaqMan™ Quantitation Kit (Thermo Fisher Scientific), is used to quantitate adapter-ligated, amplifiable Ion fragment libraries. Each library is diluted to a pM amount and pooled in equal volumes. Automated library preparation using the Ion Chef™ requires bead normalization using the Ion Library Equalizer™ Kit (Thermo Fisher Scientific). The adapter-ligated libraries are amplified using primers targeting the P1 adapter and biotin-labeled primers targeting the A/X adapters. Streptavidin is attached to the surface of the normalization beads enabling the biotin-labeled amplified library fragments to bind. The total yield of normalized libraries is 100 pM using this method.

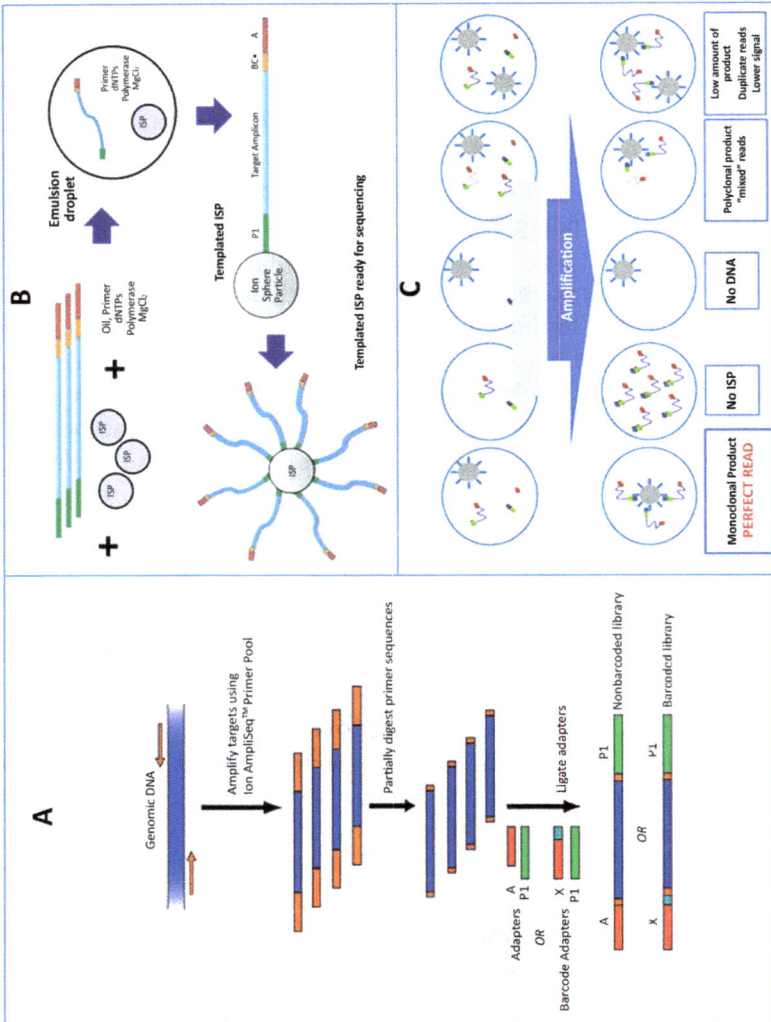

FIGURE 7.1 Ion Torrent Semiconductor Sequencing. A: library preparation – ligation of nonbarcoded (A) and barcoded (X) adapters. B: Template preparation—clonal amplification of templates onto Ion Sphere™ Particles (ISPs). C: Variations in clonal amplification products.

7.2.3.1.4 Template Preparation

Similar to 454, clonal amplification of the library fragments to generate sufficient signal for detection of nucleotide incorporation during sequencing is achieved by attaching the fragment to a bead and amplifying using emPCR. The beads used in Ion Torrent sequencing are ISPs coated in oligonucleotides complementary to the P1 adapter ligated to the library fragment. This enables binding of the library fragment to the ISP. The ISP acts as the carrier used to deposit the DNA fragments into the well as well as the solid surface on which sequencing occurs.

The emPCR reaction contains the library fragments, ISPs and reaction component such as oil, primer, dNTPs, polymerase and $MgCl_2$ forming an emulsion of microdroplets (see Figure 7.1B). Ideally, each microdroplet contains only one bead and one library fragment to ensure that a single library fragment is clonally amplified onto an ISP, that is, monoclonal amplification. A monoclonal ISP generates sufficient signal and sequencing reads. Some microdroplets may contain more than one library fragment, that is, polyclonal amplification, which generates mixed reads (see Figure 7.1C). More than one ISP generates low amount of product, duplicate reads, and lower signal. Polyclonal ISPs and ISPs with low signal are bioinformatically filtered out in the data analysis process. The absence of a library fragment in a microdroplet that contains an ISP results is a non-templated ISP. Non-templated ISPs are removed during the enrichment step. The absence of an ISP in a microdroplet results in untemplated library fragments which are removed from the templated ISPs via centrifugation and purification.

The clonal amplification process begins with denaturation of the library fragments. The reverse strand anneals to the ISP at the P1 adapter end. The forward strand is generated by polymerase extension from the P1 end. The original reverse strand then denatures leaving the amplified forward strand bound to the ISP. This annealing, denaturation, and extension cycle is repeated resulting in the ISP covered in millions of copies of the forward strand. The random ligation of the adapters in the library preparation process results in forward and reverse DNA strands (for a specific DNA target) being monoclonally amplified on different ISPs. Therefore, in a separate microdroplet, the reverse strand is monoclonally amplified on an ISP.

At the end of an application-specific number of amplification cycles, the emulsion is broken by chemical treatment and the reaction components are removed. The template-positive ISPs are enriched using immunogenic capture of templated beads. During clonal amplification, a small proportion of the PCR primers have biotin modifications. This enables biotin-labeled template-positive immunogenic enrichment of the ISPs using streptavidin-coated beads. The templated ISPs, with double stranded templates attached, are then prepared for sequencing. A test fragment [TF-A (Ion PGM) or TFC (Ion S5)], a pre-templated ISP with a synthetic target sequence, is added and acts as a positive control for templating and sequencing reactions.

7.2.3.1.5   Sequencing by Synthesis

The double stranded templates on the ISPs are denatured leaving either forward or reverse strands of target DNA attached to the ISP. Therefore, Ion Torrent enables sequencing of both strands. The sequencing primer anneals to the primer binding site on the A/X adapter. In automated preparation using the Ion Chef™, the polymerase and the sequencing primer are added and annealed to the template fragments prior to loading onto the chip. Centrifugation is used to load the ISPs into the vast array of wells on the surface of the semiconductor Ion chip. The size of the well is designed to accommodate only one ISP. Ideally, one ISP will be deposited into each of the millions of wells, however, sequencing runs often contain empty wells.

Sequencing is initiated once the chip is loaded into the instrument. In the absence of labeled nucleotides, nucleotide incorporation is determined by allowing a single, native nucleotide to flow across the surface of the chip one at a time. A "flow" is the event of one specific nucleotide being exposed to the chip followed by a wash step. The flow of nucleotides occurs in a specific order for a finite time. In addition to the use of native nucleotides, a specific order is also required because there is no detectable difference for H+ released from an A, G, C, or T bases (Buermans and den Dunnen, 2014). Ion Torrent uses the Samba flow order for SNP analysis consisting of a specific 32-base sequence   (TACGTACGTCTGAGCATCGATCGATGTACAGC)   which is repeated (IonTorrent). This flow order improves synchronicity of clonal templates (Bragg et al., 2013), therefore, it reduces phase errors, and improves sequencing accuracy of longer reads. STR sequencing was originally achieved using the Samba Gafieira flow to improve the end-to-end success ratio and signal to noise ratio for STRs (Zhang et al., 2018). However, current forensic NGS STR sequencing utilizes the Ion Samba HID2, a modified flow order consisting of over 200 nucleotides in a specific order to increase data quality.

Each time a chip is flooded with a nucleotide which is complementary to the template base directly downstream of the sequencing primer, the nucleotide is incorporated into the synthesized strand by the polymerase.

This results in hydrolysis of the incorporated nucleotide causing the release of a single H+ ion (proton) for each nucleotide incorporated during that flow. The release of the H+ ion results in a net decrease of the pH of well proportional to the number of nucleotides incorporated in the flow (0.2 pH units per single base incorporation). This results in changes in the surface potential in the metal oxide sensing layer in the chip and a voltage change in the ISFET (Rothberg et al., 2011). For a diagram of the Ion chip and wells, see (Merriman and Rothberg 2012).

In contrast to Illumina sequencing, the nucleotides do not have terminator groups, therefore, several nucleotides are incorporated after each other at a homopolymer stretch in one nucleotide flow. This results in an increase in H+ ions released and a higher pH change directly proportional to the number of nucleotides incorporated. If the nucleotide is not complementary to the template base, nucleotide incorporation will not occur, therefore, pH change and voltage changes are not detected. The chip is washed at the end of each nucleotide flow prior to the flow of the next nucleotide. The flow of the 32 nucleotides represents one cycle. Current forensic NGS kits use 500 or 650 flows for SNP and STR sequencing, respectively.

The four nucleotides at the end of the A adapter and immediately preceding the barcode sequence in the X adapter are the key sequence, AGTC. The key sequences are the first nucleotides that are read in the sequencing reaction. This is used to set baseline signal intensity. The incorporation of each complementary nucleotide to the key sequence represents a 1-mer incorporation. Sequencing of the key sequence is followed by sequencing of the barcode (X adapter) and then the DNA template.

Signal processing software is used to convert raw voltages into base calls by converting the raw data into measurements of incorporation in each well using a physical model. A base caller uses these values and corrects for phase and signal loss and normalizes to the key sequence generating corrected base calls for each flow in each well (Rothberg et al., 2011). Bioinformatic analysis applies quality filters to the data to initially remove polyclonal and low-quality reads and ultimately determine the nucleotide composition of the sequenced fragment (see Section 7.4). In addition to managing sample and run details, the onboard software, Ion Torrent™ Suite, enables real-time monitoring of key sequencing metrics during a run and performs the base-calling alignment and other primary data analysis. The Ion Torrent Variant Caller plug-in is used for variant calling of the aligned reads (Thermo Fisher Scientific).

Insertions and deletions (Indels) are the most common error type using Ion Torrent sequencing. This is the result of the imperfect scaling of the correlation between number of bases incorporated and the subsequent voltage change. An incorporation of two As, that is, AA, will have a 2-fold increase relative to a single A. However, an AAA incorporation will yield a 1.5-fold increase (3/2) in pH relative to an AA. For six As compared to five As, the relative increase is only 1.2. This disproportionate increase of the pH change relative to the nucleotide incorporations as the homopolymer length increases beyond five or six nucleotides reduces the probability that a homopolymer stretch will be sequenced correctly. Homopolymers longer than 6 bps results in increased error rates (Buermans and den Dunnen, 2014; Rothberg et al., 2011).

7.2.3.1.6   *Platforms, Assays, and Forensic Applications*

The PGM is a benchtop, medium-throughput sequencer suitable for targeted resequencing and small genome analysis. The Ion PGM has three semiconductor chips, the Ion 314, 316, and 318 chips with reads which range from 0.4 million to 5.5 million reads per chip enabling sequencing in a scalable and cost-effective manner. The first PGM generated up to 270 Mb of sequence with read lengths of up to 100 bps, slightly shorter than the 454 sequencing (van Dijk et al., 2014a). In September 2012, Thermo Fisher Scientific (then Life Technologies) launched their higher throughput sequencer the Ion Proton allowing for larger chips with higher densities suitable for exome and whole genome analysis sequencing. Ion PI chip generates 60–80 million reads per run. At the time of release, the Ion Proton's output was an order of magnitude higher (1 Gb vs. 10 Gb) than the PGM, however, its read length was 200 bp compared to 400 bp for the PGM (Reuter et al., 2015; Thermo Fisher Scientific).

The Ion GeneStudio S5 sequencer series, first released in 2015 (and updated in 2018), are the latest range of Ion Torrent sequencers, which enable throughput scalability and application flexibility. The Ion GeneStudio S5, S5 Plus, and S5 Prime System instruments have five Ion chips, which range from 3 to 130 million reads, 200–600 bp read lengths, and 0.3–50 Gb output. The Ion GeneStudio range of sequencers utilize cartridge-based consumables and buffers to reduce hands on time when preparing and running the instrument. Applications on the S5 range from targeted sequencing, 16S metagenomic sequencing, exome, and whole transcriptome sequencing (Thermo Fisher Scientific).

First released in 2016, Applied Biosystems™ Converge™ Software is a modular platform which integrates forensic DNA data management and analysis. Converge ™ enables analysis of genotype concordance between CE and NGS STR profiles, kinship, paternity, mtDNA, STR and SNP analysis, and case management (Thermo Fisher Scientific).

The lack of requirement for cameras for detection of light or fluorescent events and time-consuming imaging results in lower cost, higher portability, and shorter sequencing run times of 2–8 h. Reduced sequencing times can be utilized for forensic applications that require timely reporting of results such as DNA Intelligence (Forensic DNA Phenotyping). The multiple chip capacities provide an option for tailored usage which is scalable for cost-effective and efficient sequencing. Automation of library and template preparation with the Ion Chef™ system reduces manual handling errors and increases reproducibility in forensic DNA analysis.

Early studies utilized existing forensic SNP assays to sequence PCR amplicons on the Ion PGM in a custom approach (Daniel et al., 2014). Custom forensic assays were also developed for use with the Ion PGM for the prediction of ancestry (Phillips et al., 2014), human identification and paternity testing (Zhang et al., 2017), and STRs analysis (Zhang et al., 2018). Thermo Fisher Scientific has developed a number of commercial assays specifically for forensic applications. These assays generally require DNA template input amounts of 1 ng, however, informative profiles can often be achieved using less than 1 ng (Al-Asfi et al., 2018). The HID Ion AmpliSeq™ panels (Thermo Fisher Scientific) include the Precision ID Identity Panel (Churchill et al., 2015; Guo et al., 2016; Meiklejohn and Robertson, 2017; Seo et al., 2013), Precision ID Ancestry Panel (Al-Asfi et al., 2018; Garcia et al., 2017; Hollard et al., 2017; Pereira et al., 2017; Wang et al., 2018) and the Precision ID mtDNA Whole Genome Panel (Strobl et al., 2018). In addition, the Precision ID Globalfiler NGS STR panel can be used for STR sequencing (Li et al., 2017; Wang et al., 2017). The GeneRead DNASeq SNP panel (Qiagen), an SNP identity assay, was also successfully applied to the Ion PGM (Avent et al., 2018; de la Puente et al., 2017).

7.2.3.2 ILLUMINA/SOLEXA GENOME ANALYZER - SEQUENCING BY SYNTHESIS

Launched In 2006 by Solexa Ltd., the Genome Analyzer (GA) was developed as a low-cost DNA sequencer with wide ranging applications (Bennett 2004), producing a large number of short reads and 1 Gb of data per run. In 2007, after acquiring Solexa, the GA was further developed by Illumina (San Diego, CA, USA) as the Illumina Genome Analyzer (Illumina). The sequencing chemistry of these instruments is the basis for that of the current

Illumina instruments, including the HiSeq2500 and HiSeq X, the benchtop instruments, the MiSeq and the MiSeq FGx, and the newly released iSeq 100 Sequencing System each with their own features and performance characteristics. The key technological advances included clonal amplification of DNA fragments captured on a glass- and silicon-based flow cell surface (now made of acrylamide coated glass) (Kawashima et al., 2005) and reversible terminator chemistry (Bentley et al., 2008; Canard and Sarfati, 1994). A charge-coupled device camera records images of the fluorescently labeled, reversible terminator bases at each incorporation step, for every location on the flow cell. The dye and the terminal 3′ blocker is removed from the DNA (deprotected), allowing the next cycle to proceed.

Sequencing can be achieved by single end read, paired end (PE) reads, or mate pair sequencing. Single end sequences from one end only and is favored for small RNA molecules. PE sequences both ends of the DNA fragments and aligns the forward and reverse reads as read pairs, enabling confident and accurate alignment and detection of variants. Mate pair sequencing is used for *de novo* sequencing and the assessment of structural variation and is not widely used in forensic analysis. Mate pair sequencing is usually used in combination with PE sequencing.

The MiSeq FGx™ Forensic Genomics Solution using the ForenSeq™ DNA Signature Prep Kit (Verogen) was developed and validated for forensic purposes (Jager et al., 2017). An option to run the instrument in research mode enables sequencing of other compatible libraries such as the Nextera libraries commonly used for mtDNA sequencing (Davis et al., 2015).

7.2.3.2.1 Library Preparation

The ForenSeq™ DNA Signature Prep Kit uses a targeted sequencing approach. AmpliSeq for Illumina custom DNA panels offer alternative options for laboratories for fast targeted library preparation for all Illumina sequencers (Illumina). The PCR primers usually contain 5′ tags, which are used in the next step to attach adapters and indices (Jager et al., 2017). A similar process is tagmentation, in which enzymes simultaneously fragment and tag the DNA with adapters, an example being the Nextera® XT library method used by McElhoe et al. in 2014 to sequence whole mitochondrial genomes (McElhoe et al., 2014). After end repair and 3′ adenylation (if needed), specific adapters (i5 and i7) and indices are ligated onto each amplicon.

Single indexed libraries contain up to 48 unique 6-base Index 1 (i7) sequences for pooling up to 48 uniquely tagged libraries. Dual indexing includes 24 unique 8-base (i7) Index 1 and 16 unique 8-base (i5) Index 2 sequences, creating up to 384 unique combinations. The ForenSeq™ Signature Prep Kit contains 12 i7 and 8 i5 indices, for up to 96 uniquely indexed libraries. The additional PCR steps required during this process can lead to increased stochastic bias in the results and the requirement for short DNA fragments in some methods can make sequencing repeat sequences more difficult (Schirmer et al., 2015).

Unincorporated components of the library preparation process are removed using purification beads such as Ampure [Agencourt ® AMPure ® Agencourt Bioscience Corporation] or alternative clean-up methods such as ExoSAP-IT (Thermo Fisher Scientific).

7.2.3.2.2 Normalization

In addition to achieving even representation of libraries, normalization assists in achieving optimal cluster density on the flow cell. Bead normalization is recommended for the ForenSeq™ DNA Signature Prep Kit which is optimal for higher input amounts. However, alternative methods can be used, particularly for lower amounts as bead normalization is less effective when the capacity of the beads is not reached (Mehta et al., 2018).

The KAPA Library Quantification Kit (Roche) is a commonly used quantitative PCR (qPCR) method containing primers specific to the sequencing adapters (Guo et al., 2017). Although accurate, a limitation of qPCR methods is that adapter sequences not adequately removed prior to quantitation cause an overestimate of the amount of library present (England and Harbison, 2015). Quantitation can be achieved using the Bioanalyzer (Agilent 2100 Bioanalyzer) also providing a distribution of library fragments and an assessment of any residual free adapter/index sequences. Alternatively, the Qubit is less time consuming but also less accurate than qPCR (McElhoe et al., 2014; Robin et al., 2016).

7.2.3.2.3 Template Preparation

The pooled library is denatured, diluted and loaded onto a paired-end flow cell which is coated with oligonucleotides complementary to the P7 and P5 adapters. Clonal amplification of the library fragments is achieved using bridge amplification. Bridge amplification generates clusters on the flow cells of identical sequences in forward or reverse strand orientation. Polymerases generate a copy of every ssDNA fragment bound to the flow cell. The original strand is washed away leaving the reverse strand. This reverse DNA strand bends and attaches to a complementary oligonucleotide on the flow cell forming a bridge. Polymerase generates a new complementary strand (identical to the original DNA fragment). After denaturation, each individual strand is attached to an adapter sequence on the flow cell. This cycle is repeated across the flow cell for the thousands of DNA fragments resulting in the formation of clusters consisting of the same initial DNA fragment. At the end of clonal amplification, all of the reverse strands attached by the P5 adapter are washed leaving only forward strands attached to the flow cell by the P7 adapter. Figure 2 in both (Buermans et al., 2014) and (Heather et al., 2016) illustrates the generalized process for the generation of clusters for both bridge amplification and emPCR methods (Buermans and den Dunnen 2014; Heather and Chain 2016).

7.2.3.2.4   Sequencing by Synthesis

Sequencing by synthesis occurs in a cyclical process of nucleotide incorporation, imaging, and removal of fluorescence and protective groups. The MiSeq (FGx™) instrument uses four-dye chemistry, where each base is fluorescently labeled with a specific dye. The NextSeq™ and the MiniSeq™ instruments use two-dye sequencing chemistry, and the iSeq™ 100 has one color chemistry in two reaction steps to differentiate between the bases.

The four fluorescently labeled nucleotides are chemically modified by the incorporation of a small reversible addition to the 3' OH group (Guo et al., 2008). These act as terminators by blocking the 3' hydroxyl group on the nucleotide, restricting extension of the strand to one base in any one round (Bentley et al., 2008). Each sequencing cycle includes the incorporation of the complementary modified fluorescently labeled base, imaging of the fluorescence and then removal of the protective modification, thus enabling sequencing by synthesis to occur.

In dual indexed sequencing, the read 1 sequencing primer is annealed and extended by the polymerase (read 1), and the newly synthesized strand is washed away. The strand (with the i5 indexed adapter on it) attaches to a P5 oligo on the flow cell forming a bridge and immediately sequences (and hence identifies) the i5 index 2 sequence only, before the newly synthesized strand is again washed away.

Bridge amplification then generates the second read of the sequence. This occurs via the attachment of the DNA strands by the P7 end bend via the P5 adapter. The P5 oligonucleotide is used as the i5 sequencing primer, and the i5 index is identified by sequencing for eight cycles. The i5 index read product is then removed before P5 strands are regenerated using the P7 strand as a template, generating a P5 clonal cluster. This cluster is then sequenced using the i7 sequencing primer. Therefore, the sequencing of the DNA fragment is carried out in this order: read 1, index I7, index I5, and read 2. The sequencer knows that the P5 and P7 sequencing reactions are located in the same spot on the flow cell and associate read 1 and read 2 for each DNA fragment with the correct indices. For the ForenSeq™ system, read 2 is not complete and only 31 sequencing cycles take place.

Index hopping, first observed by Sinha et al. (2017), occurs when free adapter index fragments hybridize to single stranded library fragments and prime the extension during cluster amplification causing incorrect indices on library fragments (Sinha et al., 2017). Approaches to minimizing index hopping include stringent removal of free adapters during library preparation and using unique dual-index combinations (Costello et al., 2018).

On-instrument software controls the run and reagents, performs image analysis and base calling, and assigns a quality score to each base. A number of different options are available for further analysis of the data including BaseSpace™ or for ForenSeq™ users the Universal Analysis Software (UAS). A sequencing analysis viewer provides run metrics and quality information for each run.

7.2.3.2.5   Assays and Forensic Applications using the MiSeq™/ MiSeq FGx™

The MiSeq (FGx™) has a maximum output of 15 Gb and 25 million reads per run (sequencing kit version 3 only) and a maximum read length of 2 × 300 bp. Up to 96 samples can be run together and for detection, amplicons need to be 65 bp or greater. The following sequencing process applies to the MiSeq (FGx™) sequencer for DNA and RNA sequencing with reference to the MiSeq FGx™ Forensic Genomics Solution.

The ForenSeq™ DNA Signature Prep Kit contains a total of 231 forensic markers, 58 STRs including 27 autosomal STRs and 7 X and 24 Y haplotype markers), 94 identity-informative SNPs, 54 ancestry-informative SNPs, 22 phenotypic-informative SNPs, and 2 SNPs informative for both ancestry and phenotype plus amelogenin (Jager et al., 2017). A MiSeq reagent kit v3 600 cycle kit allows 2 × 300 bp read lengths (allowing forward and reverse sequence of 300 bases) and generates up to 25 million. The MiSeq FGx™ Forensic Genomics Solution has custom reagent kits.

Using Nextera libraries, Davis et al. (2015) sequenced mitochondrial DNA from buccal samples, tissue and bone, obtaining 100% concordance with Sanger-sequenced samples with the added advantage of resolving length heteroplasmy and new information about the homopolymer C tract in hypervariable region I (Davis et al., 2015).

A number of validation studies have been performed on ForenSeq™ DNA Signature Prep Kit for forensic analysis (Hollard et al., 2019; Jager et al., 2017; Kocher et al., 2018). Other forensic applications include sequencing of microbiomes (Jesmok et al., 2016; Lax et al., 2015), methylation studies demonstrating body fluid specificity (Forat et al., 2016), improved resolution in kinship testing (Ma et al., 2016), and mitochondrial DNA sequencing, including (King et al., 2014a), (Holland et al., 2017b), and (Peck et al., 2018).

7.3   THIRD-GENERATION SEQUENCING (SINGLE-MOLECULE SEQUENCING REAL TIME)

The relatively short read lengths achieved using second-generation sequencing technologies provide challenges for alignment and bioinformatics analysis particularly of repetitive sequences (van Dijk et al., 2014a). Some of these challenges are overcome by third-generation sequencing technologies using single-molecule DNA sequencing also allowing sequencing in real time. However, these technologies have not yet been widely adopted in forensic science (Clarke et al., 2009).

The MinION technology (Oxford Nanopore Technologies) and the Single Molecule Real Time (SMRT) platform (Pacific Biosciences) are single-molecule sequencers capable of sequencing long stretches of DNA, thousands of bases long in theory, without prior amplification.

The SMRT platform is a single-molecule sequencer based on sequencing by synthesis (Eid et al., 2009). In this technology, single DNA strands pass through a single DNA polymerase molecule anchored to the bottom of a transparent well, known as a zero-mode waveguide (ZMW) (Rhoads and Au, 2015). There are thousands of ZMWs per SMRT cell. Template DNA is prepared by the ligation of single stranded hairpin adapters onto each strand, forming a closed circular shape. As the template DNA passes through the polymerase, phospho-linked fluorescently labeled dNTPs are incorporated. The fluorescent labels are attached to the phosphate group of the dNTP rather than the base and these are cleaved naturally during the DNA synthesis process. As this happens, laser excitation of the nucleotide occurs, light is emitted and captured by a camera and the fluorophore is cleaved from the strand by the polymerase as extension continues. As there is no pause between the readings of each base, sequencing is detected in real time. The length of the continuous sequence produced is limited by the lifetime of the polymerase and it is possible for the circular DNA molecule to be sequenced many times. Individual reads are identified by bioinformatic recognition of the hair pin adapter sequences.

Fast, real time sequencing, generating long read lengths with an average of 3000 bp and up to 20,000 bp or longer, assists in assembling genomes, difficult to assemble regions such as homopolymer regions or GC rich or GC poor regions (Roberts et al., 2013). Epigenetic modifications can be detected directly without the need for bisulphite conversion as the modification causes a change in the reaction kinetics. Similarly, RNA modifications can be detected by using an RNA transcriptase instead of DNA polymerase (Vilfan et al., 2013).

Compared to other technologies, the individual reads generated using SMRT sequencing have higher error rates, however, these errors are randomly distributed and can be recovered with increasing sequencing depth (Koren et al., 2012; Roberts et al., 2013). The same random error is unlikely to be observed more than once in a sequence. To date, forensic applications of SMRT technology have been limited to microbial forensics (Eschoo et al., 2011).

Nanopore sequencing can be used to detect both nucleotide variation and also modification of bases such as methylation (Mikheyev and Tin 2014; Plesivkova et al., 2019; Schneider and Dekker 2012; Wang et al., 2014). Nanopores are typically constructed of proteins. Examples of their development and use can be found in (Laszlo et al., 2013) and (Schreiber et al., 2013). Nanopore sequencing has been further developed commercially as the MinION™ and its siblings, the GridION™ (5 flow cells) and the PromethION™ (48 flow cells) with flow cells that can be used either concurrently or individually (Leggett and Clark, 2017). The MinION™ is a small USB-powered device that does not require enzyme for the sequencing process and does not utilize a secondary signal such as light or pH.

Sequencing occurs on a disposable flow cell, which can be reused a limited number of times (Oxford Nanopore Technologies). The nanopores are ion channels in a solid semiconductor membrane substrate which is placed over a detection grid. DNA is prepared for sequencing by the addition of an adapter which interacts with a docking protein at each nanopore and guides each DNA strand through the pore electrophoretically while regulating the speed of translocation (Stoddart et al., 2009). In the R9 flowcell, a CsgG nanopore, based on the Curlin sigma S-dependent growth gene (Magi et al., 2017), is used. Each nucleotide (or modified nucleotide) disrupts the flow of ions through the pore in a characteristic way when the DNA molecule passes through the pore. Changes in the flow of ions are measured across a stretch of five bases at a time; the measurement is repeated as each DNA template passes through each pore. The measure of the electrical change of the five bases being sequenced can be observed as a "squiggle plot," with different base combinations producing a different pattern.

Novel bioinformatic solutions and new sequencing chemistry have been developed to overcome and reduce the sequence error that can occur including those caused by homopolymers (Goodwin et al., 2015; Jain et al., 2018; Koren et al., 2017; Laver et al., 2015; Zaaijer et al., 2017). Similar error correcting tools are needed for data generated by other single molecule sequencers such as those of Pacific Biosciences (Lee et al., 2014).

For a comprehensive review of the ONT technology and in particular bioinformatic tools used to access and analyze the data, see (Magi et al., 2017). Essentially, raw signal is transformed into basecalls using recurrent neural networks and presented as .FAST5 files (SimpsonLab) by the MinKnow software. These FAST5 files can be converted to FASTQ/A files bioinformatically for further processing. Much of the effort in data analysis is aimed at developing tools to overcome the sequencing errors, generally caused by the variable translocation time of the nucleotides through the pores.

In 2017, the sequencing and assembly of a complete human genome using this technology was reported for the first time (Jain et al., 2018) including the direct detection of modified bases. Nanopore sequencing technology is being evaluated for forensic applications (Cornelis et al., 2018; Cornelis et al., 2017; Cornelis et al., 2019). The direct detection of methylation, without bisulphite conversion, has implications for forensic science, where methylation status of specific sites has been shown to be a useful predictor of age and body fluid source as examples (Simpson et al., 2017). Zaaijer et al. (2017) demonstrated the utility of the technology by "reidentifying" DNA, identifying a person within 30 min. Subsequent studies included real time familial searching and the authentication of cell lines (Zaaijer et al., 2017). The long reads generated by the MinION™ were successfully used to phase variants in mixtures of mtDNA from two individuals not previously possible using other sequencing technologies (Lindberg et al., 2016). The MinION™ has also been used to successfully genotype the SNPforID consortium 52 SNP multiplex (Sanchez et al., 2006b) and the 9947A reference standard using an amplicon ligation protocol to produce DNA fragments of sufficient length for sequencing (Cornelis et al., 2017). Difficulties sequencing rs1031825 and rs1493232 loci were reported due to homopolymer stretches in the SNP flanking region also reported using other sequencing platforms (Borsting et al., 2014; Daniel et al., 2014). Similar methods have been used to successfully profile microbial communities in environmental samples such as soil and waste water (Kerkhof et al., 2017).

The ability to sequence long reads offers distinct advantages for sequencing highly repetitive sequences such as the STRs and, at a more fundamental level, enables accurate sequencing of previously difficult DNA molecules such as the Y chromosome (Oxford Nanopore Technologies). RNA can also be sequenced directly without a cDNA conversion (Keller et al., 2018). Currently, the amount and quality of DNA template required are not compatible with many current forensic applications, including metagenomics (Driscoll et al., 2017), unless whole genome amplification is applied.

7.4 DATA ANALYSIS – BIOINFORMATICS

Bioinformatics is now most closely associated with sequencing technologies but includes the analysis of all biological data, how it is collected, stored, and classified or named (Leclair et al., 2007). The large amount of sequence data generated by NGS requires processing to determine the genotype of the sample, whether for STRs, SNPs, or for less commonly used markers such as indels, epigenetic methylation markers, and Alu repetitive elements. Similar data analysis steps are also required for metagenomic analyses, single molecule sequencing and other nonhuman sequencing applications.

The bioinformatic tools required to process sequencing data generated from NGS (hereafter called tools) have largely been adopted from other areas of genomics and developed further specifically for forensic analysis. Examples are tools incorporated into software provided by the manufacturers of sequencing instruments such as the ForenSeq UAS (Verogen) and the Torrent Suite included with the Ion PGM™ and Ion GeneStudio™ S5 instruments (Thermo Fisher Scientific). For a review of bioinformatic tools relevant to forensic analysis, see (Liu and Harbison, 2018).

The following is a summary of general principles and commonly used approaches and tools.

7.4.1 RAW SEQUENCE DATA

The raw sequence output is a set of individual sequence reads each containing one or more of these sequences; adapter(s) (oligonucleotides or proteins), barcodes (indices), and/or PCR primers. The adapter and barcode sequences are removed leaving the target sequences sorted, regrouped and saved in a FASTQ file format (Cock et al., 2010). This is performed on instruments such as the Ion Torrent S5 and the Illumina MiSeq FGx™ as part of in built data processing. A FASTQ file is a text file containing the DNA sequence and a quality score for each base. [Note: a FASTA file is simply the DNA sequence with a header, i.e., a FASTQ file with the quality information removed]. FASTQ files can be recognized by the suffixes .fq or .fastq and when compressed .gz or .gzip.

Each FASTQ file for each individual sequence occupies four consecutive lines of data:

- Line 1. The sequence identifier—the name or ID of the read, preceded by a "@." For read pairs, there will be two entries with the sequence identifier, either in the same or in a second FASTQ file. PE reads may be stored in one FASTQ file (alternating) or in two different FASTQ files and have sequence identifiers ended by "/1" and "/2," respectively.
- Line 2. The sequence of the read.
- Line 3. Comments. A "+" sign.
- Line 4. Quality scores for each base of the sequence generated by the sequencer and encoded as ASCII (33+score) characters.

7.4.2 REMOVAL OF LOW-QUALITY SEQUENCE DATA

An assessment of the quality of each sequence follows with low-quality sequence either trimmed or filtered out. This is important to reduce errors in downstream processes such as genome assembly, SNP calling, or gene expression estimation. The determination of a base in a DNA sequence relies on the quality of the sequence being expressed as the probability of an incorrect base call, that is, Q scores. If errors are randomly distributed and the sequence coverage is sufficient then lower Q scores can be accommodated. Commonly used tools to assess the quality of DNA sequences include FastQC (Babraham Bioinformatics Group) and SolexaQA (Cox et al., 2010).

There are two options for removing low-quality sequence. Read/quality filtering is used to remove entire reads of overall low quality, whereas read/

quality trimming removes stretches of low-quality sequence tracts from a read and is often used to remove the low-quality sequence typically found towards the end of a read. For example, in the Torrent Suite Software, this is achieved using a sliding window of 30 bases and a quality value of 15 (Ion Torrent). Of the available tools, the FASTX-toolkit contains both a quality filter and a quality trimmer (FASTX-toolkit). Illumina sequencing platforms do not perform either a trimming or a filtering step.

7.4.3 ALIGNMENT

Unless performing *de novo* sequencing, the next analysis step is alignment of each individual read to a previously sequenced reference genome or set of DNA sequences, for example, a reference set of STR repeat sequences and flanking regions. The mapping algorithm locates the corresponding location on the reference sequence that matches each sequence read by comparing each sequence with the reference. For short reads, there may be several equally likely places in the reference sequence which may match and this is notably true for repetitive regions. A level of mismatch maybe required in order to allow for the detection of genuine sequence variation such as SNPs and for small structural variations such as indels in the sequence. By selecting appropriate quality filters, low levels of sequencing errors may be tolerated which can subsequently be separated from the true sequence variation. This process is repeated for the millions of reads in the data.

The choice of tool used depends on the most likely type of sequence error to be observed in the data and this is platform dependent. For example, when processing data from sequencers that produce mainly substitution errors such as the MiSeq FGX, Bowtie 2 (Langmead and Salzberg 2012) and Burrows-Wheeler Aligner - maximal exact matches (MEM) are most commonly selected whereas platforms that generate mainly indel errors, such as the S5, are better suited to tools such as TMAP (Caboche et al., 2014). The reference sequence, short sequence reads, or both, are often preprocessed into an indexed form for more rapid searching.

Once alignment has occurred the sequences are presented as sequence alignment map (SAM) or binary alignment map (BAM) files. SAM and BAM file formats are used to encode short read alignment, are interchangeable, and are the *de facto* standard format for short read alignments. All current alignment software can generate SAM/BAM as an alignment output. A BAM file contains the DNA sequence, the quality information, reference sequence, and alignment information in a binary format, while a SAM file is the plain text format of the BAM file. Once in BAM format, the file can be indexed, providing quick access to any region of the reference sequence. Using tools such as SAM tools, BAM files can be analyzed (e.g., for quality control), modified (e.g., for the removal of PCR duplicates, local realignment, and base quality recomputation), or used to call variation, either small (SNPs, short indels) or large (inversions, tandem duplications, deletions, and translocations) (Li et al., 2009). The BAM format without alignment position data is increasingly used as a space-saving alternative to FASTQ files for containing the short raw read data (Le Tourneau and Kamal, 2015).

Visualization of the sequence data can be carried out using many different tools, with the most common one being Integrative Genomics Viewer (IGV). Other options include Geneious (Geneious) and NextGENe (NextGENe).

7.4.3.1   ALIGNMENT TYPES

There are different forms of alignment. In whole genome sequencing, the entire DNA sequence from an organism is mapped to the appropriate reference sequence. In exome sequencing, the exonic DNA is selected prior to sequencing using array- or solution-based target enrichment techniques such as the Sequence capture human exome 2.1M array (Choi et al., 2009). Sequencing of the transcriptome (RNA-Seq) identifies which genes are transcribed in a sample and assists in fine tuning gene annotation, for example, exon boundaries. The sequence data can be mapped to a full reference sequence or to a custom transcriptome reference.

7.4.4   VARIANT CALLING

After alignment, the next step is typically variant calling for which tools such as BCFtools, GATK, and Freebayes are used. Variant calling is the process where differences between the target sequence of interest and a reference sequence are identified. The file input for variant calling is either a SAM or BAM alignment file, and the output is a .vcf file (Danecek et al., 2011). The .vcf file is then used for any further analyses that may be required.

There are two main variations on methods to perform variant calling. The first is to examine the alignment file to determine the genotype of each position of interest in the sequence. This has been used for SNPs, including mtDNA, and STRs. A number of tools have been developed for assigning STRs based on this method which are detailed in Liu and Harbison (2017).

Of the more recent developments, HipSTR has been designed for Illumina sequence data (Willems et al., 2017). HipSTR "learns" the stutter characteristics of each STR and uses this information to realign STR-containing reads and mitigate the effects of PCR stutter. An alternative, TSSV, uses semiglobal pairwise alignment and alignment scores to identify the STR flanking regions with the highest alignment score before extracting the STR allele (Anvar et al., 2014). Alignment by flanking sequence does not always locate the correct STR flank region, and it is not possible to identify sequence where the flanks are missing.

An alternative sequence-search approach has been implemented in STRait Razor (Woerner et al., 2017) and MyFLq (Van Neste et al., 2014) primarily for STR analysis. Both tools retrieve data from FASTQ files and use the flanking sequences of the STR or SNP to locate the target sequence. This solves a drawback of alignment methods; the mapping of reads to multiple or incorrect locations due to sequence similarity between repeat motifs of different STRs exacerbated by repeat complexity. Instead, string matching algorithms scan each sequence file and extract those reads that match and count them, with the possibility of including a mismatch tolerance. The most recent version of STRait Razor (V3.0) contains a method of accomplishing approximate matching, improvements from previous versions including configuration files for commercially available MPS multiplexes including SNPs and a database for the conversion of STR sequences to recommended nomenclature (Woerner et al., 2017). After trimming the flanking sequences and filtering out any reads that do not include the repeat motif, the alleles are named and defined by their length (Gettings et al., 2016; Wendt et al., 2017). The MyFlq tool uses a database of known alleles to calculate a consensus left and right flanking sequence for each STR locus, which is used to assign reads to an STR locus before removal. Each sequence is compared to a database of reference alleles for calling of the genotype. MyFlq is available as a stand alone web-based application and on Illumina BaseSpace® (Van Neste et al., 2015).

Other examples of sequence-search tools each with unique properties include STRinNGS, which identifies STRs by flanking sequence and analyzes the variation in flanking regions by aligning to a reference human genome (Friis et al., 2016). SEQ Mapper utilizes a multiple search strategy including primer sequence, flanking sequence, and repeat sequence (Lee et al., 2017). FDStools, based on TSSV, includes a model to identify likely PCR stutter products in the data, unlike other models where this interpretation step is done by the scientist using an additional interpretation method (Hoogenboom et al., 2017). A primary limitation of sequence-search methods is the reliance on setting thresholds for the matching algorithms. If set too low, sequence errors such as substitutions may lead to false inclusions. If set too high, flanking regions with genuine sequence variation may be omitted from the analysis.

7.4.5   *mtDNA SEQUENCING DATA*

Bioinformatic tools for the analysis of mtDNA align raw sequence reads to the rCRS using short read aligners. Base positions differing from the rCRS are extracted from the alignment as variants, into a .VCF file. This vcf file is translated into standardized forensic haplotype nomenclature using downstream analysis tools such as MitoSAVE (King et al., 2014b). Solutions combining various analysis tools are available such as MToolBox that combines tools for aligning reads to the reference sequence, an indel realigner, a variant caller, and a classifier for haplogroup assignment (Calabrese et al., 2014). Commercially available analysis software, including NextGENe and CLC Genomics Workbench and GeneMarker HTS, also contain all the tools necessary for quality filtering, alignment, and variant calling (Holland et al., 2017a; Peck et al., 2016; Zhou et al., 2016).

7.5   FORENSIC CONSIDERATIONS

7.5.1   *ANALYSIS AND REPORTING*

The application of NGS to forensic analysis requires the development of methods and protocols as well as analysis criteria such as analytical thresholds and method detection limits (Young et al., 2017). Stringent quality control measures must be applied to ensure stochastic effects and sequencing errors are minimized and identified. There are several sources of sequencing errors. Errors generated during PCR amplifications may appear in multiple reads if the errors originated in the initial amplifications. These errors may appear as mismatches in an alignment or as genetic variation in the sample. As sequencing errors are often random, they can be filtered out as singleton reads during variant calling. Mapping errors can occur when the mapping algorithm maps a read to the wrong location in the reference. This commonly occurs in repeat or low-complexity regions and may be present in STR data. Comparison of pipelines based on different approaches or algorithms can strengthen the validity of the sequencing data if comparable results are obtained. A limited number of studies have performed data analysis using more than one pipeline to assess concordance and reliability. Accessible, appropriately validated online or on-instrument resources and tools are an important consideration for laboratories (Gettings et al., 2016; Kim et al., 2016).

A critical aspect in the sequencing of STRs is consistency in nomenclature arising from the sequence variation within STR repeats and flanking region polymorphisms (Gettings et al., 2015). This is essential for establishing compatibility between laboratories for DNA databasing, proficiency testing, comparisons of DNA sequence profiles, and for back compatibility with existing DNA databases (van der Gaag and de Knijff, 2015). Both the International Society for Forensic Genetics and the STR Sequencing Project have raised the challenges and developed recommendations to facilitate the standardization of STR sequence nomenclature including the inclusion of complete sequence strings and flanking region variation in stored data (Gettings et al., 2017; Parson et al., 2016). SNP reporting is not complicated by nomenclature issues. However, strandedness may lead to interpretation issues, where one allele is reported for each chromosome and passed to an analysis tool. Using Snipper, the input of the SNP on the wrong strand appears as a base miscall and can compromise analysis (Santos et al., 2016). It is notable that the Ion Torrent reports all SNPs in the forward strand, while the MiSeq FGx reports SNPs consistent with dbSNP.

7.5.2 DATA STORAGE

Current DNA sequencing technologies generate vast amounts of data that must be stored and accessed when required. In contrast to less than a hundred megabytes generated from one CE STR profiling run, data generated using NGS can range from hundreds of gigabytes to terabytes of data per run, depending on the platform, application, and the number of samples and markers analyzed (Richter and Sexton, 2009). Historically, to maintain data security, most forensic laboratories are limited to on-premise storage (local servers or external hard drives). However, storage of the local hard drives must be considered as they may be subject to data loss through physical damage or destruction or through the acquisition of viruses when transferred between computers.

The forensic community has not yet reached consensus regarding the NGS files type that require retention and the length of time that files should be stored. This will be influenced by national legislation. Therefore, routine use of NGS in forensic casework may require storage of large raw data files

(FASTQ and BAM files) in addition to processed data, which will rapidly impact on the local storage capabilities. Cloud computing is an alternative to on-premise storage for NGS data. Cost savings over on-premise storage is one of the key benefits that law enforcement agencies and forensic organizations seek when they migrate data to the cloud. However, in addition to data storage, cloud-based computing can be used for bioinformatic analysis of NGS data (Bailey et al., 2017).

Storage of forensic data on the cloud requires several considerations relating to data ownership, privacy protections, data mobility, quality of service and service levels, bandwidth costs, data protection, and technical support. Understanding the encryption level and security strategy provided by cloud service provider is important. These aspects must be assessed with the security standards and the objectives of the organization and national legislation concerning genetic data.

Considerations for forensic data include the cloud deployment model, that is, public, community, hybrid, or secure private cloud. This will be influenced by whether the data is to be shared with external organizations. Sensitivity of the data and classifications (classified, sensitive, private, or data that is publicly available) and data stored in, processed in or transiting foreign countries may be subject to the legislation of the local government and data encryption technologies and information access management (Cyber Security Operations Centre 2012).

7.5.3   ETHICS – GENOME PRIVACY

The application of NGS to forensic analysis has resulted in an increase in the number of forensic loci that can be analyzed simultaneously. In addition, it enables the entire nucleotide composition of the sequenced fragment to be analyzed. This has resulted in improved mixture resolution and increased capabilities in a number of applications such as DNA Intelligence (inferring BGA and EVCs including age using methylation markers), body fluid identification, and whole mitochondrial DNA sequencing.

Although the majority of the current forensic NGS applications involve a targeted sequencing approach using specific markers, the sequence data flanking the marker of interest can be viewed. Analysis of these flanking regions may reveal genomic information about the donor previously unknown to the analyst. SNPs in the flanking regions of forensic STRs may be utilized to increase the discrimination of donors within a mixed source sample. However, issues may arise if the SNP has clinical significance.

Gettings et al. (2015) located such a SNP (rs146387238) in the intron/exon junction in the FGA gene resulting in a splice site mutation associated with a rare blood coagulation defect. As this SNP is greater than 200 bp downstream of the repeat region, the SNP may be avoided through primer design (Gettings et al., 2015).

In addition, a notable difference between CE STR profiling and these NGS applications is the region of the genome where the forensic loci of interest are located, that is, noncoding versus coding, or regulatory, regions. For example, some of these forensically relevant markers used in DNA Intelligence to predict biogeographical ancestry and externally visible characteristics are found in coding regions of the genome (Phillips et al., 2014; Walsh et al., 2014) and are located in genes known to be associated with disease (Rundshagen et al., 2004). DNA methylation is also associated with disease (Baranova et al., 2018).

The forensic community is not unfamiliar with this issue. The acceptance of current STR loci was based on the assumption that the loci were located in non-coding regions of the genome and, therefore, did not reveal medical information about the donor. This assisted in gaining public support for this methodology (Williams and Wienroth 2017). However, STRs have since been shown to contribute to the genetic architecture of quantitative human traits (Gymrek et al., 2016). Forensically relevant STRs have been shown to have specific disease associations (Courts and Madea 2011; Meraz-Rios et al., 2014).

Therefore, the expansion of the depth of the genomic information gained from NGS has major implications for genome privacy and ethical considerations which must be assessed and addressed by the forensic community. Obtaining permission to undertake expanded genome analysis, obligations to report nonforensically relevant genome data, and the retention of this information in databases are likely to be addressed through the development of legislative and/or policy frameworks (Wienroth et al., 2014; Williams and Wienroth, 2017).

7.6 CONCLUDING REMARKS

The application of DNA sequencing technologies provides tremendous scope for forensic analysis. In addition to the advantages of multiplexing markers and samples, utilization of STR sequence variation and SNP variation in the flanking region of STRs increases discrimination potential and enhances the resolution of mixtures and kinship analysis. The analysis of multiple markers, marker types and samples enables a cost-effective high-throughput approach while avoiding the depletion of valuable evidential material often occurring from multiplex analyses. Additional benefits include the potential for the simultaneous analysis of STRs with mRNAs for tissue identification (Zubakov et al., 2015). NGS offers the realistic option of sequencing the whole mtDNA genome (King et al., 2014a) or targeted subsets of the whole genome from forensic samples such as hair shafts (Parson et al., 2015), revealing useful polymorphisms outside the control region providing additional discrimination (Coble et al., 2004). An increased ability to detect low-level heteroplasmy can also be achieved (Holland et al., 2017b; Just et al., 2015). Higher resolution of related males can be achieved in Y-chromosome analysis (Qian et al., 2017). Analysis of forensically relevant SNPs analysis using NGS for biogeographic ancestry and phenotype analysis enables hundreds of SNPs to be analyzed simultaneously resulting in expanded capabilities for DNA Intelligence (Al-Asfi et al., 2018; Budowle and van Daal, 2008; Jager et al., 2017). In addition, novel markers such as microhaplotype markers can be applied to complex mixtures, ancestry, and identity analysis (Oldoni et al., 2019). Additional forensic applications include sequencing of microbial (Schmedes et al., 2016) and soil bacterial communities (Jesmok et al., 2016) and analysis of methylation markers for body fluid and tissue identification (Forat et al., 2016).

To date, RNA-Seq has been used mainly to identity transcripts/markers of interest for further assay development using quantitative or end point PCR. For example, sequencing of the whole transcriptome in this way was used by Lin et al. (2015) to investigate the impact of degradation of RNA as might be anticipated in forensic like samples on RNA-Seq (Lin et al., 2015). In other examples, stable regions of the transcriptome were identified and used to develop new mRNA markers for body fluid identification and targeted RNA sequencing combined with an STR AmpliSeq panel was used to identify body fluids and STRs from the same sample (Albani and Fleming 2018; Lin et al., 2016; Zubakov et al., 2015). In addition to mRNA body fluid markers, microRNAs have also been identified using NGS techniques (Wang et al., 2016).

A number of aspects of NGS must be considered for successful technology transfer and implementation into forensic casework. These include marker, assay and platform selection, uniform nomenclature, databases, secure storage of data, development of quality management systems, privacy, legislative and ethical issues, and admissibility of NGS-derived evidence in court. Although the adoption of NGS is accompanied by a number of challenges, its application promises to revolutionize forensic analysis.

KEYWORDS

- Sanger sequencing
- next-generation sequencing
- third-generation sequencing
- forensic DNA analysis

REFERENCES

Al-Asfi, M., et al., Assessment of the Precision ID Ancestry panel. *Int J Legal Med* **2018** 132 (6), 1581–1594.

Albani, P. P. and R. Fleming. Novel messenger RNAs for body fluid identification. *Sci Justice* **2018** 58 (2), 145–152.

Aliferi, A., et al.. DNA methylation-based age prediction using massively parallel sequencing data and multiple machine learning models. *Forensic Sci Int Genet* **2018** 37, 215–226.

Ambers, A. D., et al.. More comprehensive forensic genetic marker analyses for accurate human remains identification using massively parallel DNA sequencing. *BMC Genomics* **2016** 17 (Suppl 9), 750.

Anderson, M. W. and I. Schrijver. Next generation DNA sequencing and the future of genomic medicine. *Genes (Basel)* **2010** 1 (1), 38–69.

Anderson, S. Shotgun DNA sequencing using cloned DNase I-generated fragments. *Nucleic Acids Res* **1981** 9 (13), 3015–3027.

Anderson, S., et al. Sequence and organization of the human mitochondrial genome. *Nature* **1981** 290 (5806), 457–465.

Andreasson, H., et al. Quantification of mtDNA mixtures in forensic evidence material using pyrosequencing. *Int J Legal Med* **2006** 120 (6), 383–390.

Anvar, S. Y., et al. TSSV: A tool for characterization of complex allelic variants in pure and mixed genomes. *Bioinformatics* **2014** 30 (12), 1651–1659.

Ari, S and M Arikan. Next Generation Sequencing: Advantages, Disadvantages and Future. In K. Hakeem, H. Tombuloglu & G. Tombuloglu (Eds.) *Plant Omics: Trends and Applications*. Springer International Publishing: New York, NY, USA, **2016** 109–135.

Avent, I., et al. The QIAGEN 140-locus single-nucleotide polymorphism (SNP) panel for forensic identification using massively parallel sequencing (MPS): An evaluation and a direct-to-PCR trial. *Int J Legal Med* **2018** 133 (3), 677–688.

Babraham Bioinformatics Group. https://www.bioinformatics.babraham.ac.uk/ (accessed Mar 16, 2019).

Bailey, S. F., et al. Secure and robust cloud computing for high-throughput forensic microsatellite sequence analysis and databasing. *Forensic Sci Int Genet* **2017** 31, 40–47.

Baranova, I., et al. Aberrant methylation of PCDH17 gene in high-grade serous ovarian carcinoma. *Cancer Biomark* **2018** 23 (1), 125–133.

Barba, M., et al. Historical perspective, development and applications of next-generation sequencing in plant virology. *Viruses* **2014** 6 (1), 106–136.

Behjati, S. and P. S. Tarpey. What is next generation sequencing? *Arch Dis Child Educ Pract Ed* **2013** 98, 236–238.

Bennett, L., et al. Mixture deconvolution by massively parallel sequencing of microhaplotypes. *Int J Legal Med* **2019** 133 (3), 719–729

Bennett, S. Solexa Ltd. *Pharmacogenomics* **2004** 5 (4), 433–438.

Bentley, D. R., et al. Accurate whole human genome sequencing using reversible terminator chemistry. *Nature* **2008** 456 (7218), 53–59.

Borsting, C., et al. Evaluation of the Ion Torrent HID SNP 169-plex: A SNP typing assay developed for human identification by second generation sequencing. *Forensic Sci Int Genet* **2014** 12, 144–154.

Bragg, L. M., et al. Shining a light on dark sequencing: Characterising errors in Ion Torrent PGM data. *PLoS Comput Biol* **2013** 9 (4), e1003031.

Braslavsky, I., et al. Sequence information can be obtained from single DNA molecules. *Proc Natl Acad Sci USA* **2003** 100 (7), 3960–3964.

Budowle, B. and A. van Daal. Forensically relevant SNP classes. *Biotechniques* **2008** 44 (5), 603–608, 610.

Buermans, H.P.J. and den Dunnen J.T. Next generation sequencing technology: Advances and applications. *Biochimica et Biophys Acta* **2014** 1842, 1932–1941

Butler, John M. *Advanced Topics in Forensic DNA Typing: Methodology*. Elsevier Science Publishing Co Inc.: Amsterdam, The Netherlands **2011**.

Caboche, S., et al. Comparison of mapping algorithms used in high-throughput sequencing: Application to Ion Torrent data. *BMC Genomics* **2014** 15, 264.

Calabrese, C., et al. MToolBox: A highly automated pipeline for heteroplasmy annotation and prioritization analysis of human mitochondrial variants in high-throughput sequencing. *Bioinformatics* **2014** 30 (21), 3115–3117.

Canard, B. and R. S. Sarfati. DNA polymerase fluorescent substrates with reversible 3'-tags. *Gene* **1994** 148 (1), 1–6.

Carracedo, A., et al. DNA commission of the International Society for Forensic Genetics: Guidelines for mitochondrial DNA typing. *Forensic Sci Int* **2000** 110 (2), 79–85.

Choi, M., et al. Genetic diagnosis by whole exome capture and massively parallel DNA sequencing. *Proc Natl Acad Sci USA* **2009** 106 (45), 19096–19101.

Churchill, J. D., et al. Blind study evaluation illustrates utility of the Ion PGM system for use in human identity DNA typing. *Croat Med J* **2015** 56 (3), 218–229.

Clarke, J., et al. Continuous base identification for single-molecule nanopore DNA sequencing. *Nat Nanotechnol* **2009** 4 (4), 265–270.

Coble, M. D., et al. Single nucleotide polymorphisms over the entire mtDNA genome that increase the power of forensic testing in Caucasians. *Int J Legal Med* **2004** 118 (3), 137–146.

Cock, P. J., et al. The Sanger FASTQ file format for sequences with quality scores, and the Solexa/Illumina FASTQ variants. *Nucleic Acids Res* **2010** 38 (6). 1767–1771.

Coghlan, M. L., et al. Deep sequencing of plant and animal DNA contained within traditional Chinese medicines reveals legality issues and health safety concerns. *PLoS Genet* **2012** 8 (4), e1002657.

Consortium, Int. Hum. Genome Seq. Finishing the euchromatic sequence of the human genome. *Nature* **2004** 431 (7011), 931–945.

Cornelis, S., et al. Forensic SNP Genotyping using Nanopore MinION Sequencing. *Sci Rep* **2017** 7, 41759.

Cornelis, S., et al. Multiplex STR amplification sensitivity in a silicon microchip. *Sci Rep* **2018** 8 (1), 9853.

Cornelis, S., et al. Forensic tri-allelic SNP genotyping using nanopore sequencing. *Forensic Sci Int Genet* **2019** 38, 204–210.

Costello, M., et al. Characterization and remediation of sample index swaps by non-redundant dual indexing on massively parallel sequencing platforms. *BMC Genomics* **2018** 19 (1), 332.

Courts, C. and B. Madea. Significant association of TH01 allele 9.3 and SIDS. *J Forensic Sci* **2011** 56 (2), 415–417.

Cox, M. P., et al. SolexaQA: At-a-glance quality assessment of Illumina second-generation sequencing data. *BMC Bioinform* **2010** 11, 485.

Cummings, C. A., et al. Accurate, rapid and high-throughput detection of strain-specific polymorphisms in Bacillus anthracis and Yersinia pestis by next-generation sequencing. *Investig Genet* **2010** 1 (1), 5.

Cyber Security Operations Centre, A. S. D. (2012) Cloud computing SEcurity Considerations. https://www.acsc.gov.au/publications/protect/cloud_computing_security_considerations. htm (accessed Mar 23, 2019).

Danecek, P., et al. The variant call format and VCFtools. *Bioinformatics* **2011** 27 (15), 2156–2158.

Daniel, R., et al. A SNaPshot of next generation sequencing for forensic SNP analysis. *Forensic Sci Int Genet* **2014** 14C, 50–60.

Davis, C., et al. Sequencing the hypervariable regions of human mitochondrial DNA using massively parallel sequencing: Enhanced data acquisition for DNA samples encountered in forensic testing. *Leg Med (Tokyo)* **2015** 17 (2), 123–127.

de la Puente, M., et al. Evaluation of the Qiagen 140-SNP forensic identification multiplex for massively parallel sequencing. *Forensic Sci Int Genet* **2017** 28, 35–43.

Dorum, G., et al. Predicting the origin of stains from next generation sequencing mRNA data. *Forensic Sci Int Genet* **2018** 34, 37–48.

Dressman, D., et al. Transforming single DNA molecules into fluorescent magnetic particles for detection and enumeration of genetic variations. *Proc Natl Acad Sci USA* **2003** 100 (15), 8817–8822.

Driscoll, C. B., et al. Towards long-read metagenomics: Complete assembly of three novel genomes from bacteria dependent on a diazotrophic cyanobacterium in a freshwater lake co-culture. *Stand Genomic Sci* **2017** 12, 9.

Eduardoff, M., et al. Inter-laboratory evaluation of the EUROFORGEN Global ancestry-informative SNP panel by massively parallel sequencing using the Ion PGM. *Forensic Sci Int Genet* **2016** 23, 178–189.

Eid, J., et al. Real-time DNA sequencing from single polymerase molecules. *Science* **2009** 323 (5910), 133–138.

England, Ryan and S Harbison. Massively parallel sequencing for the forensic scientist---Sequencing archived amplified products of AmpFlSTR Identifiler and PowerPlex Y multiplex kits to capture additional information. *Aust J Forensic Sci* **2015** 49 (3), 308–325.

Ensenberger, M. G., et al. Developmental validation of the PowerPlex((R)) 21 System. *Forensic Sci Int Genet* **2014** 9, 169–178.

Eschoo, MW, et al. Microbial Forensic Analysis of Trace and Unculturable Specimens. *Microbial Forensics*. Academic Press, **2011** 155–171.

Ewing, B. and P. Green. Base-calling of automated sequencer traces using phred. II. Error probabilities. *Genome Res* **1998** 8 (3), 186–194.

Ewing, B., et al. Base-calling of automated sequencer traces using phred. I. Accuracy assessment. *Genome Res* **1998** 8 (3), 175–185.

FASTX-toolkit. http://hannonlab.cshl.edu/fastx_toolkit (accessed Mar 19, 2019).

Fierer, N., et al. Forensic identification using skin bacterial communities. *Proc Natl Acad Sci USA* **2010** 107 (14), 6477–6481.

Forat, S., et al. Methylation Markers for the Identification of Body Fluids and Tissues from Forensic Trace Evidence. *PLoS One* **2016** 11 (2), e0147973.

Fordyce, S. L., et al. High-throughput sequencing of core STR loci for forensic genetic investigations using the Roche Genome Sequencer FLX platform. *Biotechniques* **2011** 51 (2), 127–133.

Frazier, R. R., et al. Validation of the Applied Biosystems Prism 377 automated sequencer for the forensic short tandem repeat analysis. *Electrophoresis* **1996** 17 (10), 1550–1552.

Friis, S. L., et al. Introduction of the Python script STRinNGS for analysis of STR regions in FASTQ or BAM files and expansion of the Danish STR sequence database to 11 STRs. *Forensic Sci Int Genet* **2016** 21, 68–75.

Garcia, O., et al. Frequencies of the precision ID ancestry panel markers in Basques using the Ion Torrent PGM™ platform. *Forensic Sci Int Genet* **2017** 31, e1-e4.

Garrido-Cardenas, J. A., et al. DNA Sequencing Sensors: An Overview. *Sensors (Basel)* **2017** 17 (3).

Gelardi, C., et al. Second generation sequencing of three STRs D3S1358, D12S391 and D21S11 in Danes and a new nomenclature for sequenced STR alleles. *Forensic Sci Int Genet* **2014** 12, 38–41.

Geneious. https://www.geneious.com/ (accessed Mar 19, 2019).

Gettings, K. B., et al. Sequence variation of 22 autosomal STR loci detected by next generation sequencing. *Forensic Sci Int Genet* **2016** 21, 15–21.

Gettings, K. B., et al. STRSeq: A catalog of sequence diversity at human identification Short Tandem Repeat loci. *Forensic Sci Int Genet* **2017** 31, 111–117.

Gettings, Katherine Butler, et al. STR allele sequence variation: Current knowledge and future issues. *Forensic Sci Int: Genet* **2015** 18, 118–130.

Goodwin, S., et al. Oxford Nanopore sequencing, hybrid error correction, and de novo assembly of a eukaryotic genome. *Genome Res* **2015** 25 (11), 1750–1756.

Guo, F., et al. Next generation sequencing of SNPs using the HID-Ion AmpliSeq Identity Panel on the Ion Torrent PGM platform. *Forensic Sci Int Genet* **2016** 25, 73–84.

Guo, F., et al. Massively parallel sequencing of forensic STRs and SNPs using the Illumina((R)) ForenSeq DNA Signature Prep Kit on the MiSeq FGx Forensic Genomics System. *Forensic Sci Int Genet* **2017** 31, 135–148.

Guo, J., et al. Four-color DNA sequencing with 3'-O-modified nucleotide reversible terminators and chemically cleavable fluorescent dideoxynucleotides. *Proc Natl Acad Sci USA* **2008** 105 (27), 9145–9150.

Gymrek, M., et al. Abundant contribution of short tandem repeats to gene expression variation in humans. *Nat Genet* **2016** 48 (1), 22–29.

Halloran, N., et al. Sequencing reactions for the applied biosystems 373A Automated DNA Sequencer. *Methods Mol Biol* **1993** 23, 297–315.

Harris, T. D., et al. Single-molecule DNA sequencing of a viral genome. *Science* **2008** 320 (5872), 106–109.

Head, S. R., et al. Library construction for next-generation sequencing: Overviews and challenges. *Biotechniques* **2014** 56 (2), 61–64.

Heather, J. M. and B. Chain. The sequence of sequencers: The history of sequencing DNA. *Genomics* **2016** 107 (1), 1–8.

Higuchi, R., et al. DNA typing from single hairs. *Nature* **1988** 332 (6164), 543–546.

Holland, M. M., et al. Second generation sequencing allows for mtDNA mixture deconvolution and high resolution detection of heteroplasmy. *Croat Med J* **2011** 52 (3), 299–313.

Holland, M. M., et al. Evaluation of GeneMarker((R)) HTS for improved alignment of mtDNA MPS data, haplotype determination, and heteroplasmy assessment. *Forensic Sci Int Genet* **2017a** 28, 90–98.

Holland, M. M., et al. MPS analysis of the mtDNA hypervariable regions on the MiSeq with improved enrichment. *Int J Legal Med* **2017b** 131 (4), 919–931.

Hollard, C., et al. Case report: On the use of the HID-Ion AmpliSeq Ancestry Panel in a real forensic case. *Int J Legal Med* **2017** 131 (2), 351–358.

Hollard, C., et al. Automation and developmental validation of the ForenSeq() DNA Signature Preparation kit for high-throughput analysis in forensic laboratories. *Forensic Sci Int Genet* **2019** 40, 37–45.

Holley, R. W., et al. Structure of a ribonucleic acid. *Science* **1965** 147 (3664), 1462–1465.

Hoogenboom, J., et al. FDSTools: A software package for analysis of massively parallel sequencing data with the ability to recognise and correct STR stutter and other PCR or sequencing noise. *Forensic Sci Int Genet* **2017** 27, 27–40.

Hutchison, C. A., 3rd. DNA sequencing: Bench to bedside and beyond. *Nucleic Acids Res* **2007** 35 (18), 6227–6237.

Hyman, E. D. A new method of sequencing DNA. *Anal Biochem* **1988** 174 (2), 423–436.

IGV. Integrative Genomics Viewer. http://software.broadinstitute.org/software/igv/home (accessed Mar 18, 2019).

Illumina. https://www.illumina.com/ (accessed Mar 20, 2019).

Ion Torrent. https://ts-pgm.epigenetic.ru/ion-docs/ (accessed Mar 23, 2019).

Jager, A. C., et al. Developmental validation of the MiSeq FGx Forensic Genomics System for Targeted Next Generation Sequencing in Forensic DNA Casework and Database Laboratories. *Forensic Sci Int Genet* **2017** 28, 52–70.

Jain, M., et al. Nanopore sequencing and assembly of a human genome with ultra-long reads. *Nat Biotechnol* **2018**.

Jesmok, E. M., et al. Next-Generation Sequencing of the Bacterial 16S rRNA Gene for Forensic Soil Comparison: A Feasibility Study. *J Forensic Sci* **2016** 61 (3), 607–617.

Just, Rebecca S., et al. Mitochondrial DNA heteroplasmy in the emerging field of massively parallel sequencing. *Forensic Sci Int: Genet* **2015** 18, 131–139.

Kawashima, et al. Method of nucleic acid amplification. Patent U.S.2005/0100900 A1. Published May 12 2005 **2005**.

Kchouk, M, et al. Generations of Sequencing Technologies: From First to Next Generation. *Biol Med* **2017** 9, 395.

Keller, M. W., et al. Direct RNA Sequencing of the Coding Complete Influenza A Virus Genome. *Sci Rep* **2018** 8 (1), 14408.

Kerkhof, L. J., et al. Profiling bacterial communities by MinION sequencing of ribosomal operons. *Microbiome* **2017** 5 (1), 116.

Kim, E. H., et al. Massively parallel sequencing of 17 commonly used forensic autosomal STRs and amelogenin with small amplicons. *Forensic Sci Int Genet* **2016** 22, 1–7.

King, J. L., et al. High-quality and high-throughput massively parallel sequencing of the human mitochondrial genome using the Illumina MiSeq. *Forensic Sci Int Genet* **2014a** 12, 128–135.

King, J. L., et al. mitoSAVE: Mitochondrial sequence analysis of variants in Excel. *Forensic Sci Int Genet* **2014b** 12, 122–125.

Kocher, S., et al. Inter-laboratory validation study of the ForenSeq DNA Signature Prep Kit. *Forensic Sci Int Genet* **2018** 36, 77–85.

Koren, S., et al. Hybrid error correction and de novo assembly of single-molecule sequencing reads. *Nat Biotechnol* **2012** 30 (7), 693–700.

Koren, S., et al. Canu: scalable and accurate long-read assembly via adaptive k-mer weighting and repeat separation. *Genome Res* **2017** 27 (5), 722–736.

Kornberg, A. *DNA Synthesis*. W. H. Freeman and Company: San Francisco, **1974**.

Lander, E. S., et al. Initial sequencing and analysis of the human genome. *Nature* **2001** 409 (6822), 860–921.

Langmead, B. and S. L. Salzberg. Fast gapped-read alignment with Bowtie 2. *Nat Methods* **2012** 9 (4), 357–359.

Laszlo, A. H., et al. Detection and mapping of 5-methylcytosine and 5-hydroxymethylcytosine with nanopore MspA. *Proc Natl Acad Sci USA* **2013** 110 (47), 18904–18909.

Laver, T., et al. Assessing the performance of the Oxford Nanopore Technologies MinION. *Biomol Detect Quantif* **2015** 3, 1–8.

Lax, S., et al. Forensic analysis of the microbiome of phones and shoes. *Microbiome* **2015** 3, 21.

Le Tourneau, C and M Kamal. *Pan-cancer Integrative Molecular Portrait Towards a New Paradigm in Precision Medicine*. Springer: Cham, Switzerland, **2015**.

Leclair, B., et al. Bioinformatics and human identification in mass fatality incidents: The world trade center disaster. *J Forensic Sci* **2007** 52 (4), 806–819.

Lee, H., et al. Error correction and assembly complexity of single molecule sequencing reads. *bioRxiv* **2014**, 006395.

Lee, J. C., et al. SEQ Mapper: A DNA sequence searching tool for massively parallel sequencing data. *Forensic Sci Int Genet* **2017** 26, 66–69.

Leggett, R. M. and M. D. Clark. A world of opportunities with nanopore sequencing. *J Exp Bot* **2017** 68 (20), 5419–5429.

Levy, S. E. and R. M. Myers. Advancements in Next-Generation Sequencing. *Annu Rev Genomics Hum Genet* **2016** 17, 95–115.

Li, H., et al. The Sequence Alignment/Map format and SAMtools. *Bioinformatics* **2009** 25 (16), 2078–2079.

Li, H., et al. Applying massively parallel sequencing to paternity testing on the Ion Torrent Personal Genome Machine. *Forensic Sci Int Genet* **2017** 31, 155–159.

Lin, M. H., et al. Transcriptomic analysis of degraded forensic body fluids. *Forensic Sci Int Genet* **2015** 17, 35–42.

Lin, M. H., et al. Degraded RNA transcript stable regions (StaRs) as targets for enhanced forensic RNA body fluid identification. *Forensic Sci Int Genet* **2016** 20, 61–70.

Lindberg, M. R., et al. A Comparison and Integration of MiSeq and MinION Platforms for Sequencing Single Source and Mixed Mitochondrial Genomes. *PLoS One* **2016** 11 (12), e0167600.

Liu, L, et al. Comparison of Next-Generation Sequencing Systems. *J Biomed Biotechnol* **2012** 2012, 1–11.

Liu, Y. Y. and S. Harbison. A review of bioinformatic methods for forensic DNA analyses. *Forensic Sci Int Genet* **2018** 33, 117–128.

Ma, Y., et al. Next generation sequencing: Improved resolution for paternal/maternal duos analysis. *Forensic Sci Int Genet* **2016** 24, 83–85.

Magi, A., et al. Nanopore sequencing data analysis: State of the art, applications and challenges. *Brief Bioinform* **2017** 19 (6), 1256--1272.

Mardis, E. R. The impact of next-generation sequencing technology on genetics. *Trends Genet* **2008** 24 (3), 133–141.

Margulies, M., et al. Genome sequencing in microfabricated high-density picolitre reactors. *Nature* **2005** 437 (7057), 376–380.

Maxam, A. M. and W. Gilbert. A new method for sequencing DNA. *Proc Natl Acad Sci USA* **1977** 74 (2), 560–564.

McElhoe, J. A., et al. Development and assessment of an optimized next-generation DNA sequencing approach for the mtgenome using the Illumina MiSeq. *Forensic Sci Int Genet* **2014** 13, 20–29.

Meacham, F., et al. Identification and correction of systematic error in high-throughput sequence data. *BMC Bioinform* **2011** 12, 451.

Mehta, B., et al. Comparison between magnetic bead and qPCR library normalisation methods for forensic MPS genotyping. *Int J Legal Med* **2018** 132 (1), 125–132.

Meiklejohn, K. A. and J. M. Robertson. Evaluation of the Precision ID Identity Panel for the Ion Torrent() PGM() sequencer. *Forensic Sci Int Genet* **2017** 31, 48–56.

Meraz-Rios, M. A., et al. Association of vWA and TPOX polymorphisms with venous thrombosis in Mexican mestizos. *Biomed Res Int* **2014** 2014, 697689.

Merriman, B. and J. M. Rothberg. Progress in ion torrent semiconductor chip based sequencing. *Electrophoresis* **2012** 33 (23), 3397–3417.

Metzker, M. L. Sequencing technologies - the next generation. *Nat Rev Genet* **2010** 11 (1), 31–46.

Mikheyev, A. S. and M. M. Tin. A first look at the Oxford Nanopore MinION sequencer. *Mol Ecol Resour* **2014** 14 (6), 1097–1102.

Moorcraft, S. Y., et al. Understanding next generation sequencing in oncology: A guide for oncologists. *Crit Rev Oncol Hematol* **2015** 96 (3), 463–474.

Moorthie, S., et al. Review of massively parallel DNA sequencing technologies. *Hugo J* **2011** 5 (1–4), 1–12.

Mullis, K. B. and F. A. Faloona. Specific synthesis of DNA in vitro via a polymerase-catalyzed chain reaction. *Methods Enzymol* **1987** 155, 335–350.

Mullis, K., et al. Specific enzymatic amplification of DNA in vitro: the polymerase chain reaction. *Cold Spring Harb Symp Quant Biol* **1986** 51 Pt 1, 263–273.

NextGENe. http://www.softgenetics.com/NextGENe.php (accessed Mar 19, 2019).

Nyren, P. Enzymatic method for continuous monitoring of DNA polymerase activity. *Anal Biochem* **1987** 167 (2), 235–238.

Nyren, P., et al. Solid phase DNA minisequencing by an enzymatic luminometric inorganic pyrophosphate detection assay. *Anal Biochem* **1993** 208 (1), 171–175.

Ogden, R. Unlocking the potential of genomic technologies for wildlife forensics. *Mol Ecol Resour* **2011** 11 Suppl 1, 109–116.

Oldoni, F., et al. Microhaplotypes in forensic genetics. *Forensic Sci Int Genet* **2019** 38, 54–69.

Oxford Nanopore Technologies. https://nanoporetech.com/ (accessed Mar 20, 2019).

Parson, W., et al. DNA Commission of the International Society for Forensic Genetics: Revised and extended guidelines for mitochondrial DNA typing. *Forensic Sci Int Genet* **2014** 13, 134–142.

Parson, W., et al. Massively parallel sequencing of complete mitochondrial genomes from hair shaft samples. *Forensic Sci Int Genet* **2015** 15, 8–15.

Parson, W., et al. Massively parallel sequencing of forensic STRs: Considerations of the DNA commission of the International Society for Forensic Genetics (ISFG) on minimal nomenclature requirements. *Forensic Sci Int Genet* **2016** 22, 54–63.

Peck, M. A., et al. Concordance and reproducibility of a next generation mtGenome sequencing method for high-quality samples using the Illumina MiSeq. *Forensic Sci Int Genet* **2016** 24, 103–111.

Peck, M. A., et al. Developmental validation of a Nextera XT mitogenome Illumina MiSeq sequencing method for high-quality samples. *Forensic Sci Int Genet* **2018** 34, 25–36.

Pereira, V., et al. Evaluation of the Precision ID Ancestry Panel for crime case work: A SNP typing assay developed for typing of 165 ancestral informative markers. *Forensic Sci Int Genet* **2017** 28, 138–145.

Phillips, C, et al. Ancestry analysis in the 11-M Madrid bomb attack investigation. *PLoS One* **2009** 4 (8), e6583.

Phillips, C., et al. Building a forensic ancestry panel from the ground up: The EUROFORGEN Global AIM-SNP set. *Forensic Sci Int Genet* **2014** 11, 13–25.

Plesivkova, D, et al. A review of the potential of the MinION™ single-molecule sequencing system for forensic applications. *WIREs Forensic Science* **2019** 1 (1), e1323.

Qiagen. https://www.qiagen.com (accessed Mar 20, 2019).

Qian, X., et al. Next Generation Sequencing Plus (NGS+) with Y-chromosomal Markers for Forensic Pedigree Searches. *Sci Rep* **2017** 7 (1), 11324.

Reeve, M. A. and C. W. Fuller. A novel thermostable polymerase for DNA sequencing. *Nature* **1995** 376 (6543), 796–797.

Reuter, J. A., et al. High-throughput sequencing technologies. *Mol Cell* **2015** 58 (4), 586–597.

Rhoads, A. and K. F. Au. PacBio Sequencing and Its Applications. *Genomics Proteomics Bioinform* **2015** 13 (5), 278–289.

Richter, B. G. and D. P. Sexton. Managing and analyzing next-generation sequence data. *PLoS Comput Biol* **2009** 5 (6), e1000369.

Robasky, K., et al. The role of replicates for error mitigation in next-generation sequencing. *Nat Rev Genet* **2014** 15 (1), 56–62.

Roberts, R. J., et al. The advantages of SMRT sequencing. *Genome Biol* **2013** 14 (7), 405.

Robin, J. D., et al. Comparison of DNA Quantification Methods for Next Generation Sequencing. *Sci Rep* **2016** 6, 24067.

Ronaghi, M. Pyrosequencing sheds light on DNA sequencing. *Genome Res* **2001** 11 (1), 3–11.

Ronaghi, M., et al. A sequencing method based on real-time pyrophosphate. *Science* **1998** 281 (5375), 363, 365.

Rosenblum, B. B., et al. New dye-labeled terminators for improved DNA sequencing patterns. *Nucleic Acids Res* **1997** 25 (22), 4500–4504.

Rothberg, J. M., et al. Methods and Apparatus for Measuring Analytes using Large Scale FET Arrays. Patent United States 7948015. December 14 2006. **2006**.

Rothberg, J. M., et al. An integrated semiconductor device enabling non-optical genome sequencing. *Nature* **2011** 475 (7356), 348–352.

Rundshagen, U., et al. Mutations in the MATP gene in five German patients affected by oculocutaneous albinism type 4. *Hum Mutat* **2004** 23 (2), 106–110.

Saiki, R. K., et al. Enzymatic amplification of beta-globin genomic sequences and restriction site analysis for diagnosis of sickle cell anemia. *Science* **1985** 230 (4732), 1350–1354.

Sanchez, J. J., et al. A multiplex assay with 52 single nucleotide polymorphisms for human identification. *Electrophoresis* **2006a** 27 (9), 1713–1724.

Sanchez, J. J., et al. A multiplex assay with 52 single nucleotide polymorphisms for human identification. *Electrophoresis* **2006b** 27 (9), 1713–1724.

Sanger, F. and A. R. Coulson. A rapid method for determining sequences in DNA by primed synthesis with DNA polymerase. *J Mol Biol* **1975** 94 (3), 441–448.

Sanger, F., et al. Nucleotide sequence of bacteriophage phi X174 DNA. *Nature* **1977a** 265 (5596), 687–695.

Sanger, F., et al. DNA sequencing with chain-terminating inhibitors. *Proc Natl Acad Sci USA* **1977b** 74 (12), 5463–5467.

Sanger, F. and H. Tuppy. The amino-acid sequence in the phenylalanyl chain of insulin. I. The identification of lower peptides from partial hydrolysates. *Biochem J* **1951** 49 (4), 463–481.

Santos, C., et al. Inference of Ancestry in Forensic Analysis II: Analysis of Genetic Data. *Methods Mol Biol* **2016** 1420, 255–285.

Schirmer, M., et al. Insight into biases and sequencing errors for amplicon sequencing with the Illumina MiSeq platform. *Nucleic Acids Res* **2015** 43 (6), e37.

Schloss, J. A. How to get genomes at one ten-thousandth the cost. *Nat Biotechnol* **2008** 26 (10), 1113–1115.

Schmedes, S. E., et al. Expansion of Microbial Forensics. *J Clin Microbiol* **2016** 54 (8), 1964–1974.

Schneider, G. F. and C. Dekker. DNA sequencing with nanopores. *Nat Biotechnol* **2012** 30 (4), 326–328.

Schreiber, J., et al. Error rates for nanopore discrimination among cytosine, methylcytosine, and hydroxymethylcytosine along individual DNA strands. *Proc Natl Acad Sci USA* **2013** 110 (47), 18910–18915.

Seo, S. B., et al. Single nucleotide polymorphism typing with massively parallel sequencing for human identification. *Int J Legal Med* **2013** 127 (6), 1079–1086.

Shendure, J. and H. Ji. Next-generation DNA sequencing. *Nat Biotechnol* **2008** 26 (10), 1135–1145.

Shendure, J., et al. Accurate multiplex polony sequencing of an evolved bacterial genome. *Science* **2005** 309 (5741), 1728–1732.

Silva, D. S. B. S., et al. Developmental validation studies of epigenetic DNA methylation markers for the detection of blood, semen and saliva samples. *Forensic Sci Int Genet* **2016** 23, 55–63.

Simpson, J. T., et al. Detecting DNA cytosine methylation using nanopore sequencing. *Nat Methods* **2017** 14 (4), 407–410.

Simpson Lab. http://simpsonlab.github.io/2017/02/27/packing_fast5/ (accessed Mar 20, 2019).

Sinha, R., et al. Index Switching Causes "Spreading-Of-Signal" Among Multiplexed Samples In Illumina HiSeq 4000 DNA Sequencing. *bioRxiv* **2017**, 125724.

Smith, L. M., et al. Fluorescence detection in automated DNA sequence analysis. *Nature* **1986** 321 (6071), 674–679.

Srivastava, A., et al. Genetic data for PowerPlex 21 autosomal and PowerPlex 23 Y-STR loci from population of the state of Uttar Pradesh, India. *Int J Legal Med* **2019** 133 (5), 1381–1383.

Stasik, S., et al. An optimized targeted Next-Generation Sequencing approach for sensitive detection of single nucleotide variants. *Biomol Detect Quantif* **2018** 15, 6–12.

Stoddart, D., et al. Single-nucleotide discrimination in immobilized DNA oligonucleotides with a biological nanopore. *Proc Natl Acad Sci USA* **2009** 106 (19), 7702–7707.

Strobl, C., et al. Evaluation of the precision ID whole MtDNA genome panel for forensic analyses. *Forensic Sci Int Genet* **2018** 35, 21–25.

SWGDAM.SWGDAM Interpretation Guidelines for Mitochondrial DNA Analysisby Forensic DNA Testing Laboratories. **2013**.

Templeton, J. E., et al. DNA capture and next-generation sequencing can recover whole mitochondrial genomes from highly degraded samples for human identification. *Investig Genet* **2013** 4 (1), 26.

Thermo Fisher Scientific. www.thermofisher.com (accessed Mar 11, 2019).

van der Gaag, K. J., et al. Short hypervariable microhaplotypes: A novel set of very short high discriminating power loci without stutter artefacts. *Forensic Sci Int Genet* **2018** 35, 169–175.

van der Gaag, KJ and P de Knijff. Forensic nomenclature for short tandem repeats updated for sequencing. *Forensic Sci. Int. Genet. Suppl. Ser* **2015** 5, e542–e544.

van Dijk, E. L., et al. Ten years of next-generation sequencing technology. *Trends Genet* **2014a** 30 (9), 418–426.

van Dijk, E. L., et al. Library preparation methods for next-generation sequencing: Tone down the bias. *Exp Cell Res* **2014b** 322 (1), 12–20.

Van Neste, C., et al. My-Forensic-Loci-queries (MyFLq) framework for analysis of forensic STR data generated by massive parallel sequencing. *Forensic Sci Int Genet* **2014** 9, 1–8.

Van Neste, C., et al. Forensic massively parallel sequencing data analysis tool: Implementation of MyFLq as a standalone web- and Illumina BaseSpace((R))-appl cation. *Forensic Sci Int Genet* **2015** 15, 2–7.

Venter, J. C., et al. The sequence of the human genome. *Science* **2001** 291 (5507), 1304–1351.

Verogen. www.verogen.com (accessed Mar 20, 2019).

Vilfan, I. D., et al. Analysis of RNA base modification and structural rearrangement by single-molecule real-time detection of reverse transcription. *J Nanobiotechnol* **2013** 11, 8.

Walsh, S, et al. The HIrisPlex system for simultaneous prediction of hair and eye colour from DNA. *Forensic Sci Int: Genet* **2013** 7, 98–115.

Walsh, S., et al. Developmental validation of the HIrisPlex system: DNA-based eye and hair colour prediction for forensic and anthropological usage. *Forensic Sci Int Genet* **2014** 9, 150–161.

Wang, Y., et al. The evolution of nanopore sequencing. *Front Genet* **2014** 5, 449.

Wang, Z., et al. Characterization of microRNA expression profiles in blood and saliva using the Ion Personal Genome Machine^0 System (Ion PGM™ System). *Forensic Sci Int Genet* **2016** 20, 140–146.

Wang, Z., et al. Massively parallel sequencing of 32 forensic markers using the Precision ID GlobalFiler NGS STR Panel and the Ion PGM System. *Forensic Sci Int Genet* **2017** 31, 126–134.

Wang, Z., et al. Massively parallel sequencing of 165 ancestry informative SNPs in two Chinese Tibetan-Burmese minority ethnicities. *Forensic Sci Int Genet* **2018** 34, 141–147.

Watson, J. D. and F. H. Crick. Molecular structure of nucleic acids: A structure for deoxyribose nucleic acid. *Nature* **1953** 171 (4356), 737–738.

Wendt, F. R., et al. Flanking region variation of ForenSeq DNA Signature Prep Kit STR and SNP loci in Yavapai Native Americans. *Forensic Sci Int Genet* **2017** 28, 146–154.

Wienroth, M., et al. Technological innovations in forensic genetics: Social, legal and ethical aspects. *Recent Adv DNA Gene Seq* **2014** 8 (2), 98–103.

Willems, T., et al. Genome-wide profiling of heritable and de novo STR variations. *Nat Methods* **2017** 14 (6), 590–592.

Williams, R. and M. Wienroth. Social and ethical aspects of forensic genetics: A critical review. *Forensic Sci Rev* **2017** 29 (2), 145–169.

Woerner, A. E., et al. Fast STR allele identification with STRait Razor 3.0. *Forensic Sci Int Genet* **2017** 30, 18–23.

Woerner, A. E., et al. Evaluation of the precision ID mtDNA whole genome panel on two massively parallel sequencing systems. *Forensic Sci Int Genet* **2018** 36, 213–224.

Wu, R. and A. D. Kaiser. Structure and base sequence in the cohesive ends of bacteriophage lambda DNA. *J Mol Biol* **1968** 35 (3), 523–537.

Yang, X., et al. A survey of error-correction methods for next-generation sequencing. *Brief Bioinform* **2013** 14 (1), 56–66.

Young, B. A., et al. Estimating number of contributors in massively parallel sequencing data of STR loci. *Forensic Sci Int Genet* **2019** 38, 15–22.

Young, B., et al. A technique for setting analytical thresholds in massively parallel sequencing-based forensic DNA analysis. *PLoS One* **2017** 12 (5), e0178005.

Zaaijer, S., et al. Rapid re-identification of human samples using portable DNA sequencing. *Elife* **2017** 6, e27798.

Zbieć-Piekarska, R., et al. Development of a forensically useful age prediction method based on DNA methylation analysis. *Forensic Sci Int: Genet* **2015** 17, 173–179.

Zhang, J., et al. The impact of next-generation sequencing on genomics. *J Genet Genomics* **2011** 38 (3), 95–109.

Zhang, S., et al. Massively parallel sequencing of 231 autosomal SNPs with a custom panel: A SNP typing assay developed for human identification with Ion Torrent PGM. *Forensic Sci Res* **2017** 2 (1), 26–33.

Zhang, S., et al. Sequence investigation of 34 forensic autosomal STRs with massively parallel sequencing. *Sci Rep* **2018** 8 (1), 6810.

Zhou, Y., et al. Strategies for complete mitochondrial genome sequencing on Ion Torrent PGM platform in forensic sciences. *Forensic Sci Int Genet* **2016** 22, 11–21.

Zubakov, D., et al. Towards simultaneous individual and tissue identification: A proof-of-principle study on parallel sequencing of STRs, amelogenin, and mRNAs with the Ion Torrent PGM. *Forensic Sci Int Genet* **2015** 17, 122–128.

CHAPTER 8

Forensic Analysis of Externally Visible Characteristics: Phenotyping

DANIELE PODINI[1*] and KATHERINE B. GETTINGS[2]

[1]*Department of Forensic Sciences, George Washington University, 2100 Foxhall Road NW, Washington, DC 20007, USA*

[2]*US Department of Commerce, National Institute of Standards and Technology, Biomolecular Measurement Division, 100 Bureau Drive, Mail Stop 8314, Gaithersburg, MD 20899, USA*

*Corresponding author. E-mail: podini@gwu.edu

ABSTRACT

In cases where crime scene samples or human remains are not matched to known references or database samples, forensic analysis of externally visible traits can provide investigative information. The most common and straightforward analyses involve predicting pigmentation and ancestry, with the latter discussed in a separate chapter, to a general sense of an unknown individual's appearance. A large body of work now exists regarding world-wide variation in pigmentation genes. Several assays and interpretation models have been published in recent years, allowing these differences to be easily assessed with modern sequencing methods. Age-prediction methods can also help to focus an investigation. Most of these methods rely on measuring levels of methylation at specific sites in the genome which are known to change with biological age; however, other potential age-related genomic changes have also been studied. Additional externally visible traits are of interest in investigations, such as craniofacial features and height, but predictions remain challenging due to the polygenic nature of these traits and environmental influences.

8.1 INTRODUCTION

Forensic DNA analysis aimed at identifying individuals is primarily based on the analysis of polymorphisms in short tandem repeats (STRs), thoroughly discussed elsewhere in this book. These highly polymorphic markers can be effectively typed from very low amounts of DNA and a broad array of biological samples. Using a conventional single source DNA profile, generated with the latest commercially available forensic STR kits, the probability that two unrelated individuals share an identical profile is less than one divided by a number greater than the number of modern humans that have ever lived on our planet. Thus, if a person cannot be excluded as a contributor to a single source 20-STR profile obtained from a crime scene, that person (or their identical twin) is the source of that sample. This identification system though relies on a direct comparison between the profile obtained from the evidence and a profile from a reference sample, whether obtained from a suspect or from a database of DNA profiles like the combined DNA index system (CODIS), which hosts DNA profiles of convicted offenders in the United States. In cases where the STR profile obtained from a crime scene does not match any of the suspects or any of the profiles in the databases, the profile is of little use. In fact, STRs are noncoding and are purposely selected to have a homogenous distribution of alleles across all populations. Thus, no significant conclusions can be drawn on the source of the sample without a comparison to a known individual in the database. In such cases, a DNA assay targeting markers that can predict external visible characteristics (EVC) can aid investigators in providing a description of an unseen suspect. This molecular eyewitness can assist detectives in optimizing their resources, corroborate the testimony of a witness, and help researchers determine the relevance of specific evidence to the crime.

EVC prediction assays should be seen as an extra investigative tool and not as a means for direct identification of an individual. They would be applied only after the conventional STR profile yields no matches. Once a pool of suspects has been narrowed through EVC prediction, source attribution can then be confirmed with an STR profile. Moreover, a prediction of a person's appearances based on experimental data and reproducible metrics can be more reliable than the testimony of an eyewitness to a crime who may have not clear recollection of the facts and/or may have their own preexisting bias, or worse may have been "contaminated" by improper witness handling by investigators (Wells and Olson, 2003).

To date, the EVCs that can be predicted most accurately are eye, hair, and skin pigmentation, with eye color being the most accurate and skin the least of the three. This is achieved by the analysis of single-nucleotide polymorphisms (SNPs) that are associated with genes or gene expression regulating regions involved in pigmentation pathways. The next best predictable visible characteristic is age. There are also other physical characteristics that commonly used to describe a person: craniofacial features, height, male balding, and hair structure. These traits though are not yet accurately predictable either due to a lack of knowledge of their specific genetic cause or due to the fact that they are highly complex traits. In particular, traits such as height and craniofacial features are a consequence of a large number of genes interacting together where each one contributes a very small proportion of the phenotypic variance.

8.2 PIGMENTATION

8.2.1 EVOLUTION OF VARIABLE PIGMENTATION IN HUMAN POPULATIONS

The primary phenotype-informative markers with forensic predictive value are those associated with pigmentation. Selective pressures are responsible for the evolution of visibly variable pigmentation found among human populations worldwide. Significant hypotheses regarding the advantages of dark pigmentation near the equator and lighter pigmentation away from the equator have been proposed (Jablonski and Chaplin, 2010).

A longstanding popular explanation for the evolution of skin pigmentation has been the vitamin D hypothesis (Loomis, 1967). Holick (1995) postulated that early tetrapods required this vitamin to maximize calcium use in maintaining a rigid skeleton, and that the vitamin D had to either be synthesized by the organism or ingested in a sufficiently vitamin-D-rich diet (Holick, 1995). Vitamin D3 is needed for proper bone formation, and precursors of this vitamin are synthesized within the organism upon exposure to UV radiation from the sun (Wharton and Bishop, 2003). Lighter skin allows more UV penetration that works to overcome the decrease in UV radiation at higher latitudes (Jablonski and Chaplin, 2010). In equatorial regions, there is sufficient UV radiation throughout the year to allow adequate synthesis of vitamin D3 precursors, even in darkly pigmented people (Jablonski and Chaplin, 2010). Zones farther from the equator experience a corresponding increase in time of the year (depending on the tilt of the Earth on its axis), where less than adequate UV radiation exists to produce sufficient levels of vitamin D3, and there is a strong correlation between lightly pigmented skin and latitude. A deficiency in vitamin D3 leads to a bone disease known as rickets, which is characterized by the failure of developing bones to mineralize, due to poor absorption of calcium and phosphate (Wharton and Bishop, 2003). This deficiency is manifested in bowing of the legs, delay in fontanel closure, and female narrowing of pelvic bones, the last of which leads to high levels of death in childbirth (Wharton and Bishop, 2003). The significant impact of this disease on development and reproduction make it an ideal candidate for selection.

A relatively newer hypothesis in skin pigmentation research points to dark pigmentation protecting against the photodegradation of folate in regions of high UV radiation (Jablonski and Chaplin, 2000). In recent decades, folate (folic acid, a B vitamin) has been shown to significantly impact cell division during pregnancy, where a lack of folate is associated with early termination of pregnancy (Suh et al., 2001). Darker skin pigmentation would be advantageous because it would prevent UV radiation from penetrating to the highly vascularized dermis, where folate is present in the bloodstream (Jablonski, 2004). Lighter skin pigmentation would be problematic, particularly with increasing proximity to the equator. Interestingly, it is noted that in areas where there is significant seasonal change in UV radiation (on the latitude of the Mediterranean Sea) populations are most able to develop facultative pigmentation (suntan), which provides some protection (Jablonski, 2004).

These two hypotheses are not mutually exclusive and can be viewed as a merged model of ideal pigmentation balance: depending on the level of UV exposure, a population will evolve a skin pigmentation that allows sufficient vitamin D3 synthesis while protecting against folate degradation, to maximize overall fitness.

8.2.2   PIGMENTATION-INFORMATIVE MARKERS

Predicting pigmentation level from the genome begins with understanding the melanogenesis pathway and the ways in which it can be disrupted. As is the case with many such biological systems questions, the answer is complex. Melanin is synthesized in melanocytes that are located in the basal level of the skin, the hair bulb, and the iris (Parra, 2007). Differences in melanocyte density depending on body location have been described (Whiteman et al., 1999), yet they are not sufficient to explain individual differences in body pigmentation. Two factors better explain these differences: the amount and type of melanin and the shape and distribution of melanosomes (the organelles responsible for storing melanin) (Parra, 2007).

There are two types of melanin: eumelanin, brown/black in color, and phaeomelanin, red/yellow in color. The melanocortin-1 receptor gene (*MC1R*) is involved in the transfer of both types of melanin affecting human hair and skin color (Beaumont et al., 2005). The *SLC24A5* gene is another gene that codes for a putative protein shown to be strongly involved in skin pigmentation. An A to G substitution at codon 111, which determines an alanine to threonine change, is a critical polymorphism within the sequence (rs1426654). The allele frequency for the Thr111 variant ranged from 98.7% to 100% among several European-American population samples, whereas the ancestral Ala111 allele had a frequency of 93% to 100% in African, Indigenous American, and East Asian population samples (Lamason et al., 2005).

Early work studying polymorphisms associated with human pigmentation concluded that six SNPs located in five genes (*SLC24A5*, *OCA2*, *SLC45A2*, *MC1R*, and *ASIP*) track a great proportion of hair, skin, and eye pigmentation variation across populations (Branicki et al., 2011). Two other studies pointed to one particular SNP (rs12913832) in the *HERC2* gene region that is predictive of light eye color: individuals carrying the C/C genotype had only a 1% probability of having brown eyes while T/T carriers had an 80% probability of being brown eyed (Wood et al., 2014; Keyser et al., 2009; Sturm et al., 2008). With such a significant impact, it is surprising to note that this SNP is noncoding. The *HERC2* gene region encompassing rs12913832 functions as an enhancer, regulating transcription of *OCA2*, which encodes for the trans-melanosomal membrane protein "P" (Tully, 2007). In darkly pigmented human melanocytes, transcription factors HLTF, LEF1, and MITF were found binding to the *HERC2* rs12913832 enhancer carrying the T allele. Long-range chromatin loops between this enhancer and the *OCA2* promoter lead to elevated *OCA2* expression. In lightly pigmented melanocytes carrying the rs12913832 C allele, chromatin-loop formation, transcription factor recruitment, and *OCA2* expression were all reduced. Figure 8.1 shows the distribution of rs12913832 alleles, with the light eye color C allele (represented in the figure as "G" due to opposing strand being genotyped) absent in sub-Saharan Africa and becoming increasingly frequent to the north. Further elucidation of the roles of combinations of SNPs in the *HERC2*, *OCA2*, and *SLC45A2* gene regions was noted in a study of the Danish population (Mengel-From et al., 2010).

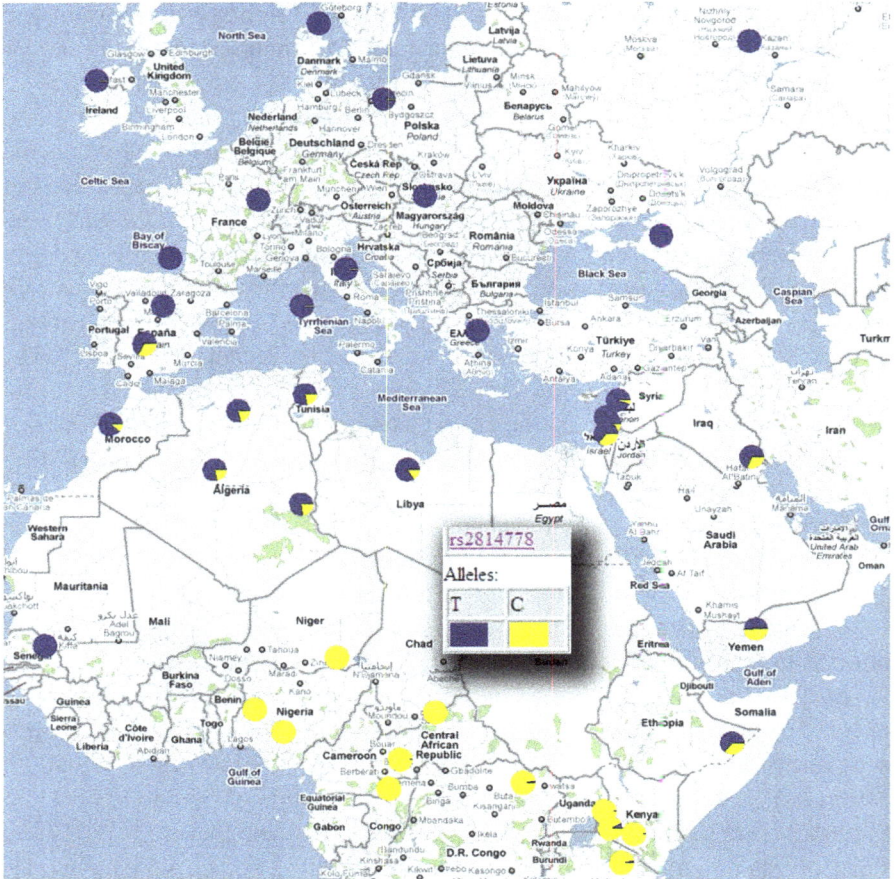

FIGURE 8.1 Data from www.alfred.med.yale.edu showing distribution of alleles at rs12913832. The A allele (associated with darker pigmentation) is monomorphic in sub-Saharan Africa, while the G allele (associated with lighter pigmentation) becomes increasingly prevalent in central to northern Europe.

8.2.3 PIGMENTATION PREDICTION TOOLS

The first pigmentation prediction assay and model was the IrisPlex system, published by a team from Erasmus University Medical Center (Walsh et al., 2011). The IrisPlex system is composed of two parts: (1) a 6-SNP assay designed for use with SNaPshot® chemistry, which employs single-base extension (SBE) primers incorporating a single fluorescently labeled nucleotide complementary to the target SNP. The SBE primers can them be resolved via capillary electrophoresis (a technology already in place in forensic DNA casework laboratories) and (2) an Excel calculator that provides the prediction probability for blue, intermediate, or brown eye color. In 2013, a research group from the University of Santiago de Compostela (USC) published a different assay and prediction model, composed of two SBE assays typing 37 SNPs in pigmentation-associated genes aimed at skin, hair, and eye color polymorphisms (under the acronym SHEP), along with an online classifier (Ruiz et al., 2013). Later in the same year, the Erasmus group expanded on their earlier system to include hair color prediction with the 24-SNP HIrisPlex system (Walsh et al., 2013). The following year, the USC group published the results of a candidate gene study for skin color prediction, along with a skin color prediction test consisting of 10 SNPs in eight genes and an online classifier (Maroñas et al., 2014). Most recently, the Erasmus group has expanded their prediction system to a 41-SNP SBE assay and Excel calculator for eye, hair, and skin pigmentation, called the HIrisPlex-S system, the output of which is exemplified in Figure 8.2 (Chaitanya et al., 2018). Table 8.1 provides a cross-reference of all 50 SNPs included in the aforementioned assays, genomic coordinates, gene regions, polymorphism types, and minor allele frequencies.

One challenge researchers have realized in European populations is the tendency for hair pigmentation darkening between childhood and adulthood sometimes appears to affect predictions, resulting in hair color predictions aligning with childhood blonde hair color, whereas the adult has brown hair. The impact of this phenomenon has also been the focus of recent work (Kukla-Bartoszek et al., 2018). Additionally, several research groups have demonstrated that females have a darker eye color than males, given the same SNP profile (Martinez-Cadenas et al., 2013; Pietroni et al., 2014; Pośpiech et al., 2016). This population-specific effect may serve to further refine eye-color prediction in some cases; however, opinions vary as to the merit of including gender in eye-color prediction models.

While all of the previously described pigmentation models were designed for use with the capillary electrophoresis technology currently available in forensic casework laboratories, adoption of these methods has been sporadic. The availability of lower cost benchtop sequencers in recent years has led manufacturers to include pigmentation prediction in commercially available assays. The Verogen ForenSeq™ system includes the 24 pigmentation SNPs from the HIrisPlex system, as well as a calculator for hair and eye color embedded in the associated software. Additionally, Thermo Fisher Scientific (Waltham, MA, USA) has two Ion AmpliSeq™ panels available for the Ion S5 sequencer, one for the HIrisPlex markers and another for the expanded HIrisPlex-S system; in both cases, users are directed to the published Excel calculators for interpretation.

a. The HIrisPlex System

	Gene	SNP	Allele	No. of Alleles
1	MC1R	rs312262906	A	0 1 2 NA
2	MC1R	rs11547464	A	0 1 2 NA
3	MC1R	rs885479	T	0 1 2 NA
4	MC1R	rs1805008	T	0 1 2 NA
5	MC1R	rs1805005	T	0 1 2 NA
6	MC1R	rs1805006	A	0 1 2 NA
7	MC1R	rs1805007	T	0 1 2 NA
8	TUBB3	rs1805009	C	0 1 2 NA
9	MC1R	rs201326893	A	0 1 2 NA
10	MC1R	rs2228479	A	0 1 2 NA
11	MC1R	rs1110400	C	0 1 2 NA
12	SLC45A2	rs28777	C	0 1 2 NA
13	SLC45A2	rs16891982	C	0 1 2 NA
14	KITLG	rs12821256	G	0 1 2 NA
15	LOC105374875	rs4959270	A	0 1 2 NA
16	IRF4	rs12203592	T	0 1 2 NA
17	TYR	rs1042602	T	0 1 2 NA
18	OCA2	rs1800407	A	0 1 2 NA
19	SLC24A4	rs2402130	G	0 1 2 NA
20	HERC2	rs12913832	T	0 1 2 NA
21	PIGU	rs2378249	C	0 1 2 NA
22	LOC105370627	rs12896399	T	0 1 2 NA
23	TYR	rs1393350	T	0 1 2 NA
24	TYRP1	rs683	G	0 1 2 NA

Display Predicted Phenotype　　　Download Predicted Phenotype

Predicted phenotype

	p-value	AUC Loss
blue eye	0.184	0
intermediate eye	0.15	0
brown eye	0.665	0
blond hair	0.33	0
brown hair	0.537	0
red hair	0.001	0
black hair	0.132	0
light hair	0.68	0
dark hair	0.32	0

b. The HIrisPlex System

	Gene	SNP	Allele	No. of Alleles
1	MC1R	rs312262906	A	0 1 2 NA
2	MC1R	rs11547464	A	0 1 2 NA
3	MC1R	rs885479	T	0 1 2 NA
4	MC1R	rs1805008	T	0 1 2 NA
5	MC1R	rs1805005	T	0 1 2 NA
6	MC1R	rs1805006	A	0 1 2 NA
7	MC1R	rs1805007	T	0 1 2 NA
8	TUBB3	rs1805009	C	0 1 2 NA
9	MC1R	rs201326893	A	0 1 2 NA
10	MC1R	rs2228479	A	0 1 2 NA
11	MC1R	rs1110400	C	0 1 2 NA
12	SLC45A2	rs28777	C	0 1 2 NA
13	SLC45A2	rs16891982	C	0 1 2 NA
14	KITLG	rs12821256	G	0 1 2 NA
15	LOC105374875	rs4959270	A	0 1 2 NA
16	IRF4	rs12203592	T	0 1 2 NA
17	TYR	rs1042602	T	0 1 2 NA
18	OCA2	rs1800407	A	0 1 2 NA
19	SLC24A4	rs2402130	G	0 1 2 NA
20	HERC2	rs12913832	T	0 1 2 NA
21	PIGU	rs2378249	C	0 1 2 NA
22	LOC105370627	rs12896399	T	0 1 2 NA
23	TYR	rs1393350	T	0 1 2 NA
24	TYRP1	rs683	G	0 1 2 NA

Display Predicted Phenotype　　　Download Predicted Phenotype

Predicted phenotype

	p-value	AUC Loss
blue eye	0.911	0
intermediate eye	0.057	0
brown eye	0.032	0
blond hair	0.657	0
brown hair	0.237	0
red hair	0.096	0
black hair	0.009	0
light hair	0.991	0
dark hair	0.009	0

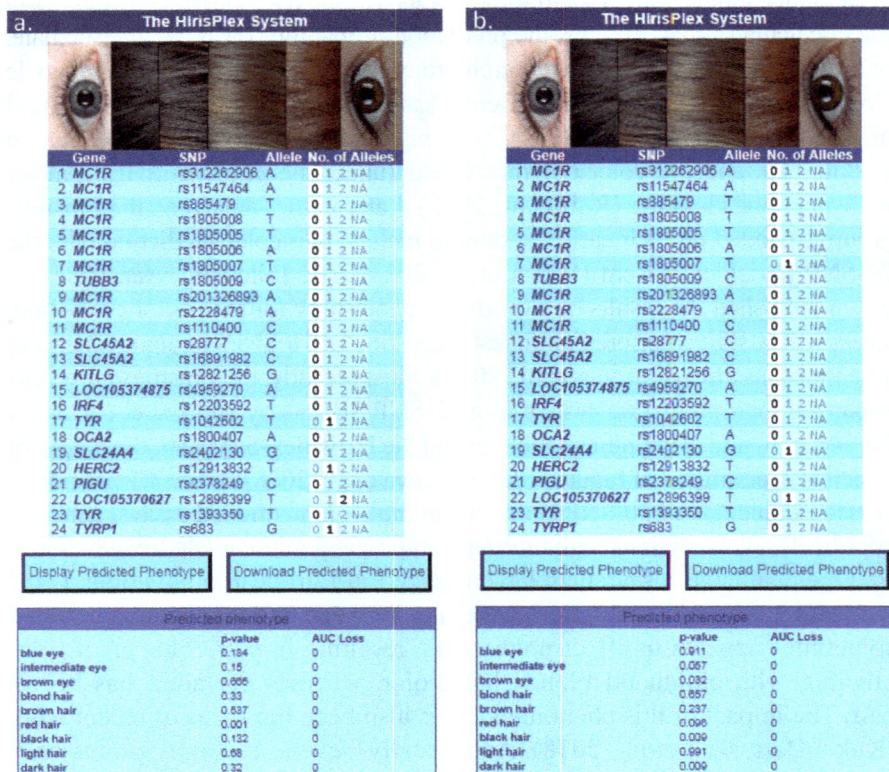

FIGURE 8.2 Example eye- and hair-color prediction outputs from HIrisPlex system web-based interface (https://hirisplex.erasmusmc.nl). The sample donor in (A) has brown eyes and dark brown hair. The predictions are correct with 0.665 probability of brown eyes and 0.537 probability of brown hair; however, the prediction probabilities for blonde hair (0.33) or, more generally, light-colored hair (0.68) are significant. The sample donor in (B) has blue eyes and light brown hair but was blonde as a child. Eye color is correctly predicted as blue (0.991). The hair color prediction is highest for blonde (0.657), followed by brown (0.237), exemplifying the phenomenon of prediction aligning with childhood hair color.

8.3　AGE

Age estimation is commonly used to describe people both in everyday life and in criminal investigations. As people age, their physical appearance changes in a somewhat objective manner, such that most people can estimate another person's approximate age with surprising accuracy (Han et al., 2013). In criminal cases an estimation of the age of the perpetrator, often obtained by

TABLE 8.1 SNPs Included in Published Forensic Pigmentation Prediction Models and Genomic Information

Panel	rs ID	Chromosome	GRCh38 Coordinate	Gene/Region	Location, Type	HGVS Protein	GMAF Frequency
I,H,S,SHEP*	rs16891982	5	33951588	SLC45A2	Exon missense	p.Phe374Leu	G=0.275
H,S	rs28777	5	33958854	SLC45A2	Intron variant		A=0.379
SHEP*	rs26722	5	33963765	SLC45A2	Exon missense	p.Glu272Lys	T=0.178
SHEP	rs13289	5	33986304	SLC45A2	Upstream variant		G=0.444
I,H,S,SHEP*	rs12203592	6	396321	IRF4	Intron variant		T=0.037
H,S	rs4959270	6	457748	IRF4	Downstream variant		A=0.337
H,S	rs683	9	12709305	TYRP1	3' UTR variant		A=0.252
S	rs10756819	9	16858086	BNC2	Intron variant		A=0.455
H,S,SHEP	rs1042602	11	89178528	TYR	Exon missense	p.Ser192Tyr	A=0.123
I,H,S	rs1393350	11	89277878	TYR	Intron variant		A=0.079
S	rs1126809	11	89284793	TYR	Exon missense	p.Arg402Gln	A=0.081
H,S	rs12821256	12	88934558	KITLG	Upstream variant		C=0.032
SHEP	rs3782974	13	94440642	DCT	Intron variant		T=0.303
I,H,S,SHEP*	rs12896399	14	92307319	SLC24A4	Intron variant		T=0.261
H,S	rs2402130	14	92334859	SLC24A4	Intron variant		G=0.269
S	rs17128291	14	92416482	SLC24A4	Intron variant		G=0.085
S	rs1800414	15	27951891	OCA2	Exon missense	p.His615Arg	C=0.121
I,H,S	rs1800407	15	27985172	OCA2	Exon missense	p.Arg419Gln	T=0.025
S	rs1470608	15	28042975	OCA2	Intron variant		G=0.412
S	rs1545397	15	27942626	OCA2	Intron variant		T=0.262

TABLE 8.1 *(Continued)*

Panel	rs ID	Chromosome	GRCh38 Coordinate	Gene/Region	Location, Type	HGVS Protein	GMAF Frequency
S	rs12441727	15	28026629	OCA2	Intron variant		A=0.139
SHEP*	rs7495174	15	28099092	OCA2	Intron variant		G=0.251
SHEP*	rs4778138	15	28090674	OCA2	Intron variant		A=0.498
SHEP*	rs4778241	15	28093567	OCA2	Intron variant		C=0.483
I,H,S,SHEP*	rs12913832	15	28120472	HERC2	Intron variant		G=0.177
S	rs2238289	15	28208069	HERC2	Intron variant		G=0.497
S	rs6497292	15	28251049	HERC2	Intron variant		G=0.328
S	rs1129038	15	28111713	HERC2	3' UTR variant		T=0.177
S,SHEP*	rs1667394	15	28285036	HERC2	Intron variant		T=0.380
SHEP*	rs11636232	15	28141480	HERC2	Exon synonymous	p.Gln3989=	T=0.086
SHEP*	rs916977	15	28268218	HERC2	Intron variant		C=0.389
SHEP*	rs12592730	15	28285213	HERC2	Intron variant		A=0.153
S	rs1426654	15	48134287	SLC24A5	Exon missense	p.Thr111Ala	A=0.438
S	rs3114908	16	89317317	ANKRD11	Intron variant		T=0.312
H,S	rs796296176	16	89919344	MC1R	Exon missense	p.Asn29fs	insA=0.001
H,S	rs1805005	16	89919436	MC1R	Exon missense	p.Val60Leu	T=0.035
H,S	rs1805006	16	89919510	MC1R	Exon missense	p.Asp84Glu	A=0.003
H,S	rs2228479	16	89919532	MC1R	Exon missense	p.Val92Met	A=0.080
H,S	rs11547464	16	89919683	MC1R	Exon missense	p.Arg142His	A=0.003
H,S,SHEP*	rs1805007	16	89919709	MC1R	Exon missense	p.Arg151Cys	T=0.019
H,S	rs201326893	16	89919714	MC1R	Exon missense	p.Tyr152Ter	A=0.000

TABLE 8.1 *(Continued)*

Panel	rs ID	Chromosome	GRCh38 Coordinate	Gene/Region	Location, Type	HGVS Protein	GMAF Frequency
H,S	rs1110400	16	89919722	MC1R	Exon missense	p.Ile155Thr	C=0.003
H,S,SHEP*	rs1805008	16	89919736	MC1R	Exon missense	p.Arg160Trp	T=0.015
H,S	rs885479	16	89919746	MC1R	Exon missense	p.Arg163Gln	A=0.191
H,S	rs1805009	16	89920138	MC1R	Exon missense	p.Asp294His	C=0.003
S	rs3212355	16	89917970	MC1R	5′ UTR variant		T=0.028
S	rs8051733	16	89957798	DEF8	Intron variant		G=0.277
S	rs6059655	20	34077942	RALY	Intron variant		A=0.013
S	rs6119471	20	34197406	ASIP	Intron variant		G=0.191
H,S	rs2378249	20	34630286	PIGU	Intron variant		G=0.184

I = IrisPlex, H = HIrisPlex, S = HIrisPlex-S

*Noted as most closely associated to eye color

HGVS nomenclature: http://varnomen.hgvs.org/

GMAF: 1000 Genomes project Global Minor Allele Frequency

witnesses and included in crime alerts, can play an important role in an investigation. Furthermore, an estimate of the age at death can be useful in human
identification cases when human remains of adult bodies have decayed to the
point that age estimation cannot be based on conventional methods. Thus,
the forensic science research community has invested significant resources
into exploring approaches to biologically predict age. These efforts have
led to the discovery of several protein and DNA epigenetic markers that
predictably change over time. These changes are correlated to time but are
also influenced by the environment. Moreover, they vary according to the
biological tissue in which they occur and are, to some extent, stochastic.

8.3.1   NON-DNA METHYLATION-BASED METHODS FOR AGE PREDICTION

Mitochondria are intracellular organelles responsible for the production of
energy with independent protein synthesis capabilities including their own
circular DNA genome. Energy is produced in the form of ATP through the
oxidation of glucose and lipids. Part of the oxygen consumed in this process
is released as free radicals like the perhydroxyl radical, superoxide, and
hydrogen peroxide (St-Pierre et al., 2002). Proteins, lipids, and DNA can
be damaged by these highly reactive molecules. Specifically, mitochondrial
DNA (mtDNA) mutagenesis is in part attributed to these molecules, and the
extent of the damage has shown to be tissue specific and correlated with a
person's age (Meissner et al., 2006; Zapico and Ubelaker, 2013). A common
mtDNA somatic mutation is a deletion of 4977 bp that has been detected
and studied in several tissues. Several methods have been developed for the
quantification of this deletion with real time PCR being the method of choice
(Ye et al., 2008). Although experimental data did not demonstrate its usefulness from typical forensic body fluids (blood, saliva, and semen), the 4977
bp deletion showed the strongest age correlation within the substantia nigra
tissue of the midbrain ($r = 0.87$), whereas it varied substantially in skeletal
muscle (0.64–0.84). Additionally mosaicism events have been observed with
neighboring tissues showing major differences in the number of mitochondria carrying the deletion, making standardization of sampling procedures a
critical factor in the effectiveness of this age-prediction approach (Meissner
and Ritz-Timme, 2010). Other studies have shown age-related increase in
heteroplasmy both coding and noncoding regions of the mtDNA genome
(Calloway et al., 2000; Lacan et al., 2009).

Telomeres are regions of repetitive sequences located at the tips of chromosomes whose function is to protect the integrity of the chromosome. Over time, in most somatic cells, the length of telomeres decreases, and this shortening is proportional to a person's age (Lingner et al., 1995). Several methods have been developed to determine telomere length, including, but not limited to, slot blot hybridization, quantitative fluorescent *in situ* hybridization (Bryant et al., 1997), or flow-fluorescence *in situ* hybridization (Poon and Lansdorp, 2001), with a quantitative PCR-based method being theoretically the most amenable to forensic samples (Cawthon, 2002). Although studies have reported a correlation coefficient between age and telomere length of up to $r = 0.832$ (Tsuji et al., 2002), individual variation, localized somatic differences, and the technical challenge of analyzing large fragments of DNA make these approaches unsuitable for forensic practices.

One of the most reliable age-prediction approaches is based on aspartic acid racemization. Mammalian proteins are synthesized exclusively with L-amino acids. Over time, there is an age-dependent increase of D-aspartic acid that, in permanent proteins such as dentin, can be used to infer the age of an individual with a high level of correlation ($r = 0.988–0.997$) (Fu et al., 1995; Ritz et al., 1990). Although reliable, this method is based on the use of gas chromatography or high-performance liquid chromatography and requires highly standardized protocols. Protein purification can be challenging, and precise calibration curves are important for trustworthy results. Age prediction based on aspartic acid racemization is a reliable method on permanent proteins making it inapplicable to typical forensic body fluid samples and limiting its application primarily to determining the age at death from human remains. Similarly, advanced glycation products accumulate over time in long-lived proteins, such as collagen, in various tissues like crystalline lens, skin, and cartilage (Verzijl et al., 2000). Enzyme-linked immunoassay has been the method of choice to detect these compounds with the highest level of correlation obtained from rib cartilage ($r = 0.90$) (Pilin et al., 2007).

8.3.2 DNA METHYLATION

The nucleotide sequence of an individual's DNA remains the same throughout his/her life and beyond, but certain DNA modifications occur over time which do not alter the sequence itself. One example is cytosine/5'-CpG-3' methylation, which is used by cells and organisms to regulate gene expression in response to a changing environment. These epigenetic modifications, when they occur in CpG islands located in transcription initiation sites, regulate downstream gene expression (Deaton and Bird, 2011). In most cases, a methylated promoter is inaccessible to its transcription factors and the gene is "turned off." Thus, given its important function in cell cycle regulation and its potential role in human diseases (i.e., cancer), DNA methylation has been the focus of studies now for quite some time (Levenson and Melnikov, 2012). As often happens in the field of human identification, knowledge initially generated for human health purposes is then adapted for forensic purposes. Specifically, the analysis of methylation sites can provide information for three forensically relevant purposes: age prediction, body fluid identification, and identical twins detection (Vidaki and Kayser, 2018).

Most of the forensically relevant methylations sites have been discovered using DNA methylation microarray screening, which allows probing thousands of sites simultaneously using the Illumina® Infinium 27 K/450 K BeadChip technology. Initially, the majority of the DNA methylation sites identified and selected for age-prediction assays were for DNA extracted from blood (Zubakov et al., 2016). More recently, other body fluids have been effectively explored for age-informative methylation sites. An example is the 7-plex SNaPshot® assay developed by Hong et al. targeting seven CpG sites: one that is specific for saliva and allows body fluid identification plus six CpG sites correlated to age in saliva. The model developed for this assay showed 94.5% correlation between predicted and chronological age with a mean absolute deviation from chronological age of 3.13 years.

Human methylation patterns can be correlated to age as well as environmental factors such as lifestyle choices or disease. These factors, the best known of which is tobacco-cigarette smoking (Rexbye et al., 2006), can make a person appear older than their biological age. Body mass index (BMI) can also affect DNA methylation. A recent study identified 187 genetic loci where alterations in DNA methylation are associated to increased obesity. These loci are found in genes involved in lipid and lipoprotein metabolism, substrate transport, and inflammatory pathways, and their methylation can predict development of type 2 diabetes (Wahl et al., 2017). Although speculative, it is possible that greater knowledge of these methylation patterns and their correlation to adiposity could enable BMI predictions.

8.3.3   METHYLATION-BASED AGE PREDICTION METHODS

Most age-prediction assays are based on bisulfite conversion of the template DNA followed by PCR amplification and sequencing. Bisulfite conversion is a chemical manipulation that changes unmethylated cytosine to uracil while methylated cytosines remain unaltered by the process. Using primers specifically designed to target bisulfite-treated DNA (i.e., with unmethylated Cs replaces by Ts), the uracil is then copied into thymine via PCR amplification, resulting in a C to T transition. Methylation is then determined by the detection of the surviving cytosines on the sequenced PCR product (Figure 8.3). Several sequencing methods have been used for this purpose including methylation site-specific SBE using the SNaPshot® kit (Hong et al., 2017), pyrosequencing (Soares Bispo Santos Silva et al., 2015; Alghanim et al., 2017), EpiTYPER™ technology (Freire-Aradas et al., 2016), Sanger sequencing (Weber-Lehmann et al., 2014), and more recently massively parallel sequencing (Vidaki et al., 2017; Richards et al., 2018). The challenging aspect of this method is that it has degrading effects on DNA and requires significant starting amounts of starting template (Holmes et al., 2014), both features that are often incompatible with forensic casework.

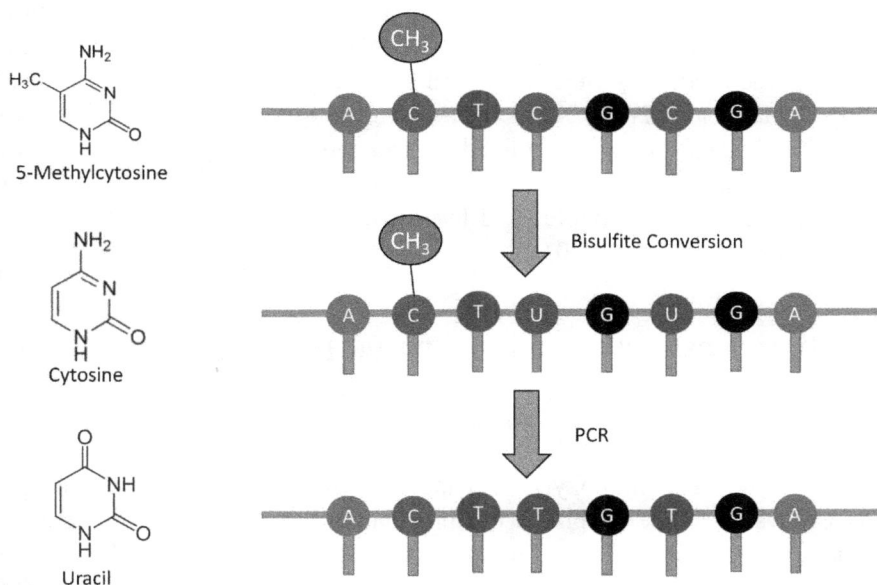

FIGURE 8.3 On the left side are shown the molecular structures of 5-methylcytosine, cytosine, and uracil. On the right side is a schematic representation of the bisulfite conversion process followed by PCR, where unmethylated cytosine is converted into uracil, then thymine, while 5-methylcytosine is simply converted into unmethylated cytosine.

Another method for detecting DNA methylation, often referred to as methylation sensitive restriction enzyme fragment analysis, is based on the use of restriction enzymes that are either inhibited by the presence of methylated cytosines or that selectively cut in presence of methylated cytosines at specific sequences like the HhaI restriction enzyme (5'-GCG^C-3'). This approach, although mostly used for methylation-based body fluid identification, has its main advantage in the absence bisulfite treatment, permitting much lower starting amounts of DNA (down to 250 pg).

Once the level of methylation at specific sites is determined, a prediction of a person's chronological age is performed. Various statistical approaches have been proposed including methods based on regression modelling, for example multivariate linear regression (Park et al., 2016) and multivariate nonlinear regression (Xu et al., 2016), or using neural networks such as generalized regression (Vidaki et al., 2017), and back-propagation (Park et al., 2016). Overall neural networks seem to outperform all other methods, as shown in a study by Vidaki et al. (2017), where age prediction based on 23 CpG sites improved from a $R^2 = 0.92$ with multiple regression analysis to $R^2 = 0.96$ when the prediction approach used a generalized regression neural network model based on a subset of 16 locations. In this latter approach, the top three predictors were located in the *NHLRC1*, *SCGN*, and *CSNK1D* genes (Vidaki et al., 2017). Alfieri et al. using a Support Vector Machine with polynomial function model obtained a mean average age-prediction error of 4.1 years on a blind test set of 33 individuals. The error was less than four years for 52% of the samples and less than 7 years for 86% of the tested individuals (Aliferi et al., 2018).

8.4   OTHER EXTERNAL VISIBLE CHARACTERISTICS (EVC)

8.4.1   *CRANIOFACIAL FEATURES*

The resemblance of monozygotic twins is a testament to the important role DNA plays in the development of appearance. In other words, "identical" twins are identical because they have the same DNA sequence, leading to the conclusion that it should be possible to derive one's facial features based on their DNA sequence. This is theoretically correct but it assumes a much deeper understanding of the mechanics of DNA expression and regulation than what is currently known. A genome-wide association study (GWAS) conducted on over 5000 individuals, targeting over 2.5 million SNPs, with facial landmarks extracted from 3D MRI, identified five independent genes (*PRDM16*, *PAX3*, *TP63*, *C5orf50*, and *COL17A1*) potentially associated with the morphology of the human face (Liu et al., 2012). A different

GWAS study of African children identified two genes (*SCHIP1* and *PDE8A*) displaying potential effects on normal human face morphology variation that had a clear effect on facial development in mice (Cole et al., 2016). Another study conducted on almost 600 individuals of mixed African and European ancestry, using a new statistical approach called bootstrapped response-based imputation modeling, identified 20 autosomal genes that significantly affect facial features. The same study determined that biogeographical ancestry, when evaluated independently from sex, explains 9.6% of the total facial variation. Conversely sex, independently from ancestry, explains 12.9% of total facial variation (Claes et al., 2014). Sex and ancestry are the major known contributors affecting normal craniofacial variation. All the other polymorphisms identified thus far contribute each only a small proportion of the variation. Similar conclusions were reached in a more recent study by Lippert et al. (2017), where whole genome sequencing was performed on 1061 individuals of diverse ancestry. Thus, it is currently not possible to use genomic data to develop an accurate sketch of a person's face, detailing traits such as shape of the nose, chin, and lips, other than what is commonly correlated to ancestry and sex. That said, as more studies are conducted on a much greater number of people and covering the entire human genome, together with the development of new statistical tools, a more accurate molecular identikit tool may be possible.

8.4.2   HEIGHT

Another important EVC commonly used when describing a suspect in a crime is height. Just like facial appearance, height is a polygenic trait with multiple variants contributing to the phenotype. In 2009 Aulchenko published the results of study aimed at predicting height based on typing 54 height-associated SNPs on a thousand Dutch people. Results showed that the prediction of the tallest 5% was just slightly more accurate than random guessing (Aulchenko et al., 2009). The International Genetics of Anthropometric Traits consortium, in a 2010 GWAS study including more than 180,000 individuals typed at almost three million SNPs, identified 180 different loci significantly associated to height. Yet, these 180 poly-morphisms only accounted for 10% of height variation (Lango Allen et al., 2010), whereas studies on twins estimate that the heritability of height is approximately 80% (McEvoy and Visscher, 2009). A more recent compre-hensive GWAS study on over 250,000 individuals identified 697 SNPs that collectively explain 16% of height variation within the studied population

(Wood et al., 2014). This study also demonstrated that by including SNPs below the GWAS significance threshold, it was possible to explain up to 29% of height variation with approximately 9500 SNPs (Wood et al., 2014).

8.4.3 BALDNESS AND HAIR STRUCTURE

Androgenic alopecia, or male pattern baldness (MPB), contributes to variation in physical appearance particularly in the European population where it is quite common. Several genes and genomic regions associated with early onset of MPB have been identified, with the strongest being the *AR/EDA2R* region on the X-chromosome, explaining why baldness is much more common in males than in females (Li et al., 2012). A more recent study identified 29 SNPs from chromosomes X, 1, 5, 7, 18, and 20 with alleles strongly associated to MPB (Marcińska et al., 2015). A prediction model based on the 20 most predictive SNPs was tested on 300 European males. Overall the accuracy of the MPB prediction in men less than 50 years of age expressed in area under the curve (AUC) was 0.657, slightly better than random guessing (which would be an AUC of 0.5), whereas in men 50 years of age or older, the AUC improved to 0.761 (Li et al., 2012).

Hair shape is also a potentially useful EVC. Pośpiech et al. through a GWAS, which included almost 27,000 individuals, developed a binary (straight vs nonstraight) prediction model on 32 SNPs from 26 genetic loci. The prediction accuracy of the assay showed an AUC of 0.664 in Europeans and 0.789 in non-Europeans. The statistically significant difference was primarily attributed to a SNP in the *EDAR* gene in non-Europeans (Pośpiech et al., 2018).

8.5 CONCLUDING REMARKS

In criminal investigations when the conventional DNA profile from crime scene evidence does not match any of the available references, a prediction of the external visible characteristics of source of the sample can help the investigation. The best predictable traits are eye, hair, and skin pigmentation and age. Traits such as height and facial morphology are very complex as they result from the interaction of hundreds, even thousands, of different genetic loci. More research is required to better understand the complexity of these interactions and phenotypic correlations. The VISible Attributes through GEnomics consortium (http://www.visage-h2020.eu/) represents one such effort. It is a collaborative European effort that aims to increase the knowledge on the relationships between DNA and appearance with the ultimate goal of enabling the development of composite sketches of unknown perpetrators from DNA evidence.

As more knowledge is generated and predictions on a greater number of traits become more accurate, there are some ethical and practical concerns that must be addressed for a sound and just implementation of this capability (Samuel and Prainsack, 2018). These tests are probabilistic; therefore, appropriate use of the results requires investigators to understand probabilities and acknowledge any preexisting bias on the specific case. Scholars in this field have raised the concern that the implementation of DNA phenotyping might increase discrimination toward minority groups within society (Koops and Schellekens, 2008), especially with relation to ancestry prediction. Even though arguably EVC are, by definition, visible, there are privacy concerns. For example, a person may have chosen to change their natural appearance by dying their hair, wearing colored contact lenses, and having plastic surgery (Ossorio, 2006) or a person may identify with a certain ancestry which may, unbeknownst to them, different from what inferred genetically. Finally, genetic data may reveal predisposition or correlation to certain diseases. In each of these cases, compromising someone's privacy may prove harmful for that individual. These concerns should be considered before implementing the systematic use of forensic DNA phenotyping in casework.

KEYWORDS

- **SNPs**
- **CpG site**
- **DNA methylation**
- **pigmentation prediction**
- **age prediction**
- **eye color**
- **skin color**
- **hair color**
- **body mass index (BMI)**
- **craniofacial features**

REFERENCES

Alghanim, H.; et al.; Detection and Evaluation of DNA Methylation Markers Found at SCGN and KLF14 Loci to Estimate Human Age. *Forensic Sci. Int. Genet.* **2017**, *31*, 81–88.

Aliferi, A.; et al.; DNA Methylation-Based Age Prediction Using Massively Parallel Sequencing Data and Multiple Machine Learning Models. *Forensic Sci. Int. Genet.* **2018**, *37*, 215–226.

Aulchenko, Y. S.; et al.; Predicting Human Height by Victorian and Genomic Methods. *Eur. J. Hum. Genet.* **2009**, *17* (8), 1070–1075.

Beaumont, K. A.; et al.; Altered Cell Surface Expression of Human MC1R Variant Receptor Alleles Associated with Red Hair and Skin Cancer Risk. *Hum. Mol. Genet.* **2005**, *14* (15), 2145–2154.

Branicki, W.; et al.; Model-Based Prediction of Human Hair Color Using DNA Variants. *Hum. Genet.* **2011**, *129* (4), 443–454.

Bryant, J. E.; et al.; Measurement of Telomeric DNA Content in Human Tissues. *BioTechniques* **1997**, *23* (3), 476–484.

Calloway, C. D.; et al.; The Frequency of Heteroplasmy in the HVII Region of MtDNA Differs Across Tissue Types and Increases with Age. *Am. J. Hum. Genet.* **2000**, *66* (4), 1384–1397.

Cawthon, R. M.; Telomere Measurement by Quantitative PCR. *Nucleic Acids Res.* **2002**, *30* (10), e47–e47.

Chaitanya, L.; et al.; The HIrisPlex-S System for Eye, Hair and Skin Colour Prediction from DNA: Introduction and Forensic Developmental Validation. *Forensic Sci. Int. Genet.* **2018**, *35*, 123–135.

Claes, P.; et al.; Modeling 3D Facial Shape from DNA. *PLoS Genet.* **2014**, *10* (3), e1004224–e1004224.

Cole, J. B.; et al.; Genomewide Association Study of African Children Identifies Association of SCHIP1 and PDE8A with Facial Size and Shape. *PLoS Genet.* **2016**, *12* (8), e1006174.

Deaton, A. M.; and Bird, A.; CpG Islands and the Regulation of Transcription. *Genes Dev.* **2011**, *25* (10), 1010–1022.

Freire-Aradas, A.; et al.; Development of a Methylation Marker Set for Forensic Age Estimation Using Analysis of Public Methylation Data and the Agena Bioscience EpiTYPER System. *Forensic Sci. Int. Genet.* **2016**, *24*, 65–74.

Fu, S.-J.; et al.; Age Estimation Using a Modified HPLC Determination of Ratio of Aspartic Acid in Dentin. *Forensic Sci. Int.* **1995**, *73* (1), 35–40.

Han, H.; et al.; Age Estimation from Face Images: Human vs. Machine Performance. In *2013 International Conference on Biometrics (ICB)*; IEEE, 2013; 1–8.

Holick, M. F.; Environmental Factors That Influence the Cutaneous Production of Vitamin D. *Am. J. Clin. Nutr.* **1995**, *61* (3), 638S–645S.

Holmes, E. E.; et al.; Performance Evaluation of Kits for Bisulfite-Conversion of DNA From Tissues, Cell Lines, FFPE Tissues, Aspirates, Lavages, Effusions, Plasma, Serum, and Urine. *PLoS One* **2014**, *9* (4), e93933.

Hong, S. R.; et al.; DNA Methylation-Based Age Prediction from Saliva: High Age Predictability by Combination of 7 CpG Markers. *Forensic Sci. Int. Genet.* **2017**, *29*, 118–125.

Jablonski, N. G.; The Evolution of Human Skin and Skin Color. *Annu. Rev. Anthr.* **2004**, *33*, 585–623.

Jablonski, N. G.; and Chaplin, G.; The Evolution of Human Skin Coloration. *J. Hum. Evol.* **2000**, *39* (1), 57–106.

Jablonski, N. G.; and Chaplin, G.; Human Skin Pigmentation as an Adaptation to UV Radiation. *Proc. Natl. Acad. Sci.* **2010**, *107* (Supp. 2), 8962–8968.

Keyser, C.; et al.; Ancient DNA Provides New Insights Into the History of South Siberian Kurgan People. *Hum. Genet.* **2009**, *126* (3), 395–410.

Koops, B.-J.; and Schellekens, M.; Forensic DNA Phenotyping: Regulatory Issues. *Colum. Sci. Tech. Law Rev.* **2008**, *9*, 158–160.

Kukla-Bartoszek, M.; et al.; Investigating the Impact of Age-Depended Hair Colour Darkening during Childhood on DNA-Based Hair Colour Prediction With the HIrisPlex System. *Forensic Sci. Int. Genet.* **2018**, *36*, 26–33.

Lacan, M.; et al.; Detection of the A189G MtDNA Heteroplasmic Mutation in Relation to Age in Modern and Ancient Bones. *Int. J. Legal Med.* **2009**, *123* (2), 161–167.

Lamason, R. L.; et al.; SLC24A5, a Putative Cation Exchanger, Affects Pigmentation in Zebrafish and Humans. *Science (80-.)* **2005**, *310* (5755), 1782–1786.

Lango Allen, H.; et al.; Hundreds of Variants Clustered in Genomic Loci and Biological Pathways Affect Human Height. *Nature* **2010**, *467* (7317), 832–838.

Levenson, V. V; and Melnikov, A. A.; DNA Methylation as Clinically Useful Biomarkers—Light at the End of the Tunnel. *Pharmaceuticals* **2012**, *5* (1), 94–113.

Li, R.; et al.; Six Novel Susceptibility Loci for Early-Onset Androgenetic Alopecia and Their Unexpected Association with Common Diseases. *PLoS Genet.* **2012**, *8* (5), e1002746.

Lingner, J.; et al.; Telomerase and DNA End Replication: No Longer a Lagging Strand Problem? *Science (80-.)* **1995**, *269* (5230), 1533–1535.

Lippert, C.; et al.; Identification of Individuals by Trait Prediction Using Whole-Genome Sequencing Data. *Proc. Natl. Acad. Sci.* **2017**, *114* (38), 10166–10171.

Liu, F.; et al.; A Genome-Wide Association Study Identifies Five Loci Influencing Facial Morphology in Europeans. *PLoS Genet.* **2012**, *8* (9), e1002932.

Loomis, W. F.; Skin-Pigment Regulation of Vitamin-D Biosynthesis in Man: Variation in Solar Ultraviolet at Different Latitudes May Have Caused Racial Differentiation in Man. *Science (80-.)* **1967**, *157* (3788), 501–506.

Marcińska, M.; et al.; Evaluation of DNA Variants Associated with Androgenetic Alopecia and Their Potential to Predict Male Pattern Baldness. *PLoS One* **2015**, *10* (5), e0127852.

Maroñas, O.; et al.; Development of a Forensic Skin Colour Predictive Test. *Forensic Sci. Int. Genet.* **2014**, *13*, 34–44.

Martinez-Cadenas, C.; et al.; Gender Is a Major Factor Explaining Discrepancies in Eye Colour Prediction Based on HERC2/OCA2 Genotype and the IrisPlex Model. *Forensic Sci. Int. Genet.* **2013**, *7* (4), 453–460.

McEvoy, B. P.; and Visscher, P. M.; Genetics of Human Height. *Econ. Hum. Biol.* **2009**, *7* (3), 294–306.

Meissner, C.; and Ritz-Timme, S.; Molecular Pathology and Age Estimation. *Forensic Sci. Int.* **2010**, *203* (1–3), 34–43.

Meissner, C.; et al.; Tissue-Specific Deletion Patterns of the Mitochondrial Genome With Advancing Age. *Exp. Gerontol.* **2006**, *41* (5), 518–524.

Mengel-From, J.; et al.; Human Eye Colour and HERC2, OCA2 and MATP. *Forensic Sci. Int. Genet.* **2010**, *4* (5), 323–328.

Ossorio, P. N.; About Face: Forensic Genetic Testing for Race and Visible Traits. *J. Law Med. Ethics* **2006**, *34* (2), 277–292.

Park, J.-L.; et al.; Identification and Evaluation of Age-Correlated DNA Methylation Markers for Forensic Use. *Forensic Sci. Int. Genet.* **2016**, *23*, 64–70.

Parra, E. J.; Human Pigmentation Variation: Evolution, Genetic Basis, and Implications for Public Health. *Am. J. Phys. Anthropol.* **2007**, *134* (S45), 85–105.

Pietroni, C.; et al.; The Effect of Gender on Eye Colour Variation in European Populations and an Evaluation of the IrisPlex Prediction Model. *Forensic Sci. Int. Genet.* **2014**, *11*, 1–6.

Pilin, A.; et al.; Changes in Colour of Different Human Tissues as a Marker of Age. *Int. J. Legal Med.* **2007**, *121* (2), 158–162.

Poon, S. S. S.; and Lansdorp, P. M.; Measurements of Telomere Length on Individual Chromosomes by Image Cytometry. *Methods Cell Biol.* **2001**, *64*, 69–96.

Pośpiech, E.; et al.; Further Evidence for Population Specific Differences in the Effect of DNA Markers and Gender on Eye Colour Prediction in Forensics. *Int. J. Legal Med.* **2016**, *130* (4), 923–934.

Pośpiech, E.; et al.; Towards Broadening Forensic DNA Phenotyping beyond Pigmentation: Improving the Prediction of Head Hair Shape from DNA. *Forensic Sci. Int. Genet.* **2018**, *37*, 241–251.

Rexbye, H.; et al.; Influence of Environmental Factors on Facial Ageing. *Age Ageing* **2006**, *35* (2), 110–115.

Richards, R.; et al.; Evaluation of Massively Parallel Sequencing for Forensic DNA Methylation Profiling. *Electrophoresis* **2018**, *39* (21), 2798–2805.

Ritz, S.; et al.; The Extent of Aspartic Acid Racemization in Dentin: A Possible Method for a More Accurate Determination of Age at Death? *Zeitschrift für Rechtsmedizin* **1990**, *103* (6), 457–462.

Ruiz, Y.; et al.; Further Development of Forensic Eye Color Predictive Tests. *Forensic Sci. Int. Genet.* **2013**, *7* (1), 28–40.

Samuel, G.; and Prainsack, B.; Forensic DNA Phenotyping in Europe: Views "on the Ground" from Those Who Have a Professional Stake in the Technology. *New Genet. Soc.* **2018**, 1–23.

Soares Bispo Santos Silva, D.; et al.; Evaluation of DNA Methylation Markers and Their Potential to Predict Human Aging. *Electrophoresis* **2015**, *36* (15), 1775–1780.

St-Pierre, J.; et al.; Topology of Superoxide Production from Different Sites in the Mitochondrial Electron Transport Chain. *J. Biol. Chem.* **2002**, *277* (47), 44784–44790.

Sturm, R. A.; et al.; A Single SNP in an Evolutionary Conserved Region Within Intron 86 of the HERC2 Gene Determines Human Blue-Brown Eye Color. *Am. J. Hum. Genet.* **2008**, *82* (2), 424–431.

Suh, J. R.; et al.; New Perspectives on Folate Catabolism. *Annu. Rev. Nutr.* **2001**, *21* (1), 255–282.

Tsuji, A.; et al.; Estimating Age of Humans Based on Telomere Shortening. *Forensic Sci. Int.* **2002**, *126* (3), 197–199.

Tully, G.; Genotype versus Phenotype: Human Pigmentation. *Forensic Sci. Int. Genet.* **2007**, *1* (2), 105–110.

Verzijl, N.; et al.; Age-Related Accumulation of Maillard Reaction Products in Human Articular Cartilage Collagen. *Biochem. J.* **2000**, *350* (2), 381–387.

Vidaki, A.; et al.; DNA Methylation-Based Forensic Age Prediction Using Artificial Neural Networks and Next Generation Sequencing. *Forensic Sci. Int. Genet.* **2017**, *28*, 225.

Vidaki, A.; and Kayser, M.; Recent Progress, Methods and Perspectives in Forensic Epigenetics. *Forensic Sci. Int. Genet.* **2018**, *37*, 180–195.

Wahl, S.; et al.; Epigenome-Wide Association Study of Body Mass Index, and the Adverse Outcomes of Adiposity. *Nature* **2017**, *541* (7635), 81.

Walsh, S.; et al.; Developmental Validation of the IrisPlex System: Determination of Blue and Brown Iris Colour for Forensic Intelligence. *Forensic Sci. Int. Genet.* **2011**, *5* (5), 464–471.

Walsh, S.; et al.; The HIrisPlex System for Simultaneous Prediction of Hair and Eye Colour from DNA. *Forensic Sci. Int. Genet.* **2013**, *7* (1), 98–115.

Weber-Lehmann, J.; et al.; Finding the Needle in the Haystack: Differentiating "Identical" Twins in Paternity Testing and Forensics by Ultra-Deep next Generation Sequencing. *Forensic Sci. Int. Genet.* **2014**, *9*, 42–46.

Wells, G. L.; and Olson, E. A.; Eyewitness Testimony. *Annu. Rev. Psychol.* **2003**, *54* (1), 277–295.

Wharton, B.; and Bishop, N.; Rickets. *Lancet* **2003**, *362* (9393), 1389–1400.

Whiteman, D. C.; et al.; Determinants of Melanocyte Density in Adult Human Skin. *Arch. Dermatol. Res.* **1999**, *291* (9), 511–516.

Wood, A. R.; et al.; Defining the Role of Common Variation in the Genomic and Biological Architecture of Adult Human Height. *Nat. Genet.* **2014**, *46* (11), 1173–1186.

Xu, C.; et al.; A Novel Strategy for Forensic Age Prediction by DNA Methylation and Support Vector Regression Model. *Sci. Rep.* **2016**, *5* (1), 17788.

Ye, C.; et al.; Quantitative Analysis of Mitochondrial DNA 4977-bp Deletion in Sporadic Breast Cancer and Benign Breast Diseases. *Breast Cancer Res. Treat.* **2008**, *108* (3), 427–434.

Zapico, S. C.; and Ubelaker, D. H.; MtDNA Mutations and Their Role in Aging, Diseases and Forensic Sciences. *Aging Dis.* **2013**, *4* (6), 364.

Zubakov, D.; et al.; Human Age Estimation From Blood Using MRNA, DNA Methylation, DNA Rearrangement, and Telomere Length. *Forensic Sci. Int. Genet.* **2016**, *24*, 33–43.

CHAPTER 9

Forensic Ancestry Inference: Data Requirements, Analysis Methods, and Interpretation of Results

OZLEM BULBUL[1] and KENNETH K. KIDD[2*]

[1]*Institute of Forensic Sciences, Istanbul University - Cerrahpasa, Istanbul, Turkey*

[2]*Department of Genetics, Yale University, New Haven, CT 06520-8005, USA*

Corresponding author. E-mail: kenneth.kidd@yale.edu

ABSTRACT

Being able to determine the biogeographic ancestry of an individual has been important in many forensic efforts to determine the identity of a partial or decayed body. Now a DNA sample can be the forensic equivalent of an unidentified individual using just some blood left at the scene of a crime or some semen left from a rape. The standard DNA markers, short tandem repeats, used globally to tie an individual to the crime scene DNA, are not good for inferring biogeographic ancestry because they do not vary much among populations. But they do vary greatly among individuals - every population has many alleles at each locus, but it is the same "many" in most populations. Single nucleotide polymorphisms (SNPs), on the other hand, can vary greatly in their frequencies among populations. Recent efforts by many researchers have begun to provide those markers. Panels of Ancestry Informative SNPs (AISNPs) have been developed by many researchers. These have been shown to vary in frequency among populations. Databases have been developed for estimating how likely it is for a DNA profile for those SNPs to occur in the different populations. Data requirements, analytic methods, and criteria for interpreting the results are all discussed.

9.1 INTRODUCTION

Over the past two decades forensic researchers have been developing panels of genetic markers for inference of the biogeographic ancestry of an individual. Multiple panels of ancestry-informative markers (AIMs) have been developed and published. One estimates an individual's ancestry using DNA polymorphisms. We note that ancestry inference is different in a forensic context from the direct to consumer companies that sell ancestry information. In a forensic context a small, highly informative panel of markers is desirable for comparisons with public databases; in the public ancestry inference context existing very large panels of single-nucleotide polymorphism (SNPs) are used and proprietary reference databases. However, similar logic underlies both: genetic similarity implies similar ancestry. In many different forensic situations the ability to estimate the ancestry of an unknown individual is a potentially valuable aid in identifying that unknown individual. It can be informative on identification of remains from a mass disaster or of remains from a single individual found "in the woods." Ancestry information can also help the police by narrowing the search for a criminal. But, in any situation, the ancestry information is helpful only to the degree it accurately narrows the likely ancestry of the unknown.

In forensic genetics, short tandem repeat (STRs) polymorphisms are the gold standards for individual identification, for example, matching a DNA profile from a crime scene with a suspect's profile. However, when it comes to ancestry estimation the primary forensic STRs do not provide sufficient ancestry information due to their high interpopulation allele sharing (Rosenberg et al., 2003). In a recent study the Rosenberg Lab tested 13 CODIS and 779 non-CODIS STR loci to determine whether or not these loci have any considerable information about ancestry (Algee-Hewitt et al., 2016). The researchers reported that despite forensic geneticists' above-mentioned common claim, the CODIS STR loci give similar ancestry information compared to 13 random non-CODIS tetranucleotide markers. This could be explained by substantial contribution of the high heterozygosity loci that could have rare alleles among populations (Algee-Hewitt et al., 2016). However, the accuracy level of ancestry information present in the STR loci is insufficient for reliable assignment. The genetic structure of populations can be analyzed better by SNPs that have known allele frequency variation among populations, than by other genomic variants (STRs or complex InDels). Consequently, most panels of AIMs use SNPs.

9.2 REQUIREMENTS FOR ANCESTRY-INFORMATIVE SNPs (AISNPs)

What are the more specifically forensic ancestry questions? In our opinion there are two. What is the best estimate of the ancestral origin of an unknown individual based on a DNA sample? How accurate is that estimate? [Note, it is always an estimate!] The AISNPs to address those questions must necessarily have allele frequencies that vary among populations. (For our purposes we lump small di-allelic insertion/deletion polymorphisms with SNPs.) A given SNP can only provide information about those populations that have different allele frequencies (Figure 9.1). If the allele frequencies are identical or nearly identical among a set of populations, that SNP will not be able to distinguish among those populations. What one often finds is that within a small biogeographic area the allele frequencies for any SNP are very similar. Thus, even though SNPs have frequencies that vary considerably around the world, they may not be able to provide ancestry information within any region but only information among distant groups of populations.

One can only estimate an individual's ancestry among the existing reference populations. Initially, a panel of SNPs is good only for the set of populations used to select the SNPs. As more populations are tested, the SNP panel may have broader applicability. Basically, the inference of ancestry can only be as good as the global coverage of the reference populations and the reference populations need to provide reasonable estimates of the allele frequencies of all the SNPs in the specific panel of SNPs.

Figure 9.1 shows several points. First, there are allele frequency differences among the continental level groups of populations in the 1000 Genomes data. Second, in the case of the specific SNP at DARC there is virtually no difference among any non-African population. Thus, while African ancestry will be suggested if the C allele is present, no specific region of non-African ancestry can be inferred if the alternative T allele is present. In contrast, the specific SNP at the EDAR locus will help differentiate East Asia and the Americas when the G allele is present but will not provide any distinction between Africa, Europe, or South Asia when the A allele is present.

Since the early 2000s many AISNPs panels have been published for the purpose of forensic ancestry assignment (Phillips et al., 2007; Kidd et al., 2014; Soundararajan et al., 2016; Mehta et al., 2017). Here we summarize the representative AISNPs panels developed for forensic applications (Table 9.1). Soundararajan et al. (2016) discussed the common SNPs, available reference populations, and the level of ancestry resolution for 21

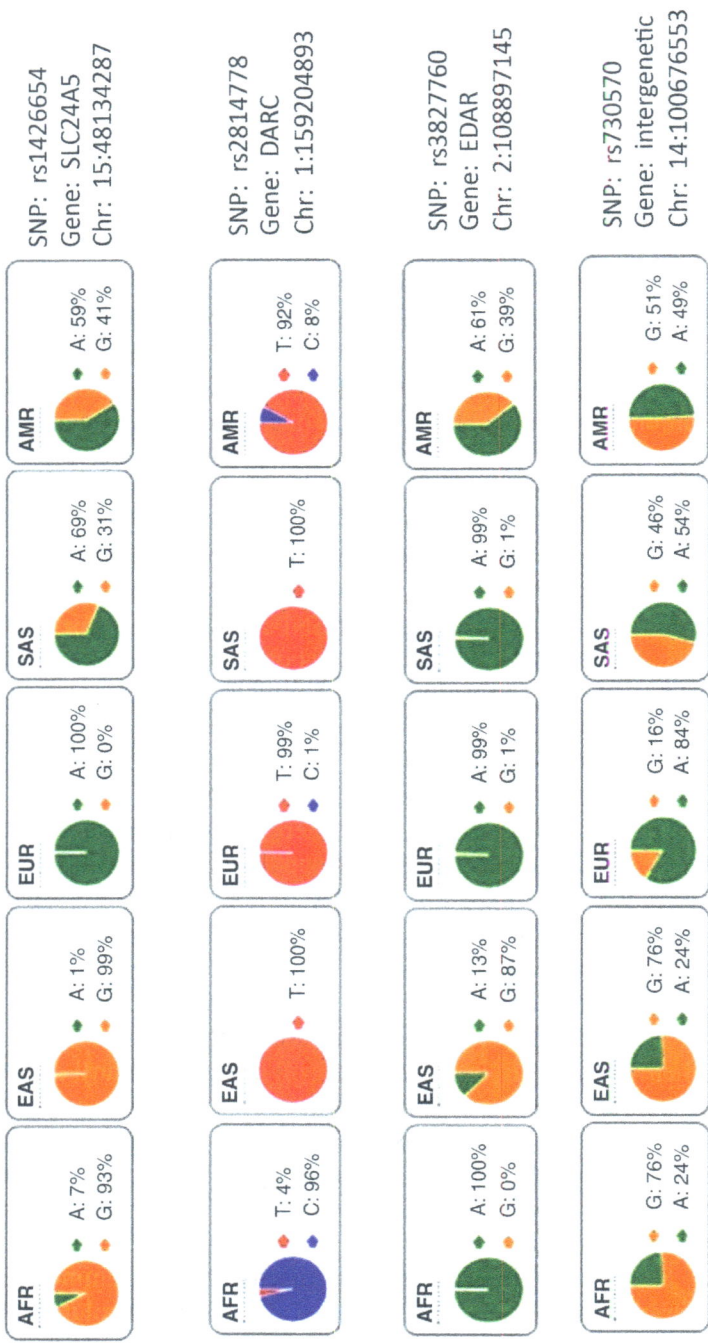

FIGURE 9.1 Four examples of highly informative ancestry informative SNPs (AISNPs) from the 1000 Genomes Phase 3 data. First three SNPs are fixed for European, African, and East Asian population, respectively. The last SNP has variation among populations.

independently published AISNP panels. That study showed that researchers put effort into selecting the best AISNPs primarily for differentiating populations at the continental level which could be achieved with only a few highly informative SNPs. A main issue has been the inadequate numbers of reference populations. The HGDP has 51 populations represented but many have small sample sizes and do not represent all regions of the world populations (Soundararajan et al., 2016). More recently the 1000 Genomes data have been used, but only 26 populations are represented and many regions of the world are not represented (Genomes Project et al., 2015). For most panels of AISNPs, it will be necessary to extend the available reference populations for finer biogeographic ancestry resolution instead of adding new panels for continental differentiations.

The panel of 55 AISNP developed by the Kidd Lab has one of the most comprehensive sets of reference populations; reference data exist for 164 populations from around the world. This panel can differentiate data on a large collection of the world's populations into at least 10 different population groups (Kidd et al., 2014; Pakstis et al., 2015). The allele frequencies of the studied populations are located in the reference database called ALlele FREquency Database (ALFRED) (https://alfred.med.yale.edu/alfred/index. asp). The inference of the biogeographic ancestry can be made using these allele frequencies on the web tool Forensic Resource/Reference on Genetics knowledge base, FROG-kb (http://frog.med.yale.edu/frogkb) (Kidd et al., 2017), which has data for many panels of AISNPs (Table 9.1).

Many different laboratory techniques can be used to genotype SNPs. However, in forensics a relatively few SNP genotyping techniques are in common use. The SNaPshot™ (Thermo Fisher Scientific, Waltham, MA, USA) minisequencing method predominates in the forensic literature. TaqMan™ hybridization probes (Thermo Fisher Scientific), hybridization microarrays, and massively parallel sequencing (MPS) are also being used.

SNaPshot™ (Thermo Fisher Scientific) method, a type of minisequencing, has been the most commonly applied to forensic DNA analysis primarily because it uses the PCR and capillary electrophoresis equipment already available in forensic laboratories. It has good sensitivity and modest multiplexing capability. SNaPshot™ (Thermo Fisher Scientific) allows genotyping of up to 30–35 SNPs in a single reaction (Mehta et al., 2017). In the reaction, the primer binds to a DNA region that is adjacent to the targeted SNP marker. Then the targeted SNP is extended with a single fluorochrome-labeled dideoxyribonucleoside triphosphate (ddNTP). The reaction mixture contains the four possible ddNTPs, each with a different fluor. Since the

TABLE 9.1 Representative Ancestry-Informative SNP (AISNP) Panels in FROG-kb.

Panel Name	No. of SNPs	SNP Type	Method	Targeted Populations/Regions	References
SNPforID 34-plex	34	AISNPs	SNaPshot™	Europe, Asia, Africa and America	Phillips et al. (2007)
128-SNPs	128	AISNPs	TaqMan	Admixed Americans	Kosoy et al. (2009)
41-SNPs	41	AISNPs	SNPlex and Sequenome iPLEX	Africa, Middle East, Europe, Central/South Asia, East Asia, the Americas and Oceania	Nievergelt et al. (2013)
Eurasiaplex	23	AISNPs	SNaPshot™	Europe and South Asia	Phillips et al. (2013)
50-SNPs	50	AISNPs and PISNPs	SNaPshot™	U.S. populations (African American, East Asian, European American, and Hispanic American/Native American)	Gettings et al. (2014)
55 AISNPs	55	AISNPs	TaqMan	Global populations	Kidd et al. (2014)
EUROFORGEN Global AIM-SNP	128	AISNPs	Sequenom iPLEX® (MPS)	Africa, Europe, East Asia, Native America and Oceania	Phillips et al. (2014)
Pacifiplex	29	AISNPs	SNaPshot™	Oceania	Santos et al. (2016)
EurEas_Gplex	14	AISNPs	SNaPshot™	Europe and East Asia	Daca-Roszak et al. (2016)
27-plex SNP	27	AISNPs	SNaPshot™	Africa, Europe, and East Asia	Wei et al. (2016)
74 AISNPs	74	AISNPs	Taqman	within East Asia	Li et al. (2016)
86 AISNPs	86	AISNPs	Taqman, MPS	Southwest Asia	Bulbul and Filoglu (2018), Bulbul et al. (2018)
HID-Ion AmpliSeq™ Ancestry Panel	165[a]	AISNPs	Ion PGM (MPS)	Continental populations (subset of Kidd lab populations)	Thermo Fisher Scientific, Kosoy et al., 2009, Kidd et al., 2014)
ForenSeq™ DNA Signature Prep Kit	164[b]	IISNPs, AISNPs, PISNPs, STRs	MiSeq FGx (MPS)	Continental populations (subset of Kidd lab populations)	The Illumina®, Churchill et al. (2016)

[a] HID-Ion AmpliSeq™ Ancestry Panel includes Kidd 55 and Seldin 128 AISNPs panels.

[b] ForenSeq™ DNA Signature Prep Kit includes Kidd 55 AISNPs panel.

ddNTP does not have a 3'OH group, the DNA polymerase enzyme cannot add a new nucleotide to the chain, resulting in only the single-base extension incorporating the specific nucleotide with its specific fluor (Phillips et al., 2007, Mehta et al., 2017).

Recent MPS, previously termed Next-Generation Sequencing, technologies allow genotyping of hundreds of SNPs in multiple samples simultaneously by employing an oligonucleotide sample barcoding strategy (Borsting and Morling, 2015). Four different methods can be used in the sequencing: pyrosequencing (Roche 454), semiconductor (Thermo Fisher Scientific Ion Torrent ™), sequencing by sequencing (Illumina), or ligation (Thermo Fisher Scientific SOLiD™). These methods differ from company to company, the most important criteria in the MPS are reading length and total number of cluster reads in each run (Ratan et al., 2013).

The MPS technology appears to have an important role in future forensic studies with high advantages in typing many DNA markers (such as STR, SNP, Indel) together and hence could provide all information in a single run. The new MPS panels have started to be produced by researchers and commercial companies, and the system has also started to be used in forensic casework (Phillips et al., 2014; Borsting and Morling, 2015; Hollard et al., 2017) (Table 9.1). This technology allows the high-throughput sequencing of DNA in an extremely rapid and streamlined fashion. Although the routine use of MPS technology in forensic laboratories is proceeding slowly; in the long term it will probably be used routinely in many labs.

9.3 REQUIREMENTS FOR REFERENCE POPULATIONS

Highly reliable ancestry assignment could be made by using the most complete possible coverage of world populations and a highly informative panel of AISNPs. The 1000 Genomes, Human Genome Diversity Project—Center d'Étude du Polymorphisme Humain (HGDP–CEPH) panel, HapMap are the most commonly preferred publicly available population data. However it is important to discuss how well reference populations represent global diversity.

Around 1000 Genomes, launched in 2008, aimed to create the largest public catalog of human variation and genotype data from a wide range of global populations, including previously characterized HapMap samples. The 1000 Genomes Phase 3 provides genetic data of the 2504 individuals from 26 populations by grouping them as Africa, Europe, East Asia, South Asia, and America (Genomes Project et al., 2015) as shown in Figure 9.1.

The HGDP–CEPH panel consists of genetic data on 1050 individuals from 52 world populations (Rosenberg, 2006). Although the global coverage of the HGDP–CEPH panel is wider, the numbers of the individuals for many populations are under 20 samples resulting in poor accuracy for individual SNP allele frequencies.

The ALFRED database contains allele frequency data of polymorphisms in human populations. The site has been developed for scientific and educational purposes and today includes 724 populations and 664,290 polymorphisms. Some of the allele frequencies on the site consist of data from Kidd Laboratory of Yale University, some published articles and selected data from some other population projects (such as the 1000 Genomes Project, HapMap) (Rajeevan et al., 2012a) to complement population data of SNP panels published for forensic purposes, which can be accessed on the site (https://alfred.med.yale.edu/alfred/snpSets.asp).

9.4 ANALYSIS METHODS

Accurate and efficient estimation of an individual ancestry depends on excellent algorithmic methods. The reliability of these analyses depends on the reference populations, the number of markers tested, the informativeness of the marker, and the degree of the admixture. STRUCTURE and principal component analysis (PCA) are commonly used for population genetics. In forensics besides these analyses, the specific programs, such as FROG-kb (http://frog.med.yale.edu/FrogKB/) and Snipper (http://mathgene.usc.es/snipper/), are designed using the likelihood approach (Phillips et al., 2007; Kidd et al., 2017). All these analysis methods require reference populations for estimating most likely ancestry of an individual based on allele frequencies. Here, we briefly explain STRUCTURE, PCA, Snipper, and FROG-kb analyses. Then we will give examples of the Snipper and FROG-kb analyses.

9.4.1 STRUCTURE ANALYSIS

STRUCTURE, the genetic similarity clustering algorithm, is the most widely used program for population analysis. The program applies a model-based Bayesian clustering approach by using genotype data to infer the presence of distinct populations, identify admixed populations, and assign individuals to specific groups based on similarity of variation patterns (Pritchard et al., 2000). Although STRUCTURE is now commonly used, there are potential

problems in how the results are interpreted. The results for the same populations can be different if different numbers of individuals are analyzed, especially if the proportions of individuals that will belong to different clusters
are very different. Differences in the actual evolutionary relationships of the
observed clusters and the different demographic histories of the populations
can easily lead to misleading patterns (Lawson et al., 2018). STRUCTURE
is often used for estimating admixture but this may cause misinterpreting
the questioned individual who may come from intermediate populations.
It could only provide reliable results when a reference set of individuals
with known admixture is included in the analysis. STRUCTURE analysis is
very useful for assessing the differentiation power of a certain marker set.
Moreover, the graphical illustrations of the results could be easily evaluated
by using CLUMPAK software (Kopelman et al., 2015).

9.4.2 PRINCIPAL COMPONENT ANALYSIS (PCA)

The PCA is used for visualizing population structure by graphically
grouping populations with similar genetic ancestry together (Cavalli-Sforza
et al., 1994). It is the most widely used type of multidimensional scaling
analyses that can be used to reduce a large set of variables to a small set
called principal components. It is a computationally efficient method if
the markers are used for controlling population substructure in association
studies. Each of the created PCs incorporates a proportion of the variation
and the proportion decreases as the number of PCs increases. Generally, the
first three PCs account for a large percentage of total variation and efficiently
represent the main patterns of genetic divergence in the dataset. The PCA of
reference population data with an individual of unknown ancestry would be
informative for defining the most likely ancestry of the individual based on
its relative position with respect to the reference populations.

9.4.3 SNIPPER

The Snipper, a web-based application, employs a Bayesian approach to calculate likelihoods of membership to ancestry groups inferred from embedded
or user-defined training sets (reference populations). The training sets can be
simply organized by using an Excel file with genotypes from HGDP–CEPH,
HapMap, or 1000 Genomes, or user-defined reference populations (Phillips
et al., 2007). The results are shown in two ways, "Bayes" and PCA analysis,

"Bayes" ranks the likelihoods and predicts the most likely ancestry; PCA illustrates the position of the unknown profile compared to the reference data and the prediction of the ancestry. Snipper estimates eigenvalues of the reference and unknown individuals' genotypes and positions them into clusters. The output illustrates PC1 and PC2 plots with individual references population clusters (in varying colors) and the position of the unknown individual (in black).

9.4.4 FROG-kb

In FROG-kb calculations, the genotype of the person is entered into the system and the program calculates the probability of that genotype arising in each of the reference populations available for the set of SNPs used. The FROG-kb calculations are based on the allele frequencies of the SNPs in the reference populations embedded in the system. The results are in the form of a list of populations, ranked by the probability of the subject's genotype occurring in each population from highest to lowest (Rajeevan et al., 2012b; Bulbul et al., 2016). Those probabilities are equivalent to population-specific random match probabilities. Those probabilities also become likelihoods when considering which population is the most likely origin of the target person. The likelihood ratios are given for each population comparing the most likely to each of the other populations.

9.5 EXAMPLES AND INTERPRETATION

How does one interpret an individual genotype for a panel of AISNPs against a set of reference populations? The assumption always made is that the reference population with the highest frequency of the individual's genotype is the population of origin. That assumption is likely false in the strictest sense but is the only possible default logic. The proper approach to implementing this assumption is to consider likelihood: the population with the highest probability of producing the genotype is the most likely population of origin *among the reference populations considered*. Then one can consider multiple populations of origin and rank their relative likelihoods.

The analysis provided by the Snipper web portal (http://mathgene.usc. es/snipper/) is based on the principle of comparing an unknown sample with reference population data based on likelihood ratios. Snipper sorts individual likelihoods in descending order and provides a prediction based on the ratio of the highest likelihoods. The reference population data (three to five major populations) are embedded for certain panels of AISNPs (e.g., 34-plex, 46 InDels). Additionally, Snipper allows construction of training sets following the function of "Binary AIM classification of individuals," classification with a custom Excel file of populations including a maximum 10,000 individual genotypes. Therefore, it can be used for any panel of SNPs for which reference genotypes are available (Phillips et al., 2007).

An example of Snipper result to analyze a EUROFORGEN Global AIM-SNP (128 AISNPs) profile is shown below (Figure 9.2). The sample is selected randomly from Toscani individual genotype in 1000 Genomes catalog (NA20806). The reference sets are available under "Forensic MPS AIMs Panel Reference Sets" for tested panel. The reference population genotypes are built from published 1000 Genomes Phase 3 and Simons Foundation Genome Diversity Project genotypes. We used the following function "Binary AIM classification of multiple individuals" with downloaded fixed reference set on Snipper web tool.

A statistical analysis of a EUROFORGEN Global AIM-SNP profile with Africa, Europe, East Asia, Oceania, South Asia, and America reference data is made immediately after the profile genotype was uploaded. The sample profile was compared to six-group reference population data. The prediction is "this profile a billion (10^9) times more likely to be European than South Asian or American, respectively." Therefore, ancestry likelihoods show the individual is much more likely to be European. Snipper also generates PCA plots showing the system of overlaying an unknown profile onto reference population data clusters. PC1 and PC2 view of populations and classified profile is shown in Figure 9.2. In the PCA plot, the black point is the tested sample profile is clustered with European reference population group (green points) and distinct from other population clusters (Figure 9.2).

The analyses provided at the FROG-kb web portal (http://frog.med. yale.edu/FrogKB/#) are also based on likelihood and likelihood ratios. The probability of the genotype of the unknown sample is calculated for each reference population. That probability is then considered the likelihood of the reference population being the ancestral origin of the unknown. Those likelihoods are then sorted and listed from most likely to least likely. The likelihood ratio for the most likely to each of the alternatives is calculated and printed. A difference from Snipper output is that reference population data are available for several different panels of SNPs and output provides the raw likelihoods are provided for each individual reference population. Dozens to over a hundred different reference populations are available, depending on the panel of SNPs considered. It is up to the user to decide

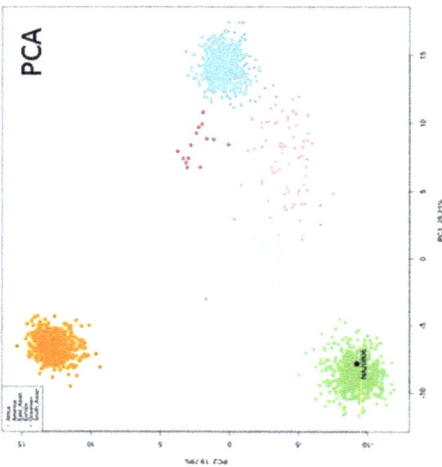

FIGURE 9.2 An example of Snipper web application (http://mathgene.usc.es/snipper/).

on the interpretation at the level of continent, region within a continent, or individual population level. The reference populations that have a likelihood ratio of less than one order of magnitude are flagged. The alternative ancestral populations within that likelihood ratio are considered not significantly different from the most likely.

The genotype of the same Toscani individual (NA20806) was also used for ancestry assignment using FROG-kb (http://frog.med.yale.edu/FrogKB/), which currently includes 164 reference populations for the 55 AISNP panel (Figure 9.3). The top 30 likelihoods are shown for Kidd 55 AISNP panel for the current reference populations. The highest population likelihood was observed for the Toscani (TSI) population. The South European and Mediterranean populations are observed within one order of magnitude. The results strongly show that this individual could be from Southern Europe. It is important to note that (as it is discussed in the previous studies) the highest likelihood is not certainly the definitive ancestry of the unknown individual and several nearby populations are likely to also have high likelihoods. While the known origin of this individual (Tuscan) was the most likely outcome, the analyses themselves could not definitively prove that over other southern European origins. Hence, a careful interpretation of the ancestry prediction should be made when reporting the results (Bulbul et al., 2016; Li et al., 2016; Kidd et al., 2017; Jin et al., 2018).

The prediction differences between Snipper and Frog-kb arise from the differences in number of and specific reference populations. This once again shows us the importance of using the most comprehensive population data as references.

9.6   THE FUTURE

Given that many panels of SNPs for forensic inference of ancestry have been published, the immediate need is not the development of a new panel of ancestry inference SNPs. Rather the field needs to improve the ability to compare how well the different SNPs can contribute to refined ancestry of an individual. The various panels involve quite diverse sets of SNPs and different reference populations. Often the SNP panels share only a relatively small number of populations restricted to resolving ancestry to only a continental level. The relative merits of the various panels or the individual SNPs within a panel cannot be readily evaluated because the individual panels have often been developed based on different sets of reference populations. As noted earlier (Soundararajan et al., 2016), there is a need for better international

238   *Forensic DNA Analysis*

KiddLab - Set of 55 AISNPs

Computed on: Wed Mar 20 2019 12:00:27 GMT+0300 (Arabistan Standart Saati)

Printed on: Wed Mar 20 2019 12:00:45 GMT+0300 (Arabistan Standart Saati)

Population likelihoods based on 55 SNPs and 164 reference populations for the DNA profile:

Print   Close

⊘ **Indicates the values are within an order of magnitude of the highest likelihood.**

Population(Region, sampleSize 2N)	Probability of Genotype in each Population	Likelihood Ratio
Toscani(TSI)(Europe,214)	⊘6.836E-13	
Iberian(IBS)(Europe,214)	⊘2.098E-13	3.26
Syriacs(Asia,250)	⊘2.071E-13	3.3
Basque(Europe,216)	⊘1.504E-13	4.55
Greek Cypriots(Europe,190)	⊘1.431E-13	4.78
Hungarians(Europe,184)	⊘7.653E-14	8.93
Ashkenazi Jews(Europe,166)	⊘7.301E-14	9.36
Turkish(Asia,154)	4.895E-14	14.0
Russians(Europe,96)	3.49E-14	19.6
Turkish Cypriots(Europe,120)	2.968E-14	23.0
Sardinian(Europe,68)	2.943E-14	23.2
Greeks(Europe,104)	2.47E-14	27.7
Yazidis(Asia,298)	1.518E-14	45.0
Norwegians(Europe,400)	1.372E-14	49.8
Adygei(Europe,108)	1.264E-14	54.1
Mixed Europeans(Europe,190)	1.184E-14	57.7
Chuvash(Europe,84)	1.005E-14	68.0
British(GBR)(Europe,182)	9.833E-15	69.5
Turks(Asia,200)	7.264E-15	94.1
Danes(Europe,284)	6.793E-15	101.0
Russians_Archangel'sk(Europe,68)	5.083E-15	134.0
Finns(FIN)(Europe,198)	4.408E-15	155.0
Palestinian Arabs(Asia,140)	4.107E-15	166.0
Kurds(Asia,296)	4.074E-15	168.0
Danes(Europe,102)	3.374E-15	203.0
Turkmen(Asia,258)	2.947E-15	232.0
Arabs from Northern Iraq(Asia,260)	2.664E-15	257.0
Mixed Europeans(CEU)(Europe,198)	2.535E-15	270.0
Roman Jews(Europe,54)	2.085E-15	328.0
Druze(Asia,212)	2.059E-15	332.0

FIGURE 9.3   An example of the Frog-kb output. Only first 30 highest likelihoods are shown.

collaboration to see if the various panels of AISNPs can be tested on the same populations to allow a direct comparison of how well different SNPs contribute to refined estimation of ancestry.

KEYWORDS

- **ancestry-informative SNPs**
- **reference populations**
- **panels of markers**
- **"continental" populations analysis methods**

REFERENCES

Algee-Hewitt, B. F.; et al.; Individual identifiability predicts population identifiability in forensic microsatellite markers. *Curr Biol* **2016**, 26 (7), 935–942.

Borsting, C.; and Morling, N.; Next generation sequencing and its applications in forensic genetics. *Forensic Sci Int Genet* **2015**, 18, 78–89.

Bulbul, O.; and Filoglu, G.; Development of a SNP panel for predicting biogeographical ancestry and phenotype using massively parallel sequencing. *Electrophoresis* **2018**, 39 (21), 2743–2751.

Bulbul, O.; et al.; Evaluating a subset of ancestry informative SNPs for discriminating among Southwest Asian and circum-Mediterranean populations. *Forensic Sci Int Genet* **2016**, 23, 153–158.

Bulbul, O.; et al.; Improving ancestry distinctions among Southwest Asian populations. *Forensic Sci Int Genet* **2018**, 35, 14–20.

Cavalli-Sforza, L. L.; et al.; *The history and geography of human genes*. Princeton University Press: Princeton, NJ, 1994.

Churchill, J. D.; et al.; Evaluation of the Illumina(®) Beta Version ForenSeq DNA Signature Prep Kit for use in genetic profiling. *Forensic Sci Int Genet* **2016**, 20, 20–29.

Daca-Roszak, P.; et al.; EurEAs_Gplex—A new SNaPshot assay for continental population discrimination and gender identification. *Forensic Sci Int Genet* **2016**, 20, 89–100.

1000 Genomes Project; et al.; *A global reference for human genetic variation. Nature* **2015**, 526 (7571), 68–74.

Gettings, K. B.; et al.; A 50-SNP assay for biogeographic ancestry and phenotype prediction in the U.S. population. *Forensic Sci Int Genet* **2014**, 8 (1), 101–108.

Hollard, C.; et al.; Case report: On the use of the HID-Ion AmpliSeq Ancestry Panel in a real forensic case. *Int J Legal Med* **2017**, 131 (2), 351–358.

Jin, S.; et al.; Implementing a biogeographic ancestry inference service for forensic casework. *Electrophoresis* **2018**, 39 (21), 2757–2765.

Kidd, K. K.; et al.; The redesigned Forensic Research/Reference on Genetics-knowledge base, FROG-kb. *Forensic Sci Int Genet* **2017**, 33, 33–37.

Kidd, K. K.; et al.; Progress toward an efficient panel of SNPs for ancestry inference. *Forensic Sci Int Genet* **2014**, 10, 23–32.

Kopelman, N. M.; et al.; Clumpak: A program for identifying clustering modes and packaging population structure inferences across K. *Mol Ecol Resour* **2015**, 15 (5), 1179–1191.

Kosoy, R.; et al.; Ancestry informative marker sets for determining continental origin and admixture proportions in common populations in America. *Hum Mutat* **2009**, 30 (1), 69–78.

Lawson, D. J.; et al.; A tutorial on how not to over-interpret STRUCTURE and ADMIXTURE bar plots. *Nat Commun* **2018**, 9 (1), 3258.

Li, C. X.; et al.; A panel of 74 AISNPs: Improved ancestry inference within Eastern Asia. *Forensic Sci Int Genet* **2016**, 23, 101–110.

Mehta, B.; et al.; Forensically relevant SNaPshot(R) assays for human DNA SNP analysis: A review. *Int J Legal Med* **2017**, 131 (1), 21–37.

Nievergelt, C. M.; et al.; Inference of human continental origin and admixture proportions using a highly discriminative ancestry informative 41-SNP panel. *Investg Genet* **2013**, 4 (1), 13.

Pakstis, A. J.; et al.; 52 additional reference population samples for the 55 AISNP panel. *Forensic Sci Int Genet* **2015**, 19, 269–271.

Phillips, C.; et al.; Eurasiaplex: A forensic SNP assay for differentiating European and South Asian ancestries. *Forensic Sci Int Genet* **2013**, 7 (3), 359–366.

Phillips, C.; et al.; Building a forensic ancestry panel from the ground up: The EUROFORGEN Global AIM-SNP set. *Forensic Sci Int Genet* **2014**, 11, 13–25.

Phillips, C.; et al.; Inferring ancestral origin using a single multiplex assay of ancestry-informative marker SNPs. *Forensic Sci Int Genet* **2007**, 1 (3–4), 273–280.

Pritchard, J. K.; et al.; Inference of population structure using multilocus genotype data. *Genetics* **2000**, 155 (2), 945–959.

Rajeevan, H.; et al.; ALFRED: An allele frequency resource for research and teaching. *Nucleic Acids Res* **2012a**, 40 (Database issue), D1010–1015.

Rajeevan, H.; et al.; Introducing the Forensic Research/Reference on Genetics knowledge base, FROG-kb. *Investig Genet* **2012b**, 3 (1), 18.

Ratan, A.; et al.; Comparison of sequencing platforms for single nucleotide variant calls in a human sample. *PLoS One* **2013**, 8 (2), e55089.

Rosenberg, N. A.; Standardized subsets of the HGDP–CEPH Human Genome Diversity Cell Line Panel, accounting for atypical and duplicated samples and pairs of close relatives. *Ann Hum Genet* **2006**, 70 (6), 841–847.

Rosenberg, N. A.; et al.; Informativeness of genetic markers for inference of ancestry. *Am J Hum Genet* **2003**, 73 (6), 1402–1422.

Santos, C.; et al.; Pacifiplex: an ancestry-informative SNP panel centred on Australia and the Pacific region. *Forensic Sci Int Genet* **2016**, 20, 71–80.

Soundararajan, U.; et al.; Minimal SNP overlap among multiple panels of ancestry informative markers argues for more international collaboration. *Forensic Sci Int Genet* **2016**, 23, 25–32.

Wei, Y. L.; et al.; A single-tube 27-plex SNP assay for estimating individual ancestry and admixture from three continents. *Int J Legal Med* **2016**, 130 (1), 27–37.

CHAPTER 10

Online Population Data Resources for Forensic SNP Analysis with Massively Parallel Sequencing: An Overview of Online Population Data for Forensic Purposes

CHRISTOPHER PHILLIPS[1*], JORGE AMIGO[2], DENNIS MCNEVIN[3],
MARIA DE LA PUENTE[1,4], ELAINE Y. Y. CHEUNG[1,5], and
MARIA VICTORIA LAREU[1]

[1] *Forensic Genetics Unit, Institute of Forensic Sciences,
Faculty of Medicine, University of Santiago de Compostela, Galicia, Spain*

[2] *Grupo de Medicina Xenómica (GMX), Faculty of Medicine,
University of Santiago de Compostela, Galicia, Spain*

[3] *Centre for Forensic Science, School of Mathematical and Physical
Sciences (MaPS), Faculty of Science, University of Technology Sydney,
Ultimo, NSW 2007, Australia*

[4] *Institute of Legal Medicine, Innsbruck Medical University,
Innsbruck, Austria*

[5] *National Centre for Forensic Studies, Faculty of Science and Technology,
University of Canberra, ACT 2617, Australia*

Corresponding author. E-mail: c.phillips@mac.com

ABSTRACT

Recently, extensive catalogs of human variation derived from whole-genome sequencing have been released as openly accessible archives of sequence variants—a resource that is highly suitable for selecting markers for new forensic tests using massively parallel sequencing. In particular, the comparison of population patterns in these databases of variants can help identify markers suitable for the inference of ancestry that can then form informative forensic assays for this purpose. This chapter outlines in detail the ancestry or co-ancestry composition, genotype data access details, and geographic distributions of the samples in the most extensive variant catalogs of: 1000 Genomes; the HGDP–CEPH panel; Simons Foundation Human Genome Diversity Project; and Estonian Biocentre Genome Diversity Panel. While 1000 Genomes systematically characterizes a large number of samples from a limted number of carefully selected populations and restricts itself to five to six populations per continent, both SGDP and EGDP have analyzed only 2–4 samples per geographic location and these are much more widely dispersed geographically. The pros and cons of each approach are discussed, and details are provided of more recently published variant compilation projects with much larger sample sizes, notably the genome aggregation database gnomAD.

10.1 INTRODUCTION

In the last five years, massively parallel sequencing (MPS; alternatively, next generation sequencing) technology has gained increasing interest in its potential use for forensic DNA analysis. With good reason, MPS not only provides much greater data depths, offering the ability to characterize the sequence variation within isometric (identical size) short tandem repeat (STR)-length alleles as well as the ability to genotype multiple SNPs on the same sequence strand (Kidd et al., 2017), but, more importantly for forensics, MPS has also enhanced sensitivity (Eduardoff et al., 2015) and works efficiently from expanded polymerase chain reaction multiplex scales that make best use of the limited DNA obtained from evidential material.

At the current stage in the development of MPS for forensic analysis, early adopting laboratories are mainly engaged in optimizing the workflows to genotype established STRs or introducing use of identification single-nucleotide polymorphisms (SNPs) to analyze highly degraded DNA. Important additional forensic analyses offered by the two main MPS system suppliers (Verogen, San Diego, USA and Thermo Fisher Scientific, Waltham, MA, USA) are SNP-based predictive tests for externally visible characteristics (EVCs) that genotype coding SNPs, and for biogeographical ancestry using ancestry-informative markers (AIMs). Verogen offers such tests as part of a large-scale, all-in-one multiplex that combines STRs and SNPs. Thermo Fisher offers their forensic tests as separate stand-alone multiplexes for sequence library preparation using multiplexes for identification SNPs, ancestry SNPs (EVC–SNPs as a custom "community panel"), and STRs. As well as potentially providing investigative leads in the absence of eyewitness testimony or a DNA database match, forensic ancestry analysis can enhance the prediction of a person's physical characteristics, inform appropriate choice of STR allele frequencies in familial search strategies, and confirm the stated ancestry of sample donors used in population allele frequency databases, to help maintain their accuracy (Phillips, 2015).

The adoption of ancestry analysis in forensic laboratories requires a step change in the approaches used for population data analysis that must aim to apply the full range of statistical ancestry tests to the SNP genotypes generated by MPS. The main analysis regimes that can help construct a picture of an unknown person's most likely ancestry include: Bayes likelihood ratio calculations, genetic cluster analysis using well established algorithms such as STRUCTURE or ADMIXTURE (which also apply Bayesian principles), genetic distance estimation, and multidimensional scaling, of which principal component analysis (PCA) and discriminant analysis of principal components are the most widely used approaches. The most reliable outcomes from all of the above analyses in terms of ancestry inference are obtained by applying comprehensive population data as the reference with which to compare the unknown casework SNP profile(s). In addition, the recent adoption of SNP analysis for identification of individuals from highly degraded remains takes the form of supplementary tests adding genetic data to failed or incomplete STR genotyping, which requires allele frequency data relevant to the populations of a laboratory's region, in order to construct appropriate kinship test statistics. Unfortunately, producing broadly based population data for use in a forensic laboratory is no easy task and is often hampered by a range of challenges—limited availability of samples from across the world that represent the full extent of human population variation, the expense and complexity of MPS analyses which may be used to generate the SNP genotypes, the possibility of disjoints between a person's actual ancestry and the location they are sampled, and making the appropriate choice of SNPs to genotype, as MPS-based forensic SNP genotyping continues to evolve.

A growing body of freely available online whole-genome variant data solves many of the challenges facing a forensic laboratory just starting to analyze ancestry with MPS and seeking to build up suitable population reference data. This chapter reviews the population and marker composition of the current major online whole-genome variant databases of 1000 Genomes (now curated in the International Genome Sample Resource: IGSR); Simons Foundation Genome Diversity Project (SGDP); and Estonian Biocentre Genome Diversity Project (EGDP). Additional genomic databases have accessible online data but also have certain limits; the most informative of these for forensic data are the genome Aggregation Database (gnomAD) that compiles SNP allele frequencies only. The commonly referenced Human Genome Diversity Project panel—Center d'Étude du Polymorphisme Humain (HGDP–CEPH) has data for a large but finite subset of SNPs, extensive in number, but sometimes lacking certain key loci used in forensic analysis (e.g., the most ancestry-informative SNP in forensic use, rs2814778).

10.2   THE 1000 GENOMES PHASE-3 VARIANT DATA FROM 2504 WHOLE GENOME SEQUENCES

Since the closure of the first genome variation collaborative program of HapMap, the 1000 Genomes project [http://www.internationalgenome.org] has been the major international consortium recording patterns of human variation from whole genome sequencing. The main project goal was to describe most of the genetic variation occurring at a population frequency greater than 1%, so deep sequencing of DNA from large-scale population samples was the defining factor in the project's framework of analysis. The project has now officially closed but the data continues to provide a rich source of variants and patterns of human variation that can be used for developing new and enhanced SNP panels for forensic applications. The project's Pilot 1 analysis, (the 1000 Genomes Low Coverage Pilot) comprised 180 individuals from four of the original HapMap populations (with acronyms: CEU European; YRI African; JPT Japanese; CHB Chinese), sequenced at 2× to 4× coverage - so an average 2–4 sequences were generated at each nucleotide position. Pilot 1 sequence data identified over nine million novel SNPs, as well as new insertions–deletion polymorphisms (Indels), and a smaller number of new structural variants, for example, segmental duplications not previously identified (the 1000 Genomes Project Consortium, 2010). An important finding from the Pilot 1 data was that a disproportionate number of the novel SNPs discovered were population specific, occurring in only one of the four populations studied. Most common variants had already been identified by HapMap, but when this project was completed the widely discussed problem of "missing heritability" turned the focus of medical genetics studies on rare rather than common variation. The 1000 Genomes successfully identified a large number of such rare variants and most were present in only one of the Pilot 1 test populations. Furthermore, HapMap used SNP arrays as the main genotyping approach, rather than sequencing; so relatively few low-frequency functional variants in coding regions were identified compared to 1000 Genomes as arrays mainly type tagSNPs closely sited to genes plus common gene variants.

The project's intermediate period comprised extensive development of precise but efficient sequencing strategies using the experience of Pilot 1 studies (i.e., calibrating the read coverage necessary for accurate reporting of a nucleotide site as a variant, not a mis-sequenced position); expansion of population sampling from the initial 4–12, then 26 discrete populations; and the analysis of variant inheritance patterns in family trios - work which formed the bulk of what is now described as Phase 1 and Phase 2 project stages. A full human variant catalog was released after Phase 1 and consisted of 28 million variants in 629 individuals from 12 populations (the 1000 Genomes Project Consortium, 2012). The Phase 1 catalog of variation can be accessed in a straightforward genomic query system called ENGINES in the SPSmart suite of SNP database browsers (Amigo et al., 2011 [http://spsmart. cesga.es]). The ENGINES browser remains the easiest and most informative way to collect data for multiple SNPs from 1000 Genomes, although Phase 1 data has now been superseded by the Phase 3 variant catalog, this final data release has not yet been adopted by SPSmart, so Phase 3 queries can only be made for individual variant sites. Therefore, when a long list of SNPs (as rs-numbers) is encountered in a population genetics publication or one reporting a new forensic SNP set, these can be uploaded directly into ENGINES and all the relevant genomic details plus full genotype lists in the 12 Phase 1 study populations can be obtained in a single query. A final important note is that multiple-allele SNPs (consisting of three or four recorded nucleotide substitution alleles at a single variant position) were not included in the Phase 1 data, presumably because most of these sites were considered to be sequencing errors and required more detailed checks of their sequence data quality during Phase 2 sequence scrutiny.

At the completion of the 1000 Genomes formal project work, an expanded variant catalog was published consisting of 79 million variants, of which 77,520,219 were simple single-nucleotide SNPs of A/C/G/T substitutions, that is, not complex nucleotide arrangements such as [A/C/-] (the 1000 Genomes Project Consortium, 2015). This enlarged variant catalog was again mainly from identification of very rare SNP variation, largely due to expansion in samples: totaling 2535 individuals in 26 populations. Readers are referred to figure 2 in the 2015 review of forensic ancestry analysis (Phillips, 2015) for the most succinct summary of the Phase 3 population sample numbers and framework. In terms of global population scope, two points should be made about the expanded populations of Phase 3. First, South

Asian populations, with origins from the Indian subcontinent, were included for the first time since HapMap (which had a single GIH Gujarati population sample). These five additional populations (GIH plus BEB Bengalis; ITU Telugu; STU Tamil; PJL Punjabis) have allowed the discovery of some population specific variation, for example the SNP rs368738705 only shows a variant allele-T in the 5 South Asian Phase 3 populations, yet all 21 other study populations are monomorphic—so this SNP remained unidentified until Phase 3 data was assessed (such late identified variants tend to carry nine-digit rs-numbers). Second, two more American populations (PEL Peruvians and ACB African Caribbeans) were added in Phase 3 to the four previous populations of Phase 1/2 from this continental region. Here, the sampling location has a fundamental disjoint with the ancestry patterns seen in the individuals sampled. As would be expected from historical patterns of migration, slavery, and colonization, almost all American continent populations have detectable proportions of Native American, European, and African co-ancestry - meaning few individuals from the Americas are without some level of admixture in their genetic heritage. The 1000 Genomes project lists these populations as admixed, but they are often used in other studies to estimate Native American population variation. However, the genetic cluster analyses detailed in the Extended Data figure 5 of the Phase 3 publication (The 1000 Genomes Project Consortium, 2015) clearly indicates that individuals of the PEL sample have the highest proportions of Native American co-ancestry (pale green cluster memberships) and the lowest of any of the American populations from other admixture contributing ancestries of European and African origin. We extended these analyses further to identify a small subset of Peruvian individuals with no or minimum admixture and these are the subject of another publication but described in the next section.

Two other details about the final Phase 3 variant catalog are important to mention. First, no fewer than 508,917 multiple-allele SNPs (approximately 1 in 152 sites) were restored to the complete set of variants released at the end of the project (Phillips et al., 2015). This subset of SNPs in the Phase 3 data provides an extensive and well-validated resource for those interested in incorporating such polymorphisms into forensic panels (see Phillips et al., 2014 for an example of the compilation of ancestry-informative tri-allelic SNPs). Second, Phase 3 studies identified 62 pairs of closely related individuals from 14 different populations within the sample set of 2535, so the figure of 2504 in total, now universally recorded in publications, represents the final dataset with 31 individuals removed (details in Table 10.1 in Phillips et al., 2015).

TABLE 10.1 Twenty-four 1000 Genomes Samples Sequenced by Simons Foundation Genome Diversity Project (SGDP)[a]

	Internal Code	SGDP Description (VCF Header Used)	Broad Regional Description	Country	Panel No. in 1000 Genomes VCF	Sex	x	y
1	X005	Esan-1	Africa	Nigeria	HG03100	M	6.5	6.0
2	X006	Esan-2	Africa	Nigeria	HG02943	F	6.5	6.0
3	X010	Gambian-1	Africa	Gambia	HG02464	M	13.4	16.7
4	X011	Gambian-2	Africa	Gambia	HG02574	F	13.4	16.7
5	X014	Mende-1	Africa	Sierra Leone	HG03078	M	8.5	−13.2
6	X015	Mende-2	Africa	Sierra Leone	HG03085	F	8.5	−13.2
7	X022	Luhya-1	Africa	Kenya	NA19023	F	1.3	36.8
8	X023	Luhya-2[b]	Africa	Kenya	**NA19044**	M	1.3	36.8
9	X012	Kinh-1	East Asia	Vietnam	HG01600	F	21.0	105.9
10	X013	Kinh-2	East Asia	Vietnam	HG01846	M	21.0	105.9
11	X024	Japanese-3	East Asia	Japan	NA18940	M	37.9	139.0
12	X001	Bengali-1	South Asia	Bangladesh	HG03006	M	23.7	90.4
13	X002	Bengali-2	South Asia	Bangladesh	HG03007	F	23.7	90.4
14	X016	Punjabi-1	South Asia	Pakistan	HG02724	M	31.5	74.3
15	X017	Punjabi-2	South Asia	Pakistan	HG02783	M	31.5	74.3
16	X018	Punjabi-3	South Asia	Pakistan	HG02790	F	31.5	74.3
17	X019	Punjabi-4	South Asia	Pakistan	HG02494	F	31.5	74.3
18	X003	English-1	West Eurasia[c]	Britain	HG00126	M	51.2	0.7
19	X004	English-2	West Eurasia	Britain	HG00128	F	51.2	0.7
20	X007	Finnish-1	West Eurasia	Finland	HG00174	F	60.2	24.9
21	X008	Finnish-2	West Eurasia	Finland	HG00190	M	60.2	24.9
22	X009	Finnish-3	West Eurasia	Finland	HG00360	M	60.2	24.9
23	X020	Spanish-1	West Eurasia	Spain	HG01503	M	39.9	−4.0
24	X021	Spanish-2	West Eurasia	Spain	HG01504	F	39.9	−4.0

[a]Internal "X" codes allow easy removal of these overlaps when arranging sample data. Note the Luhya-2 sample was removed from phase 1 as a related individual so the panel number (in bold) does not appear in phase 3 variant call format (VCF) headers.

[b]This sample was removed from Phase 1 data as a close relative.

[c]Regional description of West Eurasia in 1000 Genomes is Europe.

10.3   HGDP–CEPH PANEL VARIANT DATA EXTENDS TO 650,000 SNPs

During the period of activity of the HapMap project and before 1000 Genomes began sequence-based human variant compilation, the main worldwide population sample panel available for researchers to make their own genotyping studies was the HGDP–CEPH panel [http://www.cephb.fr/en/hgdp_panel.php]. The panel was constructed for the CEPH Foundation and this organization continues to maintain a catalog of human variation based on contributions from laboratories using the HGDP–CEPH panel for their studies. Removing close relatives from a series of related pairs reduces the original panel of more than 1000 samples from 51 populations down to 944. Details of the panel composition and a map of the population sample positions worldwide are available at SPSmart (Amigo et al., 2008), although this information is widely recorded in publications that have used the HGDP–CEPH panel. The SPSmart SNP browser accesses the variant details for two major studies of the HGDP–CEPH panel that each applied SNP arrays to genotype 650,000 loci for the 944 panel samples (studies of the Stanford University and University of Michigan). Therefore, this dataset represents a subset of genetic markers, albeit a large-scale dataset. Certain forensic SNPs are not present in the above two HGDP–CEPH SNP data, and all multiple allele SNPs are not typed by SNP arrays using one of two dyes to the two expected alleles in any one SNP. Nevertheless, the HGDP–CEPH panel has 64 Native American samples from five populations; 28 Oceanian samples from two west Pacific populations and 163 Middle East samples from one North African location and three non-Jewish populations from Israel. These population samples outside of Africa, Europe, South and East Asia, therefore, represent a significant degree of gap-filling in the geographic coverage of 1000 Genomes. The main problem is created by the missing SNPs not genotyped by the SNP array of 650,000 loci. At the latter stages of the 1000 Genomes project it was suggested that the HGDP–CEPH panel in its entirety would be sequenced to the same levels of whole genome coverage as the 2504 project samples, but this program did not come to fruition.

At the current time, the optimum approach is to query the HGDP–CEPH SNP data from Stanford University and University of Michigan genotyping projects using SPSmart and to expect a proportion of SNPs from forensic sets to be missing. In the case of the SNP*for*ID 52-plex identification SNP panel and the SNP*for*ID 34-plex ancestry panel, all SNPs are listed in separate SPSmart pages for forensic users of these panels. Although it is informative to combine 1000 Genomes and HGDP–CEPH SNP data into a compilation with the widest possible geographic scope, an important note of caution should be made. The 1000 Genomes project assigns SNP alleles to the reference sequence strand direction, whereas the SNP array allele assignments can be either the reference forward strand or the reverse strand (depending on the capture probe used for the SNP site on the array). Therefore, a significant number of SNPs in the CEPH data have the reverse allele assignments to those of 1000 Genomes (e.g., a CT SNP in one is listed as an AG SNP in the other). The compilation of symmetrical SNPs (AT and CG substitution allele sites) becomes particularly challenging, as it is usually not obvious whether the SNP array data is the reverse or the same direction as the reference strand, although as a rule of thumb, the SNP array direction for any given locus is that shown in the NCBI dbSNP database [https://www.ncbi.nlm.nih.gov/projects/SNP/].

A further limitation of HGDP–CEPH is that SNPs are not phased, again as a result of capture probes targeting different strands. This is a problem if the linkage status of SNPs in close proximity is required, as is the case for determining microhaplotype alleles (Kidd et al., 2017, 12: 215–224). Missing SNPs can be imputed and phase may be inferred using linkage disequilibrium. Both of these tasks can be performed by whole genome association analysis tools like PLINK [http://zzz.bwh.harvard.edu/plink/] (Purcell et al., 2007) but all such models are imperfect (Browning, 2008).

10.4 THE REPOSITIVE GENETIC INFORMATION REGISTRY

With many whole genome sequencing studies now publishing their sequence data and variant catalogs as part of the publication process, a website that can compile records of the data and direct researchers toward its access and use becomes an essential aid to keeping up to date with a growing body of variant data of potential relevance for forensic genetics studies. Such a service is provided by the Repositive genomic information registry [https://discover.repositive.io]. The Repositive website hosts links to a range of large-scale population studies, but at the other extreme also lists individual whole genome data from people willing to share their personal SNP information from analyses made by paid-for genomic services such as 23 and Me. In the case of individual genomes, the data has limited utility since the population of origin of most individuals is not stated while compiling SNP variant data from samples one by one is inefficient and unwieldy. Furthermore, genome analysis services tend to use genome-wide SNP arrays similar to those used to study the HGDP–CEPH population panel and represent a large-scale but limited subset of SNP data rather than the complete variant catalogs collected from sequencing whole genomes. Once logged in as a user of Repositive, researchers can receive alerts for published human variation data to help their own compilations grow and can stay up-to-date.

10.5   THE SIMONS FOUNDATION GENOME DIVERSITY PROJECT (SGDP) VARIANT DATA FROM 263 GENOMES

The SGDP [https://www.simonsfoundation.org/2013/12/23/simons-genome-diversity-project/] covers many of the geographic areas missed by 1000 Genomes' focus on populations from the main continents (Mallick et al., 2012). The regions that were clearly left unexplored by 1000 Genomes include Oceania; regions occupied by unadmixed Native American populations (with the North American Native populations and Arctic Native populations also not covered by the HGDP–CEPH panel sampling); Northeast Asia (from Siberia east toward the regions close to the Bering Straits); much of Southeast Island Asia; and Central South Asia—an ill-defined region that stretches from the Caucasus, East of the Black Sea east toward the regions north of the Himalayas into the central Asian Steppe. Although most of these regions are sparsely populated, study of peoples from such regions can help build a better picture of modern global population relationships and human population genetics in general. It should also be noted that Oceania as a continental definition covers almost half the globe but harbors population divergence between Near Oceania (Melanesia in the south and Micronesia in the north) and Far Oceania (the broad extent of islands of Polynesia that includes population variation found in Easter Islanders in the far east and Maoris in New Zealand).

The Simons Foundation describes their GDP sample panel distribution as 260 whole genome sequences from 127 populations in total: comprising samples of 39 Africans, 23 Native Americans, 27 Central Asians or Siberians, 49 East Asians, 27 Oceanians, 38 South Asians, and 71 West Eurasians. These regional definitions follow those outlined above for existing sample panels, but it should be noted that North Africans are included with sub-Saharan Africans in a single continental-region term; and West Eurasia combines European and Middle Eastern populations. An important feature of the SGDP genome data is the sampling regime used. This follows a strategy to secure the most extensive possible distribution of geographic positions, which in most cases involves just two or three samples per location. The main exception is Oceania; where 14 Papuan genomes have been sequenced and their variant data compiled. The SGDP Papuan data is already starting to be used as a point of reference where population variation from Oceania is important to include in studies comparing patterns seen in the 1000 Genomes populations. For example, a 2018 study of evidence for a double pulse of Denisovan introgression in East Asia, distinct from one such event in South Asia and Oceania (Browning et al., 2018), made use of the SGDP Papuan and African genomes.

Another important feature of SGDP sampling is overlap with both 1000 Genomes and HGDP–CEPH population samples. There are 24 samples in common with 1000 Genomes, mainly two per population (four PJL Punjabis), but not all populations are represented. These overlapping samples could have been used for sequence quality purposes and are listed in Table 10.1 with their 1000 Genomes sample codes. A further 122 samples are from the HGDP–CEPH panel and consist of mainly two samples from each of the 51 populations described earlier (1 Daur Chinese; 3 Palestinian; 3 San with the description Ju_hoan_North); and the inclusion of 14 of 17 CEPH Papuans has already been described. Table 10.2 outlines sample details and HGDP–CEPH codes for this important subset. The sample codes are particularly useful to keep on record as their data can save considerable expense and effort if laboratories choose to analyze a set of new SNPs in the HGDP–CEPH panel and no fewer than 122 of 944 samples (about 13%) do not need to be included.

Described earlier subsets leave 114 samples unique to SGDP and are detailed in Table 10.3.

Note that three additional samples, a Norwegian and two Saami, are part of the accessible variant data of SGDP (termed the C-panel of 263 samples), but their details are not included in any lists provided by Simons Foundation, so they are listed separately at the base of Table 10.3 and sampling locations are inferred. In these and all sample-detail tables, sampling locations are given as x and y values representing the global coordinates of E–W latitudes (x, positive and negative relative to east and west of the zero Greenwich meridian, respectively) and N–S longitudes (y, positive and negative relative to north and south of the equator). All population locations can be found by placing x, y values in online mapping programs, such as Google Maps. The SGDP population locations, including those of HGDP–CEPH, but not 1000 Genomes, are mapped in Figure 10.1, with location numbers identifying each population listed in Tables 10.2 and 10.3. An additional 16 samples are part of the B-panel, which are not detailed here but have accessible

SNP genotypes alongside C-panel data. Lastly, a further 21 samples did not sign a letter of consent for public sharing of their genome sequences, so the statement "300 public SGDP samples across 142 diverse populations" is explained by these additional samples.

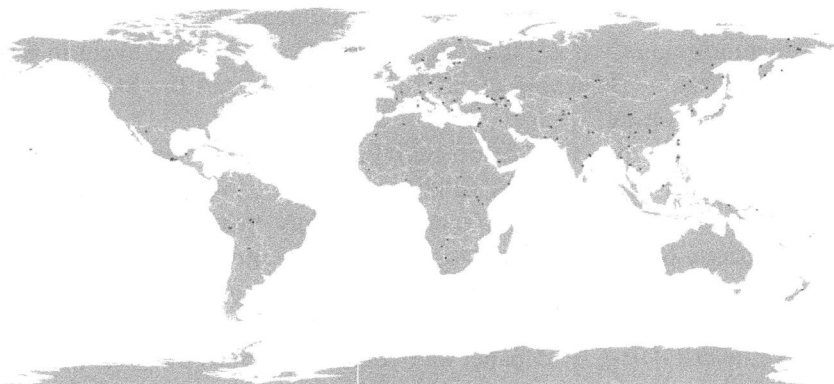

FIGURE 10.1   Geographic distribution of Simons Foundation Genome Diversity Project (SGDP) samples. Reference numbers are listed in Tables 10.2 and 10.3. The 1000 Genomes reference population locations are excluded for clarity.

10.6   THE ESTONIAN BIOCENTRE GENOME DIVERSITY PANEL (EGDP) VARIANT DATA FROM 402 GENOMES

An EGDP comprises 402 samples from 126 populations showing almost no overlap of geographic coverage with the previously described sample panels (3 Finnish, 2 Bengali could be said to mirror 1000 Genomes sampling of these populations, 3 Congo Pygmy, 3 Druze, and 6 Mongolians match HGDP-CEPH populations). Worldwide sampling coverage is particularly useful for East Europe, Central South Asia, India, and Mainland/Island Southeast Asia. These regions and the Northeast Asian regions of Siberia (which complement the extensive coverage of these areas by SGDP) reflect the original purpose of the whole genome sequencing to study the early peopling of Eurasia (Pagani et al., 2016), and readers are directed to that publication for background information on much of the population variation discovered in the EGDP samples. The large number of EGDP samples and their widespread geographic locations creates dense maps and extensive tables of population data (Figure 10.2, Table 10.4), but since so many population descriptions will be unknown to most researchers, we present the necessary details, x–y values and accompanying world map.

TABLE 10.2 A Total of 122 Human Genome Diversity Project[a]

Map No.	Internal Code	SGDP Description	Broad Regional Description	Country	HGDP–CEPH Panel No.	Sex	x	y
1	S018	BantuKenya-1	Africa	Kenya	HGDP01417	M	−3.0	37.0
	S019	BantuKenya-2	Africa	Kenya	HGDP01414	F	−3.0	37.0
2	S132	Mandenka-1	Africa	Senegal	HGDP01199	M	12.0	−12.0
	S133	Mandenka-2	Africa	Senegal	HGDP00915	F	12.0	−12.0
3	S225	Yoruba-1	Africa	Nigeria	HGDP00928	F	7.4	3.9
	S226	Yoruba-2	Africa	Nigeria	HGDP00932	M	7.4	3.9
4	S100	Ju_hoan_North-1[b]	Africa	Namibia	HGDP00991	M	−18.9	21.5
	S101	Ju_hoan_North-2	Africa	Namibia	HGDP00987	M	−18.9	21.5
	S102	Ju_hoan_North-3	Africa	Namibia	HGDP01032	M	−18.9	21.5
5	S141	Mbuti-1	Africa	Congo	HGDP00474	M	1.0	29.0
	S142	Mbuti-2	Africa	Congo	HGDP00476	F	1.0	29.0
	S143	Mbuti-3	Africa	Congo	HGDP00449	M	1.0	29.0
6	S029	Biaka-2	Africa	Central African Republic	HGDP00461	M	4.0	17.0
	S028	Biaka-1	Africa	Central African Republic	HGDP00457	M	4.0	17.0
7	S020	BantuTswana-1	Africa	Botswana or Namibia	HGDP01030	M	−28.0	24.0
	S021	BantuTswana-2	Africa	Botswana or Namibia	HGDP01034	M	−28.0	24.0
8	S016	BantuHerero-1	Africa	Botswana or Namibia	HGDP01028	M	−22.0	19.0
	S017	BantuHerero-2	Africa	Botswana or Namibia	HGDP01035	M	−22.0	19.0
9	S160	Orcadian-1	West Eurasia	Orkney Islands	HGDP00798	M	59.0	−3.0
	S161	Orcadian-2	West Eurasia	Orkney Islands	HGDP00796	F	59.0	−3.0
10	S003	Adygei-1	West Eurasia	Russia (Caucasus)	HGDP01402	M	44.0	39.0
	S004	Adygei-2	West Eurasia	Russia (Caucasus)	HGDP01401	F	44.0	39.0
11	S179	Russian-1	West Eurasia	Russia	HGDP00887	M	61.0	40.0
	S180	Russian-2	West Eurasia	Russia	HGDP00903	F	61.0	40.0
12	S022	Basque-1	West Eurasia	France	HGDP01364	M	43.0	0.0

TABLE 10.2   *(Continued)*

Map No.	Internal Code	SGDP Description	Broad Regional Description	Country	HGDP–CEPH Panel No.	Sex	x	y
	S023	Basque-2	West Eurasia	France	HGDP01365	F	43.0	0.0
13	S068	French-1	West Eurasia	France	HGDP00530	M	46.0	2.0
	S069	French-2	West Eurasia	France	HGDP00526	F	46.0	2.0
14	S026	Bergamo-1	West Eurasia	Italy (Bergamo)	HGDP01153	M	46.0	10.0
	S027	Bergamo-2	West Eurasia	Italy (Bergamo)	HGDP01172	F	46.0	10.0
15	S186	Sardinian-1	West Eurasia	Italy (Sardinia)	HGDP01079	M	40.0	9.0
	S187	Sardinian-2	West Eurasia	Italy (Sardinia)	HGDP01078	F	40.0	9.0
16	S209	Tuscan-1	West Eurasia	Italy (Tuscany)	HGDP01168	F	43.0	11.0
	S210	Tuscan-2	West Eurasia	Italy (Tuscany)	HGDP01163	M	43.0	11.0
17	S152	Mozabite-1	Africa[b]	Algeria	HGDP01253	M	32.0	3.0
	S153	Mozabite-2	Africa[b]	Algeria	HGDP01274	F	32.0	3.0
18	S024	BedouinB-1	West Eurasia	Israel (Negev)	HGDP00616	M	31.0	35.0
	S025	BedouinB-2	West Eurasia	Israel (Negev)	HGDP00650	F	31.0	35.0
19	S054	Druze-1	West Eurasia	Israel (Carmel)	HGDP00569	F	32.0	35.0
	S055	Druze-2	West Eurasia	Israel (Carmel)	HGDP00597	M	32.0	35.0
19	S164	Palestinian-1	West Eurasia	Israel (Central)	HGDP00722	M	32.0	35.0
	S165	Palestinian-2	West Eurasia	Israel (Central)	HGDP00725	M	32.0	35.0
	S166	Palestinian-3	West Eurasia	Israel (Central)	HGDP00737	F	32.0	35.0
20	S014	Balochi-1	South Asia	Pakistan	HGDP00090	M	30.5	66.5
	S015	Balochi-2	South Asia	Pakistan	HGDP00058	M	30.5	66.5
20	S034	Brahui-1	South Asia	Pakistan	HGDP00027	M	30.5	66.5
	S035	Brahui-2	South Asia	Pakistan	HGDP00019	M	30.5	66.5
21	S128	Makrani-1	South Asia	Pakistan	HGDP00160	M	26.0	64.0
	S129	Makrani-2	South Asia	Pakistan	HGDP00157	F	26.0	64.0
22	S190	Sindhi-1	South Asia	Pakistan	HGDP00208	M	25.5	69.0
	S191	Sindhi-2	South Asia	Pakistan	HGDP00195	F	25.5	69.0

TABLE 10.2 *(Continued)*

Map No.	Internal Code	SGDP Description	Broad Regional Description	Country	HGDP–CEPH Panel No.	Sex	x	y
23	S167	Pathan-1	South Asia	Pakistan	HGDP00216	M	33.5	70.5
	S168	Pathan-2	South Asia	Pakistan	HGDP00232	F	33.5	70.5
24	S040	Burusho-1	South Asia	Pakistan	HGDP00428	M	36.5	74.0
	S041	Burusho-2	South Asia	Pakistan	HGDP00338	F	36.5	74.0
25	S077	Hazara-1	South Asia	Pakistan	HGDP00124	M	33.5	70.0
	S078	Hazara-2	South Asia	Pakistan	HGDP00125	M	33.5	70.0
26	S213	Uygur-1	East Asia	China	HGDP01306	F	44.0	81.0
	S214	Uygur-2	East Asia	China	HGDP01297	M	44.0	81.0
27	S103	Kalash-1	South Asia	Pakistan	HGDP00328	M	36.0	71.5
	S104	Kalash-2	South Asia	Pakistan	HGDP00286	F	36.0	71.5
28	S074	Han-1	East Asia	China	HGDP00783	F	32.3	114.0
	S075	Han-2	East Asia	China	HGDP00785	M	32.3	114.0
29	S048	Dai-1	East Asia	China	HGDP01314	F	36.0	100.0
	S049	Dai-2	East Asia	China	HGDP01312	M	36.0	100.0
	S050	Dai-3	East Asia	China	HGDP01315	F	36.0	100.0
30	S051	Daur-2	East Asia	China	HGDP01215	F	48.5	124.0
31	S079	Hezhen-1	East Asia	China	HGDP01240	M	47.5	133.5
	S080	Hezhen-2	East Asia	China	HGDP01242	F	47.5	133.5
32	S118	Lahu-1	East Asia	China	HGDP01323	F	22.0	100.0
	S119	Lahu-2	East Asia	China	HGDP01320	M	22.0	100.0
33	S144	Miao-1	East Asia	China	HGDP01191	M	28.0	109.0
	S145	Miao-2	East Asia	China	HGDP01198	F	28.0	109.0
34	S162	Oroqen-1	East Asia	China	HGDP01203	M	50.4	126.5
	S163	Oroqen-2	East Asia	China	HGDP01211	F	50.4	126.5
35	S188	She-1	East Asia	China	HGDP01335	F	27.0	119.0
	S189	She-2	East Asia	China	HGDP01333	M	27.0	119.0
36	S205	Tujia-1	East Asia	China	HGDP01095	M	29.0	109.0
	S206	Tujia-2	East Asia	China	HGDP01098	F	29.0	109.0
37	S201	Tu-1	East Asia	China	HGDP01350	M	36.0	101.0
	S202	Tu-2	East Asia	China	HGDP01355	F	36.0	101.0
38	S215	Xibo-1	East Asia	China	HGDP01250	M	43.5	81.5
	S216	Xibo-2	East Asia	China	HGDP01246	M	43.5	81.5
39	S223	Yi-1	East Asia	China	HGDP01179	M	28.0	103.0
	S224	Yi-2	East Asia	China	HGDP01188	F	28.0	103.0
40	S150	Mongola-1	Central Asia Siberia	China	HGDP01228	M	45.0	111.0
	S151	Mongola-2	Central Asia Siberia	China	HGDP01223	F	45.0	111.0

TABLE 10.2   *(Continued)*

Map No.	Internal Code	SGDP Description	Broad Regional Description	Country	HGDP– CEPH Panel No.	Sex	x	y
41	S154	Naxi-1	East Asia	China	HGDP01338	M	26.0	100.0
	S155	Naxi-2	East Asia	China	HGDP01344	M	26.0	100.0
	S156	Naxi-3	East Asia	China	HGDP01345	F	26.0	100.0
42	S042	Cambodian-1	East Asia	Cambodia	HGDP00717	M	12.0	105.0
	S043	Cambodian-2	East Asia	Cambodia	HGDP00713	F	12.0	105.0
43	S094	Japanese-1	East Asia	Japan	HGDP00749	M	37.9	139.0
	S095	Japanese-2	East Asia	Japan	HGDP00773	F	37.9	139.0
44	S219	Yakut-1	Central Asia Siberia	Russia	HGDP00956	F	63.0	129.5
	S220	Yakut-2	Central Asia Siberia	Russia	HGDP00951	M	63.0	129.5
45	P001	Papuan-1	Oceania	Papua New Guinea	HGDP00550	F	−4.0	143.0
	P002	Papuan-2	Oceania	Papua New Guinea	HGDP00540	M	−4.0	143.0
	P003	Papuan-3	Oceania	Papua New Guinea	HGDP00541	M	−4.0	143.0
	P004	Papuan-4	Oceania	Papua New Guinea	HGDP00543	M	−4.0	143.0
	P005	Papuan-5	Oceania	Papua New Guinea	HGDP00545	M	−4.0	143.0
	P006	Papuan-6	Oceania	Papua New Guinea	HGDP00547	M	−4.0	143.0
	P007	Papuan-7	Oceania	Papua New Guinea	HGDP00548	M	−4.0	143.0
	P008	Papuan-8	Oceania	Papua New Guinea	HGDP00549	M	−4.0	143.0
	P009	Papuan-9	Oceania	Papua New Guinea	HGDP00551	M	−4.0	143.0
	P010	Papuan-10	Oceania	Papua New Guinea	HGDP00553	M	−4.0	143.0
	P011	Papuan-11	Oceania	Papua New Guinea	HGDP00555	M	−4.0	143.0
	P012	Papuan-12	Oceania	Papua New Guinea	HGDP00556	M	−4.0	143.0
	P013	Papuan-13	Oceania	Papua New Guinea	HGDP00552	F	−4.0	143.0
	P014	Papuan-14	Oceania	Papua New Guinea	HGDP00554	F	−4.0	143.0

TABLE 10.2 *(Continued)*

Map No.	Internal Code	SGDP Description	Broad Regional Description	Country	HGDP–CEPH Panel No.	Sex	x	y
46	S030	Bougainville-1	Oceania	Papua New Guinea	HGDP00660	F	−6.0	155.0
	S031	Bougainville-2	Oceania	Papua New Guinea	HGDP00656	F	−6.0	155.0
47	S107	Karitiana-1	America	Brazil	HGDP01012	M	−10.0	−63.0
	S108	Karitiana-2	America	Brazil	HGDP01018	F	−10.0	−63.0
48	S193	Surui-1	America	Brazil	HGDP00846	F	−11.0	−62.0
	S194	Surui-2	America	Brazil	HGDP00852	F	−11.0	−62.0
49	S169	Piapoco-1	America	Colombia	HGDP00702	F	3.0	−68.0
	S170	Piapoco-2	America	Colombia	HGDP00706	F	3.0	−68.0
50	S139	Mayan-1	America	Mexico	HGDP00855	F	19.0	−91.0
	S140	Mayan-2	America	Mexico	HGDP00857	F	19.0	−91.0
51	S171	Pima-1	America	Mexico	HGDP01047	M	29.0	−108.0
	S172	Pima-2	America	Mexico	HGDP01044	F	29.0	−108.0

[a]Center d'Étude du Polymorphisme Humain (HGDP–CEPH) samples sequenced by SGDP (internal "P" codes for the Papuan samples allow easy inclusion with the reference dataset)
[b]HGDP–CEPH description is San from Namibia.

TABLE 10.3 Around 114 Globally Distributed Population Samples Unique to the Simons Foundation Genome Diversity Project (SGDP) Set[a]

Map No.	Internal Code	SGDP Description (VCF header used)	Broad Regional Description	Country	Sex	x	y
52	S137	Masai-1	Africa	Kenya	M	−1.5	35.2
	S138	Masai-2	Africa	Kenya	M	−1.5	35.2
53	S124	Luo-1	Africa	Kenya	M	−0.1	34.3
	S125	Luo-2	Africa	Kenya	F	−0.1	34.3
54	S192	Somali-1	Africa	Kenya	F	5.6	48.3
55	S052	Dinka-1	Africa	Sudan	M	8.8	27.4
	S053	Dinka-2	Africa	Sudan	M	8.8	27.4
56	S109	Khomani_San-1	Africa	South Africa	F	−27.0	20.8
	S110	Khomani_San-2	Africa	South Africa	F	−27.0	20.8
57	S183	Saharawi-1	Africa[b]	Western Sahara	M	27.3	−8.9
	S184	Saharawi-2	Africa[b]	Western Sahara	M	27.3	−8.9
58	S047	Czech-2	West Eurasia	Czech Republic	M	50.1	14.4
59	S072	Greek-1	West Eurasia	Greece	M	38.0	23.7
	S073	Greek-2	West Eurasia	Greece	M	38.0	23.7

TABLE 10.3 *(Continued)*

Map No.	Internal Code	SGDP Description (VCF header used)	Broad Regional Description	Country	Sex	x	y
60	S081	Hungarian-1	West Eurasia	Hungary	F	47.5	19.1
	S082	Hungarian-2	West Eurasia	Hungary	M	47.5	19.1
61	S083	Icelandic-1	West Eurasia	Iceland	F	64.1	−21.9
	S084	Icelandic-2	West Eurasia	Iceland	F	64.1	−21.9
62	S173	Polish-1	West Eurasia	Poland	M	52.2	21.0
63	S005	Albanian-1	West Eurasia	Albania	F	41.3	19.8
64	S185	Samaritan-1	West Eurasia	Israel	M	32.2	35.3
65	S036	Bulgarian-1	West Eurasia	Bulgaria	M	42.2	24.7
	S037	Bulgarian-2	West Eurasia	Bulgaria	M	42.2	24.7
66	S001	Abkhasian-1	West Eurasia	Abkhazia	M	43.0	41.0
	S002	Abkhasian-2	West Eurasia	Russia	M	43.0	41.0
67	S045	Chechen-1	West Eurasia	Russia	M	43.3	45.7
68	S070	Georgian-1	West Eurasia	Georgia	M	42.5	41.9
	S071	Georgian-2	West Eurasia	Georgia	M	42.5	41.9
69	S120	Lezgin-1	West Eurasia	Russia	M	42.1	48.2
	S121	Lezgin-2	West Eurasia	Russia	M	42.1	48.2
70	S157	North_Ossetian-1	West Eurasia	Russia	M	43.0	44.7
	S158	North_Ossetian-2	West Eurasia	Russia	M	43.0	44.7
71	S063	Estonian-1	West Eurasia	Estonia	M	58.4	24.5
72	S064	Estonian-2	West Eurasia	Estonia	M	59.0	26.9
73	S087	Iranian-1	West Eurasia	Iran	M	35.6	51.5
	S088	Iranian-2	West Eurasia	Iran	M	35.6	51.5
74	S097	Jordanian-1	West Eurasia	Jordan	M	32.1	35.9
	S098	Jordanian-2	West Eurasia	Jordan	M	32.1	35.9
	S099	Jordanian-3	West Eurasia	Jordan	M	32.1	35.9
75	S195	Tajik-1	West Eurasia	Tajikistan	M	37.5	71.6
	S196	Tajik-2	West Eurasia	Tajikistan	M	37.5	71.6
76	S011	Armenian-1	West Eurasia	Armenia	M	39.8	46.8
77	S012	Armenian-2	West Eurasia	Armenia	M	40.6	43.1
78	S207	Turkish-1	West Eurasia	Turkey	M	38.7	35.5
	S208	Turkish-2	West Eurasia	Turkey	F	38.7	35.5
79	S089	Iraqi_Jew-1	West Eurasia	Iraq	F	33.3	44.4
	S090	Iraqi_Jew-2	West Eurasia	Iraq	M	33.3	44.4
80	S221	Yemenite_Jew-1	West Eurasia	Yemen	F	15.4	44.2
	S222	Yemenite_Jew-2	West Eurasia	Yemen	M	15.4	44.2

TABLE 10.3 *(Continued)*

Map No.	Internal Code	SGDP Description (VCF header used)	Broad Regional Description	Country	Sex	x	y
81	S032	Brahmin-1	South Asia	India	M	17.7	83.3
	S033	Brahmin-2	South Asia	India	M	17.7	83.3
82	S091	Irula-1	South Asia	India	M	13.5	80.0
	S092	Irula-2	South Asia	India	M	13.5	80.0
81	S105	Kapu-1	South Asia	India	M	17.7	83.3
	S106	Kapu-2	South Asia	India	M	17.7	83.3
83	S111	Khonda_Dora-1	South Asia	India	M	18.3	82.9
81	S126	Madiga-1	South Asia	India	M	17.7	83.3
	S127	Madiga-2	South Asia	India	M	17.7	83.3
81	S130	Mala-1	South Asia	India	M	17.7	83.3
	S131	Mala-2	South Asia	India	M	17.7	83.3
81	S177	Relli-1	South Asia	India	M	17.7	83.3
	S178	Relli-2	South Asia	India	M	17.7	83.3
81	S217	Yadava-1	South Asia	India	M	17.7	83.3
	S218	Yadava-2	South Asia	India	M	17.7	83.3
84	S114	Kusunda-1	South Asia	Nepal	M	28.1	82.5
85	S115	Kusunda-2	South Asia	Nepal	M	28.1	84.3
86	S008	Altaian-1	Central Asia Siberia	Russia	M	50.8	85.7
87	S006	Aleut-1	Central Asia Siberia	Russia	M	55.2	166.0
	S007	Aleut-2	Central Asia Siberia	Russia	F	55.2	166.0
88	S046	Chukchi-1	Central Asia Siberia	Russia	M	69.0	169.0
89	S058	Eskimo_Chaplin-1	Central Asia Siberia	Russia	M	64.5	172.9
90	S059	Eskimo_Naukan-1	Central Asia Siberia	Russia	F	66.0	169.7
	S060	Eskimo_Naukan-2	Central Asia Siberia	Russia	F	66.0	169.7
91	S061	Eskimo_Sireniki-1	Central Asia Siberia	Russia	M	64.4	173.9
	S062	Eskimo_Sireniki-2	Central Asia Siberia	Russia	F	64.4	173.9
92	S093	Itelman-1	Central Asia Siberia	Russia	F	57.0	157.0

TABLE 10.3 *(Continued)*

Map No.	Internal Code	SGDP Description (VCF header used)	Broad Regional Description	Country	Sex	x	y
93	S199	Tlingit-1	Central Asia Siberia	Russia	M	53.0	158.7
87	S200	Tlingit-2	Central Asia Siberia	Russia	F	55.2	166.0
94	S203	Tubalar-1	Central Asia Siberia	Russia	F	51.1	87.0
	S204	Tubalar-2	Central Asia Siberia	Russia	F	51.1	87.0
95	S211	Ulchi-1	Central Asia Siberia	Russia	F	52.4	140.4
95	S212	Ulchi-2	Central Asia Siberia	Russia	F	52.4	140.5
96	S065	Even-1	Central Asia Siberia	Russia	F	57.5	135.9
	S066	Even-2	Central Asia Siberia	Russia	M	57.5	135.9
	S067	Even-3	Central Asia Siberia	Russia	F	57.5	135.9
97	S134	Mansi-1	Central Asia Siberia	Russia	M	63.8	61.5
98	S135	Mansi-2	Central Asia Siberia	Russia	F	63.7	62.1
99	S116	Kyrgyz-1	Central Asia Siberia	Kyrgyzstan	M	42.9	74.6
	S117	Kyrgyz-2	Central Asia Siberia	Kyrgyzstan	F	42.9	74.6
100	S009	Ami-1	East Asia	Taiwan	M	22.8	121.2
	S010	Ami-2	East Asia	Taiwan	M	22.8	121.2
101	S013	Atayal-1	East Asia	Taiwan	M	24.6	121.3
102	S112	Korean-1	East Asia	Korea	M	37.6	127.0
	S113	Korean-2	East Asia	Korea	F	37.6	127.0
103	S197	Thai-1	East Asia	Thailand	M	13.8	100.5
	S198	Thai-2	East Asia	Thailand	F	13.8	100.5
104	S038	Burmese-1	East Asia	Myanmar	M	17.0	96.7
	S039	Burmese-2	East Asia	Myanmar	M	17.0	96.7
105	S076	Hawaiian-1	Oceania	USA	M	21.3	−157.8
106	S136	Maori-1	Oceania	New Zealand	M	−41.3	174.5
107	S085	Igorot-1	Oceania	Philippines	F	17.1	121.0

TABLE 10.3 *(Continued)*

Map No.	Internal Code	SGDP Description (VCF header used)	Broad Regional Description	Country	Sex	x	y
	S086	Igorot-2	Oceania	Philippines	M	17.1	121.0
108	S056	Dusun-1	Oceania	Brunei	F	4.7	114.7
	S057	Dusun-2	Oceania	Brunei	F	4.7	114.7
109	S174	Quechua-1	America	Peru	F	−13.5	−72.0
	S175	Quechua-2	America	Peru	M	−13.5	−72.0
	S176	Quechua-3	America	Peru	F	−13.5	−72.0
110	S146	Mixe-2	America	Mexico	F	17.0	−96.6
	S147	Mixe-3	America	Mexico	F	17.0	−96.6
111	S148	Mixtec-1	America	Mexico	M	17.0	−97.0
	S149	Mixtec-2	America	Mexico	F	17.0	−97.0
112	S227	Zapotec-1	America	Mexico	M	16.5	−97.2
	S228	Zapotec-2	America	Mexico	M	16.5	−97.2
113	S044	Chane-1	America	Argentina	M	−22.5	−63.8
114	S159	Norwegian-1	West Eurasia	Norway		60.0	11.0
115	S181	Saami-1	West Eurasia	Finland		69.0	27.0
	S182	Saami-2	West Eurasia	Finland		69.0	27.0

[a]Internal "D" codes separate these samples from 1000 Genomes Reference Data (where codes are applied: A = PEL, B = Africa; C = European; E = East Asian; F = South Asian; M = Admixed American)

[b]No sample details given but listed in variant genotype data from Simons Foundation.

TABLE 10.4 A Total of 402 Globally Distributed Population Samples Unique to the EGDP Set[a]

Map No.	Internal Code	EGDP VCF Code	Broad Regional Descriptions	Population Sample Name	Sex	x	y
116	D110	GS000035245-ASM	Sub-Saharan Africa	Congo-pygmies-1	M	0.9	15.9
	D111	GS000035246-ASM	Sub-Saharan Africa	Congo-pygmies-3	M	0.9	15.9
	D112	GS000035247-ASM	Sub-Saharan Africa	Congo-pygmies-6	M	0.9	15.9
117	D019	GS000016217-ASM	Middle East	Arabs-Israel-1	F	32.9	35.3
117	D020	GS000016885-ASM	Middle East	Arabs-Israel-2	F	33	35.2
117	D021	GS000016206-ASM	Middle East	Arabs-Israel-3	M	33.1	35.3
117	D022	GS000016212-ASM	Middle East	Arabs-Israel-4	M	32.8	35.2
117	D023	GS000016213-ASM	Middle East	Arabs-Israel-5	M	32.6	35.4

TABLE 10.4 *(Continued)*

Map No.	Internal Code	EGDP VCF Code	Broad Regional Descriptions	Population Sample Name	Sex	x	y
118	D030	GS000013749-ASM	Middle East	Assyrians-1	M	40.1	44
	D031	GS000013750-ASM	Middle East	Assyrians-3	M	40.1	44
	D032	GS000013751-ASM	Middle East	Assyrians-4	M	40.1	44
117	D124	GS000016135-ASM	Middle East	Druze-1	M	32.8	35.2
117	D125	GS000016136-ASM	Middle East	Druze-2	F	32.8	35.4
117	D126	GS000016137-ASM	Middle East	Druze-3	F	32.7	35.1
119	D193	GS000013747-ASM	Middle East	Iranians-1	M	30.4	57.1
	D194	GS000014475-ASM	Middle East	Iranians-2	M	30.4	57.1
120	D195	GS000016875-ASM	Middle East	Iranians-3	M	35.1	51.2
	D196	GS000016179-ASM	Middle East	Iranians-4	M	35.1	51.2
121	D199	GS000016181-ASM	Middle East	Jordanians-1	F	31.9	35.9
	D200	GS000014474-ASM	Middle East	Jordanians-2	M	31.9	35.9
122	D261	GS000017169-ASM	Middle East	Lebanese-1	F	33.8	35.6
123	D338	GS000016180-ASM	Middle East	Saudi-Arabians-1	M	24.8	46.7
	D339	GS000016277-ASM	Middle East	Saudi-Arabians-2	M	24.8	46.7
124	D139	GS000017199-ASM	Northern Europe	Estonians-1	F	58.1	26.8
125	D140	GS000017210-ASM	Northern Europe	Estonians-2	F	57.7	26.9
126	D141	GS000017209-ASM	Northern Europe	Estonians-3	M	57.7	27.3
127	D142	GS000017206-ASM	Northern Europe	Estonians-4	M	58.8	26.4
128	D143	GS000016919-ASM	Northern Europe	Estonians-5	M	58.5	25.9
129	D144	GS000017208-ASM	Northern Europe	Estonians-6	M	59	22.8
130	D166	GS000016894-ASM	Northern Europe	Finnish-1	F	60.9	23.4
	D167	GS000016895-ASM	Northern Europe	Finnish-2	F	60.9	23.4
	D168	GS000018756-ASM	Northern Europe	Finnish-3	M	60.9	23.4
131	D258	GS000016903-ASM	Northern Europe	Latvians-1	F	57	24.4
131	D259	GS000035027-ASM	Northern Europe	Latvians-2	M	56.9	24.5
132	D260	GS000035148-ASM	Northern Europe	Latvians-3	M	56.6	23.3
133	D270	GS000016905-ASM	Northern Europe	Lithuanians-1	F	55.3	24
	D271	GS000016904-ASM	Northern Europe	Lithuanians-2	M	55.3	24
133	D272	GS000035040-ASM	Northern Europe	Lithuanians-3	F	55.4	23.9
134	D327	GS000035024-ASM	Northern Europe	Saami-4	M	69.9	25.2
	D328	GS000035025-ASM	Northern Europe	Saami-5	M	69.9	25.2
	D329	GS000035026-ASM	Northern Europe	Saami-6	M	69.9	25.2

TABLE 10.4 *(Continued)*

Map No.	Internal Code	EGDP VCF Code	Broad Regional Descriptions	Population Sample Name	Sex	x	y
135	D346	GS000035109-ASM	Northern Europe	Swedes-1	M	59.4	18
136	D347	GS000035240-ASM	Northern Europe	Swedes-2	M	58.8	17
137	D174	GS000016892-ASM	Western Europe	Germans-1	M	52.5	10.1
	D175	GS000016893-ASM	Western Europe	Germans-2	F	52.5	10.1
	D176	GS000016891-ASM	Western Europe	Germans-3	F	52.5	10.1
138	D010	GS000035021-ASM	Southern Europe	Albanians-1	M	41.3	19.8
	D011	GS000035147-ASM	Southern Europe	Albanians-2	M	41.3	19.8
	D012	GS000035434-ASM	Southern Europe	Albanians-3	M	41.3	19.8
139	D117	GS000015872-ASM	Southern Europe	Croats-1	M	43.3	17.8
141	D118	GS000013754-ASM	Southern Europe	Croats-2	M	44.5	18
140	D119	GS000015873-ASM	Southern Europe	Croats-3	F	43.4	17.4
	D120	GS000015871-ASM	Southern Europe	Croats-6	M	44.5	18.1
141	D315	GS000015870-ASM	Southern Europe	Roma-1	F	44.4	18.1
	D316	GS000014325-ASM	Southern Europe	Roma-2	F	44.4	18.1
	D317	GS000014352-ASM	Southern Europe	Roma-5	F	44.4	18.1
142	D323	GS000016819-ASM	Eastern Europe	Russians-North-1	M	57.8	28.3
143	D324	GS000013756-ASM	Eastern Europe	Russians-North-2	M	64.7	43.4
144	D325	GS000016797-ASM	Eastern Europe	Russians-West-1	M	54.6	39.7
142	D326	GS000016796-ASM	Eastern Europe	Russians-West-2	F	57.8	28.3
145	D049	GS000019181-ASM	Eastern Europe	Bashkirs-2	F	53.3	57.5
146	D050	GS000016134-ASM	Eastern Europe	Bashkirs-3	M	51.9	58.2
147	D051	GS000016276-ASM	Eastern Europe	Bashkirs-4	M	55.3	56.1
148	D052	GS000035032-ASM	Eastern Europe	Bashkirs-6	M	54.2	56.6
149	D048	GS000035033-ASM	Eastern Europe	Bashkirs-10	F	53.3	57.9
150	D056	GS000014324-ASM	Eastern Europe	Belarusians-1	M	52.2	24.4
151	D057	GS000016104-ASM	Eastern Europe	Belarusians-2	M	52.2	27.9
150	D058	GS000014351-ASM	Eastern Europe	Belarusians-3	M	52.2	24.4
152	D059	GS000035241-ASM	Eastern Europe	Belarusians-4	F	55.1	27.7
153	D100	GS000013764-ASM	Eastern Europe	Chuvashes-1	M	53.7	54.7
	D101	GS000019182-ASM	Eastern Europe	Chuvashes-2	M	53.7	54.7
154	D102	GS000020097-ASM	Eastern Europe	Chuvashes-3	F	53.6	56.5
155	D113	GS000016186-ASM	Eastern Europe	Cossacks_Kuban-1	M	45	38.7

TABLE 10.4 *(Continued)*

Map No.	Internal Code	EGDP VCF Code	Broad Regional Descriptions	Population Sample Name	Sex	x	y
155	D114	GS000035179-ASM	Eastern Europe	Cossacks_ Kuban-2	M	45	39
156	D115	GS000035238-ASM	Eastern Europe	Cossacks-1	M	47.8	35.2
	D116	GS000035239-ASM	Eastern Europe	Cossacks-2	M	47.8	35.2
157	D180	GS000016902-ASM	Eastern Europe	Hungarians-1	F	47.4	19
158	D181	GS000016901-ASM	Eastern Europe	Hungarians-2	M	48	24.3
159	D190	GS000016896-ASM	Eastern Europe	Ingrians-1	F	60.5	29.6
160	D191	GS000017197-ASM	Eastern Europe	Ingrians-2	M	61.9	34.1
159	D192	GS000016897-ASM	Eastern Europe	Ingrians-3	F	60.5	29.6
161	D206	GS000013765-ASM	Eastern Europe	Karelians-1	M	61.2	32.4
162	D207	GS000016970-ASM	Eastern Europe	Karelians-2	M	64.2	32.2
163	D208	GS000035149-ASM	Eastern Europe	Karelians-3	M	63.1	33
164	D222	GS000014328-ASM	Eastern Europe	Komis-1	M	62.6	58
165	D223	GS000035018-ASM	Eastern Europe	Komis-2	M	64.3	54.5
166	D243	GS000015875-ASM	Eastern Europe	Kryashen-Tatars-4	M	55.9	51.2
167	D244	GS000015876-ASM	Eastern Europe	Kryashen-Tatars-5	F	55.4	49.5
168	D245	GS000015877-ASM	Eastern Europe	Kryashen-Tatars-8	F	58.5	82.2
169	D280	GS000014331-ASM	Eastern Europe	Maris-1	M	55.4	56
	D281	GS000015715-ASM	Eastern Europe	Maris-2	M	55.4	56
169	D282	GS000014332-ASM	Eastern Europe	Maris-3	M	55.5	56.1
170	D283	GS000035031-ASM	Eastern Europe	Maris-4	F	55.6	54.9
171	D285	GS000013763-ASM	Eastern Europe	Mishar-TatarM1	F	54.8	51.4
172	D286	GS000016900-ASM	Eastern Europe	Moldavians-2	F	47.1	28.7
	D287	GS000016899-ASM	Eastern Europe	Moldavians-3	M	47.1	28.7
173	D294	GS000015874-ASM	Eastern Europe	Mordvins-1	M	54.1	43.3
174	D295	GS000014330-ASM	Eastern Europe	Mordvins-2	M	54.4	45.8
175	D296	GS000013698-ASM	Eastern Europe	Mordvins-3	M	54.6	46.1
176	D310	GS000016888-ASM	Eastern Europe	Poles-1	F	52.5	20.8
	D311	GS000016889-ASM	Eastern Europe	Poles-2	F	52.5	20.8
	D312	GS000016890-ASM	Eastern Europe	Poles-3	F	52.5	20.8
177	D313	GS000015869-ASM	Eastern Europe	Poles-4	F	51.1	17

TABLE 10.4 *(Continued)*

Map No.	Internal Code	EGDP VCF Code	Broad Regional Descriptions	Population Sample Name	Sex	x	y
178	D320	GS000017202-ASM	Eastern Europe	Russians-1	F	58.9	25.7
143	D321	GS000014416-ASM	Eastern Europe	Russians-Central-1	M	64.7	43.4
179	D322	GS000035242-ASM	Eastern Europe	Russians-Central-2	M	56.4	57.2
180	D353	GS000013706-ASM	Eastern Europe	Tatars-1	M	43.3	68.2
181	D354	GS000013705-ASM	Eastern Europe	Tatars-2	M	43.3	76.9
182	D355	GS000013704-ASM	Eastern Europe	Tatars-3	F	54.6	53.8
183	D366	GS000016105-ASM	Eastern Europe	Udmurds-1	F	57.2	53.8
184	D367	GS000013694-ASM	Eastern Europe	Udmurds-2	F	57.3	54.1
184	D368	GS000035432-ASM	Eastern Europe	Udmurds-3	M	57.3	52.8
	D369	GS000035017-ASM	Eastern Europe	Udmurds-4	M	57.3	52.8
185	D370	GS000035121-ASM	Eastern Europe	Ukrainians_east-1	M	50.9	34.8
	D371	GS000035174-ASM	Eastern Europe	Ukrainians_east-2	M	50.9	34.8
186	D372	GS000035176-ASM	Eastern Europe	Ukrainians_east-3	M	50	36.2
187	D373	GS000013755-ASM	Eastern Europe	Ukrainians_north-1	M	51.5	31.4
188	D374	GS000035175-ASM	Eastern Europe	Ukrainians_west-1	M	50.6	26.2
189	D375	GS000035177-ASM	Eastern Europe	Ukrainians_west-2	M	50.3	28.7
190	D376	GS000035178-ASM	Eastern Europe	Ukrainians_west-3	M	48.3	25.9
191	D381	GS000015878-ASM	Eastern Europe	Vepsas-1	M	61.4	34.8
	D382	GS000016971-ASM	Eastern Europe	Vepsas-2	M	61.4	34.8
	D383	GS000017632-ASM	Eastern Europe	Vepsas-3	M	61.4	34.8
192	D384	GS000035244-ASM	Eastern Europe	Vepsas-4	M	61.3	35.5
193	D001	GS000014408-ASM	South Caucasus	Abkhazians-1	F	43.2	40.8
193	D002	GS000014409-ASM	South Caucasus	Abkhazians-5	M	43.1	40.6
	D003	GS000014410-ASM	South Caucasus	Abkhazians-6	M	43.1	40.6
194	D024	GS000035173-ASM	South Caucasus	Armenians-1	M	40.2	45.7
194	D025	GS000035124-ASM	South Caucasus	Armenians-2	M	40.2	44.5
195	D026	GS000013745-ASM	South Caucasus	Armenians-3	M	40.6	46.4
196	D027	GS000035126-ASM	South Caucasus	Armenians-4	M	39.9	41.3

TABLE 10.4 *(Continued)*

Map No.	Internal Code	EGDP VCF Code	Broad Regional Descriptions	Population Sample Name	Sex	x	y
197	D028	GS000035125-ASM	South Caucasus	Armenians-5	M	40.5	44.8
198	D029	GS000013746-ASM	South Caucasus	Armenians-7	M	39.9	42
199	D037	GS000013741-ASM	South Caucasus	Azerbaijanis-13	M	40.1	47.5
200	D038	GS000013742-ASM	South Caucasus	Azerbaijanis-14	F	41.5	48.8
201	D039	GS000035237-ASM	South Caucasus	Azerbaijanis-24	M	41.8	48.3
202	D172	GS000035150-ASM	South Caucasus	Georgians-1	M	43	41.4
203	D173	GS000035685-ASM	South Caucasus	Georgians-2	M	41.8	44.7
204	D034	GS000014405-ASM	North Caucasus	Avars-1	M	42.2	47
204	D036	GS000014406-ASM	North Caucasus	Avars-9	F	42.5	47.1
204	D035	GS000014407-ASM	North Caucasus	Avars-12	M	42.5	46.7
205	D045	GS000016170-ASM	North Caucasus	Balkars-1	M	43.5	43
206	D046	GS000016171-ASM	North Caucasus	Balkars-2	F	43.7	44.2
207	D047	GS000016172-ASM	North Caucasus	Balkars-4	F	43.5	43.6
208	D103	GS000013740-ASM	North Caucasus	Circassians-1	F	44.2	42.1
209	D104	GS000035113-ASM	North Caucasus	Circassians-2	M	44.7	40
	D105	GS000035114-ASM	North Caucasus	Circassians-3	M	44.7	40
207	D201	GS000014411-ASM	North Caucasus	Kabardins-1	F	43.5	43.6
207	D202	GS000014412-ASM	North Caucasus	Kabardins-2	F	43.6	43.3
207	D203	GS000035115-ASM	North Caucasus	Kabardins-3	M	43.6	43.4
207	D204	GS000014413-ASM	North Caucasus	Kabardins-4	M	43.5	43.6
210	D247	GS000014370-ASM	North Caucasus	Kumyks-1	M	42.7	47.6
210	D248	GS000014368-ASM	North Caucasus	Kumyks-2	F	43	47.5
211	D249	GS000014404-ASM	North Caucasus	Kumyks-3	F	43.3	46.6
212	D266	GS000014365-ASM	North Caucasus	Lezgins-1	M	41.4	47.8
212	D267	GS000013724-ASM	North Caucasus	Lezgins-2	F	41.6	48.3
213	D268	GS000014366-ASM	North Caucasus	Lezgins-3	M	43	47.5
214	D269	GS000035243-ASM	North Caucasus	Lezgins-4	F	41.6	48
215	D307	GS000014414-ASM	North Caucasus	North-Ossetians-2	M	43.2	43.9
216	D308	GS000013739-ASM	North Caucasus	North-Ossetians-6	M	43.2	44.5
217	D348	GS000014421-ASM	North Caucasus	Tabasarans-4	F	42	47.9
217	D349	GS000014363-ASM	North Caucasus	Tabasarans-5	M	42	48
213	D350	GS000014364-ASM	North Caucasus	Tabasarans-7	M	43	47.5
218	D197	GS000016189-ASM	Central Asia	Ishkasim-1	M	37	71.7

TABLE 10.4 *(Continued)*

Map No.	Internal Code	EGDP VCF Code	Broad Regional Descriptions	Population Sample Name	Sex	x	y
	D198	GS000016196-ASM	Central Asia	Ishkasim-2	M	37	71.7
219	D209	GS000014415-ASM	Central Asia	Kazakhs-1	M	47.5	61.5
220	D210	GS000013752-ASM	Central Asia	Kazakhs-2	M	43.6	77
221	D211	GS000035127-ASM	Central Asia	Kazakhs-3	M	51.1	71.5
222	D255	GS000016193-ASM	Central Asia	Kyrgyz_Tdj-1	F	37.8	73.3
223	D256	GS000016187-ASM	Central Asia	Kyrgyz_Tdj-2	M	38.2	74
	D257	GS000016195-ASM	Central Asia	Kyrgyz_Tdj-3	M	38.2	74
224	D251	GS000016177-ASM	Central Asia	Kyrgyz-1	M	42.2	77
225	D252	GS000016191-ASM	Central Asia	Kyrgyz-2	M	41.5	75.9
	D253	GS000016197-ASM	Central Asia	Kyrgyz-3	M	41.5	75.9
	D254	GS000013757-ASM	Central Asia	Kyrgyz-4	M	41.5	75.9
226	D318	GS000016188-ASM	Central Asia	Rushan-Vanch-1	M	38.5	71.7
	D319	GS000014417-ASM	Central Asia	Rushan-Vanch-2	M	38.5	71.7
227	D345	GS000013758-ASM	Central Asia	Shugnan-1	M	37.5	72.4
228	D351	GS000016192-ASM	Central Asia	Tajiks-1	M	38.4	68.9
229	D360	GS000035118-ASM	Central Asia	Turkmens-1	M	42.6	58.9
	D361	GS000035119-ASM	Central Asia	Turkmens-2	M	42.6	58.9
230	D362	GS000035120-ASM	Central Asia	Turkmens-3	M	42.4	59.4
231	D377	GS000016176-ASM	Central Asia	Uigurs-4	M	43.5	79.5
232	D378	GS000035028-ASM	Central Asia	Uzbek-1	F	40.3	68.2
	D379	GS000035029-ASM	Central Asia	Uzbek-2	F	40.3	68.2
233	D380	GS000035030-ASM	Central Asia	Uzbek-3	M	41	70.9
234	D401	GS000016194-ASM	Central Asia	Yaghnobi-1	M	39.5	67.6
235	D314	GS000016965-ASM	Northwest India	Punjab-1	M	17	75.9
236	D284	GS000035122-ASM	Northwest India	Marwadi	F	26.3	73
237	D356	GS000016798-ASM	Central India	Thakur-1	M	27	77.2
239	D178	GS000016799-ASM	Central India	Gupta-1	M	25.5	82.9
238	D177	GS000016803-ASM	Central India	Gond-1	M	22.2	79.9
239	D064	GS000016807-ASM	Central India	Brahmin-2	M	25.7	82.9
240	D309	GS000016808-ASM	Central India	Orissa-1	M	20.5	85.9
241	D063	GS000016809-ASM	Central India	Brahmin-1	M	25.3	83.1
242	D221	GS000016821-ASM	Central India	Kol-1	M	24.5	83.2
243	D250	GS000016966-ASM	Central India	Kurmi-1	M	25.2	83

TABLE 10.4 *(Continued)*

Map No.	Internal Code	EGDP VCF Code	Broad Regional Descriptions	Population Sample Name	Sex	x	y
244	D275	GS000017146-ASM	Central India	Madhya-Pradesh	M	23.3	77.1
239	D246	GS000035039-ASM	Central India	Kshatriya-1	M	25.7	82.7
245	D060	GS000016964-ASM	East India	Bengali-1	M	22.8	88
245	D061	GS000016801-ASM	East India	Bengali-2	M	22.9	88.3
246	D205	GS000016802-ASM	South India	Kapu-1	M	17.7	83.2
247	D044	GS000035123-ASM	South India	Balija-1	M	14.7	77.6
248	D033	GS000016805-ASM	India Austro-Asiatic	Asur-1	M	23.7	85.3
249	D337	GS000016800-ASM	India Austro-Asiatic	Santhal-1	F	22.8	85.7
250	D179	GS000016804-ASM	India Austro-Asiatic	Ho-1	M	24.1	84.2
251	D121	GS000035034-ASM	Bangladesh	Dhaka-mixed-1	M	23.7	90.4
	D122	GS000035035-ASM	Bangladesh	Dhaka-mixed-2	M	23.7	90.4
	D123	GS000035036-ASM	Bangladesh	Dhaka-mixed-3	F	23.7	90.4
252	D062	GS000035038-ASM	Nepal	Brahmin	M	28.2	84
253	D352	GS000035037-ASM	Nepal	Tamang	M	26.8	87.3
254	D072	GS000019901-ASM	Southeast Asia, Mainland	Burmese-3	M	19.7	96.2
255	D073	GS000019905-ASM	Southeast Asia, Mainland	Burmese-4	M	16.4	95.9
256	D074	GS000019902-ASM	Southeast Asia, Mainland	Burmese-8	M	22.8	95.4
257	D065	GS000019903-ASM	Southeast Asia, Mainland	Burmese-10	M	17.9	96.7
259	D067	GS000019904-ASM	Southeast Asia, Mainland	Burmese-12	M	16.8	96.2
258	D068	GS000020270-ASM	Southeast Asia, Mainland	Burmese-14	M	17.2	97.2
	D069	GS000022100-ASM	Southeast Asia, Mainland	Burmese-15	M	17.2	97.2
259	D071	GS000019906-ASM	Southeast Asia, Mainland	Burmese-20	F	16.8	96.1
260	D276	GS000016806-ASM	South India	Malayan-1	M	10.4	76.7
261	D385	GS000035110-ASM	Southeast Asia, Mainland	Vietnamese_central-1	F	16	108.2

TABLE 10.4 *(Continued)*

Map No.	Internal Code	EGDP VCF Code	Broad Regional Descriptions	Population Sample Name	Sex	x	y
262	D386	GS000035111-ASM	Southeast Asia, Mainland	Vietnamese_central-2	F	16.5	107.6
263	D387	GS000019972-ASM	Southeast Asia, Mainland	Vietnamese_north-1	F	21	105.9
264	D388	GS000019947-ASM	Southeast Asia, Mainland	Vietnamese_north-2	F	21.2	106.1
263	D389	GS000019948-ASM	Southeast Asia, Mainland	Vietnamese_north-3	M	21	105.9
265	D390	GS000019971-ASM	Southeast Asia, Mainland	Vietnamese_south-1	F	10.8	106.6
266	D391	GS000019950-ASM	Southeast Asia, Mainland	Vietnamese_south-2	F	9.8	106.3
267	D392	GS000019949-ASM	Southeast Asia, Mainland	Vietnamese_south-3	M	10	105.8
265	D393	GS000019951-ASM	Southeast Asia, Mainland	Vietnamese_south-4	F	10.8	106.6
	D394	GS000019946-ASM	Southeast Asia, Mainland	Vietnamese_south-5	M	10.8	106.6
268	D042	GS000017004-ASM	Southeast Asia, Island	Bajo-2	M	−4	122.6
	D040	GS000016941-ASM	Southeast Asia, Island	Bajo-17	M	−4	122.6
	D041	GS000017005-ASM	Southeast Asia, Island	Bajo-19	M	−4	122.6
	D043	GS000017006-ASM	Southeast Asia, Island	Bajo-21	M	−4	122.6
269	D182	GS000019966-ASM	Southeast Asia, Island	Igorot-1	F	17.1	121
	D183	GS000019963-ASM	Southeast Asia, Island	Igorot-2	M	17.1	121
	D184	GS000019907-ASM	Southeast Asia, Island	Igorot-3	F	17.1	121
	D186	GS000019908-ASM	Southeast Asia, Island	Igorot-4	F	17.1	121
	D188	GS000019909-ASM	Southeast Asia, Island	Igorot-5	F	17.1	121

TABLE 10.4 *(Continued)*

Map No.	Internal Code	EGDP VCF Code	Broad Regional Descriptions	Population Sample Name	Sex	x	y
270	D004	GS000035249-ASM	Southeast Asia, Island	Aeta-1	M	17.6	121
	D005	GS000035250-ASM	Southeast Asia, Island	Aeta-2	M	17.6	121
	D006	GS000035257-ASM	Southeast Asia, Island	Aeta-3	M	17.6	121
271	D007	GS000035392-ASM	Southeast Asia, Island	Agta-1	M	17.8	121.2
	D008	GS000035435-ASM	Southeast Asia, Island	Agta-2	M	17.8	121.2
	D009	GS000035248-ASM	Southeast Asia, Island	Agta-3	M	17.8	121.2
272	D053	GS000035251-ASM	Southeast Asia, Island	Batak-1	M	10.5	119.5
	D054	GS000035252-ASM	Southeast Asia, Island	Batak-2	M	10.5	119.5
	D055	GS000035253-ASM	Southeast Asia, Island	Batak-3	M	10.5	119.5
273	D127	GS000019954-ASM	Southeast Asia, Island	Dusun-10	F	4.7	114.8
273	D131	GS000021582-ASM	Southeast Asia, Island	Dusun-4	M	4.8	114.6
	D132	GS000019952-ASM	Southeast Asia, Island	Dusun-5	F	4.8	114.6
	D133	GS000019953-ASM	Southeast Asia, Island	Dusun-7	M	4.8	114.6
	D134	GS000020271-ASM	Southeast Asia, Island	Dusun-8	M	4.8	114.6
273	D128	GS000019978-ASM	Southeast Asia, Island	Dusun-11	F	4.8	114.8
	D129	GS000019979-ASM	Southeast Asia, Island	Dusun-12	F	4.8	114.8
273	D130	GS000019980-ASM	Southeast Asia, Island	Dusun-14	F	4.7	114.6
269	D185	GS000019964-ASM	Southeast Asia, Island	Igorot-3	F	17.1	121

TABLE 10.4 *(Continued)*

Map No.	Internal Code	EGDP VCF Code	Broad Regional Descriptions	Population Sample Name	Sex	x	y
274	D187	GS000020253-ASM	Southeast Asia, Island	Igorot-4	F	16.6	120.3
269	D189	GS000019965-ASM	Southeast Asia, Island	Igorot-6	F	17.1	121
275	D262	GS000017007-ASM	Southeast Asia, Island	Lebbo-1	M	1.7	117.2
	D263	GS000016935-ASM	Southeast Asia, Island	Lebbo-2	M	1.7	117.2
	D264	GS000016936-ASM	Southeast Asia, Island	Lebbo-3	M	1.7	117.2
	D265	GS000016937-ASM	Southeast Asia, Island	Lebbo-4	F	1.7	117.2
276	D273	GS000019967-ASM	Southeast Asia, Island	Luzon-2	F	14.6	121
277	D274	GS000019968-ASM	Southeast Asia, Island	Luzon-6	F	14.9	120.3
278	D301	GS000019981-ASM	Southeast Asia, Island	Murut-3	M	4.6	115.1
	D302	GS000019982-ASM	Southeast Asia, Island	Murut-4	M	4.6	115.1
	D303	GS000020272-ASM	Southeast Asia, Island	Murut-5	M	4.6	115.1
	D304	GS000019983-ASM	Southeast Asia, Island	Murut-6	F	4.6	115.1
	D297	GS000019984-ASM	Southeast Asia, Island	Murut-11	M	4.6	115.1
	D298	GS000019985-ASM	Southeast Asia, Island	Murut-13	F	4.6	115.1
279	D299	GS000019986-ASM	Southeast Asia, Island	Murut-19	M	4.5	114.7
	D300	GS000019987-ASM	Southeast Asia, Island	Murut-20	M	4.5	114.7
280	D395	GS000019969-ASM	Southeast Asia, Island	Vizayan-1	F	9.8	125.5
281	D396	GS000019970-ASM	Southeast Asia, Island	Vizayan-3	M	10.3	123.9

TABLE 10.4　*(Continued)*

Map No.	Internal Code	EGDP VCF Code	Broad Regional Descriptions	Population Sample Name	Sex	x	y
282	D218	GS000035686-ASM	Papua New Guinea	Koinanbe-1	M	−5.5	144.6
	D219	GS000035255-ASM	Papua New Guinea	Koinanbe-2	M	−5.5	144.6
	D220	GS000035258-ASM	Papua New Guinea	Koinanbe-3	M	−5.5	144.6
283	D240	GS000035256-ASM	Papua New Guinea	Kosipe-1	M	−8.5	147.2
	D241	GS000035260-ASM	Papua New Guinea	Kosipe-2	M	−8.5	147.2
	D242	GS000035365-ASM	Papua New Guinea	Kosipe-3	M	−8.5	147.2
284	D013	GS000016173-ASM	South Siberia	Altaians-1	F	50.8	88.3
285	D014	GS000020512-ASM	South Siberia	Altaians-2	M	51	84.6
286	D015	GS000016174-ASM	South Siberia	Altaians-3	M	51.3	85.4
284	D016	GS000016967-ASM	South Siberia	Altaians-4	M	50.8	88.3
285	D017	GS000022439-ASM	South Siberia	Altaians-5	M	51	84.6
	D018	GS000022440-ASM	South Siberia	Altaians-6	M	51	84.6
287	D070	GS000014418-ASM	South Siberia	Buryats-2	M	52.9	108.4
288	D086	GS000014629-ASM	South Siberia	Buryats-6	M	52	104.9
289	D066	GS000013761-ASM	South Siberia	Buryats-11	M	53.8	102.8
290	D075	GS000022066-ASM	South Siberia	Buryats-318	M	56.3	113
	D076	GS000022077-ASM	South Siberia	Buryats-336	M	56.3	113
	D077	GS000022090-ASM	South Siberia	Buryats-350	F	56.3	113
	D078	GS000022091-ASM	South Siberia	Buryats-355	M	56.3	113
	D079	GS000022092-ASM	South Siberia	Buryats-361	F	56.3	113
	D080	GS000020113-ASM	South Siberia	Buryats-383	M	56.3	113
	D081	GS000022093-ASM	South Siberia	Buryats-398	F	56.3	113
	D082	GS000020491-ASM	South Siberia	Buryats-406	M	56.3	113
	D083	GS000020126-ASM	South Siberia	Buryats-530	M	56.3	113
	D084	GS000022436-ASM	South Siberia	Buryats-561	M	56.3	113
	D085	GS000022094-ASM	South Siberia	Buryats-578	F	56.3	113
	D087	GS000022298-ASM	South Siberia	Buryats-636	F	56.3	113
	D088	GS000020127-ASM	South Siberia	Buryats-639	M	56.3	113
	D089	GS000022437-ASM	South Siberia	Buryats-640	M	56.3	113

TABLE 10.4 *(Continued)*

Map No.	Internal Code	EGDP VCF Code	Broad Regional Descriptions	Population Sample Name	Sex	x	y
291	D288	GS000016190-ASM	South Siberia	Mongolians-1	M	45.7	106.3
292	D289	GS000035116-ASM	South Siberia	Mongolians-2	M	43.5	104.3
293	D290	GS000035117-ASM	South Siberia	Mongolians-3	M	48	91.6
294	D291	GS000035234-ASM	South Siberia	Mongolians-4	M	48.2	96.1
295	D292	GS000035235-ASM	South Siberia	Mongolians-5	M	47.9	100.8
296	D293	GS000035236-ASM	South Siberia	Mongolians-6	M	50	106.5
297	D343	GS000022438-ASM	South Siberia	Shor-1	M	52.8	87.9
298	D344	GS000034407-ASM	South Siberia	Shor-2	F	53.2	88.4
299	D363	GS000016968-ASM	South Siberia	Tuvinians-1	M	51.5	92.8
300	D364	GS000017247-ASM	South Siberia	Tuvinians-2	M	51.2	89.5
301	D365	GS000016175-ASM	South Siberia	Tuvinians-5	F	51.2	90.5
302	D145	GS000014334-ASM	Central Siberia	Evenks-1A (Sakha)[a]	F	58.9	128.7
303	D146	GS000022096-ASM	Central Siberia	Evenks-1B (Kuyumba)[a]	F	61	97
302	D149	GS000014335-ASM	Central Siberia	Evenks-2	M	58.9	128.7
313	D160	GS000022097-ASM	Central Siberia	Evenks-3	M	64.2	93.8
302	D162	GS000014336-ASM	Central Siberia	Evenks-5	F	68.5	102.2
304	D147	GS000020004-ASM	Central Siberia	Evenks-14	F	67.5	100.4
305	D148	GS000020363-ASM	Central Siberia	Evenks-16	M	59.7	151.3
307	D151	GS000020489-ASM	Central Siberia	Evenks-22	M	64.3	100.2
309	D153	GS000020005-ASM	Central Siberia	Evenks-35	F	59.7	150.1
	D154	GS000020006-ASM	Central Siberia	Evenks-40	F	64.1	99.9
303	D155	GS000020107-ASM	Central Siberia	Evenks-41	M	64.1	99.9
310	D156	GS000020108-ASM	Central Siberia	Evenks-55	F	61	97
311	D157	GS000020109-ASM	Central Siberia	Evenks-62	M	63.6	104
312	D158	GS000020129-ASM	Central Siberia	Evens-Magadan-M1	M	61.7	96.4
	D159	GS000022293-ASM	Central Siberia	Evens_Magadan-M2	F	62	160.4
314	D161	GS000022292-ASM	Central Siberia	Evens-Magadan-M3	M	62	160.4
306	D150	GS000034297-ASM	Central Siberia	Evens-Magadan-21	F	62.2	159.1

TABLE 10.4 *(Continued)*

Map No.	Internal Code	EGDP VCF Code	Broad Regional Descriptions	Population Sample Name	Sex	x	y
308	D152	GS000020110-ASM	Central Siberia	Evens-Magadan-31	M	58.9	128.7
315	D163	GS000016165-ASM	Central Siberia	Evens-Sakha-1	M	65.3	130
316	D164	GS000016166-ASM	Central Siberia	Evens-Sakha-2	M	63.3	143.2
317	D165	GS000016167-ASM	Central Siberia	Evens-_Sakha-3	M	62.7	135.5
318	D334	GS000014402-ASM	Central Siberia	Yakuts-1	M	68.4	119
305	D330	GS000020111-ASM	Central Siberia	Yakuts-K1	M	67.5	100.4
304	D331	GS000020112-ASM	Central Siberia	Yakuts-K2	F	68.5	102.2
	D332	GS000020490-ASM	Central Siberia	Yakuts-K3	F	68.5	102.2
319	D402	GS000022441-ASM	Central Siberia	Yakuts-K4	M	65.8	105.3
320	D333	GS000022076-ASM	Central Siberia	Yakuts-M1	F	62.9	152.4
321	D335	GS000013709-ASM	Central Siberia	YakutS4	M	64.5	117.5
322	D336	GS000014333-ASM	Central Siberia	YakutS8	F	62.3	132
323	D169	GS000013714-ASM	West Siberia	Forest-Nenets	F	64.9	77.8
	D170	GS000014337-ASM	West Siberia	Forest-Nenets	F	64.9	77.8
	D171	GS000015879-ASM	West Siberia	Forest-Nenets	M	64.9	77.8
324	D212	GS000013717-ASM	West Siberia	Kets-1	M	62.5	86.3
	D213	GS000015393-ASM	West Siberia	Kets-2	M	62.5	86.3
	D214	GS000035128-ASM	West Siberia	Kets-3	F	62.5	86.3
325	D215	GS000016164-ASM	West Siberia	Khantys-1	M	65	65.8
326	D216	GS000016906-ASM	West Siberia	Khantys-2	F	61	69.1
326	D217	GS000035697-ASM	West Siberia	Khantys-3	F	61	69
	D277	GS000016184-ASM	West Siberia	Mansis-1	F	61	69
	D278	GS000016185-ASM	West Siberia	Mansis-2	M	61	69
	D279	GS000035019-ASM	West Siberia	Mansis-3	F	61	69
327	D340	GS000015392-ASM	West Siberia	Selkups-1	M	64	82
	D341	GS000013715-ASM	West Siberia	Selkups-2	F	64	82
328	D342	GS000013716-ASM	West Siberia	Selkups-3	F	65.7	87
329	D357	GS000016163-ASM	West Siberia	Tundra-Nenets-1	F	67	78.2
	D358	GS000016162-ASM	West Siberia	Tundra-Nenets-2	M	67	78.2
	D359	GS000016161-ASM	West Siberia	Tundra-Nenets-4	M	67	78.2
330	D305	GS000016159-ASM	North Siberia	Nganasans-1	F	69.4	86.2
331	D306	GS000016160-ASM	North Siberia	Nganasans-2	F	71	94.6

TABLE 10.4   *(Continued)*

Map No.	Internal Code	EGDP VCF Code	Broad Regional Descriptions	Population Sample Name	Sex	x	y
332	D095	GS000014403-ASM	Northeast Siberia	Chukchis-2	F	64.7	177.5
	D096	GS000020003-ASM	Northeast Siberia	Chukchis-3	F	64.7	177.5
	D097	GS000020001-ASM	Northeast Siberia	Chukchis-5	F	64.7	177.5
	D098	GS000014420-ASM	Northeast Siberia	Chukchis-8	F	64.7	177.5
	D099	GS000020002-ASM	Northeast Siberia	Chukchis-9	M	64.7	177.5
333	D136	GS000019997-ASM	Northeast Siberia	Eskimo-2	M	64.5	−172.9
	D138	GS000019998-ASM	Northeast Siberia	Eskimo-3	F	64.5	−172.9
	D135	GS000019999-ASM	Northeast Siberia	Eskimo-11	M	64.5	−172.9
	D137	GS000020000-ASM	Northeast Siberia	Eskimo-20	M	64.5	−172.9
334	D224	GS000022067-ASM	Northeast Siberia	Koryaks-1	F	61.9	159.2
335	D225	GS000016169-ASM	Northeast Siberia	Koryaks-2.1	F	59.1	159.9
312	D226	GS000022068-ASM	Northeast Siberia	Koryaks-2	M	62	160.4
335	D227	GS000016168-ASM	Northeast Siberia	Koryaks-3.1	M	59.1	159.9
334	D228	GS000019994-ASM	Northeast Siberia	Koryaks-3	F	61.9	159.2
	D230	GS000022071-ASM	Northeast Siberia	Koryaks-3.2	M	61.9	159.2
312	D229	GS000022069-ASM	Northeast Siberia	Koryaks-3.3	M	62	160.4
334	D231	GS000034185-ASM	Northeast Siberia	Koryaks-3.4	M	61.9	159.2
	D232	GS000019995-ASM	Northeast Siberia	Koryaks-4	F	61.9	159.2

TABLE 10.4   *(Continued)*

Map No.	Internal Code	EGDP VCF Code	Broad Regional Descriptions	Population Sample Name	Sex	x	y
	D233	GS000033948-ASM	Northeast Siberia	Koryaks-4.1	M	61.9	159.2
	D234	GS000034970-ASM	Northeast Siberia	Koryaks-4.2	M	61.9	159.2
	D235	GS000022072-ASM	Northeast Siberia	Koryaks-5	M	61.9	159.2
336	D236	GS000019992-ASM	Northeast Siberia	Koryaks-6	M	63.1	162.1
334	D237	GS000022442-ASM	Northeast Siberia	Koryaks-7	M	61.9	159.2
	D239	GS000019996-ASM	Northeast Siberia	Koryaks-9	F	61.9	159.2
	D238	GS000019993-ASM	Northeast Siberia	Koryaks-9.1	F	61.9	159.2
337	D090	GS000016938-ASM	South America	Cachi-1	F	−25.1	−66.2
	D091	GS000016939-ASM	South America	Cachi-2	M	−25.1	−66.2
	D092	GS000016940-ASM	South America	Cachi-3	M	−25.1	−66.2
	D093	GS000017077-ASM	South America	Cachi-4	M	−25.1	−66.2
	D094	GS000016942-ASM	South America	Cachi-5	F	−25.1	−66.2
338	D106	GS000016948-ASM	South America	Colla-1	F	−24.2	−66.3
	D107	GS000016949-ASM	South America	Colla-2	F	−24.2	−66.3
	D108	GS000016950-ASM	South America	Colla-3	M	−24.2	−66.3
	D109	GS000016951-ASM	South America	Colla-4	M	−24.2	−66.3
339	D397	GS000016943-ASM	South America	Wichi-1	F	−23.2	−64.1
	D398	GS000016944-ASM	South America	Wichi-2	M	-223.2	−64.1
	D399	GS000016945-ASM	South America	Wichi-3	M	-223.2	−64.1
	D400	GS000016946-ASM	South America	Wichi-4	F	-223.2	−64.1

[a]These samples have ambiguous short EGDP sample codes.

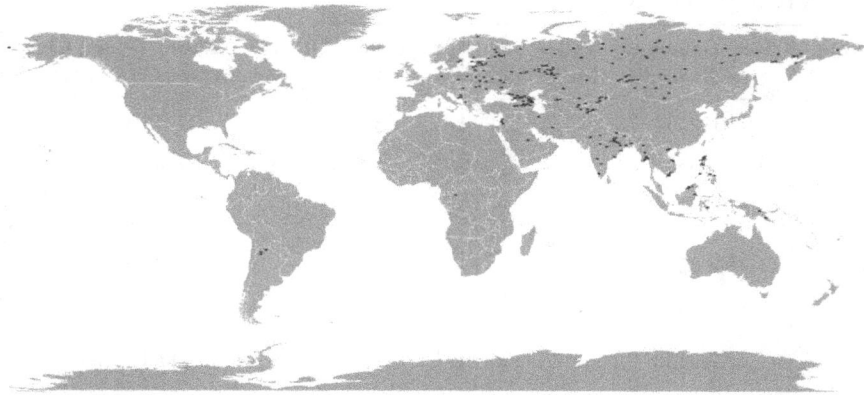

FIGURE 10.2 Geographic distribution of EGDP samples. Reference numbers are listed in Table 10.4.

Note that broad-scale regional descriptions from EGDP do not fully match those of SGDP, principally the division of Eurasia into N-, S-, W-, E-Europe and Middle East; division of Central South Asia into S-, N-Caucasus, Central Asia, and seven Indian regions; and regions of North Asia into Central-, S-, W- N- NE-Siberia.

10.7 CONSTRUCTING A SMALL NATIVE AMERICAN SUBSET FROM THE 1000 GENOMES PERUVIANS

The American sample panels in 1000 Genomes are all described as admixed, so estimating SNP allele frequencies representative of this ancestry is not accurate when European and African admixture, common to this continent's demographics, has occurred and may influence the patterns of genotypes found in an individual. In order to more precisely gauge SNP allele frequencies directly attributable to Native American ancestry alone, we analyzed the 1000 Genomes PEL Peruvians from Lima for genetic cluster membership using ADMIXTURE and a very large panel of highly differentiated SNPs, with HGDP–CEPH Surui and Karitiana as reference data. Table 10.5 lists the Native American cluster proportions obtained and their remaining proportions combined for African, European, and East Asian cluster membership. There are 18 with no detectable non-native American co-ancestry at the top of the table and these have since been used as an American ancestry reference panel that offers the full extent of SNP variation detected by 1000 Genomes.

TABLE 10.5 Eighty Five 1000 Genomes Peruvians From Lima, Peru[a]

Rank	1000 Genomes Sample Code	Native American Cluster Membership Proportion	Other Population Group Cluster Membership Proportion
1	HG02291	0.99997	0.00003
2	HG02275	0.99997	0.00003
3	HG02272	0.99997	0.00003
4	HG02271	0.99997	0.00003
5	HG02259	0.99997	0.00003
6	HG02150	0.99997	0.00003
7	HG02105	0.99997	0.00003
8	HG01974	0.99997	0.00003
9	HG01968	0.99997	0.00003
10	HG01961	0.99997	0.00003
11	HG01951	0.99997	0.00003
12	HG01938	0.99997	0.00003
13	HG01926	0.99997	0.00003
14	HG01923	0.99997	0.00003
15	HG01920	0.99997	0.00003
16	HG01572	0.99997	0.00003
17	HG02265	0.99891	0.00109
18	HG01927	0.99317	0.00683
19	HG02147	0.97418	0.02582
20	HG02266	0.95380	0.04620
21	HG02278	0.95254	0.04746
22	HG01954	0.94568	0.05432
23	HG01992	0.94243	0.05757
24	HG02104	0.93670	0.06330
25	HG02146	0.91717	0.08283
26	HG01953	0.91665	0.08335

TABLE 10.5 *(Continued)*

Rank	1000 Genomes Sample Code	Native American Cluster Membership Proportion	Other Population Group Cluster Membership Proportion
27	HG01997	0.91449	0.08551
28	HG02292	0.91423	0.08577
29	HG02299	0.90410	0.09590
30	HG01917	0.89367	0.10633
31	HG02348	0.87766	0.12234
32	HG02260	0.87383	0.12617
33	HG01942	0.87273	0.12727
34	HG02102	0.87037	0.12963
35	HG01950	0.86909	0.13092
36	HG02008	0.86085	0.13915
37	HG02003	0.84653	0.15347
38	HG01973	0.84342	0.15658
39	HG01932	0.84307	0.15694
40	HG02301	0.84051	0.15950
41	HG01941	0.83334	0.16666
42	HG01977	0.83330	0.16670
43	HG02285	0.82476	0.17524
44	HG01945	0.82327	0.17673
45	HG02262	0.81127	0.18874
46	HG02002	0.80832	0.19168
47	HG01982	0.80414	0.19586
48	HG01918	0.80213	0.19787
49	HG01939	0.79711	0.20289
50	HG02304	0.79609	0.20391
51	HG01921	0.78358	0.21642
52	HG01991	0.77745	0.22255

TABLE 10.5   *(Continued)*

Rank	1000 Genomes Sample Code	Native American Cluster Membership Proportion	Other Population Group Cluster Membership Proportion
53	HG02286	0.77597	0.22403
54	HG01935	0.76667	0.23334
55	HG01980	0.75204	0.24796
56	HG01979	0.74262	0.25738
57	HG01892	0.74161	0.25839
58	HG01976	0.70426	0.29574
59	HG01565	0.69993	0.30007
60	HG01924	0.69823	0.30177
61	HG02277	0.69664	0.30336
62	HG02089	0.68939	0.31061
63	HG02252	0.67882	0.32118
64	HG01936	0.67529	0.32471
65	HG01970	0.67346	0.32655
66	HG01948	0.67081	0.32919
67	HG01571	0.66769	0.33231
68	HG01967	0.66678	0.33323
69	HG01933	0.64122	0.35878
70	HG02298	0.63449	0.36551
71	HG02312	0.63319	0.36681
72	HG01578	0.62734	0.37266
73	HG02274	0.62272	0.37729
74	HG01947	0.61569	0.38431
75	HG01965	0.61252	0.38748
76	HG02425	0.59910	0.40090
77	HG02090	0.58286	0.41714
78	HG01971	0.57642	0.42358

TABLE 10.5 *(Continued)*

Rank	1000 Genomes Sample Code	Native American Cluster Membership Proportion	Other Population Group Cluster Membership Proportion
79	HG01893	0.57135	0.42865
80	HG02253	0.56792	0.43208
81	HG01944	0.52229	0.47772
82	HG01566	0.46398	0.53602
83	HG02345	0.46210	0.53790
84	HG01577	0.45571	0.54429
85	HG02006	0.32415	0.67585

[a]Ranked in descending proportion of Native American Co-Ancestry (cluster membership proportion), based on ADMIXTURE cluster analysis with an extensive SNP panel and HGDP–CEPH Surui and Karitiana as reference data (the top 18 indicated by the box have no detectable co-ancestry from non-American populations and are used by the authors as a representative sample set for American ancestry when analyzing 1000 Genomes SNP data)

10.8 LARGE SCALE WHOLE GENOME SEQUENCE-BASED VARIANT DATABASES

Several other genome sequencing projects which have established a much-expanded scale of sample sizes have accessible population data that provides an informative point of comparison with the more geographically focused datasets outlined above. This additional genomic data has the contrasting characteristics of a much larger sample size but limited population scope, in order to specifically identify very low frequency variation. The most widely publicized of these large-scale datasets include UK10K, aiming to sequence 10,000 genomes and analyze patterns of variation in individuals from the British Isles (https://www.uk10k.org/); and the two linked Broad Institute led international projects of the Exome Aggregation Consortium (ExAC) (Lek et al., 2016) and the Genome Aggregation Database (gnomAD). As 10KUK data concentrates on one population which is already covered by 1000 Genomes sampling, and ExAC (http://exac.broadinstitute.org) has its focus on exome-sited variants, not those across the whole genome, we describe here the gnomAD variant browser (http://gnomad.broadinstitute.org).

The gnomAD project has compiled allele frequency data for a very large set of variants (as the focus on low frequency variation can be expected to detect) in Africans (4368 genomes), Ashkenazi Jewish (151), Latino (419), East Asian (811), Finnish (1747), non-Finnish European (7509), and other (491). A larger number of exomes have been sequenced in each of these population sets plus South Asians. It is evident these population characteristics are the very opposite of those we provide in detail here for SGDP and EGDP. The Ashkenazi Jewish and Finnish samples are clearly more specific than the other groupings, but the African gnomAD samples include both African and African American individuals, which means that allele frequency estimates from this population designation will be influenced by patterns of co-ancestry within the sample set that are impossible to gauge. The Latino sample set is marked as AMR; the same label given to admixed American populations in 1000 Genomes, but the Latino sample is certain to have an even more extensive range of co-ancestry patterns than Africans, so cannot be relied on to define SNP allele frequencies applicable for one population. Furthermore, the "other" sample set completely lacks population definitions, for individuals not assignable to any of the described sample sets. Therefore, the gnomAD browser has population definition limitations but provides a useful way to check the frequency of very rare alleles in Africans, Europeans, and East Asians. This can have importance when checking whether a flanking region SNP close to the targeted site is possibly causing an allele dropout by interfering with primer binding—checks of allele frequencies in 1000 Genomes would only reveal variation of ~1% or more, but gnomAD offers the opportunity of finding much rarer polymorphisms which may explain unusual genotyping patterns. The gnomAD browser also reveals interesting additional variation in established forensic SNPs, for example, rs2156208 in the *Eurasiaplex* forensic ancestry panel (Phillips et al., 2013) has a single observation of a third G allele in Africans at an allele frequency of 0.000115. This observation also highlights the power of genome sequence-based variant catalogs to detect multiple-allele SNPs where the third allele is present in some populations at very low frequencies—multiple-allele SNPs were not detectable in any form with previous SNP array technology. It should be added that the comparison of gnomAD Ashkenazi Jewish SNP frequencies with European frequencies estimated with other data has proved to be informative for studying patterns of variation in these populations (e.g., rs10008492 and rs11779571, both from the *Eurasiaplex* panel, show high and low divergence values between each population, respectively).

10.9 ACCESSING AND ANALYZING FORENSIC SNP DATA FROM PUBLIC GENOME DATASETS

The common file format for listing SNP variation data is VCF (Variant Call Format); a text file with an arrangement in single lines of space delimited data for all the relevant information for a polymorphic site found at a specific position in the reference genome. A typical VCF file will be genome-wide or contain all variants in one chromosome when this number is very large; with the chromosome and genomic coordinates displayed in the first part of the line of data that contains the genotypes. Genomic coordinates can be for a specific build (i.e., GRCh37, or the more recently constructed GRCh38), but this is always specified by the data custodians. The build is important for a number of data checking steps. For example, the 1000 Genomes variant catalog is now referenced with GRCh38 coordinates, but to interrogate the VCF files containing the project's variant data, the tool Data Slicer tool [GRCh37.ensembl.org/Homo_sapiens/Tools/DataSlicer] can be used, but it requires a query defined by GRCh37 coordinate bounds.

All 1000 Genomes variant data is now held by the IGSR site [www.internationalgenome.org/data]. While Pilot and Phase 1 data is available, the Phase 3 data contains more than twice the number of variants (37.9 vs 84.4 million) and more populations, as well as fully annotated multiple-allele SNPs. Clicking on the VCF link and signing in as a guest gives access to compressed chromosome specific VCF files.

SGDP data is now held in the Seven Bridges Cancer Genomics Cloud [https://cgc-accounts.sbgenomics.com], which requires an account to be set up. However, a much more comprehensive explanation of the data and links to VCF variant files with SNP genotypes for the 279 publicly available samples is provided by Reich lab, Harvard at: [reichdata.hms.harvard.edu/pub/datasets/sgdp/]. This portal also has the advantage of offering extensive additional analyses of the SNP data, including phased SNP genotypes (described later) and data-processing tools, including the in-house developed SGDP-lite; suited to processing small-scale SNP queries. EGDP data is held in the Estonian Biocentre repository [evolbio.ut.ee/CGgenomes_VCF/] which provides a very large single compressed file but comprises individual chromosome specific VCF files when decompressed into the parent folder.

HGDP–CEPH variant data for 650,000 SNPs can be accessed directly in SPSmart and their genotypes downloaded as previously described. However, researchers interested in comparing these SNP genotypes to other

data for the same samples can go to the CEPH data portal [www.cephb.
fr/en/hgdp_panel.php] and explore additional variant datasets with the
option to sign in as a guest and access the genotypes directly. The Harvard
HGDP–CEPH Database Supplement 10 is recommended in particular
as this contains genotypes for the approximately 629,000 SNPs in the
Axiom Human Origins 1 SNP array [https://www.thermofsher.com/order/
catalog/901853] designed by Reich lab and containing both Denisovan/
Neanderthal specific SNP sites and a large proportion of complementary
polymorphisms to the 650,000 SNPs used in the Stanford University and
University of Michigan HGDP–CEPH studies.

Some important additional details are necessary to stress for those
willing to start exploring large-scale SNP datasets to find novel variation
of potential forensic use. First, both the EGDP and Axiom Human Origins
array HGDP–CEPH datasets were prepared using the commonly applied
PLINK software, which strips out multi-allele SNP genotypes, so this
SNP data will be found to be missing. Second, phased SNP genotypes are
becoming increasingly useful to compile when exploring microhaplotype
loci of forensic utility (Kidd et al., 2017). In VCF file formats a "pipe" (|)
denotes phased genotypes (i.e., an AG SNP will be listed as 1|0 or 0|1 for A
= reference allele and GA or AG sequence strand designations). SNP genotype data in VCF files without inferred phase uses the "forward slash" (/) as
the separator. Phased data allows haplotypes to be reconstructed from the
genotypes of closely sited SNPs, such as an example case of AG, CT, AT
SNP genotypes listed as 0|0, 1|0, 0|1 that denote haplotypes ATA and ACT.
All three main datasets have been phased, although SGDP data is separately compiled in a dedicated set of VCFs [https://sharehost.hms.harvard.
edu/genetics/reich_lab/sgdp/phased_data]. The multisampling VCFs
contain all phased SNPs per chromosome ("by sample" files are individual
phased data per SGDP sample). Third, VCF files contain the population
reference codes or descriptions on one of the top lines of data and these
need to be matched to genotypes, but more importantly, designated to their
stated population of origin or sampling location. Since small-scale SNP
data compilations are easily made in Excel, this is a simple matter of copy-
pasting into the appropriate rows. However, these will often need transposition to columns - that is, positioning SNP genotypes along the top row
and sample details listed down the leftmost column. This is the standard
format for the input of SNP data to STRUCTURE or ADMIXTURE cluster
detection algorithms (Porras-Hurtado et al., 2013); as well as uploading
data (as Excel files) into the Snipper forensic SNP classifier portal. To help

in the compilation of SNP genotypes from 1000 Genomes; HGDP–CEPH; SGDP; and EGDP project data, Excel-based lookup tables are provided in the Snipper webpage that contains MPS ancestry SNP reference data [mathgene.usc.es/snipper/forensic_mps_aims.html]. These just require the pasting of the VCF header row sample descriptions, then corresponding population details are given that can be placed into the sample rows. Note that 1000 Genomes have a mixed population order for the samples, so this resorting of rows based on population description forms an essential step. SGDP has VCF headers and codes for samples based on their population name (and as listed in Table 10.3). The 1000 Genomes has HG or NA numbers; HGDP–CEPH has HGDP numbers; and EGDP has GS numbers.

A simple form of analysis that can be performed on any compiled data from the above datasets is PCA in Snipper [http://mathgene.usc.es/snipper/analysismultipleprofiles.html]. The reference data for the three main MPS ancestry panels, described earlier, is based on 1000 Genomes data for the four main population groups, plus 18 unadmixed PEL as the Native American reference data and the SGDP Papuans as representative of Oceanian variation in these SNPs; but it is straightforward to begin to compile reference data for new forensic SNPs for the same population combinations. All SGDP and EGDP genotypes will be included as downloadable test data from the same Snipper page in the near future. When uploading files to the Snipper PCA analysis module reference genotype rows require the prefix 1 in the final column and any new SNP data obtained, including those form forensic analyses with MPS, and can be compiled into rows matching the SNP order and designated with 0 in the final column for "unknown." This returns a PCA plot with the unknown SNP profiles present as black points on the colored reference clusters in the plot, and "mouseover" information about the sample code relating to each black point. It should be noted that spatial representations in the first two or three PCA dimensions will only reflect genetic distances between genotypes when they consist only of biallelic SNPs. This is because biallelic genotypes can be coded symmetrically as −1 (homozygote), 0 (heterozygote), and +1 (alternate homozygote), whereas multi-allelic genotypes cannot. The latter can be represented by multidimensional scaling methods that use genetic distance matrices as input (e.g., principal coordinates analysis). Matched Bayes analyses are also made that perform likelihood ratio calculations to estimate the ancestry probabilities for the profiles marked as unknown.

KEYWORDS

- **massively parallel sequencing**
- **SNPs**
- **the 1000 Genomes Project Consortium**
- **ancestry-informative markers**

REFERENCES

Amigo, J.; Salas, A.; Phillips, C.; and Carracedo, Á.; SPSmart: Adapting population based SNP genotype databases for fast and comprehensive web access. BMC Bioinform. **2008**, 9, 428–433.

Amigo, J.; Salas, A.; and Phillips, C.; ENGINES: Exploring single nucleotide variation in entire human genomes. BMC Bioinform. **2011**, 12, 105–111.

Browning, S.R.; Missing data imputation and haplotype phase inference for genome-wide association studies. Hum. Genet. **2008**, 124, 439–450.

Browning, S.R.; Browning, B.L.; Zhou, Y.; Tucci, S.; and Akey, J.M.; Analysis of human sequence data reveals two pulses of archaic Denisovan admixture. Cell, **2018**, 173(1), 53–61.

Eduardoff, M.; Santos, C.; De La Puente, M.; Gross, T.E.; Fondevila, M.; Strobl, C; Sobrino, B.; Ballard, D.; Schneider, P.M.; Carracedo, Á.; Lareu, M.V.; Parson, W.; and Phillips, C.; Inter-laboratory evaluation of SNP-based forensic identification by massively parallel sequencing using the Ion PGM™. Forensic Sci. Int. Genet. **2015**, 17, 110–121.

Kidd, K.K.; Speed, W.C.; Pakstis, A.J.; Podini, D.S.; Lagacé, R.; Chang, J.; Wootton, S.; Haigh, E.; and Soundararajan, U.; Evaluating 130 microhaplotypes across a global set of 83 populations. Forensic Sci. Int. Genet. **2017**, 29, 29–37.

Lek, M.; Karczewski, K.J.; Minikel, E.V.; Samocha, K.E.; Banks, E.; Fennell, T.; O'Donnell-Luria, A.H.; Ware, J.S.; Hill, A.J.; Cummings, B.B.; et al.; Analysis of protein-coding genetic variation in 60,706 humans. Nature **2016**, 536 (7616), 285–291.

Mallick, S.; Li, H.; Lipson, M.; Mathieson, I.; Gymrek, M.; Racimo, F.; Zhao, M.; Chennagiri, N.; Nordenfelt, S.; Tandon, A.; et al.; The Simons Genome Diversity Project: 300 genomes from 142 diverse populations. Nature **2012**, 538 (7624), 201–206.

Pagani, L.; Lawson, D.J.; Jagoda, E.; Mörseburg, A.; Eriksson, A.; Mitt, M.; Clemente, F.; Hudjashov, G.; et al.; Genomic analyses inform on migration events during the peopling of Eurasia. Nature **2016**, 538 (7624), 238–242.

Phillips, C. Forensic genetic analysis of bio-geographical ancestry. Forensic Sci. Int. Genet. **2015**, 18, 49–65.

Phillips, C.; Amigo, J.; Carracedo, Á.; and Lareu, M.V.; Tetra-allelic SNPs: Informative forensic markers compiled from public whole-genome sequence data. Forensic Sci. Int. Genet. **2015**, 19, 100–106.

Phillips, C.; Freire Aradas, A.; Kriegel, A.K.; Fondevila, M.; Bulbul, O.; Santos, C.; Serrulla Rech, F.; Perez Carceles, M.D.; Carracedo, Á.; Schneider, PM.; and Lareu, M.V.;

Eurasiaplex: A forensic SNP assay for differentiating European and South Asian ancestries. Forensic Sci. Int. Genet. **2013**, 7 (3), 359–366.

Phillips, C.; Parson, W.; Lundsberg, B.; Santos, C.; Freire-Aradas, A.; Torres, M.; Eduardoff, M.; Børsting, C.; Johansen, P.; M. Fondevila, M.; Morling, N.; and Schneider, P.; EUROFORGEN-NoE Consortium; Carracedo, Á.; and Lareu, M.V.; Building a forensic ancestry panel from the ground up: The EUROFORGEN Global AIM-SNP set. Forensic Sci. Int. Genet. **2014**, 11, 13–25.

Porras-Hurtado, L.; Ruiz, Y.; Santos, C.; Phillips, C.; Carracedo, Á.; and Lareu, M.V.; An overview of STRUCTURE: applications, parameter settings, and supporting software. Front. Genet. **2013**, 4, 98.

Purcell, S.; Neale, B.; Todd-Brown, K.; Thomas, L.; Ferreira, M.A.; Bender, D.; Maller, J.; Sklar, P.; de Bakker, P.I.; Daly, M.J.; and Sham, P.C.; PLINK: A tool set for whole-genome association and population-based linkage analyses. Am. J. Hum. Genet. **2007**, 81(3), 559–575.

The 1000 Genomes Project Consortium; A map of human genome variation from population-scale sequencing. Nature **2010**, 467 (7319), 1061–1073.

The 1000 Genomes Project Consortium; An integrated map of genetic variation from 1,092 human genomes. Nature **2012**, 491 (7422), 56–65.

The 1000 Genomes Project Consortium; A global reference for human genetic variation; Nature **2015**, 526 (7571), 68–74.

CHAPTER 11

Forensic Anthropology Issues: A Synergy between Physical and Molecular Methods: The Contribution of Degraded DNA Analysis to Physical and Forensic Anthropology

ELENA PILLI[1,2*], ELISA CASTOLDI[3,4], and CRISTINA CATTANEO[4]

[1]*Molecular Anthropology and Forensic Unit, Laboratory of Anthropology, Department of Biology, University of Florence, 50122 Firenze, Italy*

[2]*Molecular Biology and Genetics Unit, Carabinieri Scientific Investigation Department, 00191 Roma, Italy*

[3]*Molecular Biology and Genetics Unit, Carabinieri Scientific Investigation Department, 43100 Parma, Italy*

[4]*LABANOF, Laboratorio di Antropologia e Odontologia Forense, Sezione di Medicina Legale, Dipartimento di Scienze Biomediche per la Salute, Università Degli Studi di Milano, 20133 Milan, Italy*

Corresponding author. E-mail: elena.pilli@unifi.it

ABSTRACT

The essential purpose of the forensic anthropological discipline is the identification of human remains when nearly or completely skeletonized remains are found and a standard soft tissue autopsy can no longer be performed. Identification of human skeletal remains is defined as the act of establishing an identity that permits an individual to be definable and recognizable. In archaeological and forensic contexts, identification involves the possibility to attribute a correct name to human remains. Different circumstances, such as those involve an unexplained natural death, homicide, accident or political, ethnic or religious violence, or mass disaster events, can require to establish the identity of a deceased individual. In all these situations, the joint use of physical and molecular methods can be effective in allowing the identification activity. This chapter will introduce the forensic anthropological activity as a fundamental tool in identification contexts of human skeletal remains and will present how a DNA analysis expert of highly degraded samples may be an important ally of physical anthropologist in challenging situations.

11.1 INTRODUCTION

Forensic anthropology has been known as *the branch of physical anthropology, which, for forensic purposes, deals with the identification of more-or-less skeletonized remains known to be, or suspected of being human* (Stewart, 1979). This definition is, however, too narrow for today's professional forensic anthropologists. A more complete definition is the one provided by *The American Board of Forensic Anthropology*, which states that: "Forensic anthropology is an applied area in the subfield of physical (i.e., biological) anthropology; it uses the science, methodology, and technology of physical/ biological anthropology and related fields to help address medicolegal issues. Forensic anthropologists use clues from the skeleton to assist medical examiners and coroners on a variety of cases, typically including those involving skeletal remains, fragmentary or decomposing remains, burned bodies, buried remains, and child abuse, as well as other trauma cases. Forensic anthropologists use their knowledge of the human skeleton, archaeological methods, and the decomposition process to help law enforcement agencies in the following key ways: (1) to determine if skeletal remains are human or nonhuman, (2) to retrieve surface remains and excavate buried remains using modified archaeological methods, (3) to assist in identifying deceased individuals who cannot be immediately identified through traditional means (such as by visual recognition, fingerprints, or dental evidence), (4) to examine remains for trauma to aid in determining what happened to the deceased individual at the time of death, and (5) to determine how long ago the individual died by examining the condition of the remains. Forensic anthropologists may work directly with forensic pathologists in a medical examiner system, or they may be consulted on an as-needed basis" (http://theabfa.org/faq/).

According to this definition, the main aim of the forensic anthropological discipline is the construction of the so-called biological profile when nearly or completely skeletonized remains are found, and a standard soft tissue autopsy can no longer be performed. The term "biological profile" refers to the identification of all the biological characteristics of the deceased (e.g., sex, age at death, stature, and ancestry), essential for a generic identification of the person who those remains belong to. Nowadays, however, the increased breadth and scope of the field includes not only these traditional analyses, but also personal identification, trauma, and taphonomic analysis, estimating the *post-mortem* interval (PMI) and the application of anthropological knowledge to the investigation of mass disasters.

Identification, however, remains a key role for physical forensic anthropologists, but more and more challenging situations as well as the advancement of DNA technology have revealed how DNA analysis and genetic anthropology (in particular forensic molecular anthropology) may be a fundamental ally of physical anthropology. As the forensic anthropologist studies the human skeleton in toto in order to identify the individual and examine trauma in the forensic context (Black, 2003; Cattaneo, 2007; Grauer, 2001), the forensic molecular anthropologist (FMA) studies skeletal element DNA in order to genetically identify individuals, provide any further genetic information about the remains, such as, for example, phenotypic characteristics and ancestry origin, and identify the skeletal elements when anthropological studies are not permitted. The ability to recover and analyze DNA from highly degraded skeletal remains represents one of the most significant challenges for molecular anthropologists and forensic ones. FMA activity is not only applied to single cases, but its expertise could also be useful in the study of war crime victims, mass disasters, and unidentified person cases (Borić et al., 2011; Budowle et al., 2005; Virkler and Lednev, 2009; Witt et al., 2012; Zupanic Pajnic et al., 2010; Dzijan et al., 2009; Lee et al., 2010; Lindblom and Montelius, 2012; Manhart et al., 2012; Marjanović et al., 2009, 2007; Pilli et al., 2018; Prinz et al., 2007). More significant and extremely valuable is the contribution of forensic molecular anthropology when severe fragmentation, decomposition, burning, or commingling has occurred, and also at scenes of crime where human remains have to be retrieved and properly collected. Unlike fingerprints and dental features, DNA-based identity testing is not restricted to any particular body part. Therefore, DNA profiling is also able to re-associate separated remains typical of mass graves or disasters such as plane crashes or explosions (Leclair et al., 2004; Olaisen et al., 1997). Molecular analysis has become a common practice for identifying human remains and providing information for kinship relationship. Bones, teeth, and hair are more durable biological material than other remains, and therefore, in many forensic cases, they represent the unique potential source of genetic material remaining after exposure to environmental conditions, traumatic events, and after a significant amount of time have passed since the death of the individual.

However, in order for DNA to be of use in the aforementioned manners, it needs to be relatively well preserved, and it needs to be extracted. Taphonomical factors can be extremely challenging; therefore, the next sections will be dedicated to the issues of extraction and DNA profiling from the calcified tissues and hair (which along with nails are the physical anthropologists' main subject of examination), before proceeding with the areas of implementation of DNA analysis in physical anthropology.

11.2 FACTORS INFLUENCING THE SUCCESS OF DNA PROFILING

When working with bone and hair samples, the main potential issues are low amount of starting molecules, degradation of DNA, and the presence of polymerase chain reaction (PCR) inhibitors (Anderung et al., 2008). DNA decay starts immediately after cells die when enzymes from the organism start breaking down cellular structures and DNA molecules (Haglund and Sorg, 1997; Latham and Madonna, 2014; Lindahl, 1993). After the initial onslaught by endogenous enzymes, the DNA is further degraded by bacteria and fungi present both within and outside the body. This biochemical degradation can be limited in certain circumstances (e.g., rapid desiccation or low temperature), but further chemical processes, such as hydrolysis and oxidation, act on the DNA regardless of the conditions affecting its structure and stability (Alaeddini et al., 2010; Haglund and Sorg, 1997; Latham and Madonna, 2014). DNA damage is a complex multifactorial process (e.g., due to chemical and physical factors), which gives rise to very challenging samples from which to gain a genetic profile for identification. Factors of DNA damage include oxidation, hydrolysis, pyrimidine dimers, cytosine deamination, and DNA–DNA and DNA–protein cross linkages. Oxidation, hydrolysis, and pyrimidine dimers are most common in forensic samples than others.

11.2.1 HYDROLYSIS

The main cause of DNA damage is the fragmentation of double helix into small pieces. The most vulnerable bond to damage in DNA is the *N*-glycosyl bond that attaches to the deoxyribose backbone. The cleavage of this bond results in the loss of a base leaving an apurinic/apyrimidinic (AP) site that forms a nick (Evans, 2007). Once a nucleotide is released, the AP can undergo a chemical rearrangement that promotes occurrence of strand breakage. Once the average DNA fragment length is reduced to below

200–250 bp, a significant loss of genetic information occurs due to the lack of suitable template DNA for amplification (Bender et al., 2004). This can result in partial or no DNA profiles. Because the reactive species is H_2O, the vast majority of forensic samples exposed to moist environmental conditions accumulate many AP sites.

11.2.2 OXIDATION

Many other lesions are mediated by free radicals. Reactive oxygen species, such as superoxide and hydrogen peroxide, are created by ionizing radiation or microbial metabolism of anaerobic bacteria that colonize *post-mortem* (PM) tissue (Alaeddini et al., 2010). Oxidative attack on the DNA bases breaks carbon–carbon double bonds of both pyrimidines and imidazole ring of purines, leading to fragmentation (Lindahl, 1993). Damage includes modifications of sugar residues, conversion of cytosine and thymine to hydantoins, removal of bases, and cross linkages (Alaeddini et al., 2010). This lesion leads to replication block during PCR: standard Taq DNA polymerase cannot bypass the lesions (Evans et al., 1993).

11.2.3 ULTRAVIOLET EXPOSURE AND ENVIRONMENTAL DNA DAMAGE

When DNA is exposed to ultraviolet light, pyrimidine dimers (pairs of adjacent thymine (T) or cytosine (C) bases) are created (Evans, 2007). Photochemical exposure induces the formation of covalent bonds between two thymines when they are close on the double helix. These linkages cause DNA polymerase to stall and arrest replication during PCR (Goodsell, 2001). Other photolesions are formed on UV exposure such as purine and pyrimidine oxidation products (Chandrasekhar and Van Houten, 2000).

Many molecular taphonomic processes [molecular taphonomy is the study of the intrinsic and extrinsic factors that impact on the degradation of the body's molecular structures, such as DNA (Latham and Madonna, 2014)] influence the preservation of biological material at macroscopic (sample) and microscopic (proteins and DNA) levels depending mainly on environmental and time factors (Brothwell and Pollard, 2001; Herrmann and Hummel, 1994; Smith et al., 2003, 2001). Degradative processes accumulate with time, while environmental conditions such as temperature, humidity, and pH modify the rate and aggressiveness of the degradation (Fondevila et al., 2008a). Diverse environmental factors can act to generate differential preservation in different skeletons, different bones within the same skeleton, and even variations in DNA quality and quantity across the same bone. Therefore, the depositional environment plays a greater role in contributing to molecule degrading than the absolute age of the DNA sample (Dobberstein et al., 2008; Hagelberg and Clegg, 1991; Haynes et al., 2002; Hochmeister et al., 1991; Leney, 2016; Meyer et al., 2000). All degradation chemical reactions are heavily influenced by temperature; as a result, the increase of 10 °C in the temperature can accelerate the reaction rate by two- to threefold (Bär et al., 1988; Gotherstrom et al., 2002; Latham and Madonna, 2014; Lindahl, 1993). Additionally, warmer temperature promotes microorganism growth, which contributes to biological decomposition. The microbes digest the protein component of bone, making the DNA more prone to damage. In addition, they produce enzyme that fragments DNA molecules (Alaeddini et al., 2010; Bär et al., 1988; Latham and Madonna, 2014). However, although some publications suggest that in some cases, mild heating could facilitate an increase in DNA yield from hard tissues (Geigl, 2002; Latham and Madonna, 2014; Reidy et al., 2009), cooler temperature is preferable to preserve the DNA integrity. In addition, the presence of humidity in the depositional environment can influence biological decomposition. Generally, water molecules participate in hydrolytic reactions that act to fragment and modify DNA molecules; therefore, the more the humidity in the depositional environment, the greater the likelihood of bone degradation, which, in turn, contributes to DNA loss (Eglinton and Logan, 1991; Latham and Madonna, 2014; Poinar and Stankiewicz, 1999). On the contrary, a burial in peat bog (a particular water environment) may be beneficial to DNA preservation due to the low presence of oxygen and high salt concentration that could slow DNA degradation by reducing microbial activity. The pH of the depositional environment also influences the biological decomposition (it occurs more rapidly in acidic and alkaline environments and influences the rate of microbial decomposition (Hedges, 2002; Hedges and Millard, 1995; Latham and Madonna, 2014; White and Hannus, 1983) and, consequently, affects the degree of DNA damage, since the rate of acid-catalyzed depurination leading to strand breaks is pH dependent (Lindahl and Nyberg, 1972). Bones and teeth reach a chemical equilibrium with the depositional environment via mineral leaching and the uptake of different solutes from the soil. This process can lead to bone degradation that can impact the rate of DNA damage. The chemical composition of the soil can interfere with the genetic analyses conducted on skeletal remains due to the presence of solutes such as tannins and humic acids that may be coextracted with the DNA and inhibit subsequent analytical steps (Collins et al., 2002; Hedges, 2002; Latham and Madonna, 2014; Pate and Hutton, 1988). In addition to the many environmental factors, intrinsic factors such as bone type and density can play a role in the process of DNA decomposition as well. Bone size and construction can impact skeletal DNA preservation. Larger bones tend to survive better and are, therefore, most available for genetic analysis. Moreover, until recently, the dense cortical portions of lower limb bones and the toughest tissues of the teeth were considered to be more reliable skeletal elements in generating DNA profiles than those spongy (Barta et al., 2014; Edson et al., 2004, 2009; Hagelberg et al., 1991; Leney, 2016; Milos et al., 2007; Mundorff et al., 2009). To date, however, several studies (Edson et al., 2009; Frisch et al., 1998; Gamba et al., 2014; Kulstein et al., 2017; Pilli et al., 2018a; Pinhasi et al., 2015; Rasmussen et al., 2014) demonstrated that petrous bone represents the better skeletal element in terms of DNA amount and preservation than femur and tooth for human identification purposes even from ancient samples, probably due to the high density of this skeletal element associated with resistance to damage and reduced bacteria-mediated DNA decay and other PM DNA decay. It is important to keep in mind that none of these environmental and intrinsic factors operate in isolation, and they may work together or in opposition regarding DNA degradation: a death scene will, therefore, be characterized by a complex interaction between these several variables.

As a result of all these different chemical and physical factors, the remaining DNA fragments that can be extracted from this biological material are short in length, and their integrity is partly lost. However, due to the fact that the rigid structure of bones and teeth provides some protection against DNA degradation (DNA molecules chemically bound to the hydroxyapatite of the hard tissues), analyzable DNA often persists in bones and teeth even after many years.

11.2.4   CONTAMINATING DNA

Another important issue associated with the analysis of (highly) degraded samples is the contamination. Exogenous DNA molecules from the environment or from people who handle the samples can easily outcompete the small amount of endogenous DNA. Contamination even with low amounts of high-quality DNA from working staff during discovery of skeletal human remains, exhumation and laboratory personnel activities, or reference samples (such as those of the victim, the suspect, and the relatives are typically available as blood stains or buccal swabs and contain large amount of high-quality DNA) can occur, and it can make it difficult to gain reliable results. Contaminating human DNA can be found in people's dead skin cells, hair, saliva, sweet, and blood. In addition, laboratory consumables and reagents can be contaminated by human DNA during production in manufacturing facility (Champlot et al., 2010; Deguilloux et al., 2011; Leonard et al., 2007). Additional DNA contamination such as cross-contamination between samples or between DNA extracts could occur during experimental processing if precautions are not in place. Therefore, as proposed by ancient approach (Willerslev and Cooper, 2005), when working with these types of samples, good practices, targeted to reduce/minimize and control contamination before and after the arrival of such specimens in the laboratory, should be mandatory. Allowing for that all DNA extractions and PCR involving the samples should be carried out in a laboratory physically separated from the laboratory in which PCR cycling and post-PCR analyses were performed, some of the precautions, which should also be applied in the high-throughput era (Llamas et al., 2017), include the following:

1. The use of protective clothing such as disposable laboratory coats (multiple gloves changes during samples handling) during excavation and when handling specimens in the laboratory.
2. Laboratory cleaning procedures with bleach and UV irradiation of hoods and laboratory bench surfaces before and after usage.
3. Processing the question samples prior to known samples and physically isolated pre-PCR facility. In addition, some laboratories control movement of laboratory personnel between spaces (a technician is not permitted on the same day to return to pre-PCR area if he/she has already entered the post-PCR area).
4. Reagent blanks and negative controls are run to monitor level of exogenous DNA in reagents, laboratory, environment, and instruments.
5. Decontamination of reagents/tools (bleach and/or UV irradiation) and specimens by removing their surface should be routine.

Two are the key points to keep in mind: protection of the samples from DNA contamination, and prevention of further endogenous DNA degradation. Therefore, it is good practice that specimens are not washed with water (water contains contaminating bacterial DNA and can deeply penetrate into the samples and cause unnecessary hydrolytic damage to the endogenous DNA) and stored correctly (samples should either be completely dried to avoid further contamination with microbial DNA or stored in a cold, dry place as soon as possible).

11.2.5 PCR INHIBITORS

Inhibitors are exogenous molecules to the samples of interest, such as humic acids, fulvic acids, tannins, and microbial DNA, or present within the sample itself such as, for example, heme in blood, melanin in hair, and fatty acids, collagen, and Ca^{2+} in bone, and are mostly coextracted with the target DNA. The presence of inhibitory molecules in a sample may offer a challenge for PCR amplification. These factors are most common causes of amplification failure even if adequate amounts of DNA are present (Alaeddini et al., 2010). Inhibitors may negatively affect cell lysis during extraction (Jacobsen and Rasmussen, 1992) or reduce polymerase activity (Wilson, 1997). Given the importance of removing PCR inhibitors from DNA extracts, it is not surprising that different strategies were developed to eliminate or overcome PCR inhibitory effects. These include dilution of the extracts (Parsons et al., 2007), the addition of more Taq DNA polymerase, and the use of different DNA polymerases (Hedman et al., 2009) and sample cleanup devices. In addition, PCR enhancers such as bovine serum albumin (Comey et al., 1994), betaine (Abu Al-Soud and Rådström, 2000), and PCRBoost™ (Marshall et al., 2015) were tested to minimize or prevent inhibition effects. The presence of inhibitors can be detected via quantitative real-time PCR (method of choice for quantifying the amount of DNA in a sample) using an internal PCR control (IPC) in the reaction. As the IPC is coamplified with DNA samples, a reduction in the reaction efficiency and a delay in amplification may be due to the presence of inhibitors in a particular sample (Kontanis and Reed, 2006).

11.3 WHAT TO SAMPLE?

The choice of which skeletal elements to sample depends on the aim of the study and obviously what is found in the burial site. If the investigation focus is on the human DNA analysis, as in the forensic field, bones, teeth, and hair are the most suitable material for genetic analysis. Otherwise, if this study focuses on infectious disease, the choice of sampling depends on the infectious agent and/or clinical manifestations. In fact, some infectious diseases, such as, for example, tuberculosis (Stone et al., 2009), leave lesions on some specific skeletal parts that can be sampled for genetic analyses. In addition, an emerging new field of anthropological and archaeological research, the study of ancient microbiome, requires specific biological samples, and sampling is carried out using calcified dental plaque (calculus) (Adler et al., 2013; Warinner et al., 2015a, 2015b, 2015c; Weyrich et al., 2015) and preserved ancient feces (coprolites) (Tito et al., 2008, 2012). As the microorganisms coevolve with the human body, this new field could provide further information on health, diet, and migration of ancient population.

The selection of specimens should be based on their good preservation and minimal diagenetic alteration. In addition, as DNA analysis is destructive, it is a good practice, also for forensic purposes, not to sample parts of the skeleton that could be informative for morphological and pathological studies, unless a DNA analysis of diseases is required.

11.3.1 BONES

When skeletonized human remains or bone elements are recovered in suspicious contexts, one of the first concerns is to distinguish whether or not the material is historical or recent. If the skeletal elements merit juridical attention, there are several visual factors, such as, for example, the compactness and density, the smooth and intact surfaces of bone fragments, and the bone weight, that can indicate good macroscopic preservation and high chances of endogenous DNA survival. The evaluation of these features can help direct the sampling. As recommended by the International Society for Forensic Genetics DNA Commission (Prinz et al., 2007), dense cortical bones such as tibia and femur should always be the first choice of sampling. Due to their density that provides a protective crystal matrix endogenous DNA, tibia and femur are less vulnerable to contaminating DNA (Campos et al., 2012; Orlando et al., 2011; Thomas P. Gilbert et al., 2005). Recently, given its extremely high density, petrous bone, located at the base of the skull between the sphenoid and occipital bones, has been shown to yield more endogenous DNA than teeth and other bones presumably due to the very high density of petrous bones associated with reduced bacteria-mediated DNA decay and other PM DNA decay (Gamba et al., 2014). Kulstein et al. (2017) and Pilli et al. (2018) demonstrated the possibility to produce remarkable and reproducible short tandem repeat (STR) typing results from petrous bone samples for forensic identification purposes even starting with ancient samples. In addition, removal of petrous bone is possible without changing the integrity of the cranium by cutting the connection between petrous and temporal bones using a surgery blade. The petrous bone was recovered from the foramen magnum, leaving a small hole visible only in basal view.

11.3.2 TEETH

Teeth are very hard tissue in the human body and are resistant to adverse conditions such as temperature, humidity, and microbial activity (Alvarez García et al., 1996; Malaver and Yunis, 2003; Marjanović et al., 2007). Therefore, the choice of sampling the teeth for genetic analysis is advantageous for several reasons. First, due to the presence of a nonporous enamel coating, teeth are more refractory to contamination by exogenous DNA than other bones (Pilli et al., 2013; Thomas P. Gilbert et al., 2005). In addition, sampling teeth is logistically less demanding than other bones, and finally, teeth can be unequivocally assigned to an individual skull. Although teeth provide a valuable source of DNA, little is known about which region is the best in terms of DNA yield (Adler et al., 2011). Different methods are described in the literature to collect material from teeth for DNA analysis. These procedures include grinding the whole tooth (Sweet and Hildebrand, 1998) or the root (Rohland and Hofreiter, 2007), sectioning of the tooth (Trivedi et al., 2002), access to pulp cavity and dentine via the crown (Tilotta et al., 2010), and incubating overnight the whole tooth, after external surface decontamination, in extraction solution (Bolnick et al., 2012). In order to obtain as maximum DNA yield as possible, tooth destruction is recommended. However, the disadvantage of this destructive activity is associated with impossibility of carrying out further analysis, which may be required. In these cases, preserving the specimens for potential subsequent morphological/radiographical or epigenetic dental trait studies is essential. Therefore, as proposed for ancient and museum remains, tooth sampling can be carried out by excising partially the root, and the inside of the tooth drilled until to produce the needed amount of powder for extraction (Pilli et al., 2018). In this way, the teeth could be placed back in the jaw socket after sampling.

11.3.3 HAIR

One of the most common evidences at the crime scene is hair sample: shed hair represents up to 90% of the hair samples collected at the crime scene (Bender and Schneider, 2006; Graham, 2007). During normal daily activities, humans and animals shed hair from their bodies, clothes, and from other objects or materials with which they make contact. Humans shed an average of 100 hairs daily particularly during physical contact, for example, between victim and suspect when a crime is being committed. While shed hairs are one of the most commonly encountered evidence types, they are most limited in terms of DNA quantity and quality. As a result, rootless hair shaft samples [the hair root, being the only living portion of the hair, contains better preserved DNA (Bengtsson et al., 2012)] submitted to a forensic laboratory for DNA analysis are reserved for mitochondrial DNA (mtDNA) analysis due to the presence of highly degraded as well as insufficient amounts of nuclear DNA. However, because mtDNA profiles do not offer the discriminatory power of nuclear DNA profiles, it could be useful to be able to assess the feasibility of recovering highly discriminatory nuclear DNA from this common evidence type. Some studies based on PCR analysis have suggested that because keratinization involves the breakdown of the nucleus, including the DNA, nuclear DNA is, by extension, simply not present in telogen hair shafts (Bengtsson et al., 2012; McNevin et al., 2005). Otherwise, some of the most recent information on the overall quantity and quality of DNA in telogen hair shafts has come from studies employing next-generation sequencing (NGS). In fact, because PCR analysis of nuclear DNA retrieved from hair is challenging, these samples are much better suited for advanced massively parallel sequencing technologies (Rasmussen et al., 2010). In addition, NGS-based shotgun sequencing may not be dependent on predefined amplicons, and the results reflect the endogenous size of the DNA. FBI researchers (Brandhagen et al., 2018) performed a high-throughput shotgun sequencing on both recently collected and aged hair samples. Results of their study showed that nuclear DNA comprised the vast majority of total DNA (99.93% and 99.88% of the reads of two freshly collected single shed hairs mapped to the human nuclear DNA, and similar results were obtained from aged hairs) in hair shafts despite high level of degradation. As a result, hair samples can provide a valuable source of nuclear DNA considering also that the hair structure provides efficient protection against exogenous contaminating DNA. As other forms of tissue often found at archaeological and forensic sites (such as bone and teeth) have been shown to be very susceptible to sources of contaminant DNA (Thomas P. Gilbert et al., 2005), hairs represent a more reliable and contaminant-resistant tissue for use in both forensic and ancient DNA analyses.

11.4 DNA ANALYSIS

11.4.1 DNA EXTRACTION

Extracting DNA from bones, teeth, and hair samples often requires modification of the DNA extraction methods used for other types of biological samples. Different techniques are utilized by laboratories to extract and purify DNA from hard tissue and hair. The focus of DNA extraction techniques is to maximize DNA yield, minimize any additional DNA damage, and remove any inhibitors that may be coextracted with the sample DNA and interfere with subsequent analyses. Initially, the first laboratory step consists of removing external contaminating DNA to the bone, teeth, and hair that would contribute to generating unreliable results. Bone and tooth decontamination can be performed mechanically using, for example, a rotary sanding tool, and/or by exposure to ultraviolet radiation (Pilli et al., 2018), or immerging the bone or tooth in a bleach solution (Kemp and Smith, 2005). Conversely, one of the ways for hair decontamination consists of sequential washes in a 5% bleach solution followed by a rinse initially in absolute ethanol and then in sterile distilled water, as proposed by Pilli et al. (2014). After surface decontamination, the hard tissues are pulverized, whereas hair samples are left to air-dry and cut into small pieces; then, all samples are incubated in extraction buffer, proteinase K and DTT (for hair samples) in order to dissolve the organic and inorganic portions of the tissue. DNA is then purified using different techniques, including also commercial kits (Cattaneo et al., 1995; Coticone et al., 2010; Johnston and Stephenson, 2016; Kemp and Smith, 2005; Kim et al., 2008; Lee et al., 2010; Rucinski et al., 2012; Silva et al., 2013). Bone/tooth pulverization allows us to obtain a greater contact surface with the different chemicals employed in the DNA extraction process, encouraging the release of a greater amount of DNA from hydroxyapatite mineral matrix. The amount of bone/tooth powder used for DNA extraction varies from laboratory to laboratory. Most published protocols call for as high as 2.5 g to as little as 0.2 g of starting bone powder. In 2013, Dabney et al. (2013) set up an improved ancient DNA extraction technique starting from 0.05 g of powder. Currently, this is the most widely used technique for DNA extraction/purification from highly degraded bone samples due to the fact that this protocol allow us to recover short fragments, even as sort as 50 bp, via the use of commercial silica columns (Chung et al., 2004; Dabney et al., 2013). A new extraction protocol suitable for highly degraded samples has been proposed by Rohland et al. (2018). The silica-based DNA extraction protocol enables the retrieval of short ($\geq$35 bp) or even very short ($\geq$25 bp) DNA fragments with minimal carryover of molecules that could inhibit library preparation for high throughput. All these extraction methods were developed in order remove and minimize the presence of inhibitors in the extracts that can cause interference with the PCR reaction. A new study has been carried out to evaluate the efficiency of various DNA extraction methods to remove high amounts of PCR inhibitors from challenging samples prior to NGS (Zeng et al., 2019). The results demonstrated that the extraction methods commonly used in most crime laboratories are compatible with NGS sequencing chemistry and platform.

In addition, several studies (Geigl, 2002; Latham and Madonna, 2014; Latham and Miller, 2018; Maciejewska et al., 2016; Madonna et al., 2015; Reidy et al., 2009; Zgonjanin et al., 2015) have investigated whether subjecting bone to mild heating may increase DNA yields, since mild heating reduces bone moisture and, therefore, damage due to hydrolytic processes, and makes the hard tissue brittle allowing to release DNA more easily during the extraction. However, high temperature is generally considered as an accelerant of DNA degradation, and for this reason, different protocols tend to remove heat from all analytical steps, including the grinding process (Courts and Madea, 2011; Morales Colón et al., 2018; Pajnič, 2016; Pilli et al., 2018; Zupanic Pajnic et al., 2012).

11.4.2   GENETIC MARKERS FOR IDENTITY TESTING

It is well known that when it comes to positive identification (e.g., through the comparison of antemortem (AM) and PM data), the main identifiers are fingerprints, teeth, DNA, medical devices, and the comparison of personal descriptors or the shape of bone (e.g., frontal sinuses). Bone anthropology can be involved when specific features of the AM and PM skeleton correspond; however, DNA analysis is very powerful.

As reported previously, DNA extraction techniques are focused on maximizing DNA yield in order to permit genetic analysis that is a crucial tool in the identification of human remains. The choice of the suitable genetic test depends upon the DNA degradation, the type of reference sample available, and the question to be addressed. Human cells contain nuclear DNA and mtDNA. Due to vast amount of variability at the DNA level between unrelated individuals, currently, portions of noncoding nuclear DNA called STRs are used routinely as genetic markers for identity testing (see Chapter 3). Despite their high power of discrimination and robustness, STR assay often fails when genotyping highly degraded samples. As expected, when analyzing extremely degraded DNA samples, signal strength was lost with larger sizes of PCR product, and a "decay curve" was observed, in which the peak height was inversely proportional to the amplicon length (Chung et al., 2004; Cotton et al., 2000; Lygo et al., 1994; Wallin et al., 1998). The development of primers that result in shorter amplicons (mini-STRs) has helped improve the profiling success of highly degraded samples. In addition, the combined use of different kits such as, for example, AmpFℓSTR® NGM SElect™ PCR Amplification Kit (Thermo-Fisher Scientific, Oyster Point, CA, USA) and PowerPlex® ESX 17 system (Promega Corporation) could help increase the number of identified loci in highly degraded samples, as described in (Pilli et al., 2018). The major disadvantage of the use of mini-STRs is that fewer loci can be simultaneously amplified in multiplex and separated by capillary electrophoresis. In addition, due to the fact that primers have been moved as close as possible to the STR targets, the wide size range of amplicons has been decreased, and all loci have the same general size (Butler et al., 2003). During capillary electrophoresis, amplicons are separated by length; therefore, a limited number of mini-STR loci can be separated in each dye channel.

Employing additional nuclear markers can prove useful for identifying highly degraded samples and offer the potential to infer the geographic ancestry and/or phenotype of human remains. In some situations, in fact, despite the reduction of amplicon sizes, it is not possible to obtain a DNA profile via STR analysis. Therefore, in such cases, single-nucleotide polymorphisms (SNPs) could be an alternative to provide more genetic data than STRs from severely fragmented DNA. SNP genotyping systems have been successfully applied to the most degraded samples such as, for example, those from World Trade Center remains (Alonso et al., 2005; Brenner and Weir, 2003) or other disasters (Biesecker et al., 2005), when STR analysis produced incomplete or no profiles. Given the valuable support provided by the SNP analysis to identification of highly degraded human remains (Børsting et al., 2012; Fondevila et al., 2008b; Phillips et al., 2007; Sanchez et al., 2006), SNPs have been proposed as complements to traditional STR and mini-STR profiling.

SNP genotyping is not a new technology for identity testing; this was the first PCR-based system to be utilized for forensic DNA testing (Comey and Budowle, 1991). However, SNPs are not as polymorphic as STRs, and SNP profiles will not be directly comparable with the profiles generated using the common STR loci (Budowle and van Daal, 2008). Therefore, a large number of SNPs must be successfully genotyped to produce a profile as discriminatory as a profile from genotyping 16-loci STR (Gill, 2001b) and estimate geographic ancestry or predict phenotypic characteristics. Microarray and primer extension assays are available for SNP analysis, even if large multiplex reactions may lead to poor amplification efficiency and make it difficult to gain accurate and reproducible profiles (Dixon et al., 2006). Until recently, a possible solution to this problem was to run tandem PCR reactions of several SNP multiplexes each consisting of a smaller subset of loci. Now, NGS technologies offer a solution for massively parallel sequencing of a large number of genetic markers, including length and sequence polymorphism. Recognizing the potential of NGS, several PCR-based kits targeting SNPs have been developed for various NGS platforms. However, PCR-based systems require intact forward and reverse primer binding sites in the template DNA and, when highly degraded samples are investigated, can result in high dropout rates (Gettings et al., 2015). Therefore, enrichment of target DNA for forensically challenging samples by using an alternative method that does not depend on the presence of intact primer binding site would improve recovery of fragmented DNA prior to deep sequencing (Avila-Arcos et al., 2011; Cummings et al., 2010; Mertes et al., 2011). An alternative strategy can be target enrichment using synthetic probes (Winters et al., 2017). This process consists of hybridizing biotinylated DNA or RNA probes to complementary DNA fragments either in solution or on solid surface (Rohland and Reich, 2012). In this case, highly degraded DNA targets can be enriched from DNA samples independent of fragment length and breakpoint (Bose et al., 2018; Gettings et al., 2015).

Unlike nuclear DNA, as generally known, mtDNA is maternally inherited [except some extraordinary cases, as proposed by (Luo et al., 2018)], and barring mutation, the sequence of all siblings and maternal relatives is identical (Giles et al., 1980). This characteristic can be exploited when supplemental genetic information is needed or when suitable autosomal STR reference is not available (Edson et al., 2018; Latham and Madonna, 2014). The lack of recombination events in the mtDNA genome can allow maternal relatives separated by several generations to serve as reference samples. This latter feature is useful in missing person identification and mass disaster cases where suitable AM and family reference samples may be unavailable. In addition, an mtDNA marker is conventionally utilized by forensic scientists to generate a profile from very difficult samples, which fail with standard STR and mini-STR analysis. As discussed in Chapter 6, mitochondrial variation is exploited for forensic identity testing by sequencing the hypervariable control region. Due to the fact that mutations in this region do not code for vital cell functions, polymorphisms between individuals are accumulate and, therefore, are abundant. mtDNA polymorphisms are usually determined by standard PCR-based sequencing approaches of mitochondrial D-loop. The concept of redesigning primer sets in order to decrease amplicon size in autosomal markers has also been applied to mtDNA analysis with success (Gabriel et al., 2001; Berger and Parson, 2009; Eichmann and Parson, 2008). Different primer sets can be used to amplify different overlapping fragments covering a target region, typically from 2 to 12 overlapping fragments of approximately 150–600 bp in length. This approach is labor intensive, consumes significant amounts of valuable DNA extract, and can be template-length dependent and costly. Moreover, due to the multiple laboratory steps required, repeated singleplex amplifications can increase the risk of contamination with exogenous human DNA. Multiplex PCR amplifications could provide a solution for exogenous contamination but require hundreds of overlapping amplicons in cases where whole mitochondrial genome sequences are needed for high-resolution identification. In addition, as previously mentioned, PCR-based systems require intact forward and reverse primer binding sites in the template DNA; therefore, an alternative method to generate complete mitochondrial genomes could be based on the probe capture enrichment process. This strategy, routinely used in ancient DNA study with human archaeological samples, as proposed, for example, by Vai et al. (2019) and Rusu et al. (2018), consists of hybridizing biotinylated DNA or RNA probes to complementary DNA fragments. This approach has potential application in forensic science, historical human identification cases, kinship analysis, and population studies. In particular, the methodology can be applied to any case where whole mitochondrial genome sequences are required to provide the highest level of maternal lineage discrimination (Shih et al., 2018; Templeton et al., 2013). In addition, using NGS technology, multiple samples can be processed in parallel (Knapp et al., 2012), reducing processing contamination risks, labor, and costs compared to classical Sanger sequencing approaches.

In addition, the strategy of typing only the mitochondrial hypervariable region could became a problem when different individuals in a population share a common haplogroup, for example, haplogroup H [the haplogroup dominates Western European mitochondrial variability (>40%)] or when distantly related individuals share a maternal ancestry that may not be known (Just et al., 2011). In fact, a study published in *Nature Communications* (Brotherton et al., 2013) showed that >70% of mtDNA variation can be located outside the control region for some haplogroups when whole mitochondrial genome is sequenced. Therefore, massively parallel sequencing of the entire mitochondrial genome allows increasing the discriminatory power (Fendt et al., 2009).

Nonetheless, with changes in the social structure and with migration events, at times, classical identification methods such as DNA alone may not be sufficient to identify human remains because the needed variables are not present in the AM set of data or in the PM one. Therefore, it is necessary to "go back" to morphological features of the face when AM photographs are available or skeletal traits when AM X-rays are available, as well as other personal descriptors. All these are domains of anthropology, which now needs to find new algorithms in order to provide identification strategies for "shapes" of the body and of the skeleton, which satisfy Daubert standards (Dirkmaat et al., 2008; Steadman et al., 2006).

11.5 MOLECULAR SOLUTIONS TO PURELY FORENSIC ANTHROPOLOGY ISSUES

The following is a brief summary of developing applications of forensic molecular anthropology to support forensic anthropology data in the study of human remains and, therefore, in different steps of the biological profile.

11.5.1 SPECIES IDENTIFICATION

The specific morphology and anatomy of complete bones permits us to distinguish among human and nonhuman skeletal remains, although the task becomes more complicated when dealing with subadult individuals (whose small bones can be easily confused with nonhuman ones); however, the task becomes even more complicated when dealing with degraded fragments. In these cases, only protein analysis (Ubelaker et al., 2004), the microscopic structure of the fragment of bone, and specifically the analysis of osteon pattern, shape, and size (Cattaneo et al., 1999, 2009; Hillier and Bell, 2007; Mulhern and Ubelaker, 2001), can help, although such methods can display limits when dealing with charred or very old and dry bones (Cattaneo, 2007). DNA can at times certainly come in handy.

The majority of molecular techniques that are used to identify species of forensic relevance use DNA markers located in mitochondrial genome for different reasons:

1. The mtDNA is present in multiple copies per cell compared to the nuclear DNA.
2. Phylogenetic trees based on mtDNA sequences tend to better reveal the species-level differentiation due to the uniparental transmission of mtDNA genome, which escapes genomic recombination.
3. Mitochondrial genes have relatively high variability and are flanked by transfer RNA genes that are conserved across species, allowing the design of "universal" primers that can be used in different taxa (GilArriortua et al., 2013; Salem et al., 2015).

Markers used for forensic species identification show little intraspecific variability (variability between members of the same species) but demonstrate sufficient interspecific variability (variability between members of different species) to discriminate between individuals of different species. In addition, markers should have a short sequence length so as to also facilitate the typing of highly degraded samples. Different markers are used to identify species of forensic relevance, such as *cytochrome b* (An et al., 2007; de Pancorbo et al., 2003; Tobe and Linacre, 2007, 2009, 2008; Wan and Fang, 2003; Wetton et al., 2004; Hsieh et al., 2003, 2006; Irwin et al., 1991;Kocher et al., 1989; Kuwayama and Ozawa, 2000; Meganathan et al., 2008; Moore et al., 2003; Rohilla and Tiwari, 2008), *cytochrome c oxidase I* -this is used in DNA barcoding and has been adopted as a marker by the Barcode for Life Consortium (Borisenko et al., 2008; Dalton and Kotze, 2011; Tavares and Baker, 2008; Hajibabaei et al., 2006; Hebert et al., 2004, 2003a, 2003b; Holmes et al., 2009; Meier et al., 2006; Santos Rojo Velasco, 2006; Smith et al., 2008)- *12S* ribosomal RNA (Balitzki-Korte et al., 2005; Kitano et al., 2007; Melton and Holland, 2007; Pilli et al., 2014), *16S* ribosomal RNA (Imaizumi et al., 2007; Mitani et al., 2009; Pilli et al., 2014; Rastogi et al., 2007), and *NDH* family (Junqueira et al., 2004; Schwenke et al., 2006). While all these genes have been investigated for species identification, the D-loop analysis has mostly been exploited for intraspecies identification (Clifford et al., 2004; Eichmann and Parson, 2007; Himmelberger et al., 2008; Mayer et al., 2007; Schneider et al., 1999; Zhang et al., 2006), though sometimes it can be applied to species identification (Fumagalli et al., 2009; Gupta et al., 2006; Kitano et al., 2007; Kocher et al., 1989; Nussbaumer and Korschineck, 2006; Pilli et al., 2014; Pun et al., 2009). In addition, a nuclear marker such as internal transcribed spacer region has been used in several studies dealing with the identification of flies of forensic relevance. Due to its high evolutionary rate, this genomic fragment has proven to be suitable for phylogenetic studies at the species and intraspecific levels (Roziah et al., 2015).

Usually, the standard analysis of species identification requires amplification of part of these genes, followed by Sanger sequencing and comparison of the obtained sequence with reference sequences saved in a database, such as GenBank. Recent studies have shown the potential of DNA metabarcoding for identifying species in wildlife forensic samples as well (Arulandhu et al., 2017). DNA metabarcoding is an approach that combines DNA barcoding (technique used to identify several species) with NGS, which enables sensitive high-throughput multispecies identification on the basis of DNA

extracted from complex samples (Taberlet et al., 2012). DNA metabarcoding uses universal primers to mass-amplify informative DNA barcode
sequences (Arulandhu et al., 2017; Fahner et al., 2016; Staats et al., 2016).
Subsequently, the obtained DNA barcodes are sequenced and compared to
a DNA sequence reference database from well-characterized species for
taxonomic assignment (Taberlet et al., 2012; Fahner et al., 2016). The main
advantage of DNA metabarcoding over other identification techniques is that
it permits the identification of species within samples that are composed of
multiple components (human/nonhuman, animal, plant, fungi, and bacteria),
which would not be possible through morphological means and would be
time consuming with traditional DNA barcoding. Furthermore, the use of
mini-barcode markers in DNA metabarcoding facilitates the identification
of species in highly processed samples containing heavily degraded DNA.

11.5.2   SEX IDENTIFICATION

Traditionally, sex determination of human skeletal material is performed by
assessing sexually dimorphic traits mainly of the pelvis and skull (Dayal
et al., 2008; Kalmey and Rathbun, 1996; MacLaughlin and Bruce, 1990;
Phenice, 1969; Steyn and Işcan, 1998; Sutherland and Suchey, 1991;
Ubelaker and Volk, 2002). A visual analysis of the pelvis is indeed typically
the preferred indicator of sex with a high degree of reliability (Phenice, 1969;
MacLaughlin and Bruce, 1990; Ubelaker and Volk, 2002), as well as specific
shapes and features of the cranium. Nevertheless, many forensic cases do
not have the possibility to rely on a complete skeleton. For this reason, many
studies aimed at developing standardized methods for sex estimation from
other postcranial bones, based on both morphological (observational) and
metric techniques (Asala, 2001; France, 1998; Gualdi-Russo, 2007; Mall
et al., 2001; Robinson and Bidmos, 2009; Spradley and Jantz, 2011). An
analysis published by Thomas et al. (2016) compared the sex determination
based on DNA and forensic anthropological estimation from 360 forensic
cases. The authors demonstrated that the overall rate of correct sex estimation from these cases is 94.7%, influenced by the amount of available
skeletal material for analysis and according to the education level of the
examiner. Morphological methods have a relatively high success rate only in
the case of remains where the pelvis is well preserved, adult skeletons and
bones are in good condition of preservation, and when the morphometric
variability in the population to which they belong is known (Daskalaki et

al., 2011; Schmidt et al., 2003). Hence, at times, skeletal sexing may result to be unreliable.

Advances in the field of molecular genetics have provided sensitive methods for sex determination that has become a valuable tool in forensic casework (Mannucci et al., 1994). Sex testing is usually performed by amplifying target intronic sequences of the human amelogenin gene, which is to be found on both genomes (Sullivan et al., 1993). In most commercially available multiplex PCR kits for human identification, the amelogenin system is included with amplicon size of 106 and 112 bp for X and Y chromosomes, respectively (Sullivan et al., 1993). However, this assay is not entirely effective (Cadenas et al., 2007; Chang et al., 2007; Ou et al., 2012; Roffey et al., 2000; Santacroce et al., 2006; Santos et al., 1998; Shadrach et al., 2004; Steinlechner et al., 2002; Takayama et al., 2009; Thangaraj et al., 2002; Chen et al., 2014; Jobling et al., 2007; Kumagai et al., 2008; Lattanzi et al., 2005; Ma et al., 2012; Maciejewska and Pawłowski, 2009; Michael and Brauner, 2004; Mitchell et al., 2006) especially for the analysis of highly degraded samples, resulting in amplification failures and incorrect sex assignments. To overcome these problems, alternative molecular-genetic assays were developed (Boonyarit et al., 2014; Esteve Codina et al., 2009; Fazi et al., 2014; Kim et al., 2010; Tschentscher et al., 2008). However, it was observed that in severely degraded DNA, such as present in ancient samples or heavily decomposed remains, also, these alternative methods failed to produce useable results. A new robust tool was developed for genetic sex determination in forensic context, especially when dealing with highly degraded human DNA (Madel et al., 2016). This method is based on real-time PCR amplification of short intergenic sequences ($\leq$50 bp) on both gonosomes. In an attempt to determine the sex of less well preserved or older archaeological samples, another strategy that involves the implementation of high-resolution melting curve analysis of PCR products after real-time PCR amplification was successfully developed (Álvarez-Sandoval et al., 2014). Exploiting NGS technology, a new method has been proposed by Skoglund et al. (2013). This method identifies sex by considering the number of reads in shotgun DNA sequencing data that align to the X and Y chromosomes. However, this approach relies on at least 100,000 sequences mapping to the human genome for accurate assignment, a prohibitive condition from many badly preserved remains. Therefore, subsequently, Mittnik et al. (2016) developed a novel approach that takes into account the ratio of sequence alignments to chromosome X compared to the autosomes and which gives accurate results with as little as several thousands of reads mapping to the human genome. This method is, therefore, suitable for light shotgun sequencing data even of samples that contain only a small percentage of endogenous DNA or that are contaminated by modern human DNA.

11.5.3   EXTERNALLY VISIBLE CHARACTERISTICS

11.5.3.1   AGE AT DEATH

Evaluation of chronological age of the donor of an unknown sample plays an important role in forensic investigations in order to identify an individual (the applicability of law depends on the age of the person in question; sometimes, the identity and age of individuals are unclear such as in the migration cases) or human skeletal remains. For forensic anthropology, age estimation involves morphological analyses of skeletal features (Meissner and Ritz-Timme, 2010). Literature provides a large amount of articles, which apply known macroscopic and microscopic techniques, divided into dental and skeletal ones, aimed at determining a range of age for the subject (Cunha et al., 2009). So long as a body is still developing, age estimation can be more accurate and provide smaller error rates, as it commonly is in the case of subadult individuals. In such cases, dental development methods as well as skeletal growth ones can furnish accurate age ranges and, thus, more precise information concerning the age at death of the subject. On the contrary, once skeletal and dental development have already settled, age estimation is much more complicated because the only parameters that can be used are based on the physiological degeneration observed in skeletal and dental structures with age. In particular, the articular degeneration of specific joints, which are not modified by pathological and occupational factors (auricular surface, pubic symphysis, ribs, as principal examples), is usually considered (Albert et al., 2010; Brooks, 1955; Rougé-Maillart et al., 2009; Suchey, 1979; Brooks and Suchey, 1990; Buckberry and Chamberlain, 2002; Cunha et al., 2009; DiGangi et al., 2009; Işcan et al., 1984, 1985, 1987; Lovejoy et al., 1985), as well as dental wear or periodontal alterations (Baccino et al., 2014; Cameriere et al., 2004, 2006, 2007; Lamendin, 1973; Lamendin et al., 1992). Microscopic methods have also been developed for such cases where macroscopy proves itself useless (Boel et al., 2007; Cho et al., 2002; Kerley, 1965; Kerley and Ubelaker, 1978; Lynnerup et al., 2006). It is, however, necessary to highlight that there are at the present virtually no reliable methods for the estimation of age at death of the elderly, and aging dead adults is still riddled with limits, large errors (Kimmerle et al., 2008), and population-specific references (Schmitt et al., 2002), limits that are necessary to be known and well explained when dealing with investigating authorities (Cunha et al., 2009).

However, these methods are only applicable to forensic cases that involve bones and teeth, and the results obtained can be ambiguous (Bauer et al., 2013). Some chemical methods such as combined aspartic acid racemization provide precise age estimation (Alkass et al., 2010), but require the presence of dental specimens. Therefore, DNA methods for age estimation were investigated (Freire-Aradas et al., 2017). The main advantage of these methods is that they can be applied to any tissue containing DNA. For more details on age estimation via DNA methods, see Chapter 8. No data from bone or teeth samples are available as of writing the book.

11.5.3.2 PREDICTING EYE AND HAIR COLOR

In disaster victim identification and other missing person identification cases, when long time has passed since the disaster event or the time when persons got missing, and the AM samples or putative relatives are not directly available, externally visible characteristics such as eye and hair color can be suitable to provide valuable guidance to locate the putative relatives for final identification of the missing via STR profiling (Chaitanya et al., 2017; Draus-Barini et al., 2013). In the next future, eye and hair color and other externally visible characteristics will become easily predictable from DNA, allowing to describe a missing person's appearance from his/her skeletal remains in a detailed manner, directing the search for AM samples or putative relatives. For more details on eye and hair color prediction, see Chapter 8. This, in general, is fused with information from the skeleton.

11.5.3.3 STATURE

Another relevant externally visible characteristic used to describe human remains and create a biological profile is stature. Stature estimation from the skeleton is relatively easy, since it is based on the length of long bones (femur and tibia mostly, but also fibula, humerus, radius, and ulna). Most of the methods require the insertion of such information in specific regression formulae. As in all other anthropological evaluations, an error range needs to be considered, as well as the population specificity of the formulae (De Mendonça, 2000; Giles, 1993; Ross and Konigsberg, 2002; Trotter and Gleser, 1952). Taking into account the rarity of the circumstances in which all the bones of a skeleton are available for the anthropological analysis, other methods were developed on other skeletal districts, such as bones of the feet and hands (Holland, 1995; Meadows and Jantz, 1992) or even from the cranium (Chiba and Terazawa, 1998; Krishan, 2008), which, however, provide wider errors.

Stature as well as other externally visible traits such as skin, eye, and hair pigmentation can currently be predicted using various SNPs (Budowle and van Daal, 2008; Draus-Barini et al., 2013; Kayser, 2015). Besides pigmentation traits, no molecular prediction tests are currently available for any other externally visible characteristics due to limited knowledge on genes and predictive DNA markers. For more details on height prediction, see Chapter 8. No data from bone or teeth samples are available as of writing the book.

11.5.4   ANCESTRY ORIGIN

A fundamental feature when building a biological profile considers the geographic origin of the individual in analysis, especially in the light of the increase in migration and the modern multicultural society. The cranium is commonly the most characterizing skeletal region for ancestry identification, according to specific characteristics that it may display when considering a specific geographic area of origin (prognatism, palate shape, and dental shape). Many studies, however, attempted to identify ethnicity from postcranial bones, such as the femur (Ballard and Trudell, 1999; Craig, 1995; Gill, 2001a).

The University of Tennessee developed a software tool for ancestry assessment based on specific cranial measurements and specific cranial points. Such points are commonly employed when creating the biological profile and especially when estimating ancestry with the use of the program FORDISC 3.1 (Elliott and Collard, 2009; Jantz and Ousley, 2005). FORDISC is, in fact, a function program that provides information on ancestry estimation through the comparison of the inserted measurements with reference population group indexes based on multivariate statistical approaches (Katherine Spradley and Jantz, 2016). Its limit, however, regards the limited groups of population considered, which make the method applicable only to American subjects. The problem of ancestry estimation is further aggravated, as previously mentioned, by the multiculturalism of modern society, where well-defined boundaries between populations are day after day more complicated to be observed, and population or ethnic groups are always more difficult to be found.

The constant awareness of the need for local methods for biological estimations created an increased diligence toward the research for skeletal collections useful for enlarging and strengthening the existing ones. The assemblage and study of human skeletal remains have indeed a longstanding scientific tradition in physical anthropology, because reference collections represent the primary source for the development of basic techniques in both forensic anthropology and bioarchaeology (e.g., (Brooks and Suchey, 1990; Byers et al., 1989; Klales et al., 2012; Lovejoy et al., 1985; Milner and Boldsen, 2012; Rougé-Maillart et al., 2009). Positive control for biological estimation is, in fact, fundamental in such disciplines, together with the awareness that physiological age indicators, growth patterns, or sexually dimorphic traits vary across populations, demanding population-specific methodologies for the assessment of basic biological profiles of skeletonized individuals (Ferreira et al., 2014; Usher, 2002). For this reason, local reference skeletal collections nowadays represent an exceptionally valuable research material (Alemán et al., 2012; Bosio et al., 2012; Cardoso, 2006; Cattaneo et al., 2018; Dayal et al., 2009; Eliopoulos et al., 2007; Ferreira et al., 2014; Hunt and Albanese, 2005; L'Abbé et al., 2005; Salceda et al., 2012) for narrowing error ranges and uncertainties of the commonly used anthropological methods.

The ancestry of a forensic evidence contributor or human remains based on ancestry informative marker analysis can also provide valuable information (Enoch et al., 2006; Fondevila et al., 2013; Kersbergen et al., 2009; Lao et al., 2006; Paschou et al., 2007; Phillips et al., 2007; Shriver et al., 2005) in aged bone samples (Romanini et al., 2015). For more details on ancestry origin, see Chapter 9.

11.5.5 CRANIOFACIAL RECONSTRUCTION

It is a well-known fact that facial reconstruction is not an identification method. It may help trigger a suspicion of identity though but does not guarantee maximum reliability. Facial reconstruction is a specialized human ability and a widely accepted identification method (Aeria et al., 2010; Smeets et al., 2010, 2012). Craniofacial reconstruction employed in the context of forensic investigation aims at estimating the facial appearance associated with an unknown skull through the reconstruction of soft tissues for victim identification. It is a technique based on facial anatomy and its relationship to the underlying skull (Claes et al., 2010a, 2010b; Wilkinson, 2010). However, several suggest that interindividual variation in facial morphology is, in most cases, primarily determined by genetic variation (Baynam et al., 2013; Claes et al., 2012; Hammond, 2007; Hopman et al., 2014; Kohn, 1991; Weinberg et al., 2013). The potential of DNA-based facial constructing is forensically of great interest in investigation activity or to progress the reinvestigation of cold cases (Claes et al., 2014). Normal facial shape is known to be highly heritable (Hair et al., 2014; Ng et al., 2017; Weinberg et al., 2013). For more details on craniofacial reconstruction, see Chapter 8. No data from bone or teeth samples are available as of writing the book.

11.5.6 TRAUMA AND PATHOLOGICAL ANALYSIS

Among the information that a skeleton can provide, of mandatory importance, in particular in the forensic context, is that concerning traumatic and pathologic markers. Anthropologists are, in fact, frequently asked to determine when skeletal fractures occurred in relation to an individual's death. The relevance of such information is double: on one hand, they can provide insight into the cause and manner of death; on the other hand, they can reveal unique characteristics necessary for personal identification. AM, perimortem and PM trauma, therefore, need to be accurately differentiated, as well as physiological and pathological bone alterations.

The diagnosis of the "vital nature" of a wound, as well as determination of the time elapsed between the production of the wound and death, is a crucial issue (Cattaneo, 2007). Bone follows similar "laws" as skin as concerns the evolution of the histological picture after the occurrence of trauma. Macroscopic, microscopic, and X-ray analyses can all help in detecting the stages of the healing process, which are periosteal bone production (woven bone) and callus formation. However, these processes require a long time and are usually not visible before one week after the trauma (Collins, 1966). Their accurate recognition is, however, fundamental for achieving personal identification: each trauma is unique, and an accurate comparison between such a PM finding and X-rays or clinical data of the person missing can provide a positive match that can unequivocally identify him.

A different issue considers the distinction between the damage occurred around death and that occurred after the deposition or skeletonization of the remains. After death, the biochemical composition of bone changes with time, especially in terms of the amount and preservation of its organic matrix (Hart, 2005). It is, therefore, still relatively easy to provide a distinction between injuries that occurred long before (AM) and long after death (PM), but it is impossible to distinguish lesions produced shortly before and shortly after death (the so-called PM injuries) (Cattaneo, 2007). The definition "PM" commonly refers to a lesion that occurred when the bone had already lost its elastic matrix, instead of to the temporal timing in which the fracture occurs (Ubelaker and Adams, 1995; Wheatley, 2008; Wieberg and Wescott, 2008). Typical PM alterations are those caused by environmental factors, such as carnivore tooth marks, surface erosion, sun bleaching, weathering, etc., and by accidental events provoked by weight of surface layers of soil, pedestrian activity, transport and fortuitous trauma, or "simple" decomposition of the remains, bone included. In the forensic anthropological setting, the term "perimortem" means either shortly before or shortly after death (Cattaneo et al., 2010). Typically, perimortem injuries are the "traumatic ones," such as sharp force trauma, gunshot wounds, and blunt force trauma. Nevertheless, according to Wieberg and Wescott (2008), the term "perimortem" results to be ineffective in a forensic anthropological context because it refers to a temporal period instead of a physical condition (fresh or dry). Studies, therefore, tried to answer those unsolved issues, thus identifying signs of hemorrhaging on bone fracture edges (Cattaneo et al., 2010) or the PMI from red blood cell modifications following decomposition (Bardale and Dixit, 2007; Cappella et al., 2015; Penttilä and Laiho, 1981). Nevertheless, macromorphological features at this moment are the main instrument in the assessments regarding fracture analysis (Cappella et al., 2014a, 2014b; Wheatley, 2008; Wieberg and Wescott, 2008).

Another important and related issue considers skeletal pathology. Despite the fact that the skeleton can sometimes be the only source of information available, it is far less informative than a fresh cadaver. First, not all pathologies are, of course, evident on bones. Additionally, the interpretation of disease from skeletal remains is biased by the uniformity and monotony of bone reaction. Bone cells, in fact, when "attacked," react by means of bone formation (osteoblasts) or bone destruction (osteoclasts), or both phenomena. For this reason, the same bone manifestation can be linked to a variety of etiologies, which makes the correct diagnosis difficult (Cunha, 2006). The accurate interpretation of skeletal pathology is, therefore, one of the most controversial and constantly investigated aspects of the forensic anthropological practice. Furthermore, several studies investigated the potential of proteins as biomarkers for pathology and disease in osseous remains (Pérez-Martínez et al., 2016; Schultz et al., 2007). In this sense, when possible, the genetic autopsy could be considered in order to verify the presence in the individual of markers of infectious or congenital disease (see Chapter 12).

11.5.7   POST-MORTEM INTERVAL (PMI)

The PMI describes the period of time elapsed between the time of death and corpse discovery. Estimation of the PMI is one of the most debated themes in forensic sciences, and despite extensive literature on this topic, its estimation still remains difficult. The complexity of estimation is due to the fact that after death, body undergoes a complicated set of physical, chemical, and biological changes depending on exogenous and endogenous factors, including body size, age, pathologies, traumas, as well as typical environmental parameters (temperature, humidity, soil composition, etc.), burial condition, and accessibility of the body to insects and/or mice or other animals (Schotsmans et al., 2017). The older human remains are, the more difficult it is to estimate the PMI. In fact, in the case of skeletal human remains, the techniques used for establishing the PMI in early PM period (e.g., temperature, PM muscle excitability, etc.) are difficult to use due to the degradation of most biological samples as a result of cadaver decomposition processes (Hostiuc et al., 2017; Kaliszan et al., 2009). Techniques used by forensic experts to estimate the PMI in the case of bone remains are based on morphological, chemical, physical, and histological methods such as citrate content (Brown et al., 2018; Schwarcz et al., 2010; Wilson and Christensen, 2017, 2017), immunological activity (Procopio and Buckley, 2017), radionuclide analysis tests (Sterzik et al., 2016), spectroscopy, luminescence (Krap et al., 2017), luminol tests (Cappella et al., 2018), UV-induced fluorescence test (Hoke et al., 2013; Sterzik et al., 2016), ultrastructural changes (Hostiuc et al., 2017), decomposition pattern (Ferreira et al., 2019; Marais-Werner et al., 2018, 2017), and, more recently, ADD, microcomputed tomography (Le Garff et al., 2017), infrared spectroscopy, Raman spectromicroscopy (Creagh and Cameron, 2017), proteomic techniques (Prieto-Bonete et al., 2019; Procopio et al., 2018; Jellinghaus et al., 2019; Fais et al., 2018), and fabric degradation patterns (Ueland et al., 2015, 2019). In addition, genetic studies were also performed. Some of them focused on RNA stability over time from blood (Bauer et al., 2003) and various tissues and organs (Fordyce et al., 2013; González-Herrera et al., 2013; Koppelkamm et al., 2011; Sampaio-Silva et al., 2013). These studies may represent a new approach to estimate the PMI and become a complementary tool for traditional methods, with the ultimate focus on increasing the accuracy of the PMI estimation. The rate of RNA degradation was successfully studied in human dental pulp as well (Poór et al., 2016). Although the teeth are already focus of forensic science, bite mark identification (Kaur et al., 2013), personal identification by dental record (Hinchliffe, 2011), or DNA-based personal identification of disaster victims (Manjunath et al., 2011), they are usually not used for PMI estimation in forensic practice. The results show that the tested method may be considered a promising tool for PMI estimation. Using RNA sequencing data generated with the Illumina NGS protocol, a group of researchers investigated the impact of PMI on gene expression using data from multiple tissues of PM donors (Ferreira et al., 2018). Their results showed that the transcriptional events triggered by death of the organism do not appear to simply reflect stochastic variation resulting from mRNA degradation but active regulation of transcription.

11.6 CONCLUDING REMARKS

At times, the information the gross anthropological analysis can provide is often limited. A clear example is easily provided by the difficulties encountered when defining the sex of unknown subadult remains. In addition, in the case of adults, many methods cannot be applied if the skeleton is extensively missing or if the remains are not intact. In such cases, in fact, both macroscopy and microscopy prove themselves often inconclusive in answering specific answers, such as those regarding pathologies or even sex and age determination. Nevertheless, in many forensic instances, bones often represent the only available material that can be used for personal identification, and for this reason, reliable and specific applied methods in degraded DNA analysis are constantly improved. Additional investigative tools are, in fact, necessary when the forensic anthropological investigation does not have valid instruments to go beyond these limits, and in such a perspective, the support of other disciplines and novel technology is essential, particularly that of molecular anthropology focusing on the analysis of degraded DNA.

KEYWORDS

- **forensic anthropology**
- **DNA profiling**
- **amplicons**
- ***post mortem* interval**

REFERENCES

Abu Al-Soud, W.; and Rådström, P.; Effects of Amplification Facilitators on Diagnostic PCR in the Presence of Blood, Feces, and Meat. *J. Clin. Microbiol.* **2000**, *38* (12), 4463–4470.

Adler, C. J.; et al.; Survival and Recovery of DNA from Ancient Teeth and Bones. *J. Archaeol. Sci.* **2011**, *38* (5), 956–964.

Adler, C. J.; et al.; Sequencing Ancient Calcified Dental Plaque Shows Changes in Oral Microbiota with Dietary Shifts of the Neolithic and Industrial Revolutions. *Nat. Genet.* **2013**, *45* (4), 450–455.

Aeria, G.; et al.; Targeting Specific Facial Variation for Different Identification Tasks. *Forensic Sci. Int.* **2010**, *201* (1–3), 118–124.

Alaeddini, R.; et al.; Forensic Implications of Genetic Analyses from Degraded DNA—A Review. *Forensic Sci. Int. Genet.* **2010**, *4* (3), 148–157.

Albert, M.; et al.; Age Estimation Using Thoracic and First Two Lumbar Vertebral Ring Epiphyseal Union. *J. Forensic Sci.* **2010**, *55* (2), 287–294.

Alemán, I.; et al.; Brief Communication: The Granada Osteological Collection of Identified Infants and Young Children. *Am. J. Phys. Anthropol.* **2012**, *149* (4), 606–610.

Alkass, K.; et al.; Age Estimation in Forensic Sciences. *Mol. Cell Proteomics* **2010**, *9* (5), 1022–1030.

Alonso, A.; et al.; Challenges of DNA Profiling in Mass Disaster Investigations. *Croat. Med. J.* **2005**, *46* (4), 540–548.

Álvarez-Sandoval, B. A.; et al.; Sex Determination in Highly Fragmented Human DNA by High-Resolution Melting (HRM) Analysis. *PLoS One* **2014**, *9* (8), e104629.

Alvarez García, A.; et al.; Effect of Environmental Factors on PCR-DNA Analysis from Dental Pulp. *Int. J. Legal Med.* **1996**, *109* (3), 125–129.

An, J.; et al.; A Molecular Genetic Approach for Species Identification of Mammals and Sex Determination of Birds in a Forensic Case of Poaching from South Korea. *Forensic Sci. Int.* **2007**, *167* (1), 59–61.

Anderung, C.; et al.; Fishing for Ancient DNA. *Forensic Sci. Int. Genet.* **2008**, *2* (2), 104–107.

Arulandhu, A. J.; et al.; Development and Validation of a Multi-Locus DNA Metabarcoding Method to Identify Endangered Species in Complex Samples. *Gigascience* **2017**, *6* (10), 1–18.

Asala, S. A.; Sex Determination from the Head of the Femur of South African Whites and Blacks. *Forensic Sci. Int.* **2001**, *117* (1–2), 15–22.

Avila-Arcos, M. C.; et al.; Application and Comparison of Large-Scale Solution-Based DNA Capture-Enrichment Methods on Ancient DNA. *Sci. Rep.* **2011**, *1* (1), 74.

Baccino, E.; et al.; Technical Note: The Two Step Procedure (TSP) for the Determination of Age at Death of Adult Human Remains in Forensic Cases. *Forensic Sci. Int.* **2014**, *244*, 247–251.

Balitzki-Korte, B.; et al.; Species Identification by Means of Pyrosequencing the Mitochondrial 12S RRNA Gene. *Int. J. Legal Med.* **2005**, *119* (5), 291–294.

Ballard, M. E.; and Trudell, M. B.; Anterior Femoral Curvature Revisited: Race Assessment from the Femur. *J. Forensic Sci.* **1999**, *44* (4), 700–707.

Bär, W.; et al.; Postmortem Stability of DNA. *Forensic Sci. Int.* **1988**, *39* (1), 59–70.

Bardale, R.; and Dixit, P. G.; Evaluation of Morphological Changes in Blood Cells of Human Cadaver for the Estimation. *Medico-Legal Update.* **2007**, *7* (2), 35–39.

Barta, J. L.; et al.; Mitochondrial DNA Preservation across 3000-Year-Old Northern Fur Seal Ribs is Not Related to Bone Density: Implications for Forensic Investigations. *Forensic Sci. Int.* **2014**, *239*, 11–18.

Bauer, C. M.; et al.; Comparison of Morphological and Molecular Genetic Sex-Typing on Mediaeval Human Skeletal Remains. *Forensic Sci. Int. Genet.* **2013**, *7* (6), 581–586.

Bauer, M.; et al.; Quantification of RNA Degradation by Semi-Quantitative Duplex and Competitive RT-PCR: A Possible Indicator of the Age of Bloodstains? *Forensic Sci. Int.* **2003**, *138* (1–3), 94–103.

Baynam, G.; et al.; The Facial Evolution: Looking Backward and Moving Forward. *Hum. Mutat.* **2013**, *34* (1), 14–22.

Bender, K.; and Schneider, P. M.; Development of a New Multiplex Assay for STR Typing of Telogen Hair Roots. *Int. Congr. Ser.* **2006**, *1288*, 654–656.

Bender, K.; et al.; Preparation of Degraded Human DNA under Controlled Conditions. *Forensic Sci. Int.* **2004**, *139* (2–3), 135–140.

Bengtsson, C. F.; et al.; DNA from Keratinous Tissue. Part I: Hair and Nail. *Ann. Anat.* **2012**, *194* (1), 17–25.

Berger, C.; and Parson, W.; Mini-Midi-Mito: Adapting the Amplification and Sequencing Strategy of MtDNA to the Degradation State of Crime Scene Samples. *Forensic Sci. Int. Genet.* **2009**, *3* (3), 149–153.

Biesecker, L. G.; et al.; Epidemiology. DNA Identifications after the 9/11 World Trade Center Attack. *Science* **2005**, *310* (5751), 1122–1123.

Black, S. M.; Forensic Anthropology—Regulation in the United Kingdom. *Sci. Justice* **2003**, *43* (4), 187–192.

Boel, L. W.; et al.; Double Lamellae in Trabecular Osteons: Towards a New Method for Age Estimation by Bone Microscopy. *HOMO* **2007**, *58* (4), 269–277.

Bolnick, D. A.; et al.; Nondestructive Sampling of Human Skeletal Remains Yields Ancient Nuclear and Mitochondrial DNA. *Am. J. Phys. Anthropol.* **2012**, *147* (2), 293–300.

Boonyarit, H.; et al.; Development of a SNP Set for Human Identification: A Set with High Powers of Discrimination Which Yields High Genetic Information from Naturally Degraded DNA Samples in the Thai Population. *Forensic Sci. Int. Genet.* **2014**, *11*, 166–173.

Borić, I.; et al.; Discovering the 60 Years Old Secret: Identification of the World War II Mass Grave Victims from the Island of Daksa near Dubrovnik, Croatia. *Croat. Med. J.* **2011**, *52* (3), 327–335.

Borisenko, A. V; et al.; DNA Barcoding in Surveys of Small Mammal Communities: A Field Study in Suriname. *Mol. Ecol. Resour.* **2008**, *8* (3), 471–479.

Børsting, C.; et al.; Typing of 49 Autosomal SNPs by Single Base Extension and Capillary Electrophoresis for Forensic Genetic Testing. *Methods Mol. Biol.* **2012**, *830*, 87–107.

Bose, N.; et al.; Target Capture Enrichment of Nuclear SNP Markers for Massively Parallel Sequencing of Degraded and Mixed Samples. *Forensic Sci. Int. Genet.* **2018**, *34*, 186–196.

Bosio, L. A.; et al.; Chacarita Project: Conformation and Analysis of a Modern and Documented Human Osteological Collection from Buenos Aires City—Theoretical, Methodological and Ethical Aspects. *Homo* **2012**, *63* (6), 481–492.

Brandhagen, M. D.; et al.; Fragmented Nuclear DNA is the Predominant Genetic Material in Human Hair Shafts. *Genes (Basel).* **2018**, *9* (12), 640.

Brenner, C. H.; and Weir, B. S.; Issues and Strategies in the DNA Identification of World Trade Center Victims. *Theor. Popul. Biol.* **2003**, *63* (3), 173–178.

Brooks, S.; and Suchey, J. M.; Skeletal Age Determination Based on the Os Pubis: A Comparison of the Acsádi-Nemeskéri and Suchey-Brooks Methods. *Hum. Evol.* **1990**, *5* (3), 227–238.

Brooks, S. T.; Skeletal Age at Death: The Reliability of Cranial and Pubic Age Indicators. *Am. J. Phys. Anthropol.* **1955**, *13* (4), 567–597.

Brotherton, P.; et al.; Neolithic Mitochondrial Haplogroup H Genomes and the Genetic Origins of Europeans Europe PMC Funders Group. *Nat. Commun.* **2013**, *4*, 1764.

Brothwell, D. R.; and Pollard, A. M.; *Handbook of Archaeological Sciences*; Wiley: Hoboken, NJ, USA, 2001.

Brown, M. A.; et al.; Citrate Content of Bone as a Measure of Postmortem Interval: An External Validation Study. *J. Forensic Sci.* **2018**, *63* (5), 1479–1485.

Buckberry, J. L.; and Chamberlain, A. T.; Age Estimation from the Auricular Surface of the Ilium: A Revised Method. *Am. J. Phys. Anthropol.* **2002**, *119* (3), 231–239.

Budowle, B.; et al.; Forensic Aspects of Mass Disasters: Strategic Considerations for DNA-Based Human Identification. *Legal Med. (Tokyo).* **2005**, *7* (4), 230–243.

Budowle, B.; and van Daal, A.; Forensically Relevant SNP Classes. *Biotechniques* **2008**, *44* (5), 603–608, 610.

Budowle, B.; and van Daal, A.; Forensically Relevant SNP Classes. *Biotechniques* **2008**, *44 Supplement* (4), 603–610.

Butler, J. M.; et al.; The Development of Reduced Size STR Amplicons as Tools for Analysis of Degraded DNA. *J. Forensic Sci.* **2003**, *48* (5), 1054–1064.

Byers, S.; et al.; Determination of Adult Stature from Metatarsal Length. *Am. J. Phys. Anthropol.* **1989**, *79* (3), 275–279.

Cadenas, A. M.; et al.; Male Amelogenin Dropouts: Phylogenetic Context, Origins and Implications. *Forensic Sci. Int.* **2007**, *166* (2–3), 155–163.

Cameriere, R.; et al.; Variations in Pulp/Tooth Area Ratio as an Indicator of Age: A Preliminary Study. J. Forensic Sci. 2004, 49 (2), 317–319.

Cameriere, R.; et al.; Reliability in Age Determination by Pulp/Tooth Ratio in Upper Canines in Skeletal Remains. *J. Forensic Sci.* **2006**, *51* (4), 861–864.

Cameriere, R.; et al.; Age Estimation by Pulp/Tooth Ratio in Canines by Mesial and Vestibular Peri-Apical X-Rays. *J. Forensic Sci.* **2007**, *52* (5), 1151–1155.

Campos, P. F.; et al.; DNA in Ancient Bone—Where Is It Located and How Should We Extract It? *Ann. Anat.* **2012**, *194* (1), 7–16.

Cappella, A.; et al.; An Osteological Revisitation of Autopsies: Comparing Anthropological Findings on Exhumed Skeletons to Their Respective Autopsy Reports in Seven Cases. *Forensic Sci. Int.* **2014a**, *244*, 315, e1–10.

Cappella, A.; et al.; The Difficult Task of Assessing Perimortem and Postmortem Fractures on the Skeleton: A Blind Text on 210 Fractures of Known Origin. *J. Forensic Sci.* **2014b**, *59* (6), 1598–1601.

Cappella, A.; et al.; The Taphonomy of Blood Components in Decomposing Bone and Its Relevance to Physical Anthropology. *Am. J. Phys. Anthropol.* **2015**, *158* (4), 636–645.

Cappella, A.; et al.; The Comparative Performance of PMI Estimation in Skeletal Remains by Three Methods (C-14, Luminol Test and OHI): Analysis of 20 Cases. *Int. J. Legal Med.* **2018**, *132* (4), 1215–1224.

Cardoso, H. F. V; Brief Communication: The Collection of Identified Human Skeletons Housed at the Bocage Museum (National Museum of Natural History), Lisbon, Portugal. *Am. J. Phys. Anthropol.* **2006**, *129* (2), 173–176.

Cattaneo, C.; et al.; A Simple Method for Extracting DNA from Old Skeletal Material. *Forensic Sci. Int.* **1995**, *74* (3), 167–174.

Cattaneo, C.; et al.; Determining the Human Origin of Fragments of Burnt Bone: A Comparative Study of Histological, Immunological and DNA Techniques. *Forensic Sci. Int.* **1999**, *102* (2–3), 181–191.

Cattaneo, C.; Forensic Anthropology: Developments of a Classical Discipline in the New Millennium. *Forensic Sci. Int.* **2007**, *165* (2–3), 185–193.

Cattaneo, C.; et al.; The Detection of Microscopic Markers of Hemorrhaging and Wound Age on Dry Bone: A Pilot Study. *Am. J. Forensic Med. Pathol.* **2010**, *31* (1), 22–26.

Cattaneo, C.; et al.; A Modern Documented Italian Identified Skeletal Collection of 2127 Skeletons: The CAL Milano Cemetery Skeletal Collection. *Forensic Sci. Int.* **2018**, *287*, 219.e1–219.e5.

Cattaneo, C.; et al.; Histological Determination of the Human Origin of Bone Fragments. *J. Forensic Sci.* **2009**, *54* (3), 531–533.

Chaitanya, L.; et al.; Bringing Colour Back after 70 Years: Predicting Eye and Hair Colour from Skeletal Remains of World War II Victims Using the HIrisPlex System. *Forensic Sci. Int. Genet.* **2017**, *26*, 48–57.

Champlot, S.; et al.; An Efficient Multistrategy DNA Decontamination Procedure of PCR Reagents for Hypersensitive PCR Applications. *PLoS One* **2010**, *5* (9), e13042.

Chandrasekhar, D.; and Van Houten, B.; In Vivo Formation and Repair of Cyclobutane Pyrimidine Dimers and 6–4 Photoproducts Measured at the Gene and Nucleotide Level in Escherichia Coli. *Mutat. Res.* **2000**, *450* (1–2), 19–40.

Chang, Y. M.; et al.; A Distinct Y-STR Haplotype for Amelogenin Negative Males Characterized by a Large Y(p)11.2 (DYS458-MSY1-AMEL-Y) Deletion. *Forensic Sci. Int.* **2007**, *166* (2–3), 115–120.

Chen, W.; et al.; Detection of the Deletion on Yp11.2 in a Chinese Population. *Forensic Sci. Int. Genet.* **2014**, *8* (1), 73–79.

Chiba, M.; and Terazawa, K.; Estimation of Stature from Somatometry of Skull. *Forensic Sci. Int.* **1998**, *97* (2–3), 87–92.

Cho, H.; et al.; Population-Specific Histological Age-Estimating Method: A Model for Known African–American and European–American Skeletal Remains. *J. Forensic Sci.* **2002**, *47* (1), 12–18.

Chung, D. T.; et al.; A Study on the Effects of Degradation and Template Concentration on the Amplification Efficiency of the STR Miniplex Primer Sets. *J. Forensic Sci.* **2004**, *49* (4), 733–740.

Claes, P.; et al.; Bayesian Estimation of Optimal Craniofacial Reconstructions. *Forensic Sci. Int.* **2010a**, *201* (1–3), 146–152.

Claes, P.; et al.; Computerized Craniofacial Reconstruction: Conceptual Framework and Review. *Forensic Sci. Int.* **2010b**, *201* (1–3), 138–145.

Claes, P.; et al.; Sexual Dimorphism in Multiple Aspects of 3D Facial Symmetry and Asymmetry Defined by Spatially Dense Geometric Morphometrics. *J. Anat.* **2012**, *221* (2), 97–114.

Claes, P.; et al.; Toward DNA-Based Facial Composites: Preliminary Results and Validation. Forensic Sci. Int. Genet. **2014**, *13*, 208–216.

Clifford, S. L.; et al.; Mitochondrial DNA Phylogeography of Western Lowland Gorillas (Gorilla Gorilla Gorilla). *Mol. Ecol.* **2004**, *13* (6), 1551–1565.

Collins, D.; Pathology of Bone. *Br. J. Surg.* **1966**, *53* (6), 563–564.

Collins, M. J.; et al.; The Survival of Organic Matter in Bone: A Review. *Archaeometry* **2002**, *44* (3), 383–394.

Comey, C. T.; and Budowle, B.; Validation Studies on the Analysis of the HLA DQ Alpha Locus Using the Polymerase Chain Reaction. *J. Forensic Sci.* **1991**, *36* (6), 1633–1648.

Comey, C. T.; et al.; DNA Extraction Strategies for Amplified Fragment Length Polymorphism Analysis. *J. Forensic Sci.* **1994**, *39* (5), 13711J.

Coticone, S.; et al.; Optimization of a DNA Extraction Method for Nonhuman and Human Bone. *J. Forensic Identif.* **2010**, *60*, 430–438.

Cotton, E. A.; et al.; Validation of the AMPFlSTR SGM plus System for Use in Forensic Casework. *Forensic Sci. Int.* **2000**, *112* (2–3), 151–161.

Courts, C.; and Madea, B.; Full STR Profile of a 67-Year-Old Bone Found in a Fresh Water Lake. *J. Forensic Sci.* **2011**, *56 Suppl 1*, S172–5.

Craig, E. A.; Intercondylar Shelf Angle: A New Method to Determine Race from the Distal Femur. *J. Forensic Sci.* **1995**, *40* (5), 777–782.

Creagh, D.; and Cameron, A.; Estimating the Post-Mortem Interval of Skeletonized Remains: The Use of Infrared Spectroscopy and Raman Spectro-Microscopy. *Radiat. Phys. Chem.* **2017**, *137*, 225–229.

Cummings, N.; et al.; Combining Target Enrichment with Barcode Multiplexing for High Throughput SNP Discovery. *BMC Genomics* **2010**, *11* (1), 641.

Cunha, E.; Pathology as a Factor of Personal Identity in Forensic Anthropology. In *Forensic Anthropology and Medicine*; Schmitt, A., Cunha, E., Pinheiro, J., Eds.; Humana Press: Totowa, NJ, USA, **2006**; pp 333–358.

Cunha, E.; et al.; The Problem of Aging Human Remains and Living Individuals: A Review. *Forensic Sci. Int.* **2009**, *193* (1–3), 1–13.

Dabney, J.; et al.; Complete Mitochondrial Genome Sequence of a Middle Pleistocene Cave Bear Reconstructed from Ultrashort DNA Fragments. *Proc. Natl. Acad. Sci. U SA.* **2013**, *110* (39), 15758–15763.

Dalton, D. L.; and Kotze, A.; DNA Barcoding as a Tool for Species Identification in Three Forensic Wildlife Cases in South Africa. *Forensic Sci. Int.* **2011**, *207* (1–3), e51–4.

Daskalaki, E.; et al.; Further Developments in Molecular Sex Assignment: A Blind Test of 18th and 19th Century Human Skeletons. *J. Archaeol. Sci.* **2011**, *38* (6), 1326–1330.

Dayal, M. R.; et al.; An Assessment of Sex Using the Skull of Black South Africans by Discriminant Function Analysis. *HOMO* **2008**, *59* (3), 209–221.

Dayal, M. R.; et al.; The History and Composition of the Raymond A. Dart Collection of Human Skeletons at the University of the Witwatersrand, Johannesburg, South Africa. *Am. J. Phys. Anthropol.* **2009**, *140* (2), 324–335.

Deguilloux, M.-F.; et al.; Analysis of Ancient Human DNA and Primer Contamination: One Step Backward One Step Forward. *Forensic Sci. Int.* **2011**, *210* (1–3), 102–109.

DiGangi, E. A.; et al.; A New Method for Estimating Age-at-Death from the First Rib. *Am. J. Phys. Anthropol.* **2009**, *138* (2), 164–176.

Dirkmaat, D. C.; et al.; New Perspectives in Forensic Anthropology. *Am. J. Phys. Anthropol.* **2008**, *137* (S47), 33–52.

Dixon, L. A.; et al.; Analysis of Artificially Degraded DNA Using STRs and SNPs—Results of a Collaborative European (EDNAP) Exercise. *Forensic Sci. Int.* **2006**, *164* (1), 33–44.

Dobberstein, R. C.; et al.; Degradation of Biomolecules in Artificially and Naturally Aged Teeth: Implications for Age Estimation Based on Aspartic Acid Racemization and DNA Analysis. *Forensic Sci. Int.* **2008**, *179* (2–3), 181–191.

Draus-Barini, J.; et al.; Bona Fide Colour: DNA Prediction of Human Eye and Hair Colour from Ancient and Contemporary Skeletal Remains. *Investig. Genet.* **2013**, *4* (1), 3.

Dzijan, S.; et al.; Evaluation of the Reliability of DNA Typing in the Process of Identification of War Victims in Croatia. *J. Forensic Sci.* **2009**, *54* (3), 608–609.

Edson, S. M.; et al.; Naming the Dead—Confronting the Realities of Rapid Identification of Degraded Skeletal Remains. *Forensic Sci. Rev.* **2004**, *16* (1), 63–90.

Edson, S. M.; et al.; Sampling of the Cranium for Mitochondrial DNA Analysis of Human Skeletal Remains. *Forensic Sci. Int. Genet. Suppl. Ser.* **2009**, *2* (1), 269–270.

Edson, S. M.; et al.; Flexibility in Testing Skeletonized Remains for DNA Analysis Can Lead to Increased Success: Suggestions and Case Studies. *New Perspect. Forensic Hum. Skelet. Identif.* **2018**, 141–156.

Eglinton, G.; and Logan, G. A.; Molecular Preservation. *Philos. Trans. R. Soc. London. Ser. B Biol. Sci.* **1991**, *333* (1268), 315–328.

Eichmann, C.; and Parson, W.; Molecular Characterization of the Canine Mitochondrial DNA Control Region for Forensic Applications. *Int. J. Legal Med.* **2007**, *121* (5), 411–416.

Eichmann, C.; and Parson, W.; "Mitominis": Multiplex PCR Analysis of Reduced Size Amplicons for Compound Sequence Analysis of the Entire MtDNA Control Region in Highly Degraded Samples. *Int. J. Legal Med.* **2008**, *122* (5), 385–388.

Eliopoulos, C.; et al.; A Modern, Documented Human Skeletal Collection from Greece. *HOMO* **2007**, *58* (3), 221–228.

Elliott, M.; and Collard, M.; F Ordisc and the Determination of Ancestry from Cranial Measurements. *Biol. Lett.* **2009**, *5* (6), 849–852.

Enoch, M.-A.; et al.; Using Ancestry-Informative Markers to Define Populations and Detect Population Stratification. *J. Psychopharmacol.* **2006**, *20* (4 Suppl), 19–26.

Esteve Codina, A.; et al.; "GenderPlex" a PCR Multiplex for Reliable Gender Determination of Degraded Human DNA Samples and Complex Gender Constellations. *Int. J. Legal Med.* **2009**, *123* (6), 459–464.

Evans, J.; et al.; Thymine Ring Saturation and Fragmentation Products: Lesion Bypass, Misinsertion and Implications for Mutagenesis. *Mutat. Res.* **1993**, *299* (3–4), 147–156.

Evans, T. C.; DNA Damage— the Major Cause of Missing Pieces from the DNA Puzzle. *NEB Expressions*. **2007**, *2.1*.

Fahner, N. A.; et al.; Large-Scale Monitoring of Plants through Environmental DNA Metabarcoding of Soil: Recovery, Resolution, and Annotation of Four DNA Markers. *PLoS One* **2016**, *11* (6), e0157505.

Fais, P.; et al.; HIF1α Protein and MRNA Expression as a New Marker for Post Mortem Interval Estimation in Human Gingival Tissue. *J. Anat.* **2018**, *232* (6), 1031–1037.

Fazi, A.; et al.; Development of Two Highly Sensitive Forensic Sex Determination Assays Based on Human DYZ1 and Alu Repetitive DNA Elements. *Electrophoresis* **2014**, *35* (21–22), 3028–3035.

Fendt, L.; et al.; Sequencing Strategy for the Whole Mitochondrial Genome Resulting in High Quality Sequences. *BMC Genomics* **2009**, *10* (1), 139.

Ferreira, M. T.; et al.; A New Forensic Collection Housed at the University of Coimbra, Portugal: The 21st Century Identified Skeletal Collection. *Forensic Sci. Int.* **2014**, *245*, 202.e1–202.e5.

Ferreira, M. T.; et al.; Application of Forensic Anthropology to Non-Forensic Issues: An Experimental Taphonomic Approach to the Study of Human Body Decomposition in Aerobic Conditions. *Aust. J. Forensic Sci.* **2019**, *51* (2), 149–157.

Ferreira, P. G.; et al.; The Effects of Death and Post-Mortem Cold Ischemia on Human Tissue Transcriptomes. *Nat. Commun.* **2018**, *9* (1), 490.

Fondevila, M.; et al.; Challenging DNA: Assessment of a Range of Genotyping Approaches for Highly Degraded Forensic Samples. *Forensic Sci. Int. Genet. Suppl. Ser.* **2008a**, *1* (1), 26–28.

Fondevila, M.; et al.; Revision of the SNPforID 34-Plex Forensic Ancestry Test: Assay Enhancements, Standard Reference Sample Genotypes and Extended Population Studies. *Forensic Sci. Int. Genet.* **2013**, *7* (1), 63–74.

Fondevila, M.; et al.; Case Report: Identification of Skeletal Remains Using Short-Amplicon Marker Analysis of Severely Degraded DNA Extracted from a Decomposed and Charred Femur. *Forensic Sci. Int. Genet.* **2008b**, *2* (3), 212–218.

Fordyce, S. L.; et al.; Long-Term RNA Persistence in Postmortem Contexts. *Investig. Genet.* **2013**, *4* (1), 7.

France, D. L.; Observation and Metric Analysis of Sex in the Skeleton," In *Forensic Osteology: Advances in the Identification of Human Remains,* K. J. Reichs, Ed.; Charles C. Thomas, Springfield, IL, USA, 1998.

Freire-Aradas, A.; et al.; Forensic Individual Age Estimation with DNA: From Initial Approaches to Methylation Tests. *Forensic Sci. Rev.* **2017**, *29* (2), 121–144.

Frisch, T.; et al.; Volume-Referent Bone Turnover Estimated from the Interlabel Area Fraction after Sequential Labeling. *Bone* **1998**, *22* (6), 677–682.

Fumagalli, L.; et al.; Simultaneous Identification of Multiple Mammalian Species from Mixed Forensic Samples Based on MtDNA Control Region Length Polymorphism. *Forensic Sci. Int. Genet. Suppl. Ser.* **2009**, *2* (1), 302–303.

Gabriel, M. N.; et al.; Improved MtDNA Sequence Analysis of Forensic Remains Using a "Mini-Primer Set" Amplification Strategy. *J. Forensic Sci.* **2001**, *46* (2), 247–253.

Gamba, C.; et al.; Genome Flux and Stasis in a Five Millennium Transect of European Prehistory. *Nat. Commun.* **2014**, *5*, 5257.

Le Garff, E.; et al.; Technical Note: Early Post-Mortem Changes of Human Bone in Taphonomy with MCT. *Int. J. Legal Med.* **2017**, *131* (3), 761–770.

Geigl, E.-M.; On the Circumstances Surrounding the Preservation and Analysis of Very Old DNA. *Archaeometry* **2002**, *44* (3), 337–342.

Gettings, K. B.; et al.; Performance of a Next Generation Sequencing SNP Assay on Degraded DNA. *Forensic Sci. Int. Genet.* **2015**, *19*, 1–9.

GilArriortua, M.; et al.; Cytochrome b as a Useful Tool for the Identification of Blowflies of Forensic Interest (Diptera, Calliphoridae). *Forensic Sci. Int.* **2013**, *228* (1–3), 132–136.

Giles, R. E.; et al.; Maternal Inheritance of Human Mitochondrial DNA. *Proc. Natl. Acad. Sci. USA.* **1980**, *77* (11), 6715–6719.

Giles, E.; Modifying Stature Estimation from the Femur and Tibia. *J. Forensic Sci.* **1993**, *38* (4), 758–763.

Gill, G. W.; Racial Variation in the Proximal and Distal Femur: Heritability and Forensic Utility. *J. Forensic Sci.* **2001a**, *46* (4), 791–799.

Gill, P.; An Assessment of the Utility of Single Nucleotide Polymorphisms (SNPs) for Forensic Purposes. *Int. J. Legal Med.* **2001b**, *114* (4/5), 204–210.

González-Herrera, L.; et al.; Studies on RNA Integrity and Gene Expression in Human Myocardial Tissue, Pericardial Fluid and Blood, and Its Postmortem Stability. *Forensic Sci. Int.* **2013**, *232* (1–3), 218–228.

Goodsell, D. S.; The Molecular Perspective: Ultraviolet Light and Pyrimidine Dimers. *Oncologist* **2001**, *6* (3), 298–299.

Gotherstrom, A.; et al.; Bone Preservation and DNA Amplification. *Archaeometry* **2002**, *44* (3), 395–404.

Graham, E. A. M.; DNA Reviews: Hair. *Forensic Sci. Med. Pathol.* **2007**, *3* (2), 133–137.

Grauer, A. L.; Human Osteology in Archaeology and Forensic Science. Edited by Margaret Cox and Simon Mays. Greenwich Medical Media Ltd., London. 2000. ISBN 1-841-100-463. 522 Pp. *Int. J. Osteoarchaeol.* **2001**, *11* (6), 447–448.

Gualdi-Russo, E.; Sex Determination from the Talus and Calcaneus Measurements. *Forensic Sci. Int.* **2007**, *171* (2–3), 151–156.

Gupta, S.; et al.; A Simple and Inexpensive Molecular Method for Sexing and Identification of the Forensic Samples of Elephant Origin. *J. Forensic Sci.* **2006**, *51* (4), 805–807.

Hagelberg, E.; et al.; Identification of the Skeletal Remains of a Murder Victim by DNA Analysis. *Nature* **1991**, *352* (6334), 427–429.

Hagelberg, E.; and Clegg, J. B.; Isolation and Characterization of DNA from Archaeological Bone. *Proc. R. Soc. London. Ser. B Biol. Sci.* **1991**, *244* (1309), 45–50.

Haglund, W. D.; and Sorg, M. H.; *Forensic Taphonomy : The Postmortem Fate of Human Remains.* CRC Press, Boca Raton, FL, USA, 1997.

Hair, J. F.; et al.; *A Primer on Partial Least Squares Structural Equation Modeling (PLS-SEM)*; Sage: Thousand Oaks, CA, USA, 2014.

Hajibabaei, M.; et al.; DNA Barcodes Distinguish Species of Tropical Lepidoptera. *Proc. Natl. Acad. Sci. USA.* **2006**, *103* (4), 968–971.

Hammond, P.; The Use of 3D Face Shape Modelling in Dysmorphology. *Arch. Dis. Child.* **2007**, *92* (12), 1120–1126.

Hart, G. O.; Fracture Pattern Interpretation in the Skull: Differentiating Blunt Force from Ballistics Trauma Using Concentric Fractures. *J. Forensic Sci.* **2005**, *50* (6), 1276–1281.

Haynes, S.; et al.; Bone Preservation and Ancient DNA: The Application of Screening Methods for Predicting DNA Survival. *J. Archaeol. Sci.* **2002**, *29* (6), 585–592.

Hebert, P. D. N.; et al.; Biological Identifications through DNA Barcodes. *Proc. Biol. Sci.* **2003a**, *270* (1512), 313–321.

Hebert, P. D. N.; et al.; Barcoding Animal Life: Cytochrome c Oxidase Subunit 1 Divergences among Closely Related Species. *Proc. Biol. Sci.* **2003b**, *270 Suppl*, S96–9.

Hebert, P. D. N.; et al.; Identification of Birds through DNA Barcodes. *PLoS Biol.* **2004**, *2* (10), e312.

Hedges, R. E. M.; and Millard, A. R.; Bones and Groundwater: Towards the Modelling of Diagenetic Processes. *J. Archaeol. Sci.* **1995**, *22* (2), 155–164.

Hedges, R. E. M.; Bone Diagenesis: An Overview of Processes. *Archaeometry* **2002**, *44* (3) 319–328.

Hedman, J.; et al.; Improved Forensic DNA Analysis through the Use of Alternative DNA Polymerases and Statistical Modeling of DNA Profiles. *Biotechniques* **2009**, *47* (5), 951–958.

Herrmann, B.; and Hummel, S.; *Ancient DNA : Recovery and Analysis of Genetic Material from Paleontological, Archaeological, Museum, Medical, and Forensic Specimens*; Springer: New York, NY, USA, 1994.

Hillier, M. L.; and Bell, L. S.; Differentiating Human Bone from Animal Bone: A Review of Histological Methods. *J. Forensic Sci.* **2007**, *52* (2), 249–263.

Himmelberger, A. L.; et al.; Forensic Utility of the Mitochondrial Hypervariable Region 1 of Domestic Dogs, in Conjunction with Breed and Geographic Information. *J. Forensic Sci.* **2008**, *53* (1), 81–89.

Hinchliffe, J.; Forensic Odontology, Part 1. Dental Identification. *Br. Dent. J.* **2011**, *210* (5), 219–224.

Hochmeister, M. N.; et al.; Typing of Deoxyribonucleic Acid (DNA) Extracted from Compact Bone from Human Remains. *J. Forensic Sci.* **1991**, *36* (6), 1649–1661.

Hoke, N.; et al.; Reconsideration of Bone Postmortem Interval Estimation by UV-Induced Autofluorescence. *Forensic Sci. Int.* **2013**, *228* (1–3), 176.e1–6.

Holland, T. D.; Brief Communication: Estimation of Adult Stature from the Calcaneus and Talus. *Am. J. Phys. Anthropol.* **1995**, *96* (3), 315–320.

Holmes, B. H.; et al.; Identification of Shark and Ray Fins Using DNA Barcoding. *Fish. Res.* **2009**, *95* (2–3), 280–288.

Hopman, S. M. J.; et al.; Face Shape Differs in Phylogenetically Related Populations. *Eur. J. Hum. Genet.* **2014**, *22* (11), 1268–1271.

Hostiuc, S.; et al.; Usefulness of Ultrastructure Studies for the Estimation of the Postmortem Interval. A Systematic Review. *Rom. J. Morphol. Embryol.* **2017**, *58* (2), 377–384.

Hsieh, H.-M.; et al.; Species Identification of Rhinoceros Horns Using the Cytochrome b Gene. *Forensic Sci. Int.* **2003**, *136* (1–3), 1–11.

Hsieh, H.-M.; et al.; Species Identification of Kachuga Tecta Using the Cytochrome b Gene. *J. Forensic Sci.* **2006**, *51* (1), 52–56.

Hunt, D. R.; and Albanese, J.; History and Demographic Composition of the Robert J. Terry Anatomical Collection. *Am. J. Phys. Anthropol.* **2005**, *127* (4), 406–417.

Imaizumi, K.; et al.; Development of Species Identification Tests Targeting the 16S Ribosomal RNA Coding Region in Mitochondrial DNA. *Int. J. Legal Med.* **2007**, *121* (3), 184–191.

Irwin, D. M.; et al.; Evolution of the Cytochrome b Gene of Mammals. *J. Mol. Evol.* **1991**, *32* (2), 128–144.

Işcan, M. Y.; et al.; Age Estimation from the Rib by Phase Analysis White Males. *J. Forensic Sci.* **1984**, *29* (4), 1094–1104.

Işcan, M. Y.; et al.; Age Estimation from the Rib by Phase Analysis: White Females. *J. Forensic Sci.* **1985**, *30* (3), 853–863.

Işcan, M. Y.; et al.; Racial Variation in the Sternal Extremity of the Rib and Its Effect on Age Determination. *J. Forensic Sci.* **1987**, *32* (2), 452–466.

Jacobsen, C. S.; and Rasmussen, O. F.; Development and Application of a New Method to Extract Bacterial DNA from Soil Based on Separation of Bacteria from Soil with Cation-Exchange Resin. *Appl. Environ. Microbiol.* **1992**, *58* (8), 2458–2462.

Jantz, R. L.; and Ousley, S. D.; *FORDISC 3.1 Personal Computer Forensic Discriminant Functions.* Forensic Anthropology Center. The University of Tennessee, Knoxville, TN, USA, 2005.

Jellinghaus, K.; et al.; Collagen Degradation as a Possibility to Determine the Post-Mortem Interval (PMI) of Human Bones in a Forensic Context—A Survey. *Legal Med.* **2019**, *36*, 96–102.

Jobling, M. A.; et al.; Structural Variation on the Short Arm of the Human Y Chromosome: Recurrent Multigene Deletions Encompassing Amelogenin Y. *Hum. Mol. Genet.* **2007**, *16* (3), 307–316.

Johnston, E.; and Stephenson, M.; DNA Profiling Success Rates from Degraded Skeletal Remains in Guatemala. *J. Forensic Sci.* **2016**, *61* (4), 898–902.

Junqueira, A. C. M.; et al.; The Mitochondrial Genome of the Blowfly Chrysomya Chloropyga (Diptera: Calliphoridae). *Gene* **2004**, *339*, 7–15.

Just, R. S.; et al.; Titanic's Unknown Child: The Critical Role of the Mitochondrial DNA Coding Region in a Re-Identification Effort. *Forensic Sci. Int. Genet.* **2011**, *5* (3), 231–235.

Kaliszan, M.; et al.; Estimation of the Time of Death Based on the Assessment of Post Mortem Processes with Emphasis on Body Cooling. *Legal Med. (Tokyo).* **2009**, *11* (3), 111–117.

Kalmey, J. K.; and Rathbun, T. A.; Sex Determination by Discriminant Function Analysis of the Petrous Portion of the Temporal Bone. *J. Forensic Sci.* **1996**, *41* (5), 865–867.

Katherine Spradley, M.; and Jantz, R. L.; Ancestry Estimation in Forensic Anthropology: Geometric Morphometric versus Standard and Nonstandard Interlandmark Distances. *J. Forensic Sci.* **2016**, *61* (4), 892–897.

Kaur, S.; et al.; Analysis and Identification of Bite Marks in Forensic Casework. *Oral Health Dent. Manag.* **2013**, *12* (3), 127–131.

Kayser, M.; Forensic DNA Phenotyping: Predicting Human Appearance from Crime Scene Material for Investigative Purposes. *Forensic Sci. Int. Genet.* **2015**, *18*, 33–48.

Kemp, B. M.; and Smith, D. G.; Use of Bleach to Eliminate Contaminating DNA from the Surface of Bones and Teeth. *Forensic Sci. Int.* **2005**, *154* (1), 53–61.

Kerley, E. R.; The Microscopic Determination of Age in Human Bone. *Am. J. Phys. Anthropol.* **1965**, *23* (2), 149–163.

Kerley, E. R.; and Ubelaker, D. H.; Revisions in the Microscopic Method of Estimating Age at Death in Human Cortical Bone. *Am. J. Phys. Anthropol.* **1978**, *49* (4), 545–546.

Kersbergen, P.; et al.; Developing a Set of Ancestry-Sensitive DNA Markers Reflecting Continental Origins of Humans. *BMC Genet.* **2009**, *10* (1), 69.

Kim, J.-J.; et al.; Development of SNP-Based Human Identification System. *Int. J. Legal Med.* **2010**, *124* (2), 125–131.

Kim, K.; et al.; Technical Note: Improved Ancient DNA Purification for PCR Using Ion-Exchange Columns. *Am. J. Phys. Anthropol.* **2008**, *136* (1), 114–121.

Kimmerle, E. H.; et al.; Inter-Observer Variation in Methodologies Involving the Pubic Symphysis, Sternal Ribs, and Teeth. *J. Forensic Sci.* **2008**, *53* (3), 594–600.

Kitano, T.; et al.; Two Universal Primer Sets for Species Identification among Vertebrates. *Int. J. Legal Med.* **2007**, *121* (5), 423–427.

Klales, A. R.; et al.; A Revised Method of Sexing the Human Innominate Using Phenice's Nonmetric Traits and Statistical Methods. *Am. J. Phys. Anthropol.* **2012**, *149* (1), 104–114.

Knapp, M.; et al.; Generating Barcoded Libraries for Multiplex High-Throughput Sequencing. *Methods Mol. Biol.* **2012**; 840, 155–170.

Kocher, T. D.; et al.; Dynamics of Mitochondrial DNA Evolution in Animals: Amplification and Sequencing with Conserved Primers. *Proc. Natl. Acad. Sci. USA.* **1989**, *86* (16), 6196–6200.

Kohn, L. A. P.; The Role of Genetics in Craniofacial Morphology and Growth. *Annu. Rev. Anthropol.* **1991**, *20* (1), 261–278.

Kontanis, E. J.; and Reed, F. A.; Evaluation of Real-Time PCR Amplification Efficiencies to Detect PCR Inhibitors. *J. Forensic Sci.* **2006**, *51* (4), 795–804.

Koppelkamm, A.; et al.; RNA Integrity in Post-Mortem Samples: Influencing Parameters and Implications on RT-QPCR Assays. *Int. J. Legal Med.* **2011**, *125* (4), 573–580.

Krap, T.; et al.; Luminescence of Thermally Altered Human Skeletal Remains. *Int. J. Legal Med.* **2017**, *131* (4), 1165–1177.

Krishan, K.; Estimation of Stature from Cephalo-Facial Anthropometry in North Indian Population. *Forensic Sci. Int.* **2008**, *181* (1–3), 52.e1–6.

Kulstein, G.; et al.; As Solid as a Rock—Comparison of CE- and MPS-Based Analyses of the Petrosal Bone as a Source of DNA for Forensic Identification of Challenging Cranial Bones. *Int. J. Legal Med.* **2017**, *132* (1), 13–24.

Kumagai, R.; et al.; DNA Analysis of Family Members with Deletion in Yp11.2 Region Containing Amelogenin Locus. *Legal Med. (Tokyo).* **2008**, *10* (1), 39–42.

Kuwayama, R.; and Ozawa, T.; Phylogenetic Relationships among European Red Deer, Wapiti, and Sika Deer Inferred from Mitochondrial DNA Sequences. *Mol. Phylogenet. Evol.* **2000**, *15* (1), 115–123.

L'Abbé, E. N.; et al.; The Pretoria Bone Collection: A Modern South African Skeletal Sample. *Homo* **2005**, *56* (2), 197–205.

Lamendin, H.; Observations on Teeth Roots in the Estimation of Age. *Int. J. Forensic Dent.* **1973**, *1* (1), 4–7.

Lamendin, H.; et al.; A Simple Technique for Age Estimation in Adult Corpses: The Two Criteria Dental Method. *J. Forensic Sci.* **1992**, *37* (5), 1373–1379.

Lao, O.; et al.; Proportioning Whole-Genome Single-Nucleotide-Polymorphism Diversity for the Identification of Geographic Population Structure and Genetic Ancestry. *Am. J. Hum. Genet.* **2006**, *78* (4), 680–690.

Latham, K.; and Madonna, M.; DNA Survivability in Skeletal Remains. In *Manual of Forensic Taphonomy*; Pokines, J. T., Symes, S. A., Eds.; CRC Press: Boca Raton, FL, USA, **2014**, 403–425.

Latham, K. E.; and Miller, J. J.; DNA Recovery and Analysis from Skeletal Material in Modern Forensic Contexts. *Forensic Sci. Res.* **2018**, *4* (1), 51–59.

Lattanzi, W.; et al.; A Large Interstitial Deletion Encompassing the Amelogenin Gene on the Short Arm of the Y Chromosome. *Hum. Genet.* **2005**, *116* (5), 395–401.

Leclair, B.; et al.; Enhanced Kinship Analysis and STR-Based DNA Typing for Human Identification in Mass Fatality Incidents: The Swissair Flight 111 Disaster. *J. Forensic Sci.* **2004**, *49* (5), 939–953.

Lee, H. Y.; et al.; DNA Typing for the Identification of Old Skeletal Remains from Korean War Victims. *J. Forensic Sci.* **2010**, *55* (6), 1422–1429.

Lee, H. Y.; et al.; Simple and Highly Effective DNA Extraction Methods from Old Skeletal Remains Using Silica Columns. *Forensic Sci. Int. Genet.* **2010**, *4* (5), 275–280.

Leney, M. D.; Sampling Skeletal Remains for Ancient DNA (ADNA): A Measure of Success. *Hist. Archaeol.* **2016**, *40* (3), 31–49.

Leonard, J. A.; et al.; Animal DNA in PCR Reagents Plagues Ancient DNA Research. *J. Archaeol. Sci.* **2007**, *34* (9), 1361–1366.

Lindahl, T.; and Nyberg, B.; Rate of Depurination of Native Deoxyribonucleic Acid. *Biochemistry* **1972**, *11* (19), 3610–3618.

Lindahl, T.; Instability and Decay of the Primary Structure of DNA. *Nature* **1993**, *362* (6422), 709–715.

Lindblom, B.; and Montelius, K.; DNA Analysis in Disaster Victim Identification. *Forensic Sci. Med. Pathol.* **2012**, *8* (2), 140–147.

Llamas, B.; et al.; From the Field to the Laboratory: Controlling DNA Contamination in Human Ancient DNA Research in the High-Throughput Sequencing Era. *STAR Sci. Technol. Archaeol. Res.* **2017**, *3* (1), 1–14.

Lovejoy, C. O.; et al.; Chronological Metamorphosis of the Auricular Surface of the Ilium: A New Method for the Determination of Adult Skeletal Age at Death. *Am. J. Phys. Anthropol.* **1985**, *68* (1), 15–28.

Luo, S.; et al.; Biparental Inheritance of Mitochondrial DNA in Humans. *Proc. Natl. Acad. Sci. USA.* **2018**, *115* (51), 13039–13044.

Lygo, J. E.; et al.; The Validation of Short Tandem Repeat (STR) Loci for Use in Forensic Casework. *Int. J. Legal Med.* **1994**, *107* (2), 77–89.

Lynnerup, N.; et al.; Assessment of Age at Death by Microscopy: Unbiased Quantification of Secondary Osteons in Femoral Cross Sections. *Forensic Sci. Int.* **2006**, *159 Suppl 1*, S100–3.

Ma, Y.; et al.; Y Chromosome Interstitial Deletion Induced Y-STR Allele Dropout in AMELY-Negative Individuals. *Int. J. Legal Med.* **2012**, *126* (5), 713–724.

Maciejewska, A.; and Pawłowski, R.; A Rare Mutation in the Primer Binding Region of the Amelogenin X Homologue Gene. *Forensic Sci. Int. Genet.* **2009**, *3* (4), 265–267.

Maciejewska, A.; et al.; The Influence of High Temperature on the Possibility of DNA Typing in Various Human Tissues. *Folia Histochem. Cytobiol.* **2016**, *53* (4), 322–332.

MacLaughlin, S. M.; and Bruce, M. F.; The Accuracy of Sex Identification in European Skeletal Remains Using the Phenice Characters. *J. Forensic Sci.* **1990**, *35* (6), 1384–1392.

Madel, M.-B.; et al.; TriXY—Homogeneous Genetic Sexing of Highly Degraded Forensic Samples Including Hair Shafts. *Forensic Sci. Int. Genet.* **2016**, *25*, 166–174.

Madonna, M.; et al.; The Utility of Baking Bone to Increase Skeletal DNA Yield.: EBSCOhost. *J. Forensic Identifiction* **2015**, *65* (2), 107–117.

Malaver, P. C.; and Yunis, J. J.; Different Dental Tissues as Source of DNA for Human Identification in Forensic Cases. *Croat. Med. J.* **2003**, *44* (3), 306–309.

Mall, G.; et al.; Sex Determination and Estimation of Stature from the Long Bones of the Arm. *Forensic Sci. Int.* **2001**, *117* (1–2), 23–30.

Manhart, J.; et al.; Disaster Victim Identification-Experiences of the "Autobahn A19" Disaster. *Forensic Sci. Med. Pathol.* **2012**, *8* (2), 118–124.

Manjunath, B. C.; et al.; DNA Profiling and Forensic Dentistry—A Review of the Recent Concepts and Trends. *J. Forensic Legal Med.* **2011**, *18* (5), 191–197.

Mannucci, A.; et al.; Forensic Application of a Rapid and Quantitative DNA Sex Test by Amplification of the X–Y Homologous Gene Amelogenin. *Int. J. Legal Med.* **1994**, *106* (4), 190–193.

Marais-Werner, A.; et al.; Decomposition Patterns of Buried Remains at Different Intervals in the Central Highveld Region of South Africa. *Med. Sci. Law* **2017**, *57* (3), 115–123.

Marais-Werner, A.; et al.; A Comparison between Decomposition Rates of Buried and Surface Remains in a Temperate Region of South Africa. *Int. J. Legal Med.* **2018**, *132* (1), 301–309.

Marjanović, D.; et al.; DNA Identification of Skeletal Remains from the World War II Mass Graves Uncovered in Slovenia. *Croat. Med. J.* **2007**, *48* (4), 513–519.

Marjanović, D.; et al.; Identification of Skeletal Remains of Communist Armed Forces Victims during and after World War II: Combined Y-Chromosome (STR) and MiniSTR Approach. *Croat. Med. J.* **2009**, *50* (3), 296–304.

Marshall, P. L.; et al.; Utility of Amplification Enhancers in Low Copy Number DNA Analysis. *Int. J. Legal Med.* **2015**, *129* (1), 43–52.

Mayer, F.; et al.; Molecular Species Identification Boosts Bat Diversity. *Front. Zool.* **2007**, *4*, 4.

McNevin, D.; et al.; Short Tandem Repeat (STR) Genotyping of Keratinised Hair. *Forensic Sci. Int.* **2005**, *153* (2–3), 237–246.

Meadows, L.; and Jantz, R. L.; Estimation of Stature from Metacarpal Lengths. *J. Forensic Sci.* **1992**, *37* (1), 147–154.

Meganathan, P. R.; et al.; Molecular Identification of Crocodile Species Using Novel Primers for Forensic Analysis. *Conserv. Genet.* **2008**, *10* (3), 767–770.

Meier, R.; et al.; DNA Barcoding and Taxonomy in Diptera: A Tale of High Intraspecific Variability and Low Identification Success. *Syst. Biol.* **2006**, *55* (5), 715–728.

Meissner, C.; and Ritz-Timme, S.; Molecular Pathology and Age Estimation. *Forensic Sci. Int.* **2010**, *203* (1–3), 34–43.

Melton, T.; and Holland, C.; Routine Forensic Use of the Mitochondrial 12S Ribosomal RNA Gene for Species Identification. *J. Forensic Sci.* **2007**, *52* (6), 1305–1307.

De Mendonça, M. C.; Estimation of Height from the Length of Long Bones in a Portuguese Adult Population. *Am. J. Phys. Anthropol.* **2000**, *112* (1), 39–48.

Mertes, F.; et al.; Targeted Enrichment of Genomic DNA Regions for Next-Generation Sequencing. *Brief. Funct. Genomics* **2011**, *10* (6), 374–386.

Meyer, E.; et al.; Extraction and Amplification of Authentic DNA from Ancient Human Remains. *Forensic Sci. Int.* **2000**, *113* (1–3), 87–90.

Michael, A.; and Brauner, P.; Erroneous Gender Identification by the Amelogenin Sex Test. *J. Forensic Sci.* **2004**, *49* (2), 258–259.

Milner, G. R.; and Boldsen, J. L.; Transition Analysis: A Validation Study with Known-Age Modern American Skeletons. *Am. J. Phys. Anthropol.* **2012**, *148* (1), 98–110.

Milos, A.; et al.; Success Rates of Nuclear Short Tandem Repeat Typing from Different Skeletal Elements. *Croat. Med. J.* **2007**, *48* (4), 486–493.

Mitani, T.; et al.; Identification of Animal Species Using the Partial Sequences in the Mitochondrial 16S RRNA Gene. *Legal Med. (Tokyo).* **2009**, *11* Suppl 1, S449–50.

Mitchell, R. J.; et al.; An Investigation of Sequence Deletions of Amelogenin (AMELY), a Y-Chromosome Locus Commonly Used for Gender Determination. *Ann. Hum. Biol.* **2006**, *33* (2), 227–240.

Mittnik, A.; et al.; A Molecular Approach to the Sexing of the Triple Burial at the Upper Paleolithic Site of Dolní Věstonice. *PLoS One* **2016**, *11* (10), e0163019.

Moore, M. K.; et al.; Use of Restriction Fragment Length Polymorphisms to Identify Sea Turtle Eggs and Cooked Meats to Species. *Conserv. Genet.* **2003**, *4* (1), 95–103.

Morales Colón, E.; et al.; Evaluation of a Freezer Mill for Bone Pulverization Prior to DNA Extraction: An Improved Workflow for STR Analysis. *J. Forensic Sci.* **2018**, *63* (2), 530–535.

Mulhern, D. M.; and Ubelaker, D. H.; Differences in Osteon Banding between Human and Nonhuman Bone. *J. Forensic Sci.* **2001**, *46* (2), 220–222.

Mundorff, A. Z.; et al.; DNA Preservation in Skeletal Elements from the World Trade Center Disaster: Recommendations for Mass Fatality Management. *J. Forensic Sci.* **2009**, *54* (4), 739–745.

Ng, M. C. Y.; et al.; Discovery and Fine-Mapping of Adiposity Loci Using High Density Imputation of Genome-Wide Association Studies in Individuals of African Ancestry: African Ancestry Anthropometry Genetics Consortium. *PLoS Genet.* **2017**, *13* (4), e1006719.

Nussbaumer, C.; and Korschineck, I.; Non-Human MtDNA Helps to Exculpate a Suspect in a Homicide Case. *Int. Congr. Ser.* **2006**, *1288*, 136–138.

Olaisen, B.; et al.; Identification by DNA Analysis of the Victims of the August 1996 Spitsbergen Civil Aircraft Disaster. *Nat. Genet.* **1997**, *15* (4), 402–405.

Orlando, L.; et al.; True Single-Molecule DNA Sequencing of a Pleistocene Horse Bone. *Genome Res.* **2011**, *21* (10), 1705–1719.

Ou, X.; et al.; Null Alleles of the X and Y Chromosomal Amelogenin Gene in a Chinese Population. *Int. J. Legal Med.* **2012**, *126* (4), 513–518.

Pajnič, I. Z.; Extraction of DNA from Human Skeletal Material. *Methods Mol. Biol.* **2016**, *1420*, 89–108.

de Pancorbo, M. M.; et al.; Cytochrome b and HVI Sequences of Mitochondrial DNA to Identify Domestic Animal Hair in Forensic Casework. *Int. Congr. Ser.* **2003**, *1239*, 841–845.

Parsons, T. J.; et al.; Application of Novel "Mini-Amplicon" STR Multiplexes to High Volume Casework on Degraded Skeletal Remains. *Forensic Sci. Int. Genet.* **2007**, *1* (2), 175–179.

Paschou, P.; et al.; PCA-Correlated SNPs for Structure Identification in Worldwide Human Populations. *PLoS Genet.* **2007**, *3* (9), 1672–1686.

Pate, F. D.; and Hutton, J. T.; The Use of Soil Chemistry Data to Address Post-Mortem Diagenesis in Bone Mineral. *J. Archaeol. Sci.* **1988**, *15* (6), 729–739.

Penttilä, A.; and Laiho, K.; Autolytic Changes in Blood Cells of Human Cadavers. II. Morphological Studies. *Forensic Sci. Int.* **1981**, *17* (2), 121–132.

Pérez-Martínez, C.; et al.; Usefulness of Protein Analysis for Detecting Pathologies in Bone Remains. *Forensic Sci. Int.* **2016**, *258*, 68–73.

Phenice, T. W.; A Newly Developed Visual Method of Sexing the Os Pubis. *Am. J. Phys. Anthropol.* **1969**, *30* (2), 297–301.

Phillips, C.; et al.; Inferring Ancestral Origin Using a Single Multiplex Assay of Ancestry-Informative Marker SNPs. *Forensic Sci. Int. Genet.* **2007**, *1* (3–4), 273–280.

Pilli, E.; et al.; Monitoring DNA Contamination in Handled vs. Directly Excavated Ancient Human Skeletal Remains. *PLoS One* **2013**, *8* (1), e52524.

Pilli, E.; et al.; Pet Fur or Fake Fur? A Forensic Approach. *Investig. Genet.* **2014**, *5* (1), 7.

Pilli, E.; et al.; Neither Femur nor Tooth: Petrous Bone for Identifying Archaeological Bone Samples via Forensic Approach. *Forensic Sci. Int.* **2018a**, *283*, 144–149.

Pilli, E.; et al.; From Unknown to Known: Identification of the Remains at the Mausoleum of Fosse Ardeatine. *Sci. Justice* **2018b**, *58*, (6) 469–478.

Pinhasi, R.; et al.; Optimal Ancient DNA Yields from the Inner Ear Part of the Human Petrous Bone. *PLoS One* **2015**, *10* (6), e0129102.

Poinar, H. N.; and Stankiewicz, B. A.; Protein Preservation and DNA Retrieval from Ancient Tissues. *Proc. Natl. Acad. Sci. USA.* **1999**, *96* (15), 8426–8431.

Poór, V. S.; et al.; The Rate of RNA Degradation in Human Dental Pulp Reveals Post-Mortem Interval. *Int. J. Legal Med.* **2016**, *130* (3), 615–619.

Prieto-Bonete, G.; et al.; Association between Protein Profile and Postmortem Interval in Human Bone Remains. *J. Proteomics* **2019**, *192*, 54–63.

Prinz, M.; et al.; DNA Commission of the International Society for Forensic Genetics (ISFG): Recommendations Regarding the Role of Forensic Genetics for Disaster Victim Identification (DVI). *Forensic Sci. Int. Genet.* **2007**, *1* (1), 3–12.

Procopio, N.; and Buckley, M.; Minimizing Laboratory-Induced Decay in Bone Proteomics. *J. Proteome Res.* **2017**, *16* (2), 447–458.

Procopio, N.; et al.; Forensic Proteomics for the Evaluation of the Post-Mortem Decay in Bones. *J. Proteomics* **2018**, *177*, 21–30.

Pun, K.-M.; et al.; Species Identification in Mammals from Mixed Biological Samples Based on Mitochondrial DNA Control Region Length Polymorphism. *Electrophoresis* **2009**, *30* (6), 1008–1014.

Rasmussen, M.; et al.; Ancient Human Genome Sequence of an Extinct Palaeo-Eskimo. *Nature* **2010**, *463* (7282), 757–762.

Rasmussen, M.; et al.; The Genome of a Late Pleistocene Human from a Clovis Burial Site in Western Montana. *Nature* **2014**, *506* (7487), 225–229.

Rastogi, G.; et al.; Species Identification and Authentication of Tissues of Animal Origin Using Mitochondrial and Nuclear Markers. *Meat Sci.* **2007**, *76* (4), 666–674.

Reidy, K. M.; et al.; Gender Identification Differences Observed For DNA Quantification versus STR Genotyping of Mummified Human Remains—How It Relates to Human Identifications in Forensic Science. *Investig. Sci. J.* **2009**, *1* (1).

Robinson, M. S.; and Bidmos, M. A.; The Skull and Humerus in the Determination of Sex: Reliability of Discriminant Function Equations. *Forensic Sci. Int.* **2009**, *186* (1–3), 86.e1–5.

Roffey, P. E.; et al.; A Rare Mutation in the Amelogenin Gene and Its Potential Investigative Ramifications. *J. Forensic Sci.* **2000**, *45* (5), 1016–1019.

Rohilla, M. S.; and Tiwari, P. K.; Restriction Fragment Length Polymorphism of Mitochondrial DNA and Phylogenetic Relationships among Five Species of Indian Freshwater Turtles. *J. Appl. Genet.* **2008**, *49* (2), 167–182.

Rohland, N.; and Reich, D.; Cost-Effective, High-Throughput DNA Sequencing Libraries for Multiplexed Target Capture. *Genome Res.* **2012**, *22* (5), 939–946.

Rohland, N.; and Hofreiter, M.; Ancient DNA Extraction from Bones and Teeth. *Nat. Protoc.* **2007**, *2* (7), 1756–1762.

Rohland, N.; et al.; Extraction of Highly Degraded DNA from Ancient Bones, Teeth and Sediments for High-Throughput Sequencing. *Nat. Protoc.* **2018**, *13* (11), 2447–2461.

Romanini, C.; et al.; Ancestry Informative Markers: Inference of Ancestry in Aged Bone Samples Using an Autosomal AIM-Indel Multiplex. *Forensic Sci. Int. Genet.* **2015**, *16*, 58–63.

Ross, A. H.; and Konigsberg, L. W.; New Formulae for Estimating Stature in the Balkans. *J. Forensic Sci.* **2002**, *47* (1), 165–167.

Rougé-Maillart, C.; et al.; Development of a Method to Estimate Skeletal Age at Death in Adults Using the Acetabulum and the Auricular Surface on a Portuguese Population. *Forensic Sci. Int.* **2009**, *188* (1–3), 91–95.

Roziah, A.; et al.; Mitochondrial and Nuclear DNA for Identification of Forensically Important Flesh Flies (Sarcophagidae: Boettcherisca Spp). *Entomol. Ornithol. Herpetol. Curr. Res.* **2015**, *04* (04), 1–4.

Rucinski, C.; et al.; Comparison of Two Methods for Isolating DNA from Human Skeletal Remains for STR Analysis. *J. Forensic Sci.* **2012**, *57* (3), 706–712.

Rusu, I.; et al.; Maternal DNA Lineages at the Gate of Europe in the 10th Century AD. *PLoS One* **2018**, *13* (3), e0193578.

Salceda, S. A.; et al.; The 'Prof. Dr. Rómulo Lambre' Collection: An Argentinian Sample of Modern Skeletons. *HOMO* **2012**, *63* (4), 275–281.

Salem, A. M.; et al.; Survey of the Genetic Diversity of Forensically Important Chrysomya (Diptera: Calliphoridae) from Egypt. *J. Med. Entomol.* **2015**, *52* (3), 320–328.

Sampaio-Silva, F.; et al.; Profiling of RNA Degradation for Estimation of Post Mortem Interval. *PLoS One* **2013**, *8* (2), e56507.

Sanchez, J. J.; et al.; A Multiplex Assay with 52 Single Nucleotide Polymorphisms for Human Identification. *Electrophoresis* **2006**, *27* (9), 1713–1724.

Santacroce, R.; et al.; Identification of Fetal Gender in Maternal Blood Is a Helpful Tool in the Prenatal Diagnosis of Haemophilia. *Haemophilia* **2006**, *12* (4), 417–422.

Santos, F. R.; et al.; Reliability of DNA-Based Sex Tests. *Nat. Genet.* **1998**, *18* (2), 103.

Santos Rojo Velasco, G. S.; Testing Molecular Barcodes: Invariant Mitochondrial DNA Sequences vs the Larval and Adult Morphology of West Palaearctic Pandasyopthalmus Species (Diptera: Syrphidae: Paragini). *Eur. J. Entomol.* **2006**, *103* (2), 443–458.

Schmidt, D.; et al.; Brief Communication: Multiplex X/Y-PCR Improves Sex Identification in ADNA Analysis. *Am. J. Phys. Anthropol.* **2003**, *121* (4), 337–341.

Schmitt, A.; et al.; Variability of the Pattern of Aging on the Human Skeleton: Evidence from Bone Indicators and Implications on Age at Death Estimation. *J. Forensic Sci.* **2002**, *47* (6), 1203–1209.

Schneider, P. M.; et al.; Forensic MtDNA Hair Analysis Excludes a Dog from Having Caused a Traffic Accident. *Int. J. Legal Med.* **1999**, *112* (5), 315–316.

Schotsmans, E. M. J.; et al.; *Taphonomy of Human Remains: Forensic Analysis of the Dead and the Depositional Environment*; John Wiley & Sons, Ltd: Chichester, UK, **2017**.

Schultz, M.; et al.; Oldest Known Case of Metastasizing Prostate Carcinoma Diagnosed in the Skeleton of a 2,700-Year-Old Scythian King from Arzhan (Siberia, Russia). *Int. J. Cancer* **2007**, *121* (12), 2591–2595.

Schwarcz, H. P.; et al.; A New Method for Determination of Postmortem Interval: Citrate Content of Bone. *J. Forensic Sci.* **2010**, *55* (6), 1516–1522.

Schwenke, P. L.; et al.; Forensic Identification of Endangered Chinook Salmon (Oncorhynchus Tshawytscha) Using a Multilocus SNP Assay. *Conserv. Genet.* **2006**, *7* (6), 983–989.

Shadrach, B.; et al.; A Rare Mutation in the Primer Binding Region of the Amelogenin Gene Can Interfere with Gender Identification. *J. Mol. Diagn.* **2004**, *6* (4), 401–405.

Shih, S. Y.; et al.; Applications of Probe Capture Enrichment Next Generation Sequencing for Whole Mitochondrial Genome and 426 Nuclear SNPs for Forensically Challenging Samples. *Genes (Basel).* **2018**, *9* (1) 49.

Shriver, M. D.; et al.; Large-Scale SNP Analysis Reveals Clustered and Continuous Patterns of Human Genetic Variation. *Hum. Genomics* **2005**, *2* (2), 81–89.

Silva, D. A.; et al.; High Quality DNA from Human Remains Obtained by Using the Maxwell® 16 Automated Methodology. *Forensic Sci. Int. Genet. Suppl. Ser.* **2013**, *4* (1), e248–e249.

Skoglund, P.; et al.; Accurate Sex Identification of Ancient Human Remains Using DNA Shotgun Sequencing. *J. Archaeol. Sci.* **2013**, *40* (12), 4477–4482.

Smeets, D.; et al.; Objective 3D Face Recognition: Evolution, Approaches and Challenges. *Forensic Sci. Int.* **2010**, *201* (1–3), 125–132.

Smeets, D.; et al.; A Comparative Study of 3-D Face Recognition Under Expression Variations. *IEEE Trans. Syst. Man, Cybern. Part C (Appl. Rev.)* **2012**, *42* (5), 710–727.

Smith, C. I.; et al.; Not Just Old but Old and Cold? *Nature* **2001**, *410* (6830), 771–772.

Smith, C. I.; et al.; The Thermal History of Human Fossils and the Likelihood of Successful DNA Amplification. *J. Hum. Evol.* **2003**, *45* (3), 203–217.

Smith, M. A.; et al.; DNA BARCODING: CO1 DNA Barcoding Amphibians: Take the Chance, Meet the Challenge. *Mol. Ecol. Resour.* **2008**, *8* (2), 235–246.

Spradley, M. K.; and Jantz, R. L.; Sex Estimation in Forensic Anthropology: Skull versus Postcranial Elements. *J. Forensic Sci.* **2011**, *56* (2), 289–296.

Staats, M.; et al.; Advances in DNA Metabarcoding for Food and Wildlife Forensic Species Identification. *Anal. Bioanal. Chem.* **2016**, *408* (17), 4615–4630.

Steadman, D. W.; et al.; Statistical Basis for Positive Identification in Forensic Anthropology. *Am. J. Phys. Anthropol.* **2006**, *131* (1), 15–26.

Steinlechner, M.; et al.; Rare Failures in the Amelogenin Sex Test. *Int. J. Legal Med.* **2002**, *116* (2), 117–120.

Sterzik, V.; et al.; Estimating the Postmortem Interval of Human Skeletal Remains by Analyzing Their Optical Behavior. *Int. J. Legal Med.* **2016**, *130* (6), 1557–1566.

Stewart, T.; *Essentials of Forensic Anthropology*. Charles C. Thomas: Springfield, IL, USA, **1979**.

Steyn, M.; and Işcan, M. Y.; Sexual Dimorphism in the Crania and Mandibles of South African Whites. *Forensic Sci. Int.* **1998**, *98* (1/2), 9–16.

Stone, A. C.; et al.; Tuberculosis and Leprosy in Perspective. *Am. J. Phys. Anthropol.* **2009**, *140* (S49), 66–94.

Suchey, J. M.; Problems in the Aging of Females Using TheOs Pubis. *Am. J. Phys. Anthropol.* **1979**, *51* (3), 467–470.

Sullivan, K. M.; et al.; A Rapid and Quantitative DNA Sex Test: Fluorescence-Based PCR Analysis of X-Y Homologous Gene Amelogenin. *Biotechniques* **1993**, *15* (4), 636–638, 640–641.

Sutherland, L. D.; and Suchey, J. M.; Use of the Ventral Arc in Pubic Sex Determination. *J. Forensic Sci.* **1991**, *36* (2), 501–511.

Sweet, D.; and Hildebrand, D.; Recovery of DNA from Human Teeth by Cryogenic Grinding. *J. Forensic Sci.* **1998**, *43* (6), 1199–1202.

Taberlet, P.; et al.; Towards Next-Generation Biodiversity Assessment Using DNA Metabarcoding. *Mol. Ecol.* **2012**, *21* (8), 2045–2050.

Takayama, T.; et al.; Determination of Deleted Regions from Yp11.2 of an Amelogenin Negative Male. *Legal Med. (Tokyo).* **2009**, *11 Suppl 1*, S578–80.

Tavares, E. S.; and Baker, A. J.; Single Mitochondrial Gene Barcodes Reliably Identify Sister-Species in Diverse Clades of Birds. *BMC Evol. Biol.* **2008**, *8*, 81.

Templeton, J. E. L.; et al.; DNA Capture and Next-Generation Sequencing Can Recover Whole Mitochondrial Genomes from Highly Degraded Samples for Human Identification. *Investig. Genet.* **2013**, *4* (1), 26.

Thangaraj, K.; et al.; Is the Amelogenin Gene Reliable for Gender Identification in Forensic Casework and Prenatal Diagnosis? *Int. J. Legal Med.* **2002**, *116* (2), 121–123.

Thomas P. Gilbert, M.; et al.; Biochemical and Physical Correlates of DNA Contamination in Archaeological Human Bones and Teeth Excavated at Matera, Italy. *J. Archaeol. Sci.* **2005**, *32* (5), 785–793.

Thomas, R. M.; et al.; Accuracy Rates of Sex Estimation by Forensic Anthropologists through Comparison with DNA Typing Results in Forensic Casework. *J. Forensic Sci.* **2016**, *61* (5), 1307–1310.

Tilotta, F.; et al.; A Comparative Study of Two Methods of Dental Pulp Extraction for Genetic Fingerprinting. *Forensic Sci. Int.* **2010**, *202* (1–3), e39–e43.

Tito, R. Y.; et al.; Phylotyping and Functional Analysis of Two Ancient Human Microbiomes. *PLoS One* **2008**, *3* (11), e3703.

Tito, R. Y.; et al.; Insights from Characterizing Extinct Human Gut Microbiomes. *PLoS One* **2012**, *7* (12), e51146.

Tobe, S.; and Linacre, A.; Species Identification of Human and Deer from Mixed Biological Material. *Forensic Sci. Int.* **2007**, *169* (2–3), 278–279.

Tobe, S. S.; and Linacre, A.; A Method to Identify a Large Number of Mammalian Species in the UK from Trace Samples and Mixtures without the Use of Sequencing. *Forensic Sci. Int. Genet. Suppl. Ser.* **2008**, *1* (1), 625–627.

Tobe, S. S.; and Linacre, A.; Identifying Endangered Species from Degraded Mixtures at Low Levels. *Forensic Sci. Int. Genet. Suppl. Ser.* **2009**, *2* (1), 304–305.

Trivedi, R.; et al.; A New Improved Method for Extraction of DNA from Teeth for the Analysis of Hypervariable Loci. *Am. J. Forensic Med. Pathol.* **2002**, *23* (2), 191–196.

Trotter, M.; and Gleser, G. C.; Estimation of Stature from Long Bones of American Whites and Negroes. *Am. J. Phys. Anthropol.* **1952**, *10* (4), 463–514.

Tschentscher, F.; et al.; Amelogenin Sex Determination by Pyrosequencing of Short PCR Products. *Int. J. Legal Med.* **2008**, *122* (4), 333–335.

Ubelaker, D. H.; and Adams, B. J.; Differentiation of Perimortem and Postmortem Trauma Using Taphonomic Indicators. *J. Forensic Sci.* **1995**, *40* (3), 509–512.

Ubelaker, D. H.; and Volk, C. G.; A Test of the Phenice Method for the Estimation of Sex. *J. Forensic Sci.* **2002**, *47* (1), 19–24.

Ubelaker, D. H.; et al.; Use of Solid-Phase Double-Antibody Radioimmunoassay to Identify Species from Small Skeletal Fragments. *J. Forensic Sci.* **2004**, *49* (5), 924–929.

Ueland, M.; et al.; The Interactive Effect of the Degradation of Cotton Clothing and Decomposition Fluid Production Associated with Decaying Remains. *Forensic Sci. Int.* **2015**, *255*, 56–63.

Ueland, M.; et al.; Understanding Clothed Buried Remains: The Analysis of Decomposition Fluids and Their Influence on Clothing in Model Burial Environments. *Forensic Sci. Med. Pathol.* **2019**, *15* (1), 3–12.

Usher, B. M.; Reference Samples: The First Step in Linking Biology and Age in the Human Skeleton. In *Paleodemography*; Hoppa, R. D., Vaupel, J. W., Eds.; Cambridge University Press: Cambridge, UK, **2002**, 29–47.

Vai, S.; et al.; A Genetic Perspective on Longobard-Era Migrations. *Eur. J. Hum. Genet.* **2019**, *27*, 647–656.

Virkler, K.; and Lednev, I. K.; Analysis of Body Fluids for Forensic Purposes: From Laboratory Testing to Non-Destructive Rapid Confirmatory Identification at a Crime Scene. *Forensic Sci. Int.* **2009**, *188* (1–3), 1–17.

Wallin, J. M.; et al.; TWGDAM Validation of the AmpFISTR Blue PCR Amplification Kit for Forensic Casework Analysis. *J. Forensic Sci.* **1998**, *43* (4), 854–870.

Wan, Q.-H.; and Fang, S.-G.; Application of Species-Specific Polymerase Chain Reaction in the Forensic Identification of Tiger Species. *Forensic Sci. Int.* **2003**, *131* (1), 75–78.

Warinner, C.; et al.; Direct Evidence of Milk Consumption from Ancient Human Dental Calculus. *Sci. Rep.* **2015a** *4* (1), 7104.

Warinner, C.; et al.; Ancient Human Microbiomes. *J. Hum. Evol.* **2015b**, *79*, 125–136.

Warinner, C.; et al.; A New Era in Palaeomicrobiology: Prospects for Ancient Dental Calculus as a Long-Term Record of the Human Oral Microbiome. *Philos. Trans. R. Soc. Lond. B. Biol. Sci.* **2015c**, *370* (1660), 20130376.

Weinberg, S. M.; et al.; Heritability of Face Shape in Twins: A Preliminary Study Using 3D Stereophotogrammetry and Geometric Morphometrics. *Dent. 3000* **2013**, *1* (1), 7–11.

Wetton, J. H.; et al.; An Extremely Sensitive Species-Specific ARMs PCR Test for the Presence of Tiger Bone DNA. *Forensic Sci. Int.* **2004**, *140* (1), 139–145.

Weyrich, L. S.; et al.; Ancient DNA Analysis of Dental Calculus. *J. Hum. Evol.* **2015**, *79*, 119–124.

Wheatley, B. P.; Perimortem or Postmortem Bone Fractures? An Experimental Study of Fracture Patterns in Deer Femora. *J. Forensic Sci.* **2008**, *53* (1), 69–72.

White, E. M.; and Hannus, L. A.; Chemical Weathering of Bone in Archaeological Soils. *Am. Antiq.* **1983**, *48* (02), 316–322.

Wieberg, D. A. M.; and Wescott, D. J.; Estimating the Timing of Long Bone Fractures: Correlation Between the Postmortem Interval, Bone Moisture Content, and Blunt Force Trauma Fracture Characteristics. *J. Forensic Sci.* **2008**, *53* (5), 1028–1034.

Wilkinson, C.; Facial Reconstruction—Anatomical Art or Artistic Anatomy? *J. Anat.* **2010**, *216* (2), 235–250.

Willerslev, E.; and Cooper, A.; Ancient DNA. *Proc. Biol. Sci.* **2005**, *272* (1558), 3–16.

Wilson, I. G.; Inhibition and Facilitation of Nucleic Acid Amplification. *Appl. Environ. Microbiol.* **1997**, *63* (10), 3741–3751.

Wilson, S. J.; and Christensen, A. M.; A Test of the Citrate Method of PMI Estimation from Skeletal Remains. *Forensic Sci. Int.* **2017**, *270*, 70–75.

Winters, M.; et al.; Are We Fishing or Catching? Evaluating the Efficiency of Bait Capture of CODIS Fragments. *Forensic Sci. Int. Genet.* **2017**, *29*, 61–70.

Witt, M.; et al.; Current Genetic Methodologies in the Identification of Disaster Victims and in Forensic Analysis. *J. Appl. Genet.* **2012**, *53* (1), 41–60.

Zeng, X.; et al.; Assessment of Impact of DNA Extraction Methods on Analysis of Human Remain Samples on Massively Parallel Sequencing Success. *Int. J. Legal Med.* **2019**, *133* (1), 51–58.

Zgonjanin, D.; et al.; Case Report: DNA Identification of Burned Skeletal Remains. *Forensic Sci. Int.: Genet. Suppl. Ser.* **2015**, *5*, e444–e446

Zhang, W.; et al.; Highly Conserved D-Loop-like Nuclear Mitochondrial Sequences (Numts) in Tiger (Panthera Tigris). *J. Genet.* **2006**, *85* (2), 107–116.

Zupanic Pajnic, I.; et al.; Molecular Genetic Identification of Skeletal Remains from the Second World War Konfin I Mass Grave in Slovenia. *Int. J. Legal Med.* **2010**, *124* (4), 307–317.

Zupanic Pajnic, I.; et al.; Highly Efficient Nuclear DNA Typing of the World War II Skeletal Remains Using Three New Autosomal Short Tandem Repeat Amplification Kits with the Extended European Standard Set of Loci. *Croat. Med. J.* **2012**, *53* (1), 17–23.

CHAPTER 12

The Molecular Autopsy: Complementary Study to Molecular Autopsy

SILVIA ZOPPIS[1*], ALEJANDRO BLANCO-VEREA[2], and MARIA BRION[2]

[1]*Florida International University, International Forensic Research Institute, 11200 SW 8th St., Miami, FL, USA 33199*

[2]*Grupo de Xenética Cardiovascular, Instituto de Investigación Sanitaria de Santiago, Complexo Hospitalario Universitario de Santiago de Compostela, 15706 Santiago de Compostela, Spain*

Corresponding author. E-mail: silvia.zoppis@alice.it

ABSTRACT

A sudden death can occur for a number of different causes and by various mechanisms but the most relevant event is the one that has a cardiac origin. As for the occurrence of a primary electrical disease that led to the fatal event, the frequent identification of normal macro- and microscopic findings (negative autopsy) represents an important issue and genetic testing of DNA extracted from *post-mortem* tissue (the "molecular autopsy") may identify a cause of death in up to 30% of sudden arrhythmic death syndrome (SADS) cases, providing essential information to the relatives. This genetic testing has moved from a candidate gene-by-gene strategy to a more comprehensive multiple gene approach and recent advances in massively parallel sequencing technologies have allowed ever-expanding panels of genes to be resequenced from comparatively small quantities of DNA, with excellent throughput capabilities and in a cost-efficient manner. This includes sequencing the whole exome, offering the technology for an "exome-wide molecular autopsy" and potentially allowing genetic testing of all major disease-associated genes, as well as genes less frequently involved in any given disease. Many forensic laboratories are implementing these techniques in their routine due to the diagnostic resolution that involves the discovery of one or several genetic variants related to the underlying cardiac pathology of the deceased individual and the possibility to search for this variant or variants in the family members; thus allowing to develop specific medical supervision protocols.

12.1   INTRODUCTION: SUDDEN CARDIAC DEATH IN THE YOUNG

A sudden death can occur for a number of different causes and by various mechanisms such as cerebral aneurysm rupture, pulmonary embolism, or cardiac diseases. Among all the possible scenarios, the most relevant is the sudden death event that has a cardiac origin. Sudden cardiac death (SCD) is defined as unexpected death that occurs from any cardiac cause in a short time, generally 1 h after the onset of symptoms. The prevalence of SCD is significant, with at least three million people worldwide dying suddenly each year (Zipes and Wellens, 1998; Liberthson, 1996; Refaat et al., 2015) and an annual incidence of one death per 1000 persons/year, affecting all ages (Saenen et al., 2015).

It is important to specify that SCD can occur in a person with or without preexisting heart disease. The majority of SCDs happen in subjects over 45 years of age (around 80% of all SCD cases) as a consequence of advanced atherosclerotic coronary artery disease that results in myocardial ischemia and fatal arrhythmias. In contrast, in young adults (<40 years of age), it is mostly caused by cardiac genetic disorders that ultimately result in lethal ventricular arrhythmias (venticular tachycardia [VC] and ventricular fibrillation [VF]).

Most of these juvenile SCDs are manifested as inherited cardiomyopathies such as hypertrophic cardiomyopathy (HCM), arrhythmogenic right ventricular cardiomyopathy (ARVC), and ion channel mutations responsible for inherited abnormalities, such as the long QT syndrome (LQTS), short QT syndrome (SQTS), Brugada syndrome (BrS), and catecholaminergic polymorphic ventricular tachycardia (CPVT) (Brion et al., 2010). In general, the four most common pathogenic categories of SCD in the young are premature atherosclerosis, primary electrical diseases, cardiomyopathies, and thoracic aortic aneurysm and dissection (TAAD). *Premature atherosclerosis* is referred to as an atherosclerotic disease, affecting subjects younger than 35 years old. Familial hereditary factors are very important, especially hypercholesterolemia. Besides, exogenous factors can contribute to the onset of the disease, as smoking and cocaine abuse. High blood pressure, autoimmune diseases, diabetes mellitus, and other rare heritable syndromes can also play a role in the disease.

Primary electrical diseases are caused by molecular defects mostly in ion channels involved in the cardiac action potential generation, under the form of "gain" or "loss of function" of one or more ionic currents that alter the balance between the depolarizing and repolarizing forces during the ventricular action potential. In general, these are diseases with autosomal dominant inheritance and variable penetrance:

LQTS: The clinical diagnosis is made by the presence of an LQTS risk score greater than or equal to 3.5 and/or when the QTc interval is 480–499 ms on serial 12-lead electrocardiogram (ECG) in a patient with unexplained syncope, or when a QTc > 500 ms is repeatedly found in asymptomatic patients. Estimated prevalence is 1:2500–1:5000. About 75% of LQTS are due to mutations of three genes, involved in the formation of K and Na ionic channels and thus in the cardiac action potential modulation: KCNQ1 (LQT1), KCNH2 (LQT2), and SCN5A (LQT3) (Ackerman et al., 2013).

SQTS: It is a rare disease. The diagnosis is performed when a QTc less than or equal to 330 ms is found, or if the QTc is < 360 ms, and there are the anamnestic data in the family of an SCD under 40 years of age, or there is a familial history of SQTS or the identification of a pathogenic mutation (Saenen et al., 2015).

BrS: Currently, 18 genes are known to be involved in the disease, explaining up to 30%–35% of all inherited cases, but the most common mutated gene is SCN5A (25%–30% of the cases). The current prevalence is 3–5:10.000, and it is more frequent in young men from Southeast Asia. Functionally, the disease is represented by a loss of function of the cardiac Na channel, and clinically, it is characterized by ST segment elevation in V1–V3 of the ECG. Incomplete penetrance and variable expressivity confound the diagnosis (Sarquella-Brugada et al., 2016).

Early repolarization syndrome: It is characterized by the occurrence of abnormal "Osborn J-waves" on the ECG during hypothermia (a J-point and ST segment elevation), and it is diagnosed by the presence of a J-point elevation greater than or equal to 1 mm in two or more contiguous inferior and/or lateral ECG leads plus VF or polymorphic VT. There are currently six genes associated. Estimated prevalence is between 6% and 13% of the general population (Saenen et al., 2015).

CPVT: It is a rare disease with an estimated prevalence of 1:10000. It is characterized by VT in conditions of elevated adrenergic tone. It is caused by a sarcoplasmic reticulum calcium overload, which leads to a rate-dependent diastolic calcium leak to the cytosol, an elevated sodium–calcium exchanger activity, and delayed afterdepolarization that finally trigger the arrhythmias. At present, five genes explain about 60% of inherited CPVT cases, and the most important gene involved is RYR2.

Idiopathic ventricular fibrillation (IVF): IVF is a group of disorders that cause cardiac arrest preferentially by documented VF in the absence of detectable cardiac, respiratory, metabolic, and toxicological reversible causes and when apparent structural or electrical heart disease could not be detected (Saenen et al., 2015). Familial IVF has been associated with mutations in SCN5A (IVF1) (Lindsay and Dietz, 2014) and in a Dutch founder population with DPP6 (IVF2). Estimated prevalence is 1%–4% of the general population.

Familial Wolff–Parkinson–White syndrome: It is caused by an accessory conduction pathway between the atrium and the ventricle, which can remain concealed or show as preexcitation of the QRS complex (PR shortening and delta-wave appearance) on the ECG. Its clinical manifestations are palpitations, syncope, and SCD. Recently, an autosomal dominant familial form associated with HCM was associated with mutations in the PRKAG2 gene (adenosine-monophosphate-activated protein kinase). Estimated prevalence is 1–3:1000 (Saenen et al., 2015).

Hereditary cardiomyopathies represent a heterogeneous group of disorders that are characterized by structural remodeling of the cardiac muscle; this can lead to a progressive loss of electrical stability of the cardiac tissue through the generation of anatomical arrhythmogenic substrate. They are mostly represented by the following diseases with autosomal dominant inheritance and variable penetrance: HCM, ARVC, dilated cardiomyopathy (DCM), restrictive cardiomyopathy, and noncompacted cardiomyopathy.

As for *TAAD*, it is important to underline that abdominal aortic aneurysm and dissection (AAAD) and TAAD represent two different diseases. Regarding the common mechanisms that lead to aortic aneurysms and dissection, there are genetic mutations that modify the contraction activity of vascular smooth muscle cells (VSMCs) and cause a degeneration of the aortic media layer by extracellular membrane damage. The final effect is the weakening of the aortic wall and the possible development of an abnormal dilatation and aneurysm formation, eventually resulting in intramural hemorrhage, aortic dissection, or rupture. As for aortic dissection, it is referred to the disruption of the media layer of the aorta with bleeding within and along the wall of the vessel, resulting in separation of the layers of the aorta wall. If left untreated, aortic aneurysms evolve toward dissection and rupture. On the one hand, AAAD has a complex multifactorial basis, in which multiple interactions between genetic and environmental factors contribute to the development of the disease. It is an asymptomatic disease in more than 60–70% of the cases and has a slow and unpredictable growing. It increases with age, and the mortality rate rises in the adult population of Europe, the USA, and Australia from 1%–2% up to more than 10% in men over 75 years old. From the genetic point of view, abdominal aortic aneurysm is complex as it does not follow a simple Mendelian inheritance because of the simultaneous presence of many genes, each of them interacting with environmental factors, determining in each individual the degree of susceptibility to the disease. Atherosclerosis, smoking, chronic inflammation, and/or infections affecting the aortic wall, respiratory distress, and high blood pressure are the most important risk factors (Saracini et al., 2012; Ryer et al., 2015). On the other hand, TAAD represents an important cause of death (1%–2%) and needs to be incorporated in the SCD work-up. Overall incidence of TAAD is 2.7 per 100.000 persons/year (Luyckx and Loeys, 2015). The mortality rate of patients with TAAD is two to three times higher than patients with AAAD. Besides, mortality after TAAD diagnosis reaches 97% with a median survival rate of three days (Saenen et al., 2015). Two major pathogenic factors for TAAD have emerged over the last decade: VSMC-specific sarcomeric protein dysfunction and dysregulation of transforming growth factor β (TGFβ) signaling. TAAD is genetically classified in two forms, depending on the association of the aortic disease with other congenital abnormalities/defects in other organs or apparatuses: nonsyndromic TAAD and syndromic TAAD. Nonsyndromic forms are caused by multiple genes coding for components of the VSMC contractile apparatus (e.g., ACTA2 and MYH11) (Saenen et al., 2015). Syndromic forms are caused by mutations in genes encoding components of the extracellular matrix (e.g., Fibrillin 1 and Collagen 3) and the TGFβ signaling cascade (e.g., TGFβR1/2 and SMAD3).

The main genetic diseases associated with TAAD are as follows:

- *Marfan syndrome (MFS):* It is caused by mutations in the FBN1 gene encoding Fibrillin 1, an important extracellular component of the microfibrils.
- *Loeys–Dietz syndrome (aneurysm-osteoarthritis syndrome):* Mutations of genes TGFBR1 and 2, SMAD3 (aneurysm-osteoarthritis syndrome), and TGFB2 (MFS-like phenotype) have been described.
- *Ehlers–Danlos syndrome (EDS):* It represents a heterogeneous group of disorders mainly characterized by skin (hyper extensibility), joint (hypermobility and luxation), and vascular (arterial rupture) findings. It is mainly caused by a deficiency of type III collagen by a COL3A1 gene mutation.

- *Bicuspid aortic valve (BAV)-related aneurysm:* So far, a few genes such as NOTCH1 (Burton and Underwood, 2007) and GATA5 (Margey et al., 2011) have been associated with nonsyndromic presentations of BAV/TAA, but they only represent a small proportion of all patients with BAV/TAA.

Approximately, 20% of patients with TAAD have a family history of the disease, and these patients are younger with more rapidly enlarging aneurysms than patients without a family history of aortic disease (Guo et al., 2011): this condition is known as familial TAAD, which can be inherited in an autosomal dominant manner with incomplete penetrance and variable expression with respect to disease presentation, age of onset, and associated features.

12.2 THE IMPORTANCE OF *POST MORTEM* EVALUATION: THE NEGATIVE AUTOPSY

For nearly half of young victims from 1 to 35–40 years of age, SCD affects people in good health and occurs without warning symptoms, pointing out the extreme importance upon medicolegal investigation and autopsy to determine the cause and manner of death (Liberthson, 1996).

The correct *post-mortem* evaluation must include the collection of appropriate samples for subsequent histological, toxicological, and genetic analyses and a precise and accurate final conclusion. In particular, it should include a detailed macroscopic and histological evaluation of the heart, as well as other key organs such as the brain, with the purpose of identifying any noncardiac causes of death (e.g., pulmonary embolism or cerebral aneurysm), before focusing on specific cardiac pathologies. Over the past few years, other imaging techniques have been studied and proposed for the diagnosis of structural causes of SCD. These noninvasive approaches appear to be useful as they may overcome some of the reservations that families have in proceeding with the traditional *post-mortem* process for many various reasons (religious, cultural, and personal). These modalities include computer tomography scanning and cardiovascular magnetic resonance imaging (Burton and Underwood, 2007).

It is necessary to specify that, if as for premature atherosclerosis, cardiomyopathies, and TAAD, the identification of the cause of death in the specific case is usually possible after an accurate and complete autopsy examination, as for the occurrence of a primary electrical disease that led to the fatal event, the frequent identification of normal macro- and microscopic findings represents an important issue that needs to be addressed. In fact, since these disorders usually do not determine any structural changes to the heart, the *post-mortem* appears to be "negative" (no cause of death is identified)—with normal histopathology and toxicology analyses results—in up to 40% of SCD cases in young populations (1–40 years old) (Margey et al., 2011; Winkel et al., 2011; Doolan et al., 2004; Corrado et al., 2001; Puranik et al., 2005; de Noronha et al., 2009). These events are often referred to as "sudden arrhythmic death syndrome" (SADS) and do not include the specific "sudden infant death syndrome" from 0 to 1 year. In these particular situations, when no cause of death is identified at the autopsy, genetic testing of DNA extracted from *post-mortem* tissue (the "molecular autopsy") may identify a cause of death in up to 30% of SADS cases (Lahrouchi et al., 2017).

Therefore, in all young SCD cases, a 5–10-mL blood sample should be collected for subsequent DNA extraction and analysis. In addition, frozen sections of the liver or spleen, which are highly cellular and rich in DNA, should also be collected and stored when possible; on the contrary, paraffin-embedded tissues are not suitable for genetic analyses because of their poor DNA quality (Doolan et al., 2008; Carturan et al., 2008). It is important to underline that obtaining a *post-mortem* blood sample in young SCD cases is now recommended by the Heart Rhythm Society/European Heart Rhythm Association guidelines (Ackerman et al., 2011) and is mandated in several countries, including Australia and New Zealand (Skinner et al., 2008).

12.3 CURRENT DEVELOPMENTS FOR IDENTIFICATION OF GENETIC PREDISPOSITION TO SCD: THE MOLECULAR AUTOPSY

To date, medicolegal investigation in cases of SCD can benefit from the so-called molecular autopsy by the analysis of genes involved in the specific condition, decreasing the percentage of negative autopsies and providing essential information to the relatives (Tester and Ackerman, 2006; Lorin de la Grandmaison, 2006; Scheiper et al., 2018).

When sudden death has occurred, the identification of the genetic basis of SCD is absolutely crucial for families (Rodriguez-Calvo et al., 2008) because many inherited cardiac diseases, with the associated risk of SCD, segregate in an autosomal dominant way so that first-degree relatives have a one in two (50%) chance of inheriting the same gene mutation.

The use of genetic testing in the setting of SCD cases (i.e., "molecular autopsy") was initiated over a decade ago (Tester et al., 2004) and involves

DNA extraction from *post-mortem* blood, followed by DNA analysis of selected candidate genes responsible for the main inherited arrhythmogenic diseases (Semsarian and Hamilton, 2012; Semsarian et al., 2015). The first four protein coding exons analyzed were the three major LQTS genes (KCNQ1, KCNH2, and SCN5A) and the CPVT gene (RYR2) (Ackerman et al., 2011; Cerrone and Priori, 2011; Wilde and Behr, 2013). Mutations in the SCN5A gene cause LQTS3 as well as BrS.

Over the last decade, the care of the patient with a potential cardio genetic disorder has tremendously evolved: the identification of an increasing number of genes and the use of advanced molecular techniques allow a molecular diagnosis, identification of high-risk relatives, and the preventive treatment or presymptomatic follow-up. These may include lifestyle modifications, pharmacological treatment, implant of a cardioverter defibrillator, or radio-frequency ablation (Saenen et al., 2015).

Over the past few years, significant advances have been developed to understand both the clinical and genetic bases of SCD (Lindsay and Dietz, 2014; Ryer et al., 2015), and genetic testing has moved from a candidate gene-by-gene strategy to a more comprehensive multiple gene approach. In many countries, recent advances in massively parallel sequencing technologies have allowed ever-expanding panels of genes (cardiac gene panels with up to 200 genes) to be resequenced from comparatively small quantities of DNA, with excellent throughput capabilities, and in a cost-efficient manner. This includes sequencing the whole exome, thus offering the technology for an "exome-wide molecular autopsy" and potentially allowing genetic testing of all major disease-associated genes, as well as genes less frequently involved in any given disease.

Whole exome sequencing (WES) and targeted sequencing have been developed as alternatives to whole genome sequencing (WGS) reducing sequencing costs, turnaround times, data storage needs, and informatics burdens compared to WGS. There are many approaches to enrich for target sequences that use different DNA preparation and capture methods that can be in solution, solid-phase, or PCR-based (Chilamakuri et al., 2014). As for WES, it often results in uneven coverage across and between genes and can particularly struggle with guanine-cytosine-rich regions such as first exons (Lan et al., 2015). In addition, the interpretation of incidental variants, as suggested by the American College of Medical Genetics and Genomics (ACMG), is also a potential issue for WES, where variants unrelated to the patient's referral condition may be detected (Green et al., 2013). In contrast, targeted sequencing of gene panels has been widely used in research and is increasingly applied in clinical settings (Voelkerding et al., 2010).

Regarding various inherited cardiac conditions (ICCs), small gene panels have been used for specific conditions, including LQTS, HCM, DCM, and ARVC (Millat et al., 2014; Akinrinade et al., 2015; Gréen et al., 2015; Kalayinia et al., 2018). Multiple workflows and bioinformatics pipelines are needed to run these various gene panels, and gene coverage is such that Sanger sequencing confirmation is still needed (Akinrinade et al., 2015; Millat et al., 2014; Glotov et al., 2015; Wilson et al., 2015).

In (Pua et al., 2016), the interesting development of a new gene panel for ICCs is described, which provides a comprehensive, single workflow assay with high levels of coverage across all ICC genes for use in research and clinical settings. Genes were chosen on the basis of reported associations of disease-causing variants with relevant ICCs identified in the Human Gene Mutation Database Professional version 2014.1, followed by addition of further genes of research interest. Pathogenic or likely pathogenic variants identified using the ICC panel in a research cohort were subjected to Sanger sequencing for confirmation. It is important to consider differences in variant calling between informatic pipelines as highlighted by the comparison of three methods that use different mapping and variant calling algorithms and data preprocessing workflows: alignment with BWA-MEM and GATK Haplotype Caller pipeline offers best sensitivity and precision (Highnam et al., 2015), while cloud-based and easily implemented pipelines on BaseSpace offer a viable alternative for those with limited in-house informatics and, based on preliminary analyses, have comparable sensitivity. As compared to the WES, deep WES, and WGS, this assay shows better performance, shorter turnaround times, lesser informatics requirements, and lower sequencing costs.

In (Bagnall et al., 2016), the genetic findings in 61 cases of sudden unexplained death in epilepsy are reported; the authors found pathogenic or probably pathogenic variants in the three common genes for the LQTS in 7% of the cases and in epilepsy genes in 25% of the cases (Bagnall et al., 2016). In contrast, as for subjects who had no history of epilepsy, the same study reports only four cases of unexplained SCD (6%), in which the person had probable pathogenic variants in epilepsy genes, suggesting that undiagnosed genetic epilepsy is uncommon in cases of unexplained SCD.

All the technologies described previously lead to a more comprehensive view of all existing genetic variation and its ability to modify phenotypes; thus, the need to develop better functional tools to study the effect of genetic variants is strongly increasing.

With the introduction of next-generation sequencing (NGS) into clinical practice, the number and size of genes investigated have increased dramatically.

Since the number of variants identified by NGS is almost proportional to the total number of DNA bases sequenced, many more variants are being identified and need to be classified as pathogenic, benign, or variant of uncertain significance (VUS) (Green et al., 2013; Lopes et al., 2013).

In order to make such distinctions, a rigorous process of interpretation is necessary to avoid misclassification and thereby ensure correct counseling; this relies on a number of complementary investigations.

1. *Frequency of variants in healthy controls*: Several public databases provide information about the frequency of variants within the coding sequence of the human genome based on WES and WGS of thousands of apparently healthy controls. Once a sequence variant has been identified in a patient, it is important to determine whether it is present or absent in such databases. A high frequency among controls indicates that the variant identified is likely to represent normal variation, while a very low frequency or complete absence suggests a potential disease-associated mutation (Hoischen et al., 2011).

2. *Published data*: It is important to clarify whether the variant has already been reported as disease causing. However, the evidence for causation needs careful evaluation since much of the published data that were generated in the pre-NGS era involved a limited number of controls. It has become evident following the introduction of NGS that a significant number of rare variants previously reported to be pathogenic are in fact likely to be benign due to their presence in the general population (Andreasen et al., 2013).

3. *Cosegregation in families*: Cosegregation of a variant with the condition in a large family with many affected individuals usually provides strong evidence for causation. However, families with multiple affected individuals are a rare occurrence, and the most common clinical scenario is that of a novel sequence variant in an individual with only few or no other clinically affected relatives. Consequently, many novel variants identified by NGS will be classified as VUS and thereby represent an inconclusive test result at present.

4. *Likely effect on the transcribed protein and evolutionary conservation*: Sequence variants exert different effects on protein structure that may or may not be pathogenic. The probable impact on protein function can be estimated from the type of mutation (nonsense, missense, and splice site) and the level of conservation through evolution by comparison to DNA-sequences of other species and by

using *in silico* prediction tools. These analyses provide information about the likelihood of pathogenicity, but cannot be used in isolation to classify a sequence variant as relevant for clinical decision making or genetic counseling (Mogensen et al., 2015).

The report by Richards S. et al. (2015) recommends the use of specific standard terminology—"pathogenic," "likely pathogenic," "uncertain significance," "likely benign," and "benign"—to describe variants identified in genes that cause Mendelian disorders. Because of the increased complexity of analysis and interpretation of clinical genetic testing described in this report, the ACMG strongly recommends that clinical molecular genetic testing should be performed in a Clinical Laboratory Improvement Amendments approved laboratory, with results interpreted by a board-certified clinical molecular geneticist or molecular genetic pathologist or the equivalent.

12.4 MANAGEMENT OF THE FAMILIES

As for the management of families following an SCD, it includes not only the correct identification of the cause of death-on the base of the clinical history of the deceased and the pathological findings at the *post-mortem*—but also the identification of relatives who may be at risk of having the same inherited heart disease and are, therefore, predisposed to SCD. Thus, a targeted clinical testing in a specialized multidisciplinary professional context in surviving family members combined with the analysis of the results from genetic testing is highly recommended (Semsarian and Ingles, 2016).

Clinical evaluation alone in families with a sudden unexplained death may identify an underlying cause in up to 50% of selected and comprehensively evaluated families in tertiary centers (Behr et al., 2008; Behr et al., 2003; Tan et al., 2005).

Offering cascade genetic testing to asymptomatic relatives should always be performed in conjunction with clinical evaluation and only alongside comprehensive pre- and post-test genetic counseling (Ingles and Semsarian, 2014). Cascade genetic testing may also reveal *de novo* cases, where the parents of the decedent do not carry the disease-causing mutation. In this case, the only at-risk relatives would be the offspring of the decedent.

If an underlying diagnosis is made using both clinical and genetic evaluation of the family, subsequent management and follow-up depend on the disease in question. This will often trigger more specific family cascade clinical screening and, if available, genetic testing (Ackerman et al., 2011).

Commonly, the relative being screened is a child, in which case regular follow-up is indicated until adulthood, with the knowledge that many genetic heart diseases most commonly manifest as clinical disease in the second decade of life (Maron et al., 2014). The multidisciplinary approach provides expertise not only in the clinical and genetic aspects of disease, but also in the integration of key links with other critical members of the team in addition to the cardiologist, including cardiac genetic counselors, geneticists, forensic pathologists, primary care physicians, nurses, clinical psychologists, and patient support groups.

The fact that to date a pathogenic genetic variant is identified only in a limited percentage of the total SADS cases (up to 30% of the cases) largely reflects a range of clinical and methodological issues relating to the type of DNA obtained, selection bias of the populations studied, the definition of sudden death, and variation in the stringency and interpretation of DNA variants in terms of pathogenicity.

12.5   NGS TECHNIQUES APPLIED TO THE MOLECULAR AUTOPSY

In recent years, parallel mass sequencing has been shown as a unique value tool in molecular autopsy for its ability to systematically identify variants on a large scale in a short period of time, allowing to look for genes that may be involved in sudden death. This search will be simpler as long as the underlying pathology has a Mendelian inheritance (Ng et al., 2010). As already described above, the most common procedure is to use a panel with all the genes that may be related to SCD; an alternative would be to perform the complete exome sequencing, which would be more oriented toward the search for new genes that may be related to the pathology.

Enrichment techniques: In order to carry out the mass sequencing on the target regions of the genes of interest, it is essential to perform an enrichment of these regions in the biological samples that will be analyzed.

There are basically two ways to accomplish this enrichment: one would be based on hybrid capture and the other on multiplexed amplification (Khodakov et al., 2016).

Hybrid capture uses oligonucleotide probes on magnetic beads to selectively capture genes/regions of interest, washing away irrelevant sequences; the main advantage is the scalability of the method, and disadvantages are the input DNA requirement and the large protocol. In this method, the first step is to design specific probes for the target region, next is shearing a genomic

DNA sample using ultra-sonication or enzyme, followed by ligation of sequencing adaptors; then, the genomic regions with ligated adaptors are PCR-amplified to increase concentration, the amplicons are exposed to the biotinylated hybrid-capture probes, and hybridization is allowed to occur. Amplicons hybridized to the probes are then captured with streptavidin-coated magnetic beads, while unbound amplicons are washed away. Bound amplicons are subsequently eluted from the beads.

Multiplexed amplification selectively amplifies the genes/regions of interest, thus increasing their concentration in comparison to irrelevant sequences. Its main advantages are low-input DNA requirements and a short protocol, while its main disadvantage is possible primer–dimer artifacts that waste sequencing reads. The general workflow is divided in four steps: primer design, target-specific multiplex PCR amplification, primer digestion, and adapter ligation.

Both enrichment techniques are offered by several commercial houses and can be used indifferently on various sequencing platforms such as the Ion Proton™ (Thermo Fisher Scientific).

It is difficult to say which method is better since there are not many studies comparing the use of two enrichment methods on the same sequencing platform; however, Samarodnitsky et al. (2015) evaluated the advantages of one method or another using Ion Torrent™ technology, and they observed that capture-based approaches showed better coverage uniformity and were less likely to exclude single-nucleotide variants (false negative) and assigned less false positives.

Ion Proton™ System sequencing platform: Once enrichment process is finished, samples are loaded onto a sequencing platform such as the Ion Proton™ System that use Ion Torrent™ technology. The system combines semiconductor sequencing technology with natural biochemistry to directly translate chemical information into digital data. Ion semiconductor sequencing is a method of DNA sequencing based on the detection of hydrogen ions that are released during the polymerization of DNA. This is a method of "sequencing by synthesis," during which a complementary strand is built based on the sequence of a template strand. The Ion Proton™ System provides sequencing run times of 2–4 h on the Ion PI™ Chip, and it is equipped with Ion Reporter™ Software, the Base calling package, providing integrated tools for tertiary data analysis. In order to locate the genetic variants, it is necessary to carry out a complete alignment process with the reference human genome, and for read alignment, commercial or open-source tools are available. It is also essential to use variant calling algorithms to detect single or multiple base variants with respect to the reference human genome: Total Variant Calling (version 5.0–7) is a specific caller for the Ion Proton System and GATK v3.5–0 (Genome Analysis Toolkit, Broad Institute) is an open-source software that can be used with other sequencing platforms. For export of raw variants and their annotations, there are several file formats (Rehm et al., 2013).

Variant prioritization process: Once the sequencing process is completed, at the moment the files with the annotations are obtained, a few hundred variants per sample are recovered in the case of sequencing a panel of genes and a few tens of thousands of variants in the case of sequencing the complete exome. In order to try to locate the variant or variants that may be related to the pathology of the analyzed individual among all these variants obtained (i.e., the ones that can be considered as mutations with a potential pathogenic significance), we must carry out a prioritization process of variants.

In the article by Gago-Diaz et al. (2017), the authors describe the steps of the prioritization process after sequencing 17 samples from individuals presenting TAAD using a panel of 22 TAAD-related genes in order to look for genetic variants that may be related to the pathology, establishing a prioritization process based on six steps, in this order:

- Focus the search on variants that may alter the function of the protein.
- Those located in exonic or splicing flanking regions were selected.
- The variants identified as synonymous will be excluded.
- A frequency filter toward rare genetic variants with minor allele frequency in the non-Finnish Europeans from the Exome Aggregation Consortium database either unknown or below 1% was then applied (ExAC, available from exac.broadinstitute.org/).
- Again focusing on rare variants, those reported more than four times in an internal database of around 100 exomes with a highly variable background were excluded.
- Finally, the genetic variants present in two or less samples from the same massive parallel sequencing run and those that seemed real during the visualization of the raw sequencing results using the integrative genomics viewer were prioritized for validation (Robinson et al., 2011; Thorvaldsdóttir et al., 2013).

Once identified, the variants should be analyzed in order to look for previous descriptions in population databases and to evaluate the clinical significance of each mutation by multiple specific databases: the authors, in fact, recommend to revise in the literature the available information of each of the prioritized genetic variants at the end of the variants prioritization process, in addition to observing their frequency in extensive reference databases such as the Exome Variant Server from the NHLBI GO Exome Sequencing Project and the Exome Aggregation Consortium (NHLBI GO Exome Sequencing Project, URL: http://evs.gs.washington.edu/EVS/). It is also useful to predict, with reservations, the pathogenicity of these variants based on the conservation score and using pathogenic prediction tools such as Polyphen-2 (Adzhubei et al., 2010), Mutation Taster (Schwarz et al., 2014), Sorting Intolerant From Tolerant (Kumar et al., 2009), and Combined Annotation Dependent Depletion (Kircher et al., 2014). Considering all the available information, candidate genetic variants should be classified according to the ACMG recommendations published in 2015 (Richards et al., 2015). Although this prioritization process is focused on a concrete work, it allows us to observe in which details, we should pay special attention when deciding to establish a protocol of prioritization of variants; hence, these steps may vary depending on the ultimate goal of the study that is going to be carried out.

12.6 CONCLUDING REMARKS

Sudden death cases are always a tragedy for families as well as an impact on society, especially when happening in apparently healthy individuals. In many cases, the causes of the sudden death are not identified after the *post-mortem* exam, and as seen in numerous studies, this is the point where molecular autopsy takes on a fundamental relevance allowing us to find the genetic causes behind the fatal event: this result is obtainable, thanks to constant cost reduction and the continuous advance in the techniques of massive sequencing in parallel that allow tracking a very high number of genes. Every day, more and more forensic laboratories are implementing these techniques in their routine due to the diagnostic resolution that involves the discovery of one or several genetic variants related to the underlying cardiac pathology of the deceased individual. This fact, in addition to giving an explanation to the family of what has happened, implies another fundamental added advantage that is represented by the search for this variant or variants in the rest of the family members and thus the possibility to develop medical supervision protocols in order to try to reduce the risks that would imply the pathology in case the relatives are found to be carriers.

ACKNOWLEDGMENTS

The authors aknowledge Dr. Bruce McCord and Dr. Sara Casado Zapico from Florida International University (Miami, FL).

KEYWORDS

- **sudden death**
- **negative autopsy**
- **molecular autopsy**

REFERENCES

Ackerman, M.J.; et al.; HRS/EHRA expert consensus statement on the state of genetic testing for the channelopathies and cardiomyopathies: This document was developed as a partnership between the Heart Rhythm Society (HRS) and the European Heart Rhythm Association (EHRA). *Heart Rhythm.* **2011**, 8(8), 1308–39. doi: 10.1016/j.hrthm.2011.05.020.

Ackerman, M.J.; Marcou, C.A. and Tester, D.J.; Personalized medicine: Genetic diagnosis for inherited cardiomyopathies/channelopathies. *Rev. Esp. Cardiol. (Engl. Ed.).* **2013**, 66(4), 298–307. doi: 10.1016/j.rec.2012.12.010.

Adzhubei, I.; et al.; A method and server for predicting damaging missense mutations. *Nat. Methods.* **2010**, 7(4), 248–9. doi:10.1038/nmeth0410-248.

Akinrinade, O.; et al.; Genetics and genotype-phenotype correlations in Finnish patients with dilated cardiomyopathy. *Eur. Heart J.* **2015**, 36(34), 2327–37. doi: 10.1093/eurheartj/ehv253.

Andreasen, C.; et al.; New population-based exome data are questioning the pathogenicity of previously cardiomyopathy-associated genetic variants. *Eur. J. Hum. Genet.* **2013**, 21, 918–28. doi: 10.1038/ejhg.2012.283.

Bagnall, R.D.; et al.; Exome-based analysis of cardiac arrhythmia, respiratory control and epilepsy genes in sudden unexpected death in epilepsy. *Ann. Neurol.* **2016**, 79, 522–34. doi: 10.1002/ana.24596.

Bagnall, R.D.; et al.; A prospective study of sudden cardiac death among children and young adults. *N. Engl. J. Med.* **2016**, 374, 2441–52. doi: 10.1056/NEJMoa1510687.

Behr, E.; et al.; Sudden Arrhythmic Death Syndrome Steering Group. Cardiological assessment of first-degree relatives in sudden arrhythmic death syndrome. *Lancet.* **2003**, 362(9394), 1457–9.

Behr, E.R.; et al.; Sudden arrhythmic death syndrome: Familial evaluation identifies inheritable heart disease in the majority of families. *Eur. Heart J.* **2008**, 29(13),1670–80. doi: 10.1093/eurheartj/ehn219.

Brion, M.; et al.; Review: New technologies in the genetic approach to sudden cardiac death in the young. *Forensic Sci. Int.* **2010**, 203(1–3), 15–24. doi: 10.1016/j.forsciint.2010.07.015.

Burton, J.L. and Underwood, J.; Clinical, educational, and epidemiological value of autopsy. *Lancet.* **2007**, 369(9571), 1471–80.

Carturan, E.; et al.; Postmortem genetic testing for conventional autopsy-negative sudden unexplained death: An evaluation of different DNA extraction protocols and the feasibility of mutational analysis from archival paraffin-embedded heart tissue. *Am. J. Clin. Pathol.* **2008**, 129(3), 391–7. doi: 10.1309/VLA7TT9EQ05FFVN4.

Cerrone, M. and Priori, S.G.; Genetics of sudden death: Focus on inherited channelopathies. *Eur. Heart J.* **2011**, 32(17), 2109–18. doi: 10.1093/eurheartj/ehr082.

Chilamakuri, C. S. R.; et al.; Performance comparison of four exome capture systems for deep sequencing. *BMC Genomics.* **2014**, 15, 449. doi:10.1186/1471-2164-15-449.

Corrado, D.; Basso, C. and Thiene, G.; Sudden cardiac death in young people with apparently normal heart. *Cardiovasc. Res.* **2001**, 50(2), 399–408.

de Noronha, S.V.; et al.; Aetiology of sudden cardiac death in athletes in the United Kingdom: A pathological study. *Heart.* **2009**, 95(17), 1409–14. doi: 10.1136/hrt.2009.168369.

Doolan, A.; Langlois, N. and Semsarian, C.; Causes of sudden cardiac death in young Australians. *Med. J. Aust.* **2004**, 180(3), 110–2.

Doolan, A.; et al.; Postmortem molecular analysis of KCNQ1 and SCN5A genes in sudden unexplained death in young Australians. *Int. J. Cardiol.* **2008**, 127(1), 138–41.

Gago-Díaz, M.; et al.; Postmortem genetics testing should be recommended in sudden cardiac death cases due to thoracic aortic dissection. *Int. J. Legal Med.* **2017**. 131(5), 1211–19. doi: 10.1007/s00414-017-1583-9.

Glotov, A.S.; et al.; Targeted next-generation sequencing (NGS) of nine candidate genes with custom AmpliSeq in patients and a cardiomyopathy risk group. *Clin. Chim. Acta.* **2015**, 446, 132–40. doi:10.1016/j.cca. 2015.04.014.

Gréen, A.; et al.; Assessment of HaloPlex amplification for sequence capture and massively parallel sequencing of arrhythmogenic right ventricular cardiomyopathy—Associated genes. *J. Mol. Diagn.* **2015**, 17(1), 31–42. doi: 10.1016/j.jmoldx.2014.09.006.

Green, R.C.; et al.; American College of Medical Genetics and Genomics. ACMG recommendations for reporting of incidental findings in clinical exome and genome sequencing. *Genet Med.* **2013**, 15(7), 565–74. doi: 10.1038/gim.2013.73.

Guo, D.C.; et al.; Familial thoracic aortic aneurysms and dissections: Identification of a novel locus for stable aneurysms with a low risk for progression to aortic dissection. *Circ. Cardiovasc. Genet.* **2011**, 4(1), 36–42. doi: 10.1161/CIRCGENETICS.110.958066.

Highnam, G.; et al.; An analytical framework for optimizing variant discovery from personal genomes. *Nat. Commun.* **2015**, 6, 6275. doi:10.1038/ ncomms7275.

Hoischen, A.; et al.; De novo nonsense mutations in ASXL1 cause Bohring–Opitz syndrome. *Nat. Genet.* **2011**, 43(8), 729–31. doi: 10.1038/ng.868.

Ingles, J. and Semsarian, C.; The value of cardiac genetic testing. *Trends Cardiovasc. Med.* **2014**, 24(6), 217–24. doi: 10.1016/j.tcm.2014.05.009.

Kalayinia, S.; et al.; Next generation sequencing applications for cardiovascular disease. *Ann. Med.* **2018**, 50(2), 91–109. doi: 10.1080/07853890.2017.1392595.

Khodakov, D.; Wang, C. and Yu Zang, D.; Diagnostics based on nucleic acid sequence variant profiling: PCR, Hybridization, and NGS approaches. *Adv. Drug Deliv. Rev.* **2016**, 105(Pt A), 3–19. doi: 10.1016/j.addr.2016.04.005.

Kircher, M.; et al.; A general framework for estimating the relative pathogenicity of human genetic variants. *Nat. Genet.* **2014**, 46(3), 310–5. doi: 10.1038/ng.2892.

Kumar, P.; Henikoff, S. and Ng, P.C.; Predicting the effects of coding non-synonymous variants on protein function using the SIFT algorithm. *Nat. Protoc.* **2009**, 4(8), 1073–82. doi:10.1038/nprot.2009.86.

Lahrouchi, N.; et al.; Utility of post-mortem genetic testing in cases of sudden arrhythmic death syndrome. *J. Am. Coll. Cardiol.* **2017**, 69(17), 2134–45. doi: 10.1016/j.jacc.2017.02.046.

Lan, J.H.; et al.; Impact of three Illumina library construction methods on GC bias and HLA genotype calling. *Human Immunol.* **2015**, 76(2/3), 166–75. doi:10.1016/j. humimm.2014.12.016.

Liberthson, R.R.; Sudden death from cardiac causes in children and young adults. *N. Engl. J. Med.* **1996**, 334(16), 1039–44.

Lindsay, M.E. and Dietz, H.C.; The Genetic Basis of Aortic Aneurysm, *Cold Spring Harb. Perspect. Med.* **2014**, 4(9), a015909. doi: 10.1101/cshperspect.a015909.

Lopes, L.R.; et al.; Genetic complexity in hypertrophic cardiomyopathy revealed by high-through put sequencing. *J. Med. Genet.* **2013**, 50, 228–39. doi: 10.1136/jmedgenet-2012-101270.

Lorin de la Grandmaison, G.; Is there progress in the autopsy diagnosis of the sudden unexplained death in adults? *Forensic Sci. Int.* **2006**, 156(2–3), 138–44.

Luyckx, I. and Loeys, B.L.; The genetic architecture of non-syndromic thoracic aortic aneurysm. *Heart.* **2015**, 101(20), 1678–84. doi: 10.1136/heartjnl-2014-306381.

Margey, R.; et al.; Sudden cardiac death in 14- to 35-year olds in Ireland from 2005 to 2007: A retrospective registry. *Europace.* **2011**, 13(10), 1411–8. doi: 10.1093/europace/eur161.

Maron, B.J.; et al.; Hypertrophic cardiomyopathy: Present and future, with translation into contemporary cardiovascular medicine. *J. Am. Coll. Cardiol.* **2014**, 64(1), 83–99.doi: 10.1016/j.jacc.2014.05.003.

Millat, G.; Chanavat, V. and Rousson, R.; Evaluation of a new high-throughput next-generation sequencing method based on a custom AmpliSeq™ Library and Ion Torrent PGM™ sequencing for the rapid detection of genetic variations in long QT syndrome. *Mol. Diagn. Ther.* **2014**, 18(5), 533–9. doi:10.1007/s40291-014-0099-y.

Millat, G.; Chanavat, V. and Rousson, R.; Evaluation of a new NGS method based on a custom AmpliSeq library and Ion Torrent PGM sequencing for the fast detection of genetic variations in cardiomyopathies. *Clin. Chim. Acta.* **2014**, 433, 266–71. doi: 10.1016/j.cca.2014.03.032.

Mogensen, J.; et al.; The current role of next-generation DNA sequencing in routine care of patients with hereditary cardiovascular conditions: A viewpoint paper of the European Society of Cardiology working group on myocardial and pericardial diseases and members of the European Society of Human Genetics. *Eur. Heart J.* **2015**, 36(22),1367–70. doi: 10.1093/eurheartj/ehv122.

Ng, S.B.; et al.; Massively parallel sequencing and rare disease. *Hum. Mol. Genet.* **2010**, 19(R2), R119–24. doi: 10.1093/hmg/ddq390.

Pua, C.J.; et al.; Development of a comprehensive sequencing assay for inherited cardiac condition Genes. *J. Cardiovasc. Transl. Res.* **2016**, 9(1), 3–11. doi: 10.1007/s12265-016-9673-5.

Puranik, R.; et al.; Sudden death in the young. *Heart-Rhythm.* **2005**, 2(12), 1277–82.

Refaat, M.M.; Hotait, M. and London, B.; Genetics of sudden cardiac death. *Curr. Cardiol. Rep.* **2015**, 17(7), 606. doi: 10.1007/s11886-015-0606-8.

Rehm, H.L.; et al.; ACMG clinical laboratory standards for next-generation sequencing. *Genet. Med.* **2013**, 15(9), 733–47. doi: 10.1038/gim.2013.92.

Richards, S.; et al.; ACMG Laboratory Quality Assurance Committee. Standards and guidelines for the interpretation of sequence variants: A joint consensus recommendation of the American College of Medical Genetics and Genomics and the Association for Molecular Pathology. *Genet Med.* **2015**, 17(5), 405–24. doi: 10.1038/gim.2015.30.

Robinson, J.T.; et al.; Integrative genomics viewer. *Nat. Biotechnol.* **2011**, 29(1), 24–6. doi: 10.1038/nbt.1754.

Rodriguez-Calvo, M.S.; et al.; Molecular genetics of sudden cardiac death. *Forensic Sci. Int.* **2008**, 182 (1–3), 1–12. doi: 10.1016/j.forsciint.2008.09.013.

Ryer, E.J.; et al.; The potential role of DNA methylation in abdominal aortic aneurysms. *Int. J. Mol. Sci.* **2015**, 16(5), 11259–75. doi: 10.3390/ijms160511259.

Saenen, J.B.; et al.; Genetics of sudden cardiac death in the young. *Clin. Genet.* **2015**, 88(2), 101–13. doi: 10.1111/cge.12519.

Samarodnitsky, E.; et al.; Evaluation of hybridization capture versus amplicon-based methods for whole-exome sequencing. *Hum. Mutat.* **2015**, 36(9), 903–14. doi: 10.1002/humu.22825.

Saracini, C.; et al.; Polymorphisms of genes involved in extracellular matrix remodeling and abdominal aortic aneurysm. *J. Vasc. Surg.* **2012**, 55(1), 171–9. doi: 10.1016/j.jvs.2011.07.051.

Sarquella-Brugada, G.; et al.; Brugada syndrome: Clinical and genetic findings. *Genet. Med.* **2016**, 18(1), 3–12. doi: 10.1038/gim.2015.35.

Scheiper, S.; et al.; Sudden unexpected death in the young—Value of massive parallel sequencing in postmortem genetic analyses. *Forensic Sci. Int.* **2018**, 293, 70–6. doi: 10.1016/j.forsciint.2018.09.034.

Schwarz, J.; et al.; MutationTaster2: Mutation prediction for the deep-sequencing age. *Nat. Methods.* **2014**, 11(4), 361–2. doi:10.1038/nmeth.2890.

Semsarian, C. and Hamilton, R.M.; Key role of the molecular autopsy in sudden unexpected death. *Heart Rhythm.* **2012**, 9(1), 145–50. doi: 10.1016/j.hrthm.2011.07.034.

Semsarian, C. and Ingles, J.; Molecular autopsy in victims of inherited arrhythmias. *J. Arrhythm.* **2016**, 32(5), 359–65.

Semsarian, C.; Ingles, J. and Wilde, A.A.; Sudden cardiac death in the young: The molecular autopsy and a practical approach to surviving relatives. *Eur. Heart J.* **2015**, 36(21), 1290–6. doi: 10.1093/eurheartj/ehv063.

Skinner, J.R.; Duflou, J.A. and Semsarian, C.; Reducing sudden death in young people in Australia and New Zealand: The TRAGADY initiative. *Med. J. Aust.* **2008**, 189(10), 539–40.

Tan, H.L.; et al.; Sudden unexplained death: Heritability and diagnostic yield of cardiological and genetic examination in surviving relatives. *Circulation.* **2005**, 112(2), 207–13.

Tester, D.J.; et al.; Targeted mutational analysis of the RyR2-encoded cardiac ryanodine receptor in sudden unexplained death: A molecular autopsy of 49 medical examiner/coroner's cases. *Mayo Clin Proc.* **2004**, 79(11), 1380–4.

Tester, D.J. and Ackerman, J.; The role of molecular autopsy in unexplained sudden cardiac death. *Curr. Opin. Cardiol.* **2006**, 21(3), 166–72.

Thorvaldsdóttir, H.; Robinson, J.T. and Mesirov, J.P.; Integrative Genomics Viewer (IGV): High-performance genomics data visualization and exploration. *Brief Bioinform.* **2013**, 14(2), 178–92. doi:10.1093/bib/bbs017.

Voelkerding, K.V.; Dames, S. and Durtschi, J.D.; Next generation sequencing for clinical diagnostics-principles and application to targeted resequencing for hypertrophic cardio-myopathy: A paper from the 2009 William Beaumont Hospital Symposium on Molecular Pathology. *J. Mol. Diagn.* **2010**, 12(5), 539–51. doi:10.2353/jmoldx.2010.100043.

Wilde, A.A. and Behr, E.R.; Genetic testing for inherited cardiac disease. *Nat. Rev. Cardiol.* **2013**, 10(10), 571–83. doi: 10.1038/nrcardio.2013.108.

Wilson, K. D.; et al.; A rapid, high-quality, cost-effective, comprehensive and expandable targeted next-generation sequencing assay for inherited heart diseases novelty and significance. *Circ. Res.* **2015**, 117(7), 603–11. doi:10.1161/CIRCRESAHA.115.306723.

Winkel, B.G.; et al.; Nationwide study of sudden cardiac death in persons aged 1–35 years. *Eur. Heart J.* **2011**, 32(8), 983–90. doi: 10.1093/eurheartj/ehq428.

Zipes, D.P. and Wellens, H.J.; Sudden cardiac death. *Circulation.* **1998**, 98(21), 2334–51.

CHAPTER 13

Wildlife Forensics: DNA Analysis in Wildlife Forensic Investigations

RITA LORENZINI* and LUISA GAROFALO

Istituto Zooprofilattico Sperimentale delle Regioni Lazio e Toscana "M. Aleandri," Centro di Referenza Nazionale per la Medicina Forense Veterinaria, Viale Europa 30, 58100 Grosseto, Italy

Corresponding author. E-mail: rita.lorenzini@izslt.it

ABSTRACT

Wildlife forensics has only recently entered the forensic scenario, but is rapidly gaining importance and is increasingly being applied to caseworks, in compliance with the laws on the conservation, protection, and welfare of wildlife and to warrant animal rights. Crimes against animals are currently widespread worldwide, being a huge source of income for criminals when wildlife trade and poaching of exotic, rare, protected or threatened species are concerned. At small geographic scale, poaching and illegal harvest of wild animals can rage on endemic populations of high conservational value; thus significantly affecting local biodiversity. DNA analysis is now becoming an essential tool available to law-enforcement authorities, and is increasingly crucial for assigning the responsibility of crimes against animals. Typically, methods and procedures of wildlife DNA analysis are originally developed for animal genetic research and only subsequently are they transferred to forensic frameworks. As in human forensics, for caseworks where wildlife is involved, investigations start with the collection of evidence on the crime scene. Biological samples are then submitted to different molecular methodologies for DNA testing, depending on the queries posed by the law enforcement. In wildlife forensics, DNA analysis is mostly requested to identify: unknown species from parts of animals that have lost their identifying morphological features; gender, when animal crimes are sex-specific; single individuals for matching DNA profiles between seized carcasses and biological traces from poaching sites; population of origin when the species is protected in one area of its distribution and not in another; paternity/maternity and family relationships to ascertain whether captive-bred individuals are possessed legally or wild-caught animals have been unlawfully removed from their habitats. Operationally, PCR-based DNA amplification, sequencing, fragment analysis and single nucleotide polymorphisms analysis are currently the most popular techniques in wildlife forensic laboratories, even though new approaches like whole-genome sequencing through next-generation sequencing technology, are rapidly making their way. Standardization and validation of procedures, quality assurance, and biostatistical treatment of molecular data, following in the footsteps of human forensics, are playing an increasingly important role in wildlife DNA forensics, especially in the view of admissibility of forensic results as scientific evidence in court.

13.1   INTRODUCTION

Maybe not all people know that animal protection, respect, and welfare is a debated issue since a long time. *Saevitia in bruta est tirocinium crudelitatis in homines*[1]. That is what Socrates (Athens 469–399 BC) said at a trial, demanding a severe punishment for a guy who had blinded a swallow just for fun. He believed that anyone who showed cruel instincts toward the weaker creatures was potentially lacking in his capacity of coexistence and civil respect for own kind, that are basic requirements for being a good citizen. In Europe, until the middle of the last century, crimes against animals were prosecuted to protect humans and their properties rather than to warrant animal rights. Animals were not considered as sentient beings, the offence concerned public morals, and the law was intended to save man from the feeling of revulsion and indignation that he might perceive when faced with cruelty to other living beings (Regan, 1983).

Nowadays, there is a great deal of international and national laws that guarantee animal rights, intended as welfare of pets and farmed animals as well as conservation of wildlife (Harrison, 1964; Dawkins, 1980; Linacre and Tobe, 2013; LINK, http://nationallinkcoalition.org), and crimes against them are prosecuted all around the world. Nevertheless, cruelty to animals and the extensive exploitation of animal resources are still frequent and often highly profitable activities. Individuals illegally taking, trading, collecting, abusing

---

[1]Being cruel to animals trains for cruelty to people.

animals only rarely are convicted, while most of times they go unidentified and easily avoid prosecution. It is difficult to obtain evidence of their guilt, and generally, penalties are low and easily sustainable by many criminals. Furthermore, financial resources to implement and enforce forensic laboratories and investigative techniques are diverted to crimes involving humans that always take higher priority.

At the global level, wildlife trade and poaching of protected species has increased dramatically in recent years, being the third source of income after the drugs and arms trafficking (Linacre and Tobe, 2013). Even though the scale of profits is difficult to quantify exactly, different sources, including the Convention on International Trade in Endangered Species of Wild Fauna and Flora (CITES), estimated that the global wildlife trafficking is worth between 8 and 20 billion US dollars annually (Alacs et al., 2010; Rosen and Smith, 2010) and, still, much remains undetected. In Europe, over 12,000 seizures of illegal wildlife products were reported by the enforcement authorities between 2005 and 2009, whereas in 2011 the value of imports into the European Union of CITES-listed animals and their derivatives was estimated at 499 million Euros (http://www.traffic.org).

Wildlife poaching for international trade is a highly lucrative criminal activity involving transnational organized crime networks (Sellar, 2009) and is combated worldwide by the unceasing efforts of different law-enforcement authorities. Illicit trafficking is currently the greatest threat to several endangered species, second only to habitat destruction. Elephants, pangolins, whales, sturgeons, rhinos, sharks, tigers, bears, and reptiles, just to make some examples, are illegally harvested from the wild every year for the smuggling of ivory, scales, meat, caviar, horns, fins, traditional medicines, gallbladders, and snakeskin (Wasser et al., 2015; Mwale et al., 2017; Ewart et al., 2018). These products leave their source countries and reach the black markets in Asia, but also in Europe (European Parliament, 2016) and the Unites States. Birds, reptiles, exotic fishes, and insects, albeit less popular to the general public than mammals, are even more impacted by wildlife trade. They are smaller, more difficult to identify, so it is easier to make them cross the international borders and sell them (the few who survive the capture and travel) as pets or collector's items.

Wildlife trafficking has a devastating impact on global biodiversity. Yet, not only iconic species are seriously threatened but also nonflag species, those who elicit low emotional impact on the public opinion, can be driven to local extinction by poaching and illegal harvest. Abundant species are taken illegally in great numbers in many European countries (Lorenzini, 2005a;

Jobin et al., 2008; Dawnay et al., 2008, 2009; Socratous et al., 2009), making the list of populations at risk more and more crowded every year. Even though regarded as minor or less important crimes with respect to homicide or injures to humans, combating wildlife crimes has become highest priority for animal conservation all around the world, and must be tackled at all levels, from international to national and regional level. It is also at the local scale that a large number of unprotected or not endangered animals are illegally killed every day, poached directly with all possible means, from weapons to snares and traps, or indirectly, through, for example, poison baits (Rendo et al., 2011). In this case, the reasons behind such illegal killings are different from the (inter)national highly lucrative trafficking mentioned earlier and deal mainly with human–animal conflicts (e.g., predation on livestock by wolf or damage to crops by wild boar), popular beliefs or local sale of food. In most countries, this illicit activity occurs frequently even in sanctuaries, national parks, and reserves where wildlife, included game species, is strictly protected by law. The majority of these poached animals, for example wild boar, roe deer, red deer, mouflon, and also many birds, neither belong to iconic species nor are listed in the CITES Appendices, so that they escape any statistics.

Procedures in DNA forensics have been originally developed for human caseworks, and only recently are they being applied in investigations where the animals are involved as victims of crimes. In the past, animal DNA testing was employed in crime scenes where animals at best served as "evidence" or "silent witness" in the offences against humans or their property. Although still in its infancy, over the last decades, and following in the footsteps of human forensics, animal DNA forensics has grown by leaps and bounds in the development and application of molecular markers and analytical techniques. On the contrary, much remains to be done regarding quality assurance, standardization, and validation of procedures among wildlife forensics laboratories.

In this chapter we will outline the genetic markers and techniques most used in wildlife forensics, and the most frequent queries posed by during the investigations of crimes against animals. A brief *excursus* on methods for the statistical treatment of genetic data will also be provided.

13.2   COLLECTION OF BIOLOGICAL EVIDENCE AND DNA ISOLATION

Investigations in forensic caseworks, involving both humans and animals as victims, always start with the assessment of the crime scene or with a search at the suspect's quarters. This is a crucial step in the investigative procedures, because all evidence (exhibits and information) that are not collected, photographed, or noted at the scene will be lost, and valuable clues could be left behind. As with human forensics, the wildlife crime scene must be "frozen," appropriate protocols should be followed during the inspection, and any kind of contamination or mistake in collecting biological evidence must be avoided (Byrd and Sutton, 2012). Guidelines for collection and handling of evidence wildlife samples have been drawn up as recommendations by qualified scientific committees (the International Society for Forensic Genetics—ISFG Commission, the European Network of Forensic Science Institutes, and the Scientific Working Group for Wildlife Forensic Sciences; Linacre et al., 2011; Linacre and Tobe, 2013) to ensure that the same standards of human forensic investigations are maintained. For example, the guidelines emphasize that the chain of custody of each evidence item (from documentation during collection to the end of processing) be maintained to avoid tampering and ensure integrity.

Biological samples for molecular analysis should be preserved and kept at proper storage temperatures (refrigeration or freezing) to prevent DNA degradation. In order to avoid contaminations with exogenous DNA, it is also important to select a proper medium for withdrawing and packaging for shipping to the laboratory (e.g., wet samples should not be stored in plastic bags, nor blood stains should be removed from substrates directly on the crime scene without sterile equipment).

In the DNA laboratory, a major concern for wildlife forensics is the potential for contamination of evidence samples with nontarget animal DNA, whereas human DNA contamination is of less concern, unless the use of universal primers. An essential requirement for each and every molecular forensics laboratory is the physical separation in different working areas (each with dedicated equipment) of pre-PCR (DNA isolation, PCR mix set up) and post-PCR (handling, analysis of amplicons) activities, following a strict workflow of operations as recommended by the ENFSI (2010a). It is also good practice that trace samples (see later), which generally contain low DNA content, be processed before high quantity DNA samples, possibly in separate rooms and sessions.

In wildlife forensics, DNA is isolated from a variety of biological samples containing DNA in different quality and quantity. Hard tissues, like teeth, bones, tusks, claws, horns, feathers, bile crystals, scales, shells, and eggs usually yield DNA in low content but more preserved over time (Figure 13.1A). Soft and fresh tissues, like frozen meat, carcasses, or blood stains on weapons and dresses (Figure 13.1B–D), hair bulbs and salivary remains, yield more DNA, but it degrades more rapidly, because physical, chemical, and bacterial decomposition acts more effectively (Ogden et al., 2009). Good-quality DNA is rarely obtained from chemically or thermally treated tissues, such as tanned leather, furs, and clothing accessories made of fur (Figure 13.1E), highly processed food, products of the traditional medicine. In this case, alternative strategies for DNA extraction may be necessary (Garofalo et al., 2018; Pilli et al., 2014).

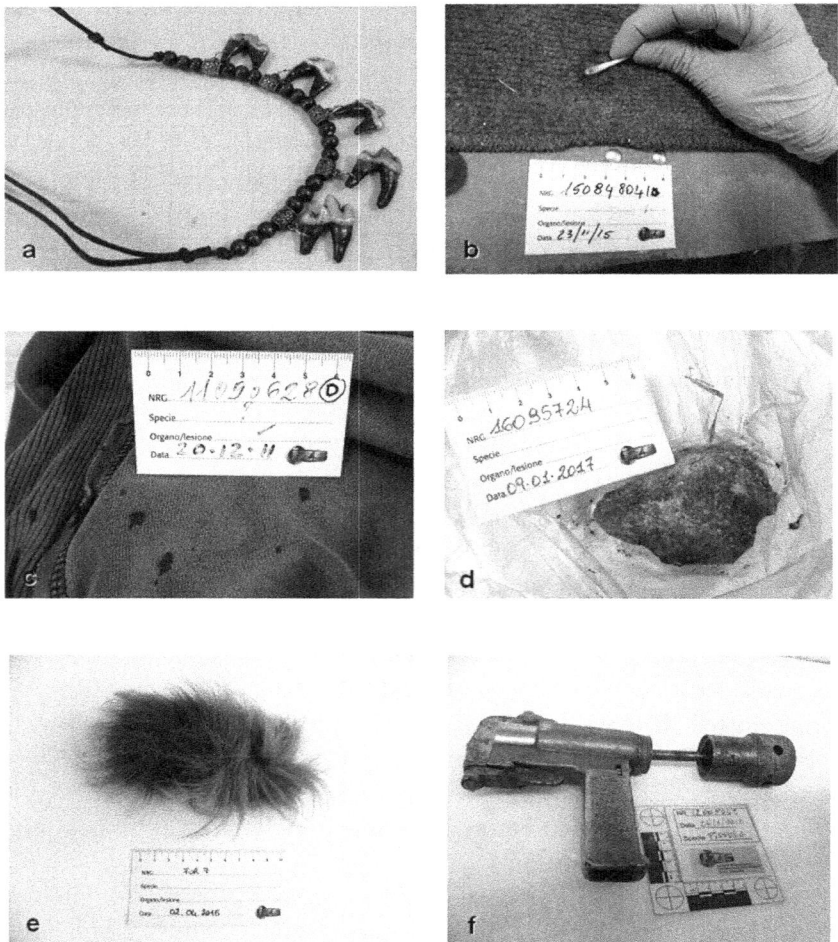

FIGURE 13.1   Evidence samples from wildlife forensic caseworks. (A) necklace made with dogs teeth; (B) bloodstain in the trunk of a car; (C) bloodstains on clothes; (D) blood on a stone collected on a poaching site; (E) dyed animal fur from an illegally traded species; (F) captive bolt pistol seized in an illegal abattoir.

Manual methods to isolate DNA usually consist in three main phases: lysis/digestion of proteins with proteinase K, DNA binding, and DNA elution. The lysis/digestion step allows for analytical adjustments according to the type of sample (longer time of digestion for hard tissues, addition of detergents and/or dithiothreitol for hairs and feathers, etc.). Silica-based columns and Chelex beads are widely used for DNA binding, while eluting buffers containing Tris and EDTA are commonly used for DNA storage. Traditional organic isolation according to chloroform/phenol/isopropanol-based procedures is also used. Howsoever, commercial kits and automated instruments are currently preferred by wildlife forensic labs to minimize manual handling and the risk of contamination for evidence samples. After isolation, the DNA is quantified. Accuracy in the estimate of DNA concentration is a critical factor, because it allows to load a proper DNA amount in downstream analyses. For example, DNA overloading in Short Tandem Repeats (STRs) amplifications produces off-scale peaks that make the interpretation of results challenging. Conversely, loading too little DNA can lead to low signals and loss of alleles (allele dropout), due to stochastic amplifications in a low copy number regime. DNA quantification is frequently carried out using spectrometry or fluorescence. However, alternative techniques are currently available that measure the total DNA amount with higher accuracy (real-time PCR) or quantify precisely low abundance DNA targets from known species in mixtures (droplet digital PCR, Floren et al., 2015).

13.3 IDENTIFICATION OF SPECIES

Identification of unknown species is a basic DNA test for a wildlife forensic laboratory and a common request from law-enforcement. This analysis is only occasionally applied in human forensics, where species other than human are rarely involved. On the contrary, species assignment can sometimes be crucial to provide scientific evidence that a crime against animals has been committed, such as the illegal trade of the wildlife species listed in the appendices of CITES. Species identification is also required in poaching cases, to verify which species has been illegally hunted for food, fun or for collecting. The species composition of meat in poisoned baits can be useful information to direct forensic investigations when wild or domestic animals are designedly poisoned.

Genetic identification of species becomes necessary when the questioned sample has lost its identifying morphological features. In wildlife forensics, biological matrices from evidence samples are often made up of small parts of an animal, and these can be further masked by processing methods, like cooking, tanning, and mixing. In these instances, the species can be identified only by DNA analysis. A method that is widely used to identify species is the amplification and sequencing of a variable DNA segment (either coding or neutral) showing conserved flanking sequences for binding of universal primers, followed by comparison of the obtained sequence with in-house known reference specimens and/or with data from public online databases. A general criterion for selecting a diagnostic segment of this kind is to focus on DNA regions which maximize interspecific genetic diversity, while minimizing intraspecific diversity. Some mitochondrial genes meet perfectly these criteria and are currently the most popular markers for the identification of species in animal forensics, unanimously approved by the scientific community (Bär et al., 2000; Carracedo et al., 2000; Wilson et al., 1995). The attractiveness of mitochondrial DNA (mtDNA) for species testing is basically due to its small genome, an almost exclusively uniparental mode of inheritance, the lack of recombination, and the presence of mitochondria in multiple copies per single cell, which, coupled with the protective role of mitochondrial membranes toward the DNA, increases the chance to amplify the target genes from scarce and highly degraded DNA of forensic samples. Furthermore, a mutation rate for mitochondrial genes that is from 10 to 25 higher than that of nuclear genes allows the genetic differentiation of phylogenetically close species (Pereira et al., 2010).

Cytochrome b (Cytb) is one of the most popular markers for species identification and phylogenetic reconstructions, both in research and forensics. First validation procedures in wildlife forensic testing have been focused just on this gene (e.g., Ahlers et al., 2017; Branicki et al., 2003; Hsieh et al., 2001; Parson et al., 2000). Encoding a structural protein of the electron transport chain, Cytb is under evolutionary constrains, and rates of nucleotide mutation roughly correspond to rates of speciation. Some regions, however, show high degree of sequence homology among species, which is used for binding of universal primers, and low intraspecific variation, that ensures a correct delimitation of most species. Cytochrome oxidase I (COI) gene is also widely used to identify species. It was first adopted for the Barcoding project, proposed in 2003 with the aim to create a databank of all extant species catalogued for the same DNA region (Dawnay et al., 2007; Hebert et al., 2003). However, the application of COI on routine testing proved effective for species identification within certain taxonomic groups (e.g., insects, fishes, birds, and some mammals; Dalton and Kotze, 2011; Wilson-Wilde et al., 2010; Kerr et al., 2007), but it revealed unsuitable when applied to particular mammal and bird species (Boonseub et al., 2009; Tobe et al., 2009). Furthermore, being the original COI amplicon nearly 650 bp in length, shorter segments can be amplified from degraded and fragmented DNA of many forensic samples (Ogden, 2011; Hajibabaei et al., 2006). Ribosomal genes (12S and 16S) have proven informative at the species level for some taxa (e.g., parrots and cockatoos, Coghlan et al., 2012a). In others, genes of the NADH dehydrogenase (ubiquinone) complex revealed a good amount of interspecific differences, like the subunit ND1 in the monitor lizards (genus *Varanus*; Welton et al., 2013), ND2 in birds (Boonseub et al., 2009), and ND5 in fishes (Birstein et al., 2000).

Interspecific sequence variation at coding genes, like COI and Cytb, however, may fail to distinguish closely related species (e.g., the critically endangered sturgeons of the genus *Acipenser*, Birstein et al., 2000), and the use of a second, highly variable DNA sequence, like the noncoding displacement loop (D-loop or control region), in these cases can help disentangling species similarity (Iyengar, 2014 and references herein; Gupta et al., 2011; Dalebout et al., 2008). For example, the D-loop has been used to distinguish the species within the Hierofalcon complex (the so-called desert falcons, genus *Falco*), where taxa display para- or polyphyletic phylogenetic patterns due to incomplete lineage sorting or hybridization of natural or anthropogenic origin (Wink et al., 2004). In any case, the use of two markers for species identification from degraded samples is a good practice that minimizes the possibility of false negatives caused by PCR failure: if one primer pair fails to bind for some reasons, a second chance of succeeding with the second pair will still stand. However, amplification of both markers adds confidence and reliability to diagnosis.

Recently, techniques other than amplification and sequencing have been used to identify species in wildlife forensics. Kitpipit et al. (2016) identified elephant species through a multiplex real-time PCR assay based on differences in melting temperatures at Cytb and ND5, demonstrating the accuracy, sensitivity, specificity, and absence of cross-reactivity with nontarget species of their protocol. Robust tests and thorough validations (see below) are actually good practices when species-specific primers are used in the melting - curve-based analyses, and especially when intraspecific polymorphism is high or melting temperatures in closely related species overlap (Berry and Sarre, 2007).

In wildlife forensics, identification of species in mixtures is a major challenge, mainly because universal primers are not applicable, due to overlapping sequences and uninterpretable results. In this instance, species-specific primers can be used to *detect* species (not to *identify*), which means to verify that some ex(sus)pected species are actually present in the sample (Tobe and Linacre, 2008). Currently, new approaches based on high-throughput sequencing, that is, Next-Generation Sequencing (NGS), are promising and represent a valuable resource to resolve mixtures in a variety of complex substrates. NGS technology has been successfully used, for example, to identify endangered mammal species in products of the traditional Chinese medicine (Coghlan et al., 2012b) and in illegal food mixtures (Tillmar et al., 2013).

In human forensics, standardization and validation of methods are essential for court admissibility of forensic results as scientific evidence. Conversely, in wildlife forensics, routine standardization of molecular protocols is not always possible, due to different factors, such as the variety of animal species, difference in the national legislations, legal protection of species according to geographical regions, etc. Furthermore, wildlife DNA forensic tests are performed with different techniques in different laboratories, according to equipment, expertise, and money availability. Despite these actual difficulties, some general requirements and indications for species identification have been suggested by the ISFG Commission (recommendations 1–5; Linacre et al., 2011), and by the ENFSI (2010b). For example, they strongly recommend that molecular markers be validated prior to application in evidence samples by including on reports information on marker specificity, sensitivity, reproducibility, robustness, amplification conditions, and data quality (Pereira et al., 2010; Ogden et al., 2009; Budowle et al., 2005; SWGDAM, 2003). Recently, interlaboratory comparison tests for species identification are also being organized by the working group for Animal Plant and Soil Traces of ENFSI, and by the US Fish and Wildlife Service Forensics Laboratory in Ashland, Oregon. Although extremely useful to test laboratories capabilities, international wildlife proficiency tests, however, are not easy to plan, due to both the huge number of animal species that can be involved and specific expertise of each laboratory (Johnson et al., 2014).

In order to identify the species from unknown evidence samples, the sequences obtained using universal primers are compared for matching to reference sequences from in-house known specimens (if available) and/or with the sequences registered in open repositories such as NCBI/EMBL/DDBJ (www.insdc.org) and BOLD (www.barcodinglife.com) databases. As a general rule, sequence homology with published online sequences is evaluated through some parameters, like the query coverage, E-value (a measure of the likelihood that a given sequence match occurs purely by chance) and bit score (a measure of sequence homology independent from query sequence and database size). The BLAST algorithm lists the similarity between the submitted sequence and the homologous sequences of the database in descending order of bit score (Branicki et al., 2003; Parson et al., 2000). Generally, 100% sequence homology is obtained with species that are well represented on the online database and show on average low intraspecific genetic variability. Conversely, if a genetically highly variable species is present with few sequences, the algorithm can return lower percentages of sequence identity. The species may also not be present in the database (a frequent situation when dealing with rare species; Dalton and Kotze, 2011). In this case, the next closest sequence anyway appears in the results screen (usually showing low similarity values), but obviously species assignment is highly doubtful and should be avoided. Although the access to free published resources is indeed an invaluable opportunity for wildlife forensic scientists, it should be emphasized, however, that data submitted to the online databases are unauthenticated, in the sense that everyone can lodge a sequence without external review, and errors or misidentifications are quite common (Dawnay et al., 2007). Some general rules have been suggested to obtain confident results when using online databases, regarding for example the minimum length of submitted sequences and statistical thresholds of similarity values (Linacre and Tobe, 2013). However, there are no strict guidelines that state what constitutes an exclusion or, conversely, what constitutes an inclusion. When the level of homology is questionable, much is based on the expertise of single wildlife forensic geneticist. This is one of the reasons why the comparison of unknown sequences with those from online repositories should be supported by building phylogenetic trees (or dendrograms) based on sequence alignments from reference species. Once the unknown sequence is included in the alignment, the tree shows the most likely source species as the species that is placed closer to the sample tested (Ogden et al., 2009). Several statistical methods can be used to generate phylogenetic trees, depending on the underlying theoretical approach: unweighted pair group with arithmetic mean, neighbor-joining, maximum parsimony, minimum evolution, Bayesian analysis, and haplotype networks are the most common. An in-depth and detailed treatment of methods to infer phylogenies (which is beyond the scope of this chapter) can be found in Felsenstein (2004) and Huson et al. (2010).

Despite their wide use, mtDNA-based assays, however, may exhibit some drawbacks that confuse the identification, like the co-amplification of nontarget nuclear copies (pseudogenes or Numts) when universal primers are used, heteroplasmy, incomplete lineage sorting and introgression. In such cases, robust standardizations and validations of tests, as well use of supplementary nuclear markers (the latter rarely used in wildlife so far), can overcome potential misidentifications (Alacs et al., 2010). Additionally, when evidence samples appear from very closely related taxa (e.g., subspecies), the use of mitochondrial genes as diagnostic markers may be ineffective, due to insufficient inter-taxa variability. For example, some wild species are genetically closely related to their domestic counterparts (e.g., wolf vs dog, mouflon vs sheep, wild boar vs pig), due to their evolutionary recent common ancestor, and usually mitochondrial variability within taxon is higher than that between taxa. In this case, the application of highly polymorphic nuclear loci, like STRs and single-nucleotide polymorphisms (SNPs), associated with population assignment tests are successfully used to distinguish close taxa both in wildlife forensics (Lorenzini et al., 2020) and research (see below).

13.4   SEXING

Molecular identification of gender in wildlife forensic samples is required when animal crimes are sex specific, that is, when a male can be legally harvested, but a female cannot (or vice versa), and morphologic integrity is compromised, or the species shows no sexual dimorphism. In North America, for example, hunting regulations allow differential harvest of male and female white-tailed deer (*Odocoileus virginianus,* according to regions and seasons (Lindsay and Belant, 2008). Sex-typing test is also requested for some CITES-listed species, for which one of the two sexes is particularly at risk if some of its body parts are much in demand, for example, on the black market (horns as trophies, testicles as aphrodisiacs, elephant tusks for ivory, etc.). Knowing the gender of a forensic animal sample can be a useful, additional information in complex investigations involving individual identification (Caniglia et al., 2010), reconstruction of parentage relationships (Abe et al., 2012) and hybridization mechanisms (Vilà et al., 2003).

Protocols for DNA-based identification of sex in wildlife forensic caseworks were originally developed for molecular ecology and conservation genetic studies of wild populations (Shaw et al., 2003; Bradley et al., 2001). For instance, methods for the analysis of noninvasive samples (feces, hairs, tooth, feathers) collected in the field completely meet the workflow standards used in processing highly degraded samples (good laboratory practices, amplification of short DNA fragments, protocols validation, etc.), and therefore they can be easily transferred to forensic frameworks.

Different markers on the Y and X chromosomes are currently used for sexing forensic samples of mammal species, like the amelogenin gene, sex-determining region and zinc-finger protein gene (ZFX/Y). These sequences are highly conserved across mammals and can be successfully amplified using the same primers in many species. Two different intronic sizes in the chromo-helicase-DNA binding protein gene on the Z and W sexual chromosomes are used for sexing avian samples (An et al., 2007). In mammals, males are heterogametic (XY), while females are homogametic (XX). In birds, conversely, females bear different sexual chromosomes (ZW), while males are homogametic (ZZ). DNA tests are usually based on the selective amplification of gender-specific fragments on the Y and W chromosomes (Morinha et al., 2012, 2013; Morin et al., 2005). Amplicons are visualized as bands on agarose gels after end-point PCRs, as peaks in fragment-based analysis, or as curves in real-time PCRs, depending on the method. Absence of the Y/W-specific bands is diagnostic for the homogametic sex, but it may also signify failure of amplification. To exclude this possibility, an additional marker, for example a nuclear biparental STR or a mtDNA gene, is included as positive control in the PCR reaction (Gupta et al., 2006; Lorenzini et al., 2004). Alternative methods can also be applied according to groups of taxa. In many felid species, sex-typing tests have been set up using concurrently the zinc-finger and amelogenin regions, that both contain deletions on the Y chromosome, but not in the homologous regions on the X chromosome (Pilgrim et al., 2005). Sex-linked markers can be included as single loci in species-specific STR panels for individual identification in canids (Sundqvist et al., 2001), but they can also be amplified as Y chromosome haplotypes containing multiple STR loci, as routinely used in our laboratory in forensic cases involving the wolf (*Canis lupus*).

13.5 INDIVIDUAL IDENTIFICATION

In human forensics, the DNA match between an individual profile and the biological traces left on the crime scene is the most frequent query to a forensic laboratory. In wildlife forensics, individual identification is often used in poaching caseworks where a carcass or body parts (e.g., meat, trophies, skins) from illegally killed animals are found at a suspect, and blood stains, hairs, excrements or other biological materials are retrieved on the crime scene, that is, the place where the animal/s has/have been poached. In these cases, the role of DNA match between the genetic profiles is crucial for assigning the responsibility of the offence.

As for humans, DNA profiling systems in animals are currently based on highly polymorphic STR loci. However, commercial kits have been developed and validated only for some domestic animals, such as dogs, cats, horses, and cows, but they are unavailable for wildlife species. Every wildlife forensic laboratory sets up and validates its own home-made STR amplification panel for individual identification in each of the species targeted by wildlife criminals (Dicks et al., 2017; Socratous et al., 2009). The types and numbers of STR markers are chosen based on their ease-to-interpret and level of polymorphism in the population source of the unknown sample. Variability at single selected loci should be high enough to provide sufficient assignment power for individual identification, and, importantly, a reference population database of allele frequencies should be set up on a reasonable number of representative individuals (Butler, 2005). Databases are used to estimate the genetic parameters for population structure and to verify that loci from a forensic STR panel are either on different chromosomes or not genetically tightly linked (linkage disequilibrium), so that they are inherited independently. In other words, population data are essential to derive the relevant genetic parameters required to assess the strength of the DNA evidence through a proper statistical approach (Weir, 2012).

Unfortunately, population genetic data are scarce for most wildlife species, or they even do not exist. The reason is that many wild animals are rare, endangered, highly protected, or simply elusive; therefore, collecting samples for population genetic data can be difficult or even impossible in practice. Furthermore, it is noteworthy that such databases are relative to one single population and may not be fit to other populations of the same species, if their genetic structures are different. Indeed, the lack of population genetic data is a major challenge for wildlife forensic scientists.

An additional difficulty in the application of STRs in wildlife forensics is the use of dinucleotide repeats, instead of tetranucleotide repeats, as routinely employed in human forensics. Loci with two base repeats are not recommended in human as well as in wildlife forensic genetics (Linacre et al., 2011), because they are highly prone to the amplification of stutter bands, broken repeats, and unbalanced alleles in heterozygotes, which makes their interpretation and standardization difficult. Dinucleotide loci, however, can be the only STRs available in the literature for a particular wild species (Andreassen et al., 2012; Dicks et al., 2017). Methods to isolate species-specific STR markers, either di- or tetranucleotides, are complex, requiring expertise, time, and funding, so that when dealing with wild species, STRs specific to the taxon of interest may not be available, or may their isolation be unfeasible to a forensic wildlife laboratory. Consequently, it is often necessary to use markers that were previously isolated from other species (e.g., Lorenzini, 2005b), often from domestic animals, either pets or livestock. This can lead to levels of genetic variability that are lower than those observed in the source species, and to the presence of null or false alleles, due to mutations or mismatches in the binding sites of primers. The repeatability of forensic results must therefore be monitored closely. Finally, following the international standards and guidelines of the SWGWILD (2012), STR alleles should be sequenced and allelic ladders be generated to designate accurately alleles from questioned samples. Validation studies on forensic applications of STRs in wild species are also recommended (Linacre et al., 2011), but this is done only rarely (Dicks et al., 2017). Despite these drawbacks, examples of population databases used in wildlife forensics do exist and, indeed, they are increasingly growing. Applications in caseworks can be found that regard the mouflon (*Ovis aries musimon*; Guerrini et al., 2015; Lorenzini et al., 2011), wild boar (*Sus scrofa*; Lorenzini et al., 2005a), wolf (*Canis lupus*; Caniglia et al., 2010), badger (*Meles meles*; Dawnay et al., 2008), and red deer (*Cervus elaphus*; Frantz et al., 2006).

Individual identification can be also assessed through the analysis of SNPs. Their use, however, is currently very limited in wild animals (Kitpipit et al., 2012), because they are difficult to isolate and classify, and a large number is required to achieve a sufficient level of discriminatory and statistical power. SNP isolation and validation in nonmodel species (not to mention the application in wildlife DNA forensics) is still an area of novel research (Ogden, 2011; Garvin et al., 2010).

As in human forensic investigations, the interpretation of matching DNA profiles needs a statistical support to evaluate the weight-of-evidence. Foremost, it is necessary to know how common the DNA profile in question is within the population: the frequency of the genetic profile is estimated by the random match probability (RMP), which is defined as the probability that an individual randomly chosen from the population shows that profile, or, in other words, the probability that two individuals randomly chosen from the population show the same genotype by chance. RMP calculation can accommodate for the existence of subpopulations, rare alleles, inbreeding, and relatedness through adjustments that depend on the population structure. In the evaluation of DNA evidence according to the frequentist approach, the RMP value is used to provide indication on how many individuals in the population might be expected to share by chance the same genetic profile. A more logic way to present the information about the DNA profile frequency and to provide significance of two matching profiles is the likelihood approach. Likelihood ratios (LRs) are odds values that compare probabilities of the profiles under two competing hypotheses that are generally the following: (1) the two genetic profiles match because they belong to the same animal, and (2) the two genetic profiles match by chance, and belong to different animals. The profile frequency in terms of RMP is used to derive LRs as 1/RMP. Large LR values indicate stronger evidence for hypothesis 1 than for hypothesis 2 and indicate how many times more likely it is that the genetic profile (e.g., obtained from a trace on the poaching site) matches that particular animal (a carcass found at a suspect), compared to coming from any other unrelated animal in the population. Finally, a fully Bayesian approach that includes nongenetic or nonscientific evidence (e.g., testimony of an eyewitness, cause of death for the animal, or circumstantial evidence) in the context of a logical framework can also be used including prior odds in the calculation of LRs. This method, however, has not currently gained widespread usage, neither in human nor in wildlife forensics (Linacre and Tobe, 2013). For an in-depth analysis of the statistical methods applied to forensic genetic data (Linacre and Tobe, 2013; Balding, 2005; Butler, 2005; Buckleton et al., 2004; Evett and Weir, 1998).

Operationally, there are many free open sources that assist wildlife scientists in the statistical treatment of genetic data. We point out the most common: GENEPOP (Rousset, 2008), GDA (Lewis and Zaykin, 2001), Arlequin (Excoffier and Lischer, 2010), API-Calc (Ayres and Overall, 2004), Genetix (Belkhir et al., 2004), and Gimlet (Valière, 2002).

13.6   POPULATION OF ORIGIN

When a species is protected across its whole range, knowing the geographic provenance of a specimen illegally harvested or traded is not essential, because in any case it is a crime. It becomes of paramount importance if the species is protected in one area and not in another or if there are geographical populations that are under protection as evolutionary significant units (ESUs *sensu* Moritz, see Crandall et al., 2000 and references therein), even in the absence of a recognized taxonomic status (Zachos et al., 2014). In this case, the identification of species may not be sufficient to assess that a crime has been committed, rather it is crucial to determine where that particular seized sample comes from and what is its source population.

The assignment of a wild animal to a given population is similar to tracing the genetic ancestry in human identification, and population membership can be assessed, provided that the candidate populations show different, detectable genetic structures. Wild species are commonly subdivided into local populations dwelling in different areas of the distribution that can be genetically highly divergent, due to prolonged geographical isolation, bottlenecks, and random genetic drift (Frankham et al., 2004). Such discrete differences can be detected at the mtDNA level, often as different population frequencies of haplotypes in the Cytb gene and D-loop. Subsequently, the distribution of mitochondrial lineages is analyzed with classical clustering methods for phylogeny reconstructions (see Section 13.3 in this chapter) and the source population for a questioned sample can be determined with high confidence (Kitpipit et al., 2016; Jobin et al., 2008).

When geographic populations bear same genetic structures at the mitochondrial genes, they can instead show different allele frequencies at STR loci, and private alleles may also be present. The analysis of a panel of specie-specific STRs with enough resolution is used in this case as the molecular method of choice for a statistically based distinction of populations. It has been suggested (Manel et al., 2005, 2002) from both empirical and simulated data sets that high statistical certainty (99.9%) in the assignment of individuals can be achieved if two populations are highly differentiated (F_{ST} values in the range of 0.15–0.20) when 10 STR loci with heterozygosity $H >$ 0.60 are used and 30–50 individuals per population are collected to construct the databases. Once population data are obtained from multiple geographic areas and the differences are defined, proper statistical analyses are used to provide the likelihood of an individual originating from a given population or geographic area (see below). As mentioned earlier in this chapter regarding the DNA match between genetic profiles, even for population membership appropriate databases (in terms of both type/number of loci and number of reference individuals) are essential to compare putative source populations and draw reliable conclusions as to the assignment of unknown samples (Ogden and Linacre, 2015). Unfortunately, online or public repositories of data are not available for wild populations, and wildlife forensic scientists can only relay on their in-house databases. Scientific journals, however, are increasingly requiring authors to make their genotype data freely available at the moment of publication, and this will be of great benefit for the scientific wildlife forensic community.

The source population (i.e., the original reproductive population) of an unknown individual is commonly identified through Bayesian assignment tests that use STR alleles or, less frequently, SNP panels. Widely applied in genetics and ecology of wild populations, this approach is increasingly being used in wildlife forensic contexts, where, however, a consensus statistical approach for forensic assignment of the geographic origin has yet to be proposed by the insiders. In simple terms, the Bayesian tests compare the alleles of the questioned DNA profile with the allele frequencies in the candidate populations, assigning the individual to the population from which it most likely came from. One of the most popular software programs used for population assignment is STRUCTURE (Falush et al., 2003; Pritchard et al., 2000), a model-based clustering algorithm that uses multilocus genotypes to identify clusters of genetically similar individuals without assuming a particular mutation process. The software infers a number of theoretical panmictic populations from the estimated posterior likelihood of the data and derives the average proportional membership (q) for each population. Simulations based on real data are used to set a q-threshold for the correct assignment of individuals to their own population, even in case of genotypes with admixed ancestry (Lorenzini et al., 2011, 2013). Under this approach, the true source population is assumed to be sampled, and questioned genetic profiles will always be assigned, even when data from the real population of origin are absent. Other programs (like GeneClass2, Piry et al., 2004) are available that can accommodate for the possibility that none of the candidate populations is the source of the unknown genotype, but their assignment power seems lower (Manel et al., 2002). Likelihood ratios can also be employed as an alternative method for population assignment, although they remain mostly used in DNA matches. LRs provide the probability of observing a genetic profile under two competing hypotheses, through a quantitative estimate. The advantages consist in the direct assessment of an alternative source population, instead of the simple identification of the most probable population, and in the statistic q-threshold that no longer needs to be established. The disadvantage lies in the errors estimated from the distribution of the individual likelihoods that can be very large if the candidate populations show high genetic variability (Ogden and Linacre, 2015).

In wildlife forensics, the assignment of single individuals to their geographic areas is not common due to the difficulty of collecting large reference databases for each candidate population. It has been applied in tracking the areas of origin for ivory (Wasser et al., 2015; 2004). Using sophisticated statistical methods and an extensive population database based on allele frequencies from hundreds elephants across the entire African range, researchers successfully assigned tons of ivory tusks from the largest seizure ever made to their (sub)populations or single locations (Wasser et al., 2007). Population assignment was also applied in forensic caseworks involving poaching of mouflon (*Ovis aries musimon*) from the islands of Sardinia (Lorenzini et al., 2011) and Cyprus (Guerrini et al., 2015), and the illegal trade of Mediterranean land tortoise (*Testudo hermanni hermanni*; Biello et al., 2018), American gopher tortoise (*Gopherus polyphemus;* Schwartz and Karl, 2008), Indian leopard (*Panthera pardus*; Mondol et al., 2014), and Hyacinth macaws (*Anodorhynchus hyacinthinus*; Presti et al., 2015).

The possibility exists that neutral nuclear markers (like STRs) are not able to discriminate between genetically very closely related populations, when they show weak genetic structure. In this case, markers under selection can be used to reach higher geographic resolution. Nielsen et al. (2012) provided evidence for the association of some SNP markers with functional genes under selective pressure in cod (*Gadus morhua*), herring (*Clupea harengus*), sole (*Solea solea*), and hake (*Merluccius merluccius*). They used differences in allele frequencies at selected SNPs to identify the geographic origin of fish catches for forensic purposes, both illegal fishing and mislabeling in food frauds. Although being an alluring opportunity, the application of genome-wide approaches to wildlife forensics is still at its very early stage and, currently, it is used to unveil commercial frauds rather than to assess wildlife crimes.

13.7   PARENTAGE

Establishing family relationships among individuals, either first or next-degree kinship, is frequently requested to human forensics laboratories. In wildlife forensics, relatedness among animals is mostly assessed to distinguish between wild-caught and captive-bred individuals (Dawnay et al., 2009). Many wild species are protected worldwide and their possession or sale is never legal, whereas individuals from other species can be kept or sold only if they are born in captivity. However, traffickers often harvest animals from the wild and trade them as captive reared, showing off false documentation. During these operations, many animals die for capture, while others do not survive stressful travels. Wildlife criminals find it much simpler and cheaper to catch animals in the wild than to rear them according to current laws. On the other hand, this is the only viable way for them, if the species does not reproduce in captivity, which holds true particularly for exotic birds and large mammals. In this case, paternity/maternity DNA test and kinship analysis is an effective method to unmask this illegal activity, as described in the forthcoming caseworks.

High-resolution paternity testing was conducted in the Australian endemic black-cockatoos (*Calyptorhynchus* spp.): forensic scientists (White et al., 2012) managed to matched a red-tailed black-cockatoo nestling to a tree hollow from which it was poached through the use of DNA from eggshell recovered from the nest. In order to control the trade of endemic species in South Africa, Coetzer et al. (2017) successfully applied a 16 locus STR panel for parentage analyses in the Cape parrot (*Poicephalus robustus*) to determine if birds had been bred in captivity, and so could be legally traded, or if they had been illegally removed from the wild. Feline STR markers were used for parentage assessment in a poaching case involving the African lion (*Panthera leo*) to trace the pride of origin from seized lion parts (Miller et al., 2014). Although not currently endangered, the lion in Africa is seriously threatened with extinction in the near future, due to pitiless poaching for its bones to supply a growing market in Asia. Reptile species, especially if rare, are also greatly affected by illegal traffic because they are highly prized as pets (TRAFFIC, http://www.traffic.org). Currently, the issue of wild-caught reptiles being mis-declared as captive-bred is a major challenge to wildlife forensics laboratories. Paternity testing was used to investigate a robbery case involving the Greek tortoise (*Testudo graeca*, Mucci et al., 2014). Six individuals were allegedly stolen from a private breeder and offered for sale on the web by a suspected thief. In order to reconstruct their pedigree, paternity test and kinship analysis were performed using a panel of 14 STR loci. Eventually, the captive origin of the stolen tortoises, as declared by the owner, was clearly ascertained and the theft was proven.

Genetic variants at STR loci are inherited from one generation to the next following the rules of Mendelian segregation: all the alleles present in an individual's profile must be also present in its true parents. Consequently, establishing parent–offspring relationships can be done through the method of parental exclusion, in the sense that if one or more STR loci show inconsistency in the inheritance of alleles between parent and offspring, then the parentage can be excluded. In this case, reference population databases are not essential. If, however, there is compatibility between the profiles, or, in other words, if the putative parent cannot be excluded as being the true parent of an offspring, then statistical significance of nonexclusion should be provided through the use of population genetic data. Just like in human forensics, likelihood ratios, LRs, are usually applied to provide the significance of nonexclusion in terms of paternity index or probability of paternity. In both cases, the two alternative hypotheses being compared are as follow: (1) the putative father is the true father, and (2) the true father is another animal, that is, the two genetic profiles are compatible only by chance. Paternity index indicates how many times is more likely if the tested individual is the true father of an offspring than if the true father is another individual taken at random from the population. LR takes high values when hypothesis 1 is favored. This statement, however, is not intuitive and can be difficult to interpret by nonscientists. Often, LR values are more accessibly presented as probability of paternity using a Bayesian formula according to Essen-Möller (Balding, 2005; Butler, 2005; Evett and Weir, 1998), and quoting it as percentage of paternity. In contrast to human forensics, where a value greater than 99.7% (Gjertson et al., 2007) indicates proven paternity, in wildlife forensics this threshold is not formally established.

In parentage testing, discrepancy occurring at many loci most probably means the exclusion of paternity or maternity. However, a single or few inconsistencies may also occur, which can be due to mutations rather than to false parentage. In order to account for such occurrence, mutation rate should be known per each locus per generation in the presence of detailed multigenerational pedigrees (Städele and Vigilant, 2016), following the guidelines that the ISFG highly recommends for human forensics. It should be said, however, that carrying out family studies in wild animal genetics to derive mutation rates at STR loci goes widely beyond the possibilities of any forensic laboratory.

In order to determine whether an animal is of wild or captive origin, it may be necessary to know familial relationships beyond the parent-offspring parentage. Molecular-based reconstructions of pedigrees are sometimes used in the field of conservation, behavior, and evolution of wild species (*e.g.,* Lorenzini et al., 2004), but rarely in wildlife forensics, mainly because large amount of data (in terms of both reference population size and number/informativeness of STR loci) are essential to apply kinship statistical methods other than parent–offspring relationships (Jones et al., 2010).

A good number of user-friendly, powerful genetic software for paternity testing and kinship analysis are freely available on the web (see Jones et al., 2010 for a review). Some of them follow the likelihood ratio approach and allow for genotyping errors, mutations, null alleles, and the appraisal of a set of candidate parents. CERVUS (Marshal et al., 1998), KINGROUP (Konovalov et al., 2004), ML-relate (Kalinowski et al., 2006), Colony (Jones and Wang, 2010), Familias (Egeland et al., 2000), EasyDNA (Fung, 2003) are the most used.

The analysis of STR loci is currently (and probably will still be in the near future) the dominant approach for parentage and kinship testing in wild animal populations. However, use of large-scale data from SNP arrays or whole-genome sequencing (using even low-quality DNA from forensic and noninvasive samples) is potentially the future direction for wildlife forensics, especially when pedigree reconstructions need to resolve accurately the relationships of distantly related dyads (Snyder-Mackler et al., 2016).

13.8 CONCLUDING REMARKS

The interest in animal conservation, protection, and welfare is currently shared at the global level, and the number of laws that guarantee animal rights is increasingly growing. Wildlife forensic science, although being still in its infancy, opens many opportunities to assist law enforcement in criminal investigations. Animal DNA analysis, in particular, can be crucial in forensic caseworks where molecular identification of species, individual, gender, or source population is required. Genetic data from a huge amount of animal species and the most recent molecular techniques have been borrowed by research and successfully applied to animal forensics. In the last decades, hundreds of wildlife forensic caseworks were passed through the scrutiny of molecular tools, allowing the ascertainment of numerous crimes. This demonstrates the great value of animal DNA forensics to combat wildlife crime by prosecuting and, at the same time, deterring potential animal criminals. Wildlife forensic procedures are currently available at great numbers for the scientific community through papers and data submitted to free online databases. Much, however, still remains to be done regarding the achievement of highest standards of quality assurance, standardization, and validation of procedures among wildlife forensics laboratories, contrary to what is a well-established practice in human forensics. However, the efforts that forensic DNA scientists are making in this regard will certainly be an invaluable added value for the conservation of animal species and improvement of investigations of crimes against wildlife.

KEYWORDS

- wildlife crimes
- animal DNA analysis
- molecular markers
- endangered species
- poaching
- illegal animal trading

REFERENCES

Abe, H.; Hayano, A.; and Inoue-Murayama, M.; Forensic species identification of large macaws using DNA barcodes and microsatellite profiles. *Mol. Biol. Rep.* **2012**, *39*(1), 693–699.

Ahlers, N; ForCyt DNA database of wildlife species. *Forensic Sci. Int. Genet. Suppl. Ser.* **2017**, *6*, e466–e468.

Alacs, E.; et al.; DNA detective: A review of molecular approaches to wildlife forensics. *Forensic Sci. Med. Pathol.* **2010**, *6*, 180–194.

An, J.; et al.; A molecular genetic approach for species identification of mammals and sex determination of birds in a forensic case of poaching from South Korea. *Forensic Sci. Int.* **2007**, *167*, 59–61.

Andreassen, R.; et al.; A forensic DNA profiling system for Northern European brown bears (*Ursus arctos*). *Forensic Sci. Int. Genet.* **2012**, *6*, 798–809.

Ayres, K.L.; and Overall, A.D.J.; API-Calc 1.0: A computer program for calculating the average probability of identity allowing for substructure, inbreeding and the presence of close relatives. *Mol. Ecol. Notes* **2004**, *4*, 315–318.

Balding, D.J.; *Weight-of-evidence for forensic DNA profiles*, John Wiley & Sons, United Kingdom, **2005**.

Bär, W.; et al.; DNA Commission of the International Society for Forensic Genetics: Guidelines for mitochondrial DNA typing. *Int. J. Legal Med.* **2000**, *113*(4), 193–196.

Belkhir, K.; et al.; 1996–2004 GENETIX 4.05, logiciel sous Windows TM pour la génétique des populations. Laboratoire Génome, Populations, Interactions, CNRS UMR 5171, Université de Montpellier II, Montpellier (France), **2004**.

Berry, O.; and Sarre, S.D.; Gel-free species identification using melt-curve analysis. *Mol. Ecol. Notes* **2007**, *7*, 1–4.

Biello, R.; Who's who in the western Hermann's tortoise conservation: a STR toolkit and reference database for wildlife forensic genetic analyses. *BioRxiv* **2018**, 484030.

Birstein, V.J.; Doukakis, P.; and DeSalle, R.; Polyphyly of mtDNA lineages in the Russian sturgeon, *Acipenser gueldenstaedtii*: Forensic and evolutionary implications. *Conserv. Genet.* **2000**, *1*(1), 81–88.

Boonseub, B.; Tobe, S.S.; and Linacre, A.M.T.; The use of mitochondrial DNA genes to identify closely related avian species. *Forensic Sci. Int. Genet. Suppl. Ser.* **2009**, *2*, 275–277.

Bradley, B.J.; Chambers, K.E.; and Vigilant, L.; Accurate DNA-based sex identification of apes using non-invasive samples. *Conserv. Genet.* **2001**, *2*, 179–181.

Branicki, W.; Kupiec, T.; and Pawlowski, R.; Validation of cytochrome b sequence analysis as a method of species identification. *J. Forensic Sci.* **2003**, *48*(1), 1–5.

Buckleton, J.S.; Triggs, C.M.; and Walsh, S.J.; *Forensic DNA evidence interpretation*, CRC Press, London, **2004**.

Budowle, B; et al.; Recommendations for animal DNA forensic and identity testing. *Int. J. Legal Med.* **2005**, *119*: 295–302.

Butler, J.M.; *Forensic DNA typing: Biology, technology, and genetics of STR Markers*. Elsevier Academic Press, London, **2005**.

Byrd, J.H.; and Sutton, L.K.; Defining a crime scene and physical evidence collection. In: *Wildlife forensics: Methods and applications*; Huffman, J.E. and Wallace, J.R., Eds.; John Wiley & Sons, United Kingdom, 51, **2012**.

Caniglia, R.; et al.; Forensic DNA against wildlife poaching: Identification of a serial wolf killing in Italy. *Forensic Sci. Int. Genet.* **2010**, *4*(5), 334–338.

Carracedo, A.; et al.; DNA commission of the international society for forensic genetics, guidelines for mitochondrial DNA typing. *Forensic Sci. Int.* **2000**, *110*, 79–85.

Coetzer, W.G.; et al.; Testing of microsatellite multiplexes for individual identification of Cape Parrots (*Poicephalus robustus*): Paternity testing and monitoring trade. *PeerJ* **2017**, *5*, e2900.

Coghlan, M.L.; et al.; Egg forensics: An appraisal of DNA sequencing to assist in species identification of illegally smuggled eggs. *Forensic Sci. Int. Genet.* **2012a**, *6*(2), 268–273.

Coghlan, M.L.; et al.; Deep sequencing of plant and animal DNA contained within Traditional Chinese Medicines reveals legality issues and health safety concerns. *PLoS Genet.* **2012b**, *8*(4), e1002657.

Crandall, K.A.; et al.; Considering evolutionary processes in conservation biology. *Trends Ecol. Evol.* **2000**, *15*, 290–295.

Dalebout, M.L.; et al.; DNA identification and the impact of illegal, unregulated, and unreported (IUU) fishing on rare whales in Micronesian waters. *Micronesica* **2008**, *40*(1/2), 139–147.

Dalton, D.L.; and Kotze, A; DNA barcoding as a tool for species identification in three forensic wildlife cases in South Africa. *Forensic Sci. Int.* **2011**, *207*, e51–e54.

Dawkins, M.S.; *Animal suffering: The science of animal welfare*. Chapman & Hall, London, **1980**.

Dawnay, N.; et al.; Validation of the barcoding gene COI for use in forensic genetic species identification. *Forensic Sci. Int.* **2007**, *173*(1), 1–6.

Dawnay, N.; et al.; A forensic STR profiling system for the Eurasian badger: A framework for developing profiling systems for wildlife species. *Forensic Sci. Int. Genet.* **2008**, *2*, 47–53.

Dawnay, N.; et al.; Genetic data from 28 STR loci for forensic individual identification and parentage analyses in six bird of prey species. *Forensic Sci. Int.* **2009**, *3*(2), e63–e69.

Dicks, K.L.; et al.; Validation studies on dinucleotide STRs for forensic identification of black rhinoceros *Diceros bicornis*. *Forensic Sci. Int. Genet.* **2017**, e25–e27.

Egeland, T.; et al.; Beyond traditional paternity and identification cases. Selecting the most probable pedigree. *Forensic Sci. Int.* **2000**, *110*(1), 47–59.

ENFSI, Contamination prevention guidelines. **2010a**. http://enfsi.eu/wp-content/uploads/2016/09/dna_contamination_prevention_guidelines_for_the_file_contamantion_prevention_final_-_v2010_0.pdf

ENFSI (*European Network of Forensic Science Institutes*), Recommended minimum criteria for the validation of various aspects of the DNA profiling process. **2010b**. http://enfsi.eu/wp-content/uploads/2016/09/minimum_validation_guidelines_in_dna_profiling_-_v2010_0.pdf

European Parliament. **2016**. http://ec.europa.eu/environment/cites/pdf/WAP_EN_WEB.PDF

Evett, I.; and Weir, B.S.; *Interpreting DNA evidence: Statistical genetics for forensic scientists*; Sinauer Associates, Sunderland, MA, **1998**.

Ewart, K.M.; et al.; An internationally standardized species identification test for use on suspected seized rhinoceros horn in the illegal wildlife trade. *Forensic Sci. Int. Genet.*, **2018**, *32*, 33–39.

Excoffier, L.; and Lischer, H.E.L.; Arlequin suite ver 3.5: A new series of programs to perform population genetics analyses under Linux and Windows. *Mol. Ecol. Res.* **2010**, *10*, 564–567.

Falush, D.; Stephens, M.; and Pritchard, J.K.; Inference of population structure using multilocus genotype data: linked loci and correlated allele frequencies. *Genetics* **2003**, *164*, 1567–1587.

Felsenstein, J.; *Inferring phylogenies*. Sinauer Associates, Sunderland, MA, **2004**.

Floren, C.; et al.; Species identification and quantification in meat and meat products using droplet digital PCR (ddPCR). *Food Chem.* **2015**, *173*, 1054–1058.

Frankham, R.; Ballou, J.D.; and Briscoe, D.A.; *A primer of conservation genetics*. Cambridge University Press, Cambridge, UK, **2004**.

Frantz, A.C.; et al.; Genetic structure and assignment tests demonstrate illegal translocation of red deer (*Cervus elaphus*) into a continuous population. *Mol. Ecol.* **2006**, *15*, 3191–3203.

Fung, W.K.; User-friendly programs for easy calculations in paternity testing and kinship determinations. *Forensic Sci. Int.* **2003**, *136*, 22–34.

Garofalo, L.; et al.; Hindering the illegal trade in dog and cat furs through a DNA-based protocol for species identification. *PeerJ* **2018**, *6*, e4902.

Garvin, M.R.; Saitoh, K.; and Gharrett, A.J.; Application of single nucleotide polymorphisms to non-model species: A technical review. *Mol. Ecol. Res.* **2010**, *10*, 915–934.

Gjertson, D.W.; et al.; ISFG: Recommendations on biostatistics in paternity testing. *Forensic Sci. Int. Genet.* **2007**, *1*(3), 223–231.

Guerrini, M.; et al.; Molecular DNA identity of the mouflon of Cyprus (*Ovis orientalis ophion*, Bovidae): Near Eastern origin and divergence from Western Mediterranean conspecific populations. *Syst. Biodivers.* **2015**, *13*(5), 472–483.

Gupta, S.K.; Thangaraj, K.; and Singh, L.; A simple and inexpensive molecular method for sexing and identification of the forensic samples of elephant origin. *J. Forensic Sci.* **2006**, *51*(4): 805–807.

Gupta, S.K.; Thangaraj, K.; and Singh, L.; Case report. Identification of the source of ivory idol by DNA analysis. *J. Forensic Sci.* **2011**, *56*(5), 1343–1345.

Hajibabaei, M.; et al.; A minimalist barcode can identify a specimen whose DNA is degraded. *Mol. Ecol. Res.* **2006**, *6*(4), 959–964.

Harrison, R.; *Animal machines: The new factory farming industry.* Vincent Stuart, London, **1964**.

Hebert, P.D.; Ratnasingham, S.; and de Waard, J.R.; Barcoding animal life: Cytochrome c oxidase subunit 1 divergences among closely related species. *Proc. R. Soc. Lond. Ser. B. Biol. Sci.* **2003**, *270*(Suppl. 1), S96–S99.

Hsieh, H.M.; et al.; Cytochrome b gene for species identification of the conservation animals. *Forensic Sci. Int.* **2001**, *122*(1), 7–18.

Huson, D. H.; et al; Phylogenetic networks. Concepts, algorithms and applications. Cambridge University Press, Cambridge, UK. **2010**.

Iyengar, A.; Forensic DNA analysis for animal protection and biodiversity conservation: A review. *J. Nat. Conserv.* **2014**, *22*, 195–205.

Jobin, R.M.; Patterson, D.; and Zhang, Y.; DNA typing in populations of mule deer for forensic use in the Province of Alberta. *Forensic Sci. Int.* **2008**, *2*, 190–197.

Johnson, R.; Wilson-Wilde, L.; and Linacre, A.; Current and future directions of DNA in wildlife forensic science. *Forensic Sci. Int. Genet.* **2014**, *10*, 1–11.

Jones, O.R.; and Wang, J.; COLONY: A program for parentage and sibship inference from multilocus genotype data. *Mol. Ecol. Res.* **2010**, *10*, 551–555.

Jones, A.G.; et al.; A practical guide to methods of parentage analysis. *Mol. Ecol. Res.* **2010**, *10*, 6–30.

Kalinowski, S.T.; Wagner, A.P.; and Taper, M.L.; ML-RELATE: A computer program for maximum likelihood estimation of relatedness and relationship. *Mol. Ecol. Notes* **2006**, *6*, 576–579.

Kerr, K.C.; et al.; Comprehensive DNA barcode coverage of North American birds. *Mol. Ecol. Res.* **2007**, *7*(4), 535–543.

Kitpipit, T.; et al.; The development and validation of a single SNaPshot multiplex for tiger species and subspecies identification—Implications for forensic purposes. *Forensic Sci. Int. Genet.* **2012**, *6*(2), 250–257.

Kitpipit, T.; et al.; A novel real time PCR assay using melt curve analysis for ivory identification. *Forensic Sci. Int.* **2016**, *267*, 210–217.

Konovalov, D.A.; Manning, C.; and Henshaw, M.T.; KINGROUP: A program for pedigree relationship reconstruction and kin group assignment using genetic markers. *Mol. Ecol. Notes* **2004**, *4*, 779–782.

Lewis, P.O.; and Zaykin, D.; Genetic Data Analysis: Computer program for the analysis of allelic data. **2001**. Available free from http://phylogeny.uconn.edu/software/

Linacre, A.M.T.; and Tobe, S.S.; *Wildlife DNA analysis. Applications in forensic science*. John Wiley & Sons, Chichester, United Kingdom, **2013**.

Linacre, A.; et al.; ISFG: Recommendations regarding the use of non-human (animal) DNA in forensic genetic investigations. *Forensic Sci. Int. Genet.* **2011**, *5*, 501–505.

Lindsay, A.R.; and Belant J.L.; A simple and improved PCR-based technique for white-tailed deer (*Odocoileus virginianus*) sex identification. *Conserv. Genet.* **2008**, *9*(2), 443–447.

Lorenzini, R.; DNA forensics and the poaching of wildlife in Italy: A case study. *Forensic Sci. Int.* **2005a**, *153*, 218–221.

Lorenzini, R.; A panel of polymorphic microsatellites in the threatened Apennine chamois (*Rupicapra pyrenaica* ornata). *Mol. Ecol. Notes* **2005b**, *5*, 372–374.

Lorenzini, R.; et al.; Noninvasive genotyping of the endangered Apennine brown bears: A case study not to let one's hair down. *Anim. Conserv.* **2004**, *7*, 199–209.

Lorenzini, R.; et al.; Wildlife molecular forensics: Identification of the Sardinian mouflon STR profiling and the Bayesian assignment test. *Forensic Sci. Int. Genet.* **2011**, *5*, 345–349.

Lorenzini, R.; et al.; Wolf–dog crossbreeding: "Smelling" a hybrid may not be easy. *Mammal. Biol.* **2013**, *5*(4), 345–349.

Lorenzini et al.; Matching STR and SNP genotyping to discriminate between wild boar, domestic pigs and their recent hybrids for forensic purposes. *Sci. Rep.* **2020**, *10*, 3188.

Manel, S.; Berthier, P.; and Luikart, G.; Detecting wildlife poaching: identifying the origin of individuals with Bayesian assignment tests and multilocus genotypes. *Conserv. Genet.* **2002**, *16*(3), 650–659.

Manel, S.; Gaggiotti, O.E.; and Waples, R.S.; Assignment methods: Matching biological questions with appropriate techniques. *Trends Ecol. Evol.* **2005**, *20*(3), *136–142*.

Marshall, T.C.; et al.; Statistical confidence for likelihood-based paternity inference in natural populations. *Mol. Ecol.* **1998**, *7*, 639–655.

Miller, S.M.; et al.; Evaluation of microsatellite markers for populations studies and forensic identification of african lions (*Panthera leo*). *J. Heredity* **2014**, *105*(6), 856–866.

Mondol, S.; et al.; Tracing the geographic origin of traded leopard body parts in the Indian subcontinent with DNA-based assignment tests. *Conserv. Biol.* **2014**, *29*(2), 556–564.

Morin, P.A.; et al.; Interfamilial characterization of a region of the ZFX and ZFY genes facilitates sex determination in cetaceans and other mammals. *Mol. Ecol.* **2005**, *14*(10): 3275–3286.

Morinha, F.; Cabral, J.A.; and Bastosa, E.; Molecular sexing of birds: A comparative review of polymerase chain reaction (PCR)-based methods. *Theriogenology* **2012**, *78*(4): 703–714.

Morinha, F.; et al.; High-resolution melting analysis for bird sexing: A successful approach to molecular sex identification using different biological samples. *Mol. Ecol. Res.* **2013**, *13*(3): 473–483.

Mucci, N.; Mengoni, C.; and Randi, E.; Wildlife DNA forensics against crime: Resolution of a case of tortoise theft. *Forensic Sci. Int. Genet.* **2014**, *8*(1), 200–202.

Mwale, M.; et al.; Forensic application of DNA barcoding for identification of illegally traded African pangolin scales. *Genome* **2017**, *60*(3), 272–284.

Nielsen, E.E.; et al.; Gene-associated markers provide tools for tackling illegal fishing and false eco-certification. *Nat. Commun.* **2012**, *3*, 851–856.

Ogden, R.; Unlocking the potential of genomic technologies for wildlife forensics. *Mol. Ecol. Resour.* **2011**, *11*(1), 109–116.

Ogden, R.; and Linacre, A.; Wildlife forensic science: A review of genetic geographic origin assignment. *Forensic Sci. Int. Genet.* **2015**, *18*, 152–159.

Ogden, R.; Dawnay, N.; and McEwing, R.; Wildlife DNA forensics—Bridging the gap between conservation genetics and law enforcement. *Endanger. Species Res.* **2009**, *9*, 179–195.

Parson, W.; et al.; Species identification by means of the cytochrome b gene. *Int. J. Legal Med.* **2000**, *114*(1), 23–28.

Pereira, F.; Carneiro, J.; and van Asch, B.; A guide for mitochondrial DNA analysis in non-human forensic investigations. *Open Forensic Sci. J.* **2010**, *3*, 33–44.

Pilgrim, K.L.; et al.; Felid sex identification based on noninvasive genetic samples. *Mol. Ecol. Notes* **2005**, *5*: 60–61.

Pilli, E.; et al.; Pet fur or fake fur? A forensic approach. *Invest. Genet.* **2014**, *5*, 7.

Piry, S. et al.; GENECLASS2: A software for genetic assignment and first-generation migrant detection. *J. Hered.* **2004**, *95*(6), 536–539.

Presti, F.T.; et al.; Population genetic structure in Hyacinth Macaws (*Anodorhynchus hyacinthinus*) and identification of the probable origin of confiscated individuals. *J. Hered.* **2015**, *106*(S1), 491–502.

Pritchard, J.K.; Stephens, M.; and Donnelly, P.; Inference of population structure using multilocus genotype data. *Genetics* **2000**, *155*, 945–959.

Regan, T.; *The case for animal rights*. University of California Press, Berkeley, LA, **1983**.

Rendo, F.; et al.; Microsatellite based ovine parentage testing to identify the source responsible for the killing of an endangered species. *Forensic Sci. Int. Genet.* **2011**, *5*(4), 333–335.

Rosen, G.E.; and Smith, K.F.; Summarizing the evidence on the international trade in illegal wildlife. *EcoHealth* **2010**, *7*(1), 24–32.

Rousset, F.; GENEPOP'007: A complete re-implementation of the GENEPOP software for Windows and Linux. *Mol. Ecol. Res.* **2008**, *8*, 103–106.

Schwartz, T.S.; and Karl, S.A.; Population genetic assignment of confiscated gopher tortoises. *J. Wildlife Manage.* **2008**, *72*(1), 254–259.

Sellar, J.M.; Illegal trade and the Convention on International Trade in Endangered Species of Wild Fauna and Flora (CITES). In: *Wildlife forensic investigation*; Linacre, A.M.T., Ed.; Taylor and Francis, London, 11–18, **2009**.

Shaw, C.N.; Wilson, P.J.; and White, B.N.; A reliable molecular method of gender determination for mammals. *J. Mammal.* **2003**, *84*(1), 123–128.

Snyder-Mackler, N.; et al.; Efficient genome-wide sequencing and low coverage pedigree analysis from non-invasively collected samples. *Genetics* **2016**, *203*, 699–714.

Socratous, E.; Graham, A.M.; and Rutty, G.N.; Forensic DNA profiling of *Cervus elaphus* species in the United Kingdom. *Forensic Sci. Int. Genet. Suppl. Ser.* **2009**, *2*, 281–282.

Städele, V.; and Vigilant, L.; Strategies for determining kinship in wild populations using genetic data. *Ecol. Evol.* **2016**, *6*(17), 6107–6120.

Sundqvist, A.K.; et al.; Y chromosome haplotyping in Scandinavian wolves (*Canis lupus*) based on microsatellite markers. *Mol. Ecol.* **2001**, *10*, 1959–1966.

SWGDAM; Revised validation guidelines. **2003**. http://www.cstl.nist.gov/div831/strbase/validation/SWGDAM_Validation.doc

SWGWILD (Scientific Working Group for Wildlife Forensic Sciences); Standards and Guidelines. **2012**. https://www.wildlifeforensicscience.org/wp-content/uploads/2016/07/swgwild-standards_and_guidelines_2–0_12192012.pdf

Tillmar, A.O.; et al.; A universal method for species identification of mammals utilizing Next Generation Sequencing for the analysis of DNA mixtures. *PLoS One* **2013**, *8*(12): e83761.

Tobe, S.S.; Kitchener, A.; and Linacre, A.; Cytochrome b or cytochrome c oxidase subunit I for mammalian species identification—An answer to the debate. *Forensic Sci. Int. Genet. Suppl. Ser.* **2009**, *2*(1), 306–307.

Tobe, S.S.; and Linacre, A.M.; A multiplex assay to identify 18 European mammal species from mixtures using the mitochondrial cytochrome b gene. *Electrophoresis* **2008**, *29*, 340–347.

Valière, N.; GIMLET: A computer program for analysing genetic individual identification data. *Mol. Ecol. Notes* **2002**, *2*(3), 377–379.

Vilà, C.; et al.; Combined use of maternal, paternal and biparental genetic markers for the identification of wolf-dog hybrids. *Heredity* **2003**, *90*, 17–24.

Wasser, S.K.; et al.; Assigning elephant DNA to geographic region of origin: Applications to the ivory trade. *Proc. Natl. Acad. Sci. USA* **2004**, *101*(41), 14847–14852.

Wasser, S.K.; et al.; Using DNA to track the origin of the largest ivory seizure since the 1989 trade ban. *Proc. Natl. Acad. Sci. USA* **2007**, *104*(10), 4228–4223.

Wasser, S.K.; et al.; Genetic assignment of large seizures of elephant ivory reveals Africa's major poaching hotspots. *Science* **2015**, *349*(6243), 84–87.

Weir, B.S.; Statistics for wildlife forensic DNA. In: *Wildlife forensics: Methods and applications*; Huffman, J. E.; and Wallace, J. R., Eds.; John Wiley & Sons, United Kingdom, *237*, **2012**.

Welton, L.J.; et al.; Dragons in our midst: Phyloforensics of illegally traded Southeast Asian monitor lizards. *Biol. Conserv.* **2013**, *159*, 7–15.

White, Nicole E.; et al.; Application of STR markers in wildlife forensic casework involving Australian black-cockatoos (*Calyptorhynchus* spp.). *Forensic Sci. Int. Genet.* **2012**, *6*(5), 664–670.

Wilson, M.R.; et al.; Validation of mitochondrial DNA sequencing for forensic casework analysis. *Int. J. Legal Med.* **1995**, *108*(2), 68–74.

Wilson-Wilde, L.; et al.; Current issues in species identification for forensic science and the validity of using the cytochrome oxidase I (COI) gene. *Forensic Sci. Med. Pathol.* **2010**, *6*(3), 233–241.

Wink, M.; et al.; Phylogenetic relationships in the hierofalco complex (saker-, gyr-, lanner-, laggar falcon). *Raptors Worldw.* **2004**, 499504.

Zachos, F.E.; et al.; The unique Mesola red deer of Italy: Taxonomic recognition (*Cervus elaphus italicus* nova ssp., Cervidae) would endorse conservation. *Ital. J. Zool.* **2014**, *81*(1), 136–143.

USEFUL LINKS

CITES Convention on International Trade of Endangered Species https://www.cites.org

International Society for Animal Genetics: www.isag.us

International Society for Forensic Genetics: www.isfg.org

International Union for Conservation of Nature (Red List of Threatened Species): www.iucnredlist.org

SWFS Society for Wildlife Forensic Science https://www.wildlifeforensicscience.org

TRACE Tools and Resources for Applied Conservation and Enforcement https://www.tracenetwork.org

TRAFFIC https://www.traffic.org

European Union of Environment Directorate http://ec.europa.eu/environment/cites/home_en.htm

UNODC United Nations Office on Drugs and Crime https://www.unodc.org

CHAPTER 14

Forensic Entomology: The Utility of Insects at Court and in Human Identification

SIMONETTA LAMBIASE[1*] and AARON M. TARONE[2]

[1]*Department of Public health, Experimental and Forensic Medicine, Pavia University, 27100 Pavia, Italy*

[2]*Department of Entomology, Texas A&M University, College Station, TX 77843-2475, USA*

Corresponding author. E-mail: s.lambiase@unipv.it

ABSTRACT

Knowledge of insects can be used to resolve a variety of issues that are litigated in the courtroom. A common use of entomology applied to the medico-legal field, traditionally, provides temporal information to death investigations and sometimes the location of death. The synergy of the entomology with toxicology may be very useful to resolve problems related to the cause of the death. Genetics can be used to help identify insect specimens, especially when immature stages are difficult to identify by morphology, but vertebrate DNA derived from insects can also be used to identify humans (victims or offenders in according to the evidences and the crime scenes). In this chapter, we discuss basic medical–legal entomology, the most common involved insects, their behaviors, and potential uses of entomology in investigations.

14.1 INTRODUCTION

Insects and other arthropods live everywhere in the world, having adapted over time to many types of habitats, even the most inhospitable habitats like Antarctica (Baust and Edwards, 1979; Lopez-Martinez et al., 2008). Given their ubiquity, it is no surprise that some of them interact very closely with humans and their activities (Bertone et al., 2016). Insects can affect humanity in a variety of ways, some of which are not typically considered by the general public, whereas some others are well known for the damage they cause as carriers of pathogens, for other impacts on human health, and for their effects in agriculture. Others are known to many in the public because they are useful, as in the case of bees or silkworms, or are known as being particularly beautiful, as in the case of some butterflies and beetles. We could continue to describe extensively the general influence that insects have in every aspect of our lives, but we prefer to focus our attention toward the most important thing about these insects: understanding their role in the habitat, their ecological and reproductive behavior, their dietary needs, and their relationship with us. This means, on the one hand, defending us from the damage they could cause us and, on the other hand, being able to interpret their importance on a deductive basis when encountered in legal settings. The field that studies insects, and other arthropods, in the courtroom is forensic entomology.

Because of the omnipresence of insects in our lives they can be informative in legal settings; therefore, forensic entomology is a large field of applications of entomology to legal investigations. It may concern urban health aspects, for example, infestations of places of service to human communities (schools, canteens, hospitals, etc.), infestation of food storage warehouses (flours, corn, meat, fish) or other manufactured goods, and possibly museums. In urban and storage infestation, the entomological approach may contribute to individuate the origin of the infestation, both in terms of its period of insurgence and geographic origin, and to limit and / or to prevent the damages. Moreover, entomology is applied to criminal (or medicolegal) investigations in case of violent or suspicious death, because it provides information about the time elapsed from the death, the cadaver displacement, the cause of the death, the identification of the victim and, in some cases, of the guilty.

The first need of the specialists is to identify the involved species and obtain all other information otherwise meaningless in the absence of the first. In the following pages, we will try to summarize the application of forensic entomology, especially in the medical–legal field, with emphasis on the genetic identification, which is also the least used approach in the investigations. Given the focus of this text, the introduction of the topic is necessarily superficial and reports general observations that can include exceptions and assumptions known to experts, which may not be apparent to the readers of this chapter. For readers broadly interested in the topic area of forensic entomology and related topics, greater detail is provided in additional material (Amendt et al., 2007; Byrd and Castner, 2010; Gennard, 2012; Tomberlin and Benbow, 2015; Rivers and Dahlem, 2014; Benbow et al., 2015). The contents of this chapter is intended to give a general overview of how different insects may be used in forensic entomology as a means to assist geneticists and toxicologists in understanding how to aid or augment current applications.

14.2 INSECTS AND THEIR NUTRITIONAL AND REPRODUCTIVE SUBSTRATES

Feeding and reproduction represent fundamental aspects of existence that contribute to the evolutionary fitness of organisms (De Block and Stoks, 2005; Wilder et al., 2016); when offspring and adults have the same nutritional needs, it can happen that the extended trophic substrate is also chosen for reproduction, so that the neonate insects immediately find a source of nourishment. In other cases, when the adult diet is different from that of the progeny, it is possible for a certain substrate to mainly provide a reproductive function and for another to serve as the neonate resource. Different types of insects exhibit different development patterns relevant to this concern (Bybee et al., 2015). Insects are generally oviparous (Séguy, 1950). Some of them develop immature specimens with morphology very similar to the parents and are called nymphs; they cannot reproduce and lack the wings. In other cases, the immature specimens are completely different from the parents in morphology and physiology and are called larvae, and in the case of flies (commonly encountered as evidence) they are also called maggots.

The development of insects passes through a series of stages through a phenomenon called a moult that allows them to grow in size, thanks to the loss of the external cuticle after the synthesis of a newer and bigger one (Schwalman, 1988). The number of the immature stages varies with taxonomic group and species and the nature of their last is depending on the species and the environmental conditions. To complete their cycle and to pass from the last immature stage to the adult stage, some insects (e.g., butterflies, beetles, and flies) must undergo complete metamorphosis within an apparently static structure that is the pupa or the chrysalis; this complex development pathway is indicative of an evolutionary advantage in insects, because it avoids competition for food between adults and immatures. This kind of development pattern is called holometabolous developmental cycle.

The relationship between insects and the environment, and consequently the relationship between insects and the substrate upon which they feed or on which they reproduce themselves, is often strong and not casual. Given this relationship between reproductive and nutritional substrates and insects entomological knowledge can act as a tool in the justice system. In Europe the medical–legal application of forensic entomology underwent formal study less than a century ago; whereas in other parts of the world, starting from ancient societies, entomology was well known (McKnight, 1981) and used by the justice in case of murders.

In Europe, medicolegal forensic entomology can be traced back to the work of Jean Pierre Mégnin who systematically identified relationships between insects and cadavers (Michaud et al., 2015). He noted that remains exhibited eight decomposition stages and defined eight groups of insect families attracted from each of them (Mégnin, 1894). These first observations lead to the thought that not all the necrophilous insects are attracted at the same time by the cadaver; on the contrary, waves of colonizer insects follow each other on a corpse. This relationship is believed to be based on the great specificity of the necrophagous insect olfactory system and aspects of interspecific competition. There have been many studies assessing insect colonization patterns and correlation between the decomposition phases and insect colonization since Mégnin's original work and from the end of the 18th century to today, many others have followed (e.g., Bornemissza, 1957; Reed, 1958; Payne, 1965; Hewadikaram and Goff, 1991; Perez et al., 2014). One particularly notable development in recent years is the establishment of anthropological research facilities to study human taphonomy, which have also enabled entomological research on human remains across a range of conditions. Bass was the first to establish such a facility in Tennessee and noted different observations than discovered by Megnin. He stated that the *post-mortem* transformation could be divided in four successive phases (fresh, chromatic, decay, and dehydration) associated to four waves of insect colonization and, mainly, the decomposition was interpreted as a continuous process and no longer as a sequence of discrete stages (Rodriguez and Bass, 1983). Moreover, there is evidence that insect successional processes are not tied directly to decomposition stages (Schoenly and Reid, 1987). Indeed, in the same cadaver we can appreciate at the same moment different coexisting stages, according to the natural differences in anatomic districts of the body and to the environment. This observation resulted in an accumulated degree based total body score in forensic anthropology, which is currently a focus of research for death investigation (Megyesi et al., 2005). Given the complexity of the decomposition process, it should come as no surprise that while there are clear patterns in insect occurrence on human and animal remains (Perez et al., 2014), there are also examples of exceptions to the generalities (Byrd and Castner, 2010) necessitating a greater dissection of successional processes on remains (Michaud et al., 2015, Michaud and Moreau, 2017).

Despite the progress in entomological data and their applications, while in Europe and around most parts of the world entomology is fully developed, in Italy the professional partners that work at a crime scene often lack the information, ability, and conditions to use this resource. This is a pity because insects can provide valuable information to the legal system, sometimes in ways that are unexpected and do not reflect traditional forensic entomological applications. Examples highlighting this point (as well as traditional casework applications) can be found in various publications noted in the introduction, including Byrd and Castner (2010) who published a report about a murder disguised as a road accident. The victim, a woman, was found into a car recovered from the bottom of a river during the spring. The remains were very well preserved from the cold water. Her husband declared a recent communication with her, but the surface of the car was covered by larvae of aquatic insects which made contact with the river bottoms during the autumn. The species was not necrophagous, but their seasonal developmental patterns indicated that the car was in the water for a much longer period of time than the husband had indicated. Thus, the insects collected in that case were equivalent in their use as necrophagous insects in their indication of the period of the death and indictment of the husband of the victim.

Other similar examples could be reported, but this description is just to focus on the idea that each naturalistic observation would be taken in account to perform the best investigation of a crime scene and not only on what insect closely related to the corpse is found. Moreover, other kinds of insects or other arthropods are detectable on carrion as opportunistic feeders: they sometimes are scavengers that feed on the remains, sometimes they are predators of the species colonizing the corpse. It is fundamental, in any case, to obtain information from these observations in order to identify the species and their relevant biological features.

Thus, the complexity of the picture provided by the corpses, ephemeral ecosystems, may contribute to the investigations. Indeed, the French experience, in particular the partnership of the Gendarmerie with the French University and the realization of a certificated forensic lab ISO 17025, make the entomological findings scientific evidence at court more valuable (Charabidze, 2014).

14.3   GENERAL CONCEPTS RELATED TO SPECIES IDENTITY IN FORENSIC ENTOMOLOGY

One important aspect of forensic entomology is the identification of insects that are of forensic interest. This knowledge is critical to unlocking the information that may be relevant to casework because the forensically relevant biology of the insect is linked to its identity. For example, some species have very specific dietary requirements (e.g., wood destroying insects), whereas others are generalists that can feed on a variety of resources (e.g., ants). A common group of insects of forensic importance are necrophagous and saprophagous insects, as they are often associated with decomposing organic matter. In addition, since a subset of these insects utilize decomposing remains as a resource for their developing offspring, knowledge regarding their development can be useful in providing temporal information about a death, if environmental conditions associated with remains are known (or correctly assumed) and the development of the insect in question has been studied.

In the urban entomology the involved insects are often opportunistic and belong to the first group (i.e., cockroaches). But in case of infestation of stored food it is common to find colonizer species such as the Lepidoptera (butterflies and moths) and Coleoptera (beetles) in all the immature stages and as adults. In case of the medicolegal entomology insects are often necrophagous.

In this last field the opportunistic insects often belong especially to the order of Coleoptera, whereas those that reproduce themselves on human or animal carrion belong to the order of Diptera; exceptions do exist, such as the Dermestidae beetles that not only feed on (dehydrated) remains but also reproduce on them, because both adults and their progeny have the same dietary needs. The beetles are highly species rich among insects and other animals, whereas Diptera are less so and, in particular our interest is generally focused on the terrestrial species belonging to the flies (Diptera: Brachycera), in contrast to the other groups with aquatic larvae, as the mosquitos, for example (Diptera: Nematocera). Fortunately, the species of common interest in forensic entomology are only a few dozen (Byrd and Castner, 2010). It is to be noted that some species, such as black soldier flies (Tomberlin et al., 2002) can feed on plant and animal substances and so they may be present on the food and on corpses as well. Thus, the identity of a species found in evidence can lead investigators to investigative valuable information. The examples provided here focused on feeding habits, but other behaviors, seasonality, and regional occurrence (among others) are features of an insect that may be linked to its identity that could be useful to investigators. Below some common orders of insects are described with respect to their forensic usefulness.

14.3.1 LEPIDOPTERA

Within the approximately 165,000 species (Regier et al., 2009) that make up this *taxon*, fortunately, only a small part is associated with foodstuffs or remains. The buccal apparatus of the adult Lepidoptera is always a siphon, therefore the adult does not cause direct damage. However, the immature stages have strong jaws and can masticate stored food products or animal remains. The eggs are laid directly on the foodstuffs, and from these larvae hatch that are responsible for the damage caused to the foodstuffs which can also be contaminated by excrements, silk webs, and exuviae. Among the Lepidoptera, we list the more common families (and their species) involved in food contamination as Pyralidae (*Pyralis farinalis*), Gelechiidae (*Sitotroga cerealella*), Phycitidae (*Plodia interpunctella, Ephestia kuehniella*), Liposcelidae (*Liposcelis divinatorius*), and Tineidae (*Nemapogon granella*) (Süss and Gelosi, 1991; Suss et al., 2001).

These insects are easily recognizable through their morphology and the kind of damage they produce. A small subset of these insects is also capable of utilizing carrion (Payne and King, 1969). They are distinct in their use of animal remains, typically found on drier older remains, with some like the Tineidae completing their lifecycle on animal remains. Several taxa can metabolize keratin, allowing them to use hair and fingernails that are inaccessible to other insects as a food resource (Hughes and Vogler, 2006). Lepidoptera in this group, such as clothes moths in the genus *Tineola*, are capable of feeding on animal remains (typically in more advanced states of decay) and can also cause damage to goods (e.g., wool sweaters). Recently, problems correlated to insect infestation have been identified in the field of the green building because of the organic matter (both vegetal and animal) used in building materials.

14.3.2   COLEOPTERA

The beetles are a highly diverse taxon with as many as approximately 400,000 described species (Lawrence et al., 2011). Beetles, adults, and larvae are insects equipped with strong jaws; therefore, their diet is solid. Due to their strong jaws, species are found damaging structures made of wood, they feed on stored products, and are commonly found on animal remains feeding on the remains themselves or predating other insects on the remains.

Among the families (and species) that feed on food we list, that is, Curculionidae (*Sitophilus granaries, Sitophilus oryzae*), Tenebrionidae (*Triboliunm confusum, Tenebrio molitor*), Silvanidae (*Oryzephilus surinamensis, O. mercator*), Dermestidae (*Dermestes lardarius, Trogoderma granarium*), Ptinidae (*Anobium puncatum*). The wood-destroying insects include the Buprestidae, Cerambycidae, Bostrichidae, and Curcuionidae (Suss, 1990; Süss and Gelosi, 1991; Suss et al., 2001). As with the Lepidoptera, while adult specimens can help provide information about the species of concern; the kind of the damage is often enough to recognize the species involved. For example, in wood destroying cases, the fine powdery piles of frass found near the entrances to their galleries is indicative of recognition of the powder post beetles (Bostrichidae: Lyctinae), being typical of them.

With respect to medico/legal entomology, the most common opportunistic families of beetles that interact with the corpses, to feed on it or to prey the eggs or maggots growing on it, are Geotrupidae, Histeridae, Staphylinidae, Silphidae, and Cleridae. Their predatory ability could cause mistakes in *post mortem* interval (PMI) calculation if they are numerous in the death scene. For example, Wall et al. (2001) reported 0%–97% larval fly mortality for the blow fly *Lucilia sericata* due in part to predation primarily by beetles from the family Carabidae at their field site.

Some beetles from the families Scarabaeidae, Silphidae, Staphylinidae, and Dermestidae are often found feeding and developing on animal remains. These species, especially the *Dermestes* genus in Italy, may be of interest because they are commonly encountered and can complete their developmental cycle on the remains. The females lay eggs on them and both adults and larvae feed on the same dehydrated tissues. That means that we can recover both the immature stages and the adults on the same corpse. Because their generally late colonization and their eating habit (they eat dehydrated food) in medical-legal field their utility is often in cases of longer decomposition timelines where the faster developing flies have already completed development.

The frass of these beetles is also reported to yield DNA and toxicological information from the feeding substrate (Byrd and Castner 2010).

The timing of arrival of adult beetles to animal remains has also been studied (Matuszewski, 2011; Matuszewski and Szafalowicz, 2013; Matuszewski and Madra-Bielewicz, 2016). For several beetle species, the pre-appearance interval (the period of time from death/placement of remains to when a species arrives) has been studied with respect to temperature. Results suggest that there is a predictable and thermally dependent curve that can describe arrival times of beetles visiting animal remains.

14.3.3 HYMENOPTERA

The Hymenoptera, which includes bees, wasps, and ants, include over 140,000 species (Klopfstein et al., 2013). Many are important in forensic investigations for several reasons. First, many species possess stingers and can inject a venom into prey or as a defense against potential predators. Second, many species live in social or semisocial colonies and can cooperate with one another. This lifestyle can sometimes result in very successful colonies comprised of thousands (or more) of individuals. These two traits lead to a variety of interactions with humans that could be of interest in the courtroom.

They can be involved directly in the deaths of humans and animals when they sting, especially when an entire social group attacks. For instance when their nest is disturbed a colony will defend itself against a perceived attack. When the infirm (e.g., infants, the elderly) are exposed to attack by colonies, they may be unable to extract themselves from attack quickly, making them most susceptible to death and injury in such cases. Allergies to venom can also lead to lethality even if only one sting occurs.

The sociality of these insects can lead to nests with large numbers that can disrupt or enhance human activities and which may forage in human environments. In these cases, civil litigation related to the control of these insects may occur. These types of cases may range from litigation related to the protection of bees to the management of ant infestations in buildings.

Many of the Hymenoptera are predatory. This means that their presence in casework may need to be accounted for in forensic casework. For instance, fire ants (*Solenopsis invicta*) are reported to impact the observation of blow-flies on remains by predating larvae and eggs (Wells and Greenberg, 1994; Stoker et al., 1995). Some wasps are parasitoids, which lay their eggs in a host. Those eggs hatch and then feed on the internal organs of the host, ultimately killing it when development is completed. Parasitoids infest a wide variety of insects, thus it is not surprising that they can also be associated with insects that are pests or which feed on carrion. Parasitoids on remains can alter the rates of successful emergence. They also have their own development rates, which can be used to estimate timelines associated with a death alongside the development of their hosts (Grassberger and Frank, 2003).

Finally, a wide variety of ants in particular are noted for scavenging human and animal remains (recently reviewed in Eubanks et al., 2019). Their feeding can alter the appearance of remains, requiring knowledge of their feeding to avoid misinterpreting ant feeding as perimortem wounds (Byard, 2005). They are also known to feed on remains throughout the process of decomposition, both above and belowground. Given their ubiquity, the authors noted a potential combination of ant biology and genetic technology that could be leveraged to identify clandestine graves. This concept hinged on the fact that ants are widely distributed, in some cases (e.g., fire ants in the Southeastern USA) can reach high densities, forage the environment for food regularly (both above and belowground), and are known to return protein meals to their larvae. These combinations of behaviors make ants a likely environmental sampler that could be subjected to a colony-wide gut content analysis via genetic analysis that could identify the presence of human remains in an area via identification of human DNA in ant larval samples. They noted that the current development of next-generation sequencing technologies that are field deployable (Parker et al., 2017; Johnson et al., 2017), in combination with advanced field deployable DNA isolation (Priye et al., 2016) and PCR techniques (Krishnan et al., 2002), could potentially allow real-time on-site analysis of ant samples in an area suspected of harboring a human grave.

14.3.4   DIPTERA

Among the flies, the species belonging to the order Diptera that are of most interest to forensic work colonize decomposing matter; including food (fruits, vegetables, cheese, and meat), feces, wounds, and corpses. Accordingly, they can be encountered as evidence in a variety of forensically relevant situations ranging from food contamination to abuse and neglect to death investigations. Adult saprophagous flies typically have sponging mouthparts, with larvae that are vermiform. Many fly families are encountered as pests and will not be recounted in detail here but may be of relevance to casework. Common families in medicolegal entomology include the Muscidae, Sarcophagidae, Calliphoridae, Phoridae, and Piophilidae.

The most useful families in criminal investigation are those that commonly enter our houses or are encountered in towns or fields. Their livery is metallic (green and blue bottleflies—Calliphoridae), black (latrine flies - Fanniidae), brown (house flies—Muscidae), and black with gray longitudinal stripes on the thorax and black and white chessboard on the abdomen (flesh flies - Sarcophagidae). The Calliphoridae family is ubiquitous and is often the first group to detect a recent death (fresh cadaver) in a very short time and to lay eggs on the corpse, sometimes in less than an hour. The Muscidae and Sarcophagidae can also be found on remains in early stages of decomposition.

The Sarcophagidae family is also attracted to carrion throughout the decomposition process and for that reason, it can provide information similar to that provided by blowflies; moreover, while the blowflies lay eggs, the flesh flies are generally larviparous depositing larvae at the first larval instar. The problem is that not all the species have this behavior and some of them can lay older maggots or eggs and maggots, or only eggs. This is the case, for example, of *Sarcophaga argyrostoma* (personal observation S. Lambiase) and *Blaesoxipha plinthopyga* (Pimsler et al., 2014). When encountered, this peculiar reproductive behavior reduces their usefulness in providing information regarding *post-mortem* colonization timing; nevertheless, such species could also be indicative of the displacement of a corpse in some cases. For example, the presence of *Blaesoxipha plinthopyga* on remains (along with *Megaselia scalaris, Lucilia cuprina*, and *Synthesiomyia nudiseta*) is highly associated with indoor death investigations in Harris County, TX, USA (Sanford, 2017).

Following the first wave of colonization, we could collect species belonging to the Muscidae, Fanniidae, and Piophilidae. These species may not be useful themselves as indicators of death, but may provide other useful information. Piophilidae are considered to indicate how much time elapsed from the saponification. Likewise, the Fanniidae and Muscidae have been reported as indicators of premortem abuse and neglect (Byrd and Castner, 2010). Many other families develop on remains (like Sepsidae and Phoridae) in according to the environment and the decomposition stage. For instance, the Phoridae are noted for their ability to access remains in crypts, that are buried, and are otherwise inaccessible to many other flies.

Flies are generally a common type of insect found in medicolegal forensic entomology. They are also considered important because many, like the blow flies and flesh flies, are primary colonizers of remains. This behavior allows investigators to estimate a minimum *post-mortem* interval by estimating the timing of insect colonization, which is described in detail below.

14.3.4.1   *TIMING OF COLONIZATION*

To understand why insects can be so useful to rebuild the history of a cadaver it is important to consider two described aspects of the necrophilous insect reproductive ethology. The first aspect of insect biology of interest is that they can detect the decomposing matter in a very short time and over relatively long distances—in a species-specific manner. The second aspect of insect biology important to *post-mortem* timing is that their developmental time is considered species-specific and temperature-dependent, as explained below. Flies, and any other primary colonizers of remains, can be particularly useful in forensic entomology due these two traits. As the females detect a corpse, they often immediately lay their eggs on the cadaver that will feed their offspring. The rapidity in oviposition is explained by the fact that, as in the most insect taxa, only one coupling is enough to guarantee to the female the amount of sperm to cover the entire female reproductive life. So, in 15–60 min the corpse may be colonized if environmental conditions allow it.

> But what does "if environmental conditions allow it" mean?
> What could be the reason if that does not happen?

To answer to these questions, we need to take in account a variety of situations. One of these is the exposition of the corpse to the environment: it depends on the habitat (high mountains, desert areas, open fields, woods, but also apartment or other indoor locations) and on the meteorology because in the dark or windy/rainy day flies do not undergo oviposition. Moreover, in certain seasons or weather conditions, for example, flies are not active (e.g., below certain species-specific temperatures, or for adverse weather, or because it is night). This delay in colonization can last only a few hours (e.g., because it is night or because it is raining) or many days/weeks (because it is in the middle of winter in a country with a harsh climate). The cause of death and the variables are very numerous and some of them are related to the condition of the corpse and its exposure to the environment (isolation from mechanical barrier such as burial, package with different kinds of envelops, freezer compartment, or other chemical means and equipment of concealment of the corpse) could slow down a lot (if not prevent in some cases) the colonization of the remains; more commonly, even a body found in a closed apartment could be colonized after death though possibly with a delay for insects to discover the remains.

Biotic factors affect the colonization process too. For example, the environmental presence of large amount of predators feeding on the eggs laid from the Diptera or their maggots (as described due to predation by ants or beetles above) has an effect on colonization patterns and may impact estimates of the *post mortem* interval as it relates to estimates of insect age. Similarly, genetic and microbiological analyses indicate that bacteria are known to produce important molecules that colonizing blowflies evaluate when arriving at a resource (Ma et al., 2012; Tomberlin et al., 2012; Liu et al., 2016; Rhinesmith-Carranza et al., 2018). Thus, in some instances (e.g., antibiotics treatment premortem) there may by impacts on the microbiome that could alter attractiveness of remains to colonizing insects. This is supported by the observation that experimental removal of flies from colonization alters carrion microbiome constituents as well as the taxa willing to colonize those remains (Pechal et al., 2013).

Another situation that should not be underestimated is the possibility that the deceased was affected by myiasis, a parasitosis of live animals by flies; such cases are usually linked to the environmental degradation of neglected patients, plagued by decubitus or who have undergone surgery. In these extreme situations it is possible that their wounds are colonized while they are still alive, leading to the hypothesis that their insect-estimated timelines will not line up with the actual *post-mortem* interval (Gherardi and Lambiase, 2006). While it is tempting to think that such cases are rare enough for the scenario to not be considered, there are clear examples in the literature that indicate the relevance of this situation. In Harris County, TX, USA, an individual was found behind a business with a severe and advanced case of myiasis. They died several hours later in the hospital, demonstrating that had the person succumbed to their wounds a few hours earlier there was potential for a wildly different interpretation of the insect evidence found with the body (Sanford et al., 2014).

> The examples until now described refer to exposed environments. What happens in case of buried corpses or underwater corpses?

With buried corpses, the colonization is slower than in open air. The most part of first colonizer flies are not scavengers and for this reason are not able to reach the buried remains. However, the maggots of some other families (some species belonging to Muscidae and Sarcophagidae) (Szpila et al., 2010; Pastula, 2013), or adults themselves of very small flies (Phoridae) can lay eggs just on the corpse in according to its depth and the composition of the soil.

These different abilities of the flies allow us to decipher the immediately *post-mortem* events: to find entomological evidences belonging to certain taxa or others or both of them lead to consider, for example, a premeditated murder or not. Also, in this case, and regardless of the need for PMI calculation, the identification of the colonizer species is fundamental.

In case of aquatic findings, we must distinguish the fresh water from salt water. In this second case, aquatic insects do not exist (though Anderson (Anderson, 2009; Anderson and Bell, 2016) has described comparable processes with noninsect arthropods in the Pacific Ocean), but in case of fresh water, as it has been described before, some species can be helpful (Byrd and Caster, 2010). Moreover, in both the environments the terrestrial necrophilous flies may colonize floating or beached bodies, giving the emersion/beach period and possibly the environment of origin of a body carried by currents. In addition, in this case it would be necessary to establish the species and to know their geographical distribution.

It is evident that the "ifs" are not lacking and make the assessment of the PMI a delicate calculation. For these reasons it also becomes very important for the entomologists to have any kind of information about the corpse conditions and the crime scene to understand if or why the colonization does not indicate the time of death. In short, the process of evaluating *post-mortem* timelines with insect evidence requires making assumptions. It is worth noting that genetic theory is contributing to forensic entomology literature in this area. Tarone and Sanford (2017), recognizing presence of a core assumption that could be violated for a variety of reasons, consider *post-mortem* estimates with insect evidence to share features with Hardy–Weinberg equilibrium and the neutral theory of evolution. They advocate for the development of empirical tests for assumptions related to analyses. For instance, for species that have members that are more or less prone to colonizing in a myiasis event, could a genetic test be developed to inform investigators of the probability that remains were likely colonized pre- or *post-mortem*? Similarly, there are numerous environments that may impact insect development (temperature, diet, drugs, etc.)—are there gene expressions or other molecular markers that could identify such conditions (Tarone et al., 2015)? In the case of diapause (a hibernation-like state triggered by the onset of winter conditions) gene expression has been identified as a marker of potential delays in insect development in a forensically relevant fly (Fremdt et al., 2014). Specifically, they identified three heat shock proteins (*hsp23*, *hsp24*, and *hsp70*) that were significantly upregulated in diapausing *Calliphora vicina*. They also noted that high variance in *anterior fat body protein* expression in pooled samples could be a reliable marker of diapause.

This area of identifying molecular markers of assumptions in forensic entomology is likely to expand considerably with the introduction of next-generation sequencing technologies (Tarone et al., 2015). There now a variety of transcriptome and genome studies published for forensically relevant blowflies and flesh flies (Hahn et al., 2009; Lee et al., 2011; Sze et al., 2012; Zhang et al., 2013; Anstead et al., 2015; Andere et al., 2016; Martinson et al., 2019). These publications, and similar subsequent projects, will enhance the ability of researchers to screen for mRNA (and subsequently protein or other molecular) markers of any condition of concern to forensic entomology analyses. Thus, in the future, following the strategy of Tarone and Sanford (2017) one could collect a fly in evidence, calculate its age given a set of assumptions, and test the specimen for molecular markers that would allow an investigator to identify likely violations of those assumptions (temperature exposure, drug exposure, etc.). As an example, consider the blow fly *Chrysomya rufifacies*. Its larvae are facultative predators of other blow flies and in some cases the species can have devastating impacts on competing species by predating its competitors (Wells and Greenberg, 1992; Baumgartner, 1993; Brundage et al., 2014). Pimsler et al. (2019) have analyzed the transcriptomes of predating and nonpredating siblings and identified several genes that are markers of predation (i.e., they are significantly up- or downregulated when facultative predation is initiated compared to the expression of those genes in nonpredating siblings of predators in the same arena) including genes that share sequence similarity with the *Drosophila melanogaster* genes *asterix*, *glass bottom boat*, *arginase*, *Host cell factor*, and *silver*. Such genes, or metabolic products implied by their known functions in other species (e.g., *N*-aceyldopamine levels are altered in *silver* mutants (Walter et al., 1996)) could be used in the future to determine if *Chrysomya rufifacies* on a body were likely to have impacted the other species feeding on the remains through their predatory behavior, allowing forensic entomologists to determine when care should be taken with interpretation of evidence in cases when this facultative predator is in evidence. Investigators can ask if in a specific case, facultative predation was likely to have occurred and subsequently if that predation was likely to impact results. While there will be a period of time between identification of potential markers of forensically relevant conditions (e.g., predation, myaisis, and diapause), their validation, and subsequent development of standard operating procedures for forensic laboratories; all of the components for such assays are beginning to appear in the literature and are likely to be an active area of research in the coming years.

14.4   THE APPLICATION OF THE DEVELOPMENTAL CYCLE OF INSECTS TO THE FORENSIC FIELD

In the previous section, two main aspects of insect biology were noted as relevant to death investigation. The *second* aspect, common to all insects, regards the fact that the developmental time is considered species specific and temperature dependent.

This means that a given species takes a different time to complete its ontogeny depending on the temperature at which it is exposed; at the same time, different species require different times to develop at the same growth temperature. It follows that in order to know the age of the specimens feeding on a corpse we need to consider the temperature of the scene where we think the cadaver decomposed itself and the species to which the specimens belong to. Studies on the life cycle of insects developed since the end of the last century and the application of this knowledge to the forensic environment allowed the integration of the successional method to assign the time death of somebody. The life cycle of insects, being correlated to the environmental conditions, is like a biologic clock, so it is useful in calculation of the PMI if the recovered species are the first colonizers and all assumptions are appropriate.

It is important to note that during insect development, there are stadia that last considerably longer than others, such that, if gross morphology is considered a broad (and potentially uninformative) timeline may be reported (Tarone and Foran, 2008, 2011). As an example, metamorphosis for flies often occupies the last half of immature development. Thus, if a puparium is collected, there will be an imprecise estimate of insect age as the insect could be ~50%–100% through its immature lifecycle. A similar, though lesser, challenge can exist for third instar larvae of the Calliphoridae - especially if evidence is collected in a way that does not allow the investigator to differentiate between a feeding or wandering (in preparation of pupariation) third instar. There are ways to decrease this imprecision however. If one has a detailed knowledge of development of the species, it is possible to dissect or image the puparium and report a more refined age estimate. Here, genetic analyses can help expand the accessibility of such assesments as genetic knowledge now outstrips detailed insect development knowledge in the pool of biology trained students today. Genetics can assist in dissecting development because during the developmental process genes are being up- and downregulated. Gene expression has been used to identify egg masses that are early versus late in the process of development of forensically

relevant flies (Tarone et al., 2007) and to refine larval and pupal development (Tarone and Foran, 2011; Boehme et al., 2013, 2014; Wang et al.,
2018). As an example, for developing embryos the genes *bicoid* (anterior
determinant in early development), *slalom* (a dorsoventral patterning and
salivary gland expressed gene), and *chitin synthase* (important to the production of a component of larval cuticle late in embryogenesis) were evaluated and shown to be useful in identifying distinct portions of embryonic
development in *Lucilia sericata* samples, with the first two expressed at their
highest levels early in development and the other expressed at its highest
levels later in development. These studies were based on quantitative PCR
analyses and have demonstrated the principle that the strategy is feasible.
However, it is worth noting that the best genes for such an approach will
not be obvious until considerable validation research is done. As genomic
technologies have advanced, the ability to screen entire transcriptomes for
the most informative markers is advancing. Several transcriptomic studies of
development of forensically important flies have been published (Sze et al.,
2012; Zajac et al., 2018; Martinson et al., 2019). These studies have followed
different strategies that, in part, reflect the technology available at the time
of their experiments to determine differentially expressed portions of the
transcriptome during development. Some have sequenced a portion (3' ends)
of a transcriptome, the whole transcriptome, or implemented a joint genome
and transcriptome sequencing strategy. In all cases, there are clear examples
of differential expression in multiple genes that can be used to separate flies
of different ages. These screens and the genomic resources associated with
them are identifying genes that should be further evaluated for their ability to
robustly predict (and refine) the age estimates of forensically important flies.

Literature is quite rich in terms of growth curves of the species of insects
remarkable in forensic field. However, on the basis of the Grassberger's
observations (2007) all available data are not yet sufficient. This is because
the traits used to make estimates of insect age, size, and development time
are quantitative traits, which are known for responding to the environment,
genetic variation, and the interaction between the two (Tomberlin et al.,
2011; Tarone et al., 2015; Tarone, 2015; Blanckenhorn, 2015). Accordingly,
forensically important traits may be impacted by a variety of environmental
factors (some noted earlier), many of which have been studied in experiments of forensically important insects (reviewed in Tomberlin et al., 2011).
However, genetic factors and the interaction between the environment and
genetics may also alter insect sizes or development rates (Gallagher et al.,
2010; Tarone et al., 2011; Owings et al., 2014), meaning the biological clock

may tick a little faster or slower depending on the environmental and genetic conditions relevant to a particular case. Any of these factors may explain why authors from different countries obtain different results, even while working on the same species at the same conditions. For this reason, maybe, it could be useful that each country has its own literature obtained from its strains of the species of interest. It is worth noting that Tarone et al. (2015) note a long-term strategy to address this issue. Just as they advocated to determine gene expression markers of environmental exposure, they also advocated using genomic technologies to determine expression and DNA variants to identify sequences that are markers fast or slow/large or small individuals of a species. Such experiments have been done to determine alleles of genes associated with variation in flowering time in *Arabidopsis thaliana* (Atwell et al., 2010) and body size in *Drosophila melanogaster* (Turner et al., 2011). Genetic analyses of forensically important flies to address such issues have occurred. Tarone (2015) and Hjelmen et al. (2020) reported the results of a selection experiment on development time of *Cochliomyia macellaria*. Results from that experiment indicate that sufficient genetic variation is segregating in that species to drive >5 days variation in development time at 25 °C. In addition, information from the selection response could be used to calculate narrow sense heritability of the trait (Tarone et al., 2016), indicating that ~10%–30% of the variation in development time in that species could be due to additive genetic variation (variation within strains in that species was ~100 h). Sequencing experiments with those strains, or similar experiments, will help to resolve genetic contributors to blow fly developmental variation.

The two fundamental observations previously exposed have laid the foundations of the forensic entomology: the insect cycles are temperature dependent and species specific; in case of the medicolegal entomology we also know that the colonization may occur as soon as people die: for this reason, in all those cases in which the recovered corpses are actively colonized, to apply data from the developmental cycle of the immature stages collected on the them (and not more the thanatology or the colonizing species only) give us answers around the *post-mortem* interval.

If the remains have been decomposing for relatively longer periods of time, then possibly only late waves of colonization will be in evidence. In these cases, the successional method is still useful to state the time of death. This has been the case of the recovery of a skeletonized man that showed only a small piece of part of his body still covered by saponified tissue colonized by a late colonizer fly; other entomological evidences were puparial cases of the previous colonizers. In this case it was possible to place the species in accordance with their climatic needs and verify the compatibility in terms of colonization time with the only alive species. The calculation was so precise that the entomological results, that indicated the time of death 5 months before the recovery of the skeleton, were confirmed after the recognition of the victim (S. Lambiase, personal data).

In any case it follows that it is necessary to assign the species to the specimens feeding on the substrate and to know the environmental parameters, especially the temperature, in particular in the goods storage centers or at the crime scene, to define their age.

To assign the age of the specimens collected is crucial to define when the infestation started. In case of stored food, for example, knowing the age of the immature specimens indicates if those products were infested before or after their arrival in that center. This is possible comparing the age of the collected specimens with the information about the import/export documents. On the contrary, in case of the recovery of a colonized corpse, the maggots can be used for the calculation of the PMI often corresponding to the death moment. To identify the species, and knowing the environmental conditions at which they developed, allows us to trace back to the date of the oviposition that generated it. In case of medical–legal entomology, the picture is more complex than in case of infested food: in this last case only, a few species are usually collected while a lot are recognizable on a cadaver. Moreover, storage environments are very similar each to the other and very stable from a thermic point of view and the infestation is an exception; on the contrary, the recovery of a corpse can occur everywhere, and it is associated to a multitude of variables. For all these reasons, remembering the phenomena of the successional waves of colonization and the colonizer species vary in according to the environment and to the thanatology, the species belonging to the first wave would be the most significant for the assessment of the PMI.

This assessment tool can be used for the evaluation of the *post-mortem* interval on the assumption that the first wave of dipterans immediately decomposes after the death of the individual, if the environmental conditions allow it.

14.5   PROBLEMS IN IDENTIFICATION

14.5.1   IDENTIFICATION OF ENTOMOLOGICAL EVIDENCE

Typically, insect identification is done through the use of a morphological key that can allow for the determination of species by its physical structures (e.g., Whitworth, 2006). However, in some cases, these keys may not be informative. For example, keys are needed for each developmental stadium because immature and adult structures differ. If a larval or pupal key does not exist (e.g., Szpila, 2009), then it is not possible to identify the insect without rearing specimens to adulthood. Giving a look at the general morphology of the Diptera maggots, growth is accomplished with little differences in morphology. In particular, the stigmata of the posterior *spiracula* pass from one opening to three shifting from the first stage to the third one and only this last stage is useful to identify the species. In these cases, the differences in larval structures among members of the same genus can be subtle. Similarly, even with adult specimens, it may not be possible to identify sister taxa within a genus reliably without an expert. Despite the potential utility in forensic field of Sarcophagidae (they are active in early decomposition stage, colonize indoor, and buried remains) we still need to improve the knowledge about the morphological markers useful in maggots and adult identification. Some species are identifiable only analyzing the male genitalia (adult specimens) and very few specialists around the world are capable of that (e.g., Pape and Richet). For these reasons many authors are interested in the genetic identification of this *taxon* of flies using different methods (Stamper et al., 2013; Chimeno et al, 2019; Buenaventura et al., 2018; Chen et al., 2018). Thus, molecular methods can be useful in determining species identification in forensic entomology.

For the reasons noted above, forensic entomologists engage in several practices to aid in identification of specimens. If possible, they will raise part of the collected specimens to maturity (thus aiding in physical identification). Often the samples delivered to the forensic laboratory are preserved in EtOH. In this case, if they are too young for the morphological analysis, they lose their utility both in PMI evaluation and in the dislocation of the corpse. Since ethanol is a DNA preservative, these specimens can be analyzed with PCR and gene sequencing to determine species identity.

The identification of insects for forensic purposes has been well studied for several taxa (Stevens et al., 2002; Wells and Stevens, 2008). A full description of the process of molecular identification of forensically important insects can be found in Tarone et al. (2015). The general strategy is to amplify through PCR a genetic locus that is found in all species, with conserved enough sequences to allow primer binding, but also divergent enough among species to differentiate among them by sequence. The ideal markers separate species into monophyletic groups. With the availability of a database of known sequences, DNA from an unknown specimen can be sequenced and it will cluster with a clade of known sequences in a monophyletic group - thus identifying the specimen. The *Cytochrome Oxidase I* and *II* loci are common targets for this analysis in insects of forensic importance. However, in some instances, they are insufficient to separate sister taxa. In those cases, other genes, such as *bicoid* (Park et al., 2013), have been used to resolve some species identifications more effectively. For example, several taxa in the *Chrysomya* and *Lucilia* are similar both morphologically and genetically and various strategies have been employed to differentiate among them as mitochondrial sequences are insufficient to resolve the relationships among related species (Stevens et al., 2002; Picard et al., 2012, 2018; Park et al., 2013; Grzywacz et al, 2017; Sontigun et al, 2018; Federico et al., 2018). With the arrival of genomic tools, there is an opportunity for resolution of some issues associated with closely related taxa, as has been done in other taxa with numerous closely related species that exhibit phylogenies that are difficult to resolve with a handful of genetic sequences (Rokas et al., 2003; Delsuc et al., 2006; Johnson et al., 2013; Gillung et al., 2018). These resources can be screened for loci that are present in all taxa of interest, but which diverge clearly among them and create clear monophyletic clusters.

14.5.2   GUT CONTENT ANALYSES TO IDENTIFY SPECIES AND INDIVIDUALS FED ON BY INSECTS

Literature refers of cases in which the identification of somebody throughout analysis of their tissue is not possible, for example because the corpse has been moved and is undetectable. In these rare cases it is possible to extract the human profile from detected insect evidence, for example, Diptera maggots and Dermestidae larvae or frass. A patricide occurred some years ago in northern Italy: the son occulted the dead father in his garage and only some days later he moved him to the place where he was discovered a couple of weeks later (Lambiase, personal data). In such cases the analysis of the entomological evidence found on the first crime scene might confirm the displacement of the cadaver.

Traditionally encountered insects in forensic entomology are not the only potential identification tools. Note the proposal by Eubanks et al. (2019) in the Hymenoptera section to leverage field deployable DNA analysis, genomic sequencing technology, and the analysis of ant colonies to identify locations of clandestine graves. Similarly, Spitaleri et al. (2006) described how they identified the victim killed in a certain house and later transported and abandoned at a beach, by analyzing a dead mosquito found in that house. Thus, a hematophagous insect may transport and preserve the human DNA of the people from which they take a bloodmeal. This property could be applied in those cases of sexual assaults where the guilty is affect by parasitosis—lice or mites for example. They are hematophagous arthropods and they are transmitted very easily and quickly from person to person. The identification of such a specimen on a healthy sexually abused victim could address to the identification of the guilty.

While the identification of an individual through their DNA in a forensically important tool, it is also important to confirm if an insect in evidence was feeding on human tissue in some cases. In instances where decedents passed away, or are hidden, in filthy locations (e.g., a body found in a dumpster or an apartment full of refuse), it is possible that an insect collected from a body may not have been feeding on human remains. This situation may impact interpretation of entomological analyses and can also be addressed by gut content analysis of evidentiary insects (Linville et al., 2004). Genetic analyses of insect gut contents, typically with *cytochrome b* primers targeting vertebrates in general and humans specifically, can be used to determine if an insect was feeding on human versus animal remains. As genomic technologies are developed, it is possible that these applications may be done in the field. For instance, nanopore sequencing technologies have enabled field sampling of Antarctic microbial mats (Johnson et al., 2017), *Arabidopsis* specimens in the United Kingdom (Parker et al., 2017), and herpetological samples in the rainforest (Pomeranz et al., 2018).

The history of the entomogenetic methods applied to the human identification shows that the interest in this field of the forensic entomology has grown quite closed to the use of the traditional entomology in criminal investigations (Boakye, 1999; Wells et al., 2001; Zehner, 2004) and today it could represent the future of the forensic entomology itself. Successful human DNA extraction is possible when sample is degraded and, in according to the kind of insect, also at many hours from their last meal (Pilli et al, 2016; Schal, 2018).

14.5.3   *ENTOMOTOXICOLOGY*

The analysis of DNA from insect evidence is not the only molecular information that can be gleaned from them. Another important form of molecular evidence that can be found in insect specimens is toxicological. As insects feed, they ingest and metabolize the compounds endogenous to the remains. Such compounds can include any drugs (licit or illicit) ingested by a decedent. This information could be helpful directly in death investigations in rare instances where tissue from the decedent is not available for analysis but insects from them are, by providing information regarding the presence (but not dose) of drugs in their system at the moment of death. However, this information is also important for interpreting results from the analyses of insect age from specimens collected off of remains. Drugs can impact insect growth and development. Thus, their presence can affect any estimate insect of insect age relying on size or developmental progress. A detailed description of the field can be found in Goff and Lord (2010). However, an important point from this field that relates to concepts presented here is worth discussing. While some carrion feeding insects are impacted by the presence of chemicals in the human body – not all of them are impacted by all compounds, nor are they necessarily affected in the same way. For example, *Boettscherina peregrina* increases development rate when fed morphine (Goff et al., 1991), but evidence for *Lucilia sericata* suggests a slowing of development (Hedouin et al., 1999). Thus, the interpretation of results from entomotoxicological analyses is linked to species identity.

Entomotoxicological analysis could also be used for the detection of the Ethyl glucuronide (EtG) and ethyl sulfate (EtS), specific and sensitive biomarkers for the diagnosis of acute or chronic alcohol abuse (Lambiase et al., 2017).

In addition, a concept not generally considered in discussions of ento-motoxicology is the presence of antibiotics. As noted earlier, bacteria play an important role in the recruitment of some species known to be primary colonizers of remains. Thus, the presence of antibiotics could alter the micro-biome of a decedent and alter the attractiveness of remains to one or more potential colonizers. One type of case known to be challenging in forensic entomology are instances where insects have not colonized a decedent, espe-cially under circumstances where they would be expected to do so (Greenberg and Kunich, 2002). In these scenarios, the presence of antibiotics (or other compounds expected to alter the microbiome of a decedent) may be impor-tant information that could help to explain these atypical cases. In addition, genomic technologies have enhanced the ability to evaluate microbes and their correlations with features of interest (e.g., time of death) in death inves-tigations (Pechal et al., 2014, 2018; Metcalf et al., 2016). These studies iden-tify common taxa (e.g., the *Proteus* and *Ignatzschineria* genera) in relatively high or low abundance at different points in the decomposition process. At the moment, such analyses rely heavily on 16S or meta-genomic sequencing strategies, which provide community-wide information regarding microbial taxa associated with remains. Microbes are also associated with variation in development and survival of forensically relevant fly species (Ahmad et al., 2006; Barnes and Gennard, 2011; Crooks et al., 2016), thus treatment with antibiotics may alter microbial communities, and the resulting phenotypes of flies feeding on those communities. Current technologies have set the stage for a deeper understanding of when (or if) such effects are expected to be common, and of large or small effect, in realistic conditions.

14.6 CONCLUSIONS

Forensic entomology uses entomological (or other arthropod) evidence to provide information to the court regarding a variety of types of cases. Experts can be called to address questions as varied as when someone died, how someone died, when a food supply was infested, or if the protective measures to prevent insect damage to a building were sufficient. In all of these instances, the identity of the insect in question is critical to determining answers to those questions. While some insects can be identified easily by their morphological traits, some cannot - or cannot be easily identified without obtaining the services of a highly specialized expert. In addition, some developmental stages of insects are easier to identify than others. In these cases genetic technologies can be useful in determining the identities of insects in evidence. However, this is not the only use for genetic applications in forensic entomology. Gene expression and related markers are being identified for a variety of forensically important points in development and environmental conditions. The next-generation sequencing is being used to dissect the relationship between insects and the microbiome. In addition, gut content analyses of insects can be important in making forensically important linkages between individuals and specific scenarios or locations while also confirming that insects in evidence were feeding on what they are assumed to be feeding on. Thus, forensic analysts should not overlook insects and arthropods present at their investigations and should be aware of the potential genetic approaches that can enhance such applications.

KEYWORDS

- forensic entomology
- identification
- entomotoxicology
- gut content genetic analysis
- clandestine grave

REFERENCES

Ahmad, A., A. Broce, L. Zurek. Evaluation of significance of bacteria in larval development of *Cochliomyia macellaria* (Diptera: Calliphoridae). *J. Med. Entomol.* **2006**, 43, 1129–1133.

Amendt, J., C. P. Campobasso, E. Gaudry, C Reiter, H. N. LeBlanc, M. J. Hall. Best practice in forensic entomology—Standards and guidelines. *Int. J. Legal Med.* **2007**, 121, 90–104.

Andere, A. A., R. N. Platt, D. A. Ray, C. J. Picard. Genome sequence of *Phormia regina* Meigen (Diptera: Calliphoridae): Implications for medical, veterinary and forensic research. *BMC Genomics* **2016**, 17, 842.

Anderson, G.S. Decomposition and invertebrate colonization of cadavers in coastal marine environments. *Current Concepts in Forensic Entomology.* Springer, **2009**, pp. 223–272.

Anderson, G.S., L.S. Bell. Impact of marine submergence and season on faunal colonization and decomposition of pig carcasses in the Salish Sea. *PLoS One.* **2016**, 11, e0149107.

Anstead, C. A., P. K. Korhonen, N. D. Young, R. S. Hall, A. R. Jex, S. C. Murali, D. S. Hughes, S. F. Lee, T. Perry, A. J. Stroehlein. *Lucilia cuprina* genome unlocks parasitic fly biology to underpin future interventions. *Nat. Commun.* **2015**, 6, 7344.

Atwell, S., Y. S. Huang, B. J. Vilhjalmsson, G. Willems, M. Horton, Y. Li, D. Meng, A. Platt, A. M. Tarone, T. T. Hu, R. Jiang, N. W. Muliyati, X. Zhang, M. A. Amer, I. Baxter, B. Brachi, J. Chory, C. Dean, M. Debieu, J. de Meaux, J. R. Ecker, N. Faure, J. M. Kniskern, J. D. Jones, T. Michael, A. Nemri, F. Roux, D. E. Salt, C. Tang, M. Todesco, M. B. Traw, D. Weigel, P. Marjoram, J. O. Borevitz, J. Bergelson, M. Nordborg. Genome-wide association study of 107 phenotypes in *Arabidopsis thaliana* inbred lines. *Nature* **2010**, 465, 627–631.

Barnes, K. M., D. E. Gennard. The effect of bacterially-dense environments on the development and immune defences of the blowfly *Lucilia sericata*. *Physiol. Entomol.* **2011**, 36, 96–100.

Baumgartner, D. L. Review of *Chrysomya rufifacies* (Diptera: Calliphoridae). *J. Med. Entomol.* **1993**, 30, 338–352.

Baust, J. G., J. S. Edwards. Mechanisms of freezing tolerance in an Antarctic midge, *Belgica antarctica*. *Physiol. Entomol.* **1979**, 4, 1–5.

Benbow, M. E., J. K. Tomberlin, A. M. Tarone. *Carrion ecology, evolution, and their applications.* CRC Press, Boca Raton, FL, USA, **2015**.

Bertone, M. A., M. Leong, K. M. Bayless, T. L. Malow, R. R. Dunn, M. D. Trautwein. Arthropods of the great indoors: Characterizing diversity inside urban and suburban homes. *PeerJ.* **2016**, 4, e1582.

Blanckenhorn, W. Quantitative genetics of life history traits in coprophagous and necrophagous insects. In: *Carrion ecology, evolution, and their applications*; M.E. Benbow, J.K. Tomberlin, A.M. Tarone (Eds.), CRC Press, pp. 333–352, **2015**.

Boakye, D. A., J. Tang, P. Truc, A. Merriweather, T. R. Unnasch. Identification of bloodmeals in haematophagous Diptera by *cytochrome B* heteroduplex analysis. *Med. Vet. Entomol.* **1999**, 13, 282–7.

Boehme, P., P. Spahn, J. Amendt, R. Zehner. Differential gene expression during metamorphosis: a promising approach for age estimation of forensically important *Calliphora vicina* pupae (Diptera: Calliphoridae). *Int. J. Legal Med.* **2013**, 127, 243–249.

Boehme, P., P. Spahn, J. Amendt, R. Zehner. The analysis of temporal gene expression to estimate the age of forensically important blow fly pupae: Results from three blind studies. *Int. J. Legal Med.* **2014**, 128, 565–573.

Bornemissza, G. F. An analysis of arthropod succession in carrion and the effect its decomposition on the soil fauna. *Aust. J. Zool.* **1957**, 5, 1–12.

Brundage, A., M. E. Benbow, J. K. Tomberlin. Priority effects on the life-history traits of two carrion blow fly (Diptera, Calliphoridae) species. *Ecol. Entomol.* **2014**, 39, 539–547.

Buenaventura, E., C. Valverde-Castrob, M. Wolffb, O. Triana-Chavezc, A. Gómez-Palaciod. DNA barcoding for identifying synanthropic flesh flies (Diptera, Sarcophagidae) of Colombia. *Acta Tropica* **2018**, 182, 291–297.

Byard, R. W. Autopsy problems associated with postmortem ant activity. *Forensic Sci. Med. Pathol.* **2005**, 1, 37–40.

Bybee, S. M., Q. Hansen, S. Buesse, H. M. Cahill Wightman, M. A. Branham. For consistency's sake: The precise use of larva, nymph and naiad within Insecta. *Syst. Entomol.* **2015**, 40, 667–670.

Byrd, J. H., J. L. Castner. *Forensic entomology: The utility of arthropods in legal investigations.* CRC Press, **2010**.

Charabidze, D., M. Gosselin. *Insectes, Cadavres, Scènes de Crime. Principes et Applications de l'Entomologie Medico-Legale.* De Boeck Supérieur Ed., p. 261, **2014**.

Chena, W., Y. Shanga, L. Rena, K. Xieb, X. Zhanga, C. Zhanga, S. Suna, Y. Wanga, L. Zhaa, Y. Guoa. Developing a MtSNP-based genotyping system for genetic identification of forensically important flesh flies (Diptera: Sarcophagidae). *Forensic Sci. Int.* **2018**, 290, 178–188.

Chimeno, C., J. Moriniére, J. Podhorna, L. Hardulak, A. Hausmann, F. Reckel, J. E. Grunwald, R. Penning, G. Haszprunar. DNA barcoding in forensic entomology—Establishing a DNA reference library of potentially forensic relevant arthropod species. *J. Forensic Sci.* **2019**, 64, 593–601.

Crooks, E. R., M. T. Bulling, K. M. Barnes. Microbial effects on the development of forensically important blow fly species. *Forensic Sci. Int.* **2016**, 266, 185–190.

De Block, M., R. Stoks. Fitness effects from egg to reproduction: Bridging the life history transition. *Ecology* **2005**, 86, 185–197.

Delsuc, F., H. Brinkmann, D. Chourrout, H. Philippe. Tunicates and not cephalochordates are the closest living relatives of vertebrates. *Nature* **2006**, 439, 965.

Eubanks, M. D., C. Lin, A. M. Tarone. The role of ants in vertebrate carrion decomposition. *Food Webs* **2019**, 10, e00109.

Federico C., D. Lombardo, N. La Porta, A. M. Pappalardo, V. Ferritc, F. Lombardo, S. Saccone. Rapid molecular identification of necrophagous Diptera by means of variable-length intron sequences in the wingless gene. *J. Forensic Legal Med.* **2018**, 56, 66–72.

Fremdt, H., J. Amendt, R. Zehner. Diapause-specific gene expression in *Calliphora vicina* (Diptera: Calliphoridae)—A useful diagnostic tool for forensic entomology. *Int. J. Legal Med.* **2014**, 128, 1001–1011.

Gallagher, M. B., S. Sandhu, R. Kimsey. Variation in developmental time for geographically distinct populations of the common green bottle fly, *Lucilia sericata* (Meigen). *J. Forensic Sci.* **2010**, 55, 438–442.

Gennard, D. *Forensic entomology: An introduction.* John Wiley & Sons, **2012**.

Gherardi, M., Lambiase S. Miasi ed entomologia forense: segnalazione casistica. *La riv. italiana di med. Leg.* **2006**, 28, 617–628.

Gillung, J. P., S. L. Winerton, K. M. Bayless, Z. Khouri, M. L. Borowiec, D. Yeates, L. S. Kimsey, B. Mishof, S. Shin, X. Zhou, C. Mayer. Anchored phylogenomics unravels the evolution of spider flies (Diptera: Acroceridae) and reveals discordance between nucleotides and amino acids. *Mol. Phylogenetics Evol.* **2018**, 128, 233–245.

Goff, M., W. D. Lord. Insect as toxicological indicator and the impact of drugs and toxin on insect development. In: *Forensic entomology: The utility of using arthropods in legal investigations*, J.H. Byrd and J. L. Castner (Eds.), 427–434, **2010**.

Goff, M. L., W. A. Brown, K. Hewadikaram, A. Omori. Effect of heroin in decomposing tissues on the development rate of *Boettcherisca peregrina* (Diptera, Sarcophagidae) and implications of this effect on estimation of postmortem intervals using arthropod development patterns. *J. Forensic Sci.* **1991**, 36, 537–542.

Grassberger, M., C. Frank. Temperature-related development of the parasitoid wasp *Nasonia vitripennis* as forensic indicator. *Med. Vet. Entomol.* **2003**, 17, 257–262.

Grassberger, M., et al. *C. vicina* from Austria, Spain, Greece and Scotland—Are there any differences in development. 5th EAFE meeting, 2nd–5th May 2007, Brussels (Belgium).

Greenberg, B., J. C. Kunich. *Entomology and the law: Flies as forensic indicators.* Cambridge University Press, **2002**.

Grzywacz, A., D. Wyborska, M. Piwczyński. DNA barcoding allows identification of European Fanniidae (Diptera) of forensic interest. *Forensic Sci. Int.* **2017**, 278, 106–114.

Hahn, D. A., G. J. Ragland, D. D. Shoemaker, D. L. Denlinger. Gene discovery using massively parallel pyrosequencing to develop ESTs for the flesh fly *Sarcophaga crassipalpis*. *BMC Genomics* **2009**, 10, 234.

Hedouin, V., B. Bourel, L. Martin-Bouyer, A. Becart, G. Tournel, M. Deveaux, D. Gosset. Determination of drug levels in larvae of *Lucilia sericata* (Diptera: Calliphoridae) reared on rabbit carcasses containing morphine. *J. Forensic Sci.* **1999**, 44, 351–353.

Hjelmen, C.E., J.J. Parrott, S.P. Srivastav, A.S. McGuane, L.L. Ellis, A.D. Stewart, J.S. Johnston, A.M. Tarone. Effect of phenotype selection on genome size variation in two species of diptera. *Genes* **2020**, 11, 218.

Hewadikaram, K. A., M. L. Goff. Effect of carcass size on rate of decomposition and arthropod succession patterns. *Am. J. Forensic Med. Pathol.* **1991**, 12(3), 235–240.

Hughes, J., A. P. Vogler. Gene expression in the gut of keratin-feeding clothes moths *Tineola* and keratin beetles *Trox* revealed by subtracted cDNA libraries. *Insect Biochem. Mol. Biol.* **2006**, 36, 584–592.

Johnson, B. R., M. L. Borowiec, J. C. Chiu, E. K. Lee, J. Atallah, P. S. Ward. Phylogenomics resolves evolutionary relationships among ants, bees, and wasps. *Curr. Biol.* **2013**, 23, 2058–2062.

Johnson, S. S., E. Zaikova, D. S. Goerlitz, Y. Bai, S. W. Tighe. Real-time DNA sequencing in the Antarctic dry valleys using the Oxford Nanopore sequencer. *J. Biochem. Technol.* **2017**, 28, 2.

Klopfstein, S., L. Vilhelmsen, J. M. Heraty, M. Sharkey, F. Ronquist. The hymenopteran tree of life: Evidence from protein-coding genes and objectively aligned ribosomal data. *PLoS One* **2013**, 8, e69344.

Krishnan, M., V. M. Ugaz, M. A. Burns. PCR in a Rayleigh-Benard convection cell. *Science* **2002**, 298, 793.

Lambiase, S., A. Groppi, D. Gemmellaro, L. Luca Morini. Evaluation of ethyl glucuronide and ethyl sulfate in *Calliphora vicina* as potential biomarkers for ethanol intake. *J. Anal. Toxicol.* **2017**, 41, 17–21.

Lawrence, J. F., A. Slipinski, A. E. Seago, M. K. Thayer, A. F. Newton, and A. E. Marvaldi. Phylogeny of the *Coleoptera* based on morphological characters of adults and larvae. *Ann. Zool.* **2011**, 61, 1–217.

Lee, S. F., Z. Z. Chen, A. McGrath, R. T. Good, P. Batterham. Identification, analysis, and linkage mapping of expressed sequence tags from the Australian sheep blowfly. *BMC Genomics* **2011**, 12, 406.

Linville, J. G., J. Hayes, J. D. Wells. Mitochodrial DNA and STR analyses of maggot crop contents: Effect of specimen preservation technique. *J. Forensic Sci.* **2004**, 49, 1–4.

Liu, W., M. Longnecker, A. M. Tarone, J. K. Tomberlin. Responses of *Lucilia sericata* (Diptera: Calliphoridae) to compounds from microbial decomposition of larval resources. *Anim. Behav.* **2016**, 115, 217–225.

Lopez-Martinez, G., M. A. Elnitsky, J. B. Benoit, R. E. Lee Jr, D. L. Denlinger. High resistance to oxidative damage in the Antarctic midge *Belgica antarctica*, and developmentally linked expression of genes encoding superoxide dismutase, catalase and heat shock proteins. *Insect Biochem. Mol. Biol.* **2008**, 38, 796–804.

Ma, Q., A. Fonseca, W. Q. Liu, A. T. Fields, M. L. Pimsler, A. F. Spindola, A. M. Tarone, T. L. Crippen, J. K. Tomberlin, T. K. Wood. *Proteus mirabilis* interkingdom swarming signals attract blow flies. *ISME J.* **2012**, 6, 1356–1366.

Martinson, E. O., J. Peyton, Y. D. Kelkar, E. C. Jennings, J. B. Benoit, J. H. Werren, D. L. Denlinger. Genome and ontogenetic-based transcriptomic analyses of the flesh fly, *Sarcophaga bullata*. *G3: Genes Genomes Genet.* **2019**, 9, 1313–1320.

Matuszewski, S. Estimating the pre-appearance interval from temperature in *Necrodes littoralis* L.(Coleoptera: Silphidae). *Forensic Sci. Int.* **2011**, 212, 180–188.

Matuszewski, S., A. Mądra-Bielewicz. Validation of temperature methods for the estimation of pre-appearance interval in carrion insects. *Forensic Sci. Med. Pathol.* **2016**, 12, 50–57.

Matuszewski, S., M. Szafałowicz. Temperature-dependent appearance of forensically useful beetles on carcasses. *Forensic Sci. Int.* **2013**, 229, 92–99.

McKnight, B. E. *The washing away of wrongs (Sung Tz'u, 1186–1249): Forensic medicine in thirteenth-century China.* Brian E. McKnight (Trans. and Ed.). United States: Center for Chinese Studies, University of Michigan, p. 181, **1981**.

Mégnin, J. P. *La faune des cadavres: application de l'entomologie à la medicine légale.* *L'Encyclopédie Scientifique des Aide-mémoire*, Paris: Masson et Gauthier-Villaars, **1894**.

Megyesi, M., S. P. Nawrocki, N. H. Haskell. Using accumulated degree-days to estimate the postmortem interval from decomposed human remains. *J. Forensic Sci.* **2005**, 50, 1–9.

Metcalf, J. L., Z. Z. Xu, S. Weiss, S. Lax, W. Van Treuren, E. R. Hyde, S. J. Song, A. Amir, P. Larsen, N. Sangwan. Microbial community assembly and metabolic function during mammalian corpse decomposition. *Science* **2016**, 351, 158–162.

Michaud, J.-P., G. Moreau. Facilitation may not be an adequate mechanism of community succession on carrion. *Oecologia* **2017**, 183, 1143–1153.

Michaud, J.-P., K. G. Schoenly, G. Moreau. Rewriting ecological succession history: Did carrion ecologists get there first? *Quart. Rev. Biol.* **2015**, 90, 45–66.

Owings, C. G., C. Spiegelman, A. M. Tarone, J. K. Tomberlin. Developmental variation among *Cochliomyia macellaria* Fabricius (Diptera: Calliphoridae) populations from three ecoregions of Texas, USA. *Int. J. Legal Med.* **2014**, 128, 709–717.

Park, S. H., C. H. Park, Y. Zhang, H. Piao, U. Chung, S. Y. Kim, K. S. Ko, C. H. Yi, T. H. Jo, J. J. Hwang. Using the developmental gene *bicoid* to identify species of forensically important blowflies (Diptera: Calliphoridae). *BioMed Res. Int.* **2013**, 2013, 538051.

Parker, J., A. J. Helmstetter, D. Devey, T. Wilkinson, A. S. Papadopulos. Field-based species identification of closely-related plants using real-time nanopore sequencing. *Sci. Rep.* **2017**, 7, 8345.

Pastula, E. C., R. W. Merritt. Insect arrival pattern and succession on buried carrion in Michigan. *J. Med. Entomol.* **2013**, 50, 432–439.

Payne, J. A. A summer carrion study on the baby pig *Sus scrofa* Linnaeus. *Ecology* **1965**, 46, 592–602.

Payne, J. A., E. W. King. Lepidoptera associated with pig carrion. *J. Lepidopterists' Soc.* **1969**, 23, 191–195.

Pechal, J. L., T. L. Crippen, M. E. Benbow, A. M. Tarone, S. Dowd, J. K. Tomberlin. The potential use of bacterial community succession in forensics as described by high throughput metagenomic sequencing. *Int. J. Legal Med.* **2014**, 128, 193–205.

Pechal, J. L., T. L. Crippen, A. M. Tarone, A. J. Lewis, J. K. Tomberlin, M. E. Benbow. Microbial community functional change during vertebrate carrion decomposition. *PLoS One* **2013**, 8, e79035.

Pechal, J. L., C. J. Schmidt, H. R. Jordan, M. E. Benbow. A large-scale survey of the postmortem human microbiome, and its potential to provide insight into the living health condition. *Sci. Rep.* **2018**, 8, 5724.

Perez, A. E., N. H. Haskell, J. D. Wells. Evaluating the utility of hexapod species for calculating a confidence interval about a succession based postmortem interval estimate. *Forensic Sci. Int.* **2014**, 241, 91–95.

Picard, C. J., M. H. Villet, J. D. Wells. Amplified fragment length polymorphism confirms reciprocal monophyly in *Chrysomya putoria* and *Chrysomya chloropyga*: A correction of reported shared mtDNA haplotypes. *Med. Vet. Entomol.* **2012**, 26, 116–119.

Picard, C. J., J. D. Wells, A. Ullyot, K. Rognes. Amplified fragment length polymorphism analysis supports the valid separate species status of *Lucilia caesar* and *L. illustris* (Diptera: Calliphoridae). *Forensic Sci. Res.* **2018**, 3, 60–64.

Pilli, E., et al. Human identification by lice: A next generation sequencing challenge. *Forensic Sci. Int.* **2016**, 266, e71–e78.

Pimsler, M. L., T. Pape, J. S. Johnston, R. A. Wharton, J. J. Parrott, D. Restuccia, M. R. Sanford, J. K. Tomberlin, and A. M. Tarone. Structural and genetic investigation of the egg and first-instar larva of an egg-laying population of *Blaesoxipha plinthopyga* (Diptera: Sarcophagidae), a species of forensic importance. *J. Med. Entomol.* **2014**, 51, 1283–1295.

Pimsler, M. L., S.-H. Sze, S. Saenz, S. Fu, J. K. Tomberlin, A.M. Tarone. Gene expression correlates of facultative predation in the blow fly *Chrysomya rufifacies* (Diptera: Calliphoridae). *Ecol. Evol.* **2019**, 9(15), 8690–8701.

Pomerantz, A., N. Penafiel, A. Arteaga, L. Bustamante, F. Pichardo, L. A. Coloma, C. L. Barrio-Amoros, D. Salazar-Valenzuela, S. Prost. Real-time DNA barcoding in a rainforest using nanopore sequencing: Opportunities for rapid biodiversity assessments and local capacity building. *GigaScience* **2018**, 7, giy033.

Priye, A., S. Wong, Y. Bi, M. Carpio, J. Chang, M. Coen, D. Cope, J. Harris, J. Johnson, A. Keller. Lab-on-a-drone: Toward pinpoint deployment of smartphone-enabled nucleic acid-based diagnostics for mobile health care. *Anal. Chem.* **2016**, 88, 4651–4660.

Reed, H. B. A study of dog carcass communities in Tennessee, with special references to insect. *Am. Midl. Nat.* **1958**, 59, 213–245.

Regier, J. C., A. Zwick, M. P. Cummings, A. Y. Kawahara, S. Cho, S. Weller, A. Roe, J. Baixeras, J. W. Brown, C. Parr. Toward reconstructing the evolution of advanced moths and butterflies (Lepidoptera: Ditrysia): An initial molecular study. *BMC Evol. Biol.* **2009**, 9, 280.

Rhinesmith-Carranza, J., W. Liu, J. K. Tomberlin, M. Longnecker, A. M. Tarone. Impacts of dietary amino acid composition and microbial presence on preference and performance of immature *Lucilia sericata* (Diptera: Calliphoridae). *Ecol. Entomol.* **2018**, 43, 612–620.

Rivers, D. B., G. A. Dahlem. *The science of forensic entomology*. John Wiley & Sons, **2014**.

Rodriguez, W., W. Bass. Insect activity and its relationship to decay rates of human cadavers in east Tennessee. *J. Forensic Sci.* **1983**, 28 (2), 423–432.

Rokas, A., B. L. Williams, N. King, S. B. Carroll. Genome-scale approaches to resolving incongruence in molecular phylogenies. *Nature* **2003**, 425, 798.

Sanford, M.R., T.L. Whitworth, D.R. Phatak. Human wound colonization by *Lucilia eximia* and Chrysomya rufifacies (Diptera: Calliphoridae): myiasis, perimortem, or postmortem colonization? *J. Med. Entomol.* **2014**, 51, 716–719.

Sanford, M. R. Insects and associated arthropods analyzed during medicolegal death investigations in Harris County, Texas, USA: January 2013-April 2016. *PLoS One* **2017**, 12, e0179404.

Schal, C., N. Czado, R. Gamble, A. Barrett, K. Weathers, K. M. Lodhi. Isolation, identification, and time course of human DNA typing from bed bugs, *Cimex lectularius*. *Forensic Sci. Int.* **2018**, 293, 1–6.

Schoenly, K., W. Reid. Dynamics of heterotrophic succession in carrion arthropod assemblages: Discrete seres or a continuum of change? *Oecologia* **1987**, 73, 192–202.

Schwalman, F. Insect morphogenesis. *Monograph in developmental biology*; vol 20. Sauer (Ed.). Karger, p. 356, **1988**.

Seguy, E. *La biologie des Diptéres*. Paris: Paul Lechevelier, p. 609, **1950**.

Sontigun, N., K. L. Sukontason, J. Amendt, B. K. Zajac, R. Zehner, K. Sukontason, T. Chareonviriyaphap, A. Wannasan. Molecular analysis of forensically important blow flies in Thailand. *Insects* **2018**, 9, 159.

Spitaleri, S., C. Romano, E. Di Luise, E. Ginestra, L. Saravo. Genotyping of human DNA recovered from mosquitoes found on a crime scene. *Int. Congr. Ser.* **2006**, 1288, 574–576.

Stamper, T., G. A. Dahlem, C. Cookman, R. W. DeBry. Phylogenetic relationships of flesh flies in the subfamily Sarcophaginae based on three mtDNA fragments (Diptera: Sarcophagidae). *Syst. Entomol.* **2013**, 38, 35–44.

Stevens, J.R., R. Wall, J.D. Wells. Paraphyly in Hawaiin hybrid blowfly populations and the evolutionary history of anthropophilic species. *Insect Mol. Biol.* **2002**, 11, 141–148.

Stoker, R. L., W. E. Grant, S. B. Vinson. *Solenopsis invicta* (Hymenoptera: Formicidae) effect on invertebrate decomposers of carrion in central Texas. *Environ. Entomol.* **1995**, 24, 817–822.

Suss, L. Gli intrusi. *Guida di entomologia urbana*. Bologna: Calderini Edagricole, pp. 226, **1990**.

Suss, L., A. Gelosi. *Insetti e acari dei cereali in magazzino*. Bologna: Calderini Edagricole, pp. 108, **1991**.

Suss, L., D. P. Locatelli. *I parassiti delle derrate*. Bologna: Calderini Edagricole, pp. 363, **2001**.

Sze, S. H., J. P. Dunham, B. Carey, P. L. Chang, F. Li, R. M. Edman, C. Fjeldsted, M. J. Scott, S. V. Nuzhdin, A. M. Tarone. A de novo transcriptome assembly of *Lucilia sericata* (Diptera: Calliphoridae) with predicted alternative splices, single nucleotide polymorphisms and transcript expression estimates. *Insect Mol. Biol.* **2012**, 21, 205–221.

Szpila, K. Key for the identification of third instars of European blowflies (Diptera: Calliphoridae) of forensic importance. In: *Current concepts in forensic entomology*. Springer, pp. 43–56, **2009**.

Szpila, K., J. G. Voss, T. Pape. A new Dipteran forensic indicator in buried bodies. *Med. Vet. Entomol.* **2010**, 24, 278–283.

Tarone, A. M. Ecological genetics. In: *Carrion ecology, evolution, and their applications*. CRC Press, pp. 308–347, **2015**.

Tarone, A.M., D. R. Foran. Generalized additive models and *Lucilia sericata* growth: Assessing confidence intervals and error rates in forensic entomology. *J. Forensic Sci.* **2008**, 53, 942–948.

Tarone, A. M., D. R. Foran. Gene expression during blow fly development: Improving the precision of age estimates in forensic entomology. *J. Forensic Sci.* **2011**, 56 (1), S112–122.

Tarone, A. M., K. C. Jennings, D. R. Foran. Aging blow fly eggs using gene expression: A feasibility study. *J. Forensic Sci.* **2007**, 52, 1350–1354.

Tarone, A. M., C. J. Picard, S.-H. Sze. *Genomic tools to reduce error in PMI estimates derived from entomological evidence*. National Institute of Justice, **2016**.

Tarone, A. M., M. R. Sanford. Is PMI the hypothesis or the null hypothesis? *J. Med. Entomol.* **2017**, 54, 1109–1115.

Tarone, A. M., B. Singh, C. J. Picard. *Molecular biology in forensic entomology*. In: *Forensic entomology: International dimensions and frontiers*; J. K. Tomberlin, M. E. Benbow (Eds.), pp. 297–316, **2015**.

Tomberlin, J. K., M. E. Benbow. *Forensic entomology: International dimensions and frontiers*. CRC Press, **2015**.

Tomberlin, J. K., M. E. Benbow, A. M. Tarone, R. M. Mohr. Basic research in evolution and ecology enhances forensics. *Trends Ecol. Evol.* **2011**, 26, 53–55.

Tomberlin, J. K., T. L. Crippen, A. M. Tarone, B. Singh, K. Adams, Y. H. Rezenom, M. E. Benbow, M. Flores, M. Longnecker, J. L. Pechal, D. H. Russell, R. C. Beier, T. K. Wood. Interkingdom responses of flies to bacteria mediated by fly physiology and bacterial quorum sensing. *Anim. Behav.* **2012**, 84, 1449–1456.

Turner, T. L., A. D. Stewart, A. T. Fields, W. R. Rice, A. M. Tarone. Population-based resequencing of experimentally evolved populations reveals the genetic basis of body size variation in *Drosophila melanogaster*. *PLoS Genet.* **2011**, 7(3), e1001336.

Wall, R., K. Pitts, K. Smith. Pre-adult mortality in the blowfly *Lucilia sericata*. *Med. Vet. Entomol.* **2001**, 15, 328–334.

Walter, M. F., L. L. Zeineh, B. C. Black, W. E. McIvor, T. R. Wright, H. Biessmann. Catecholamine metabolism and in vitro induction of premature cuticle melanization in wild type and pigmentation mutants of *Drosophila melanogaster*. *Arch. Insect Biochem. Physiol.* **1996**, 31, 219–233.

Wang, Y., Z. Y. Gu, S. X. Xia, J. F. Wang, Y. N. Zhang, L. Y. Tao. Estimating the age of *Lucilia illustris* during the intrapuparial period using two approaches: Morphological changes and differential gene expression. *Forensic Sci. Int.* **2018**, 287, 1–11.

Wells, J., B. Greenberg. Interaction between *Chrysomya rufifacies* and *Cochliomyia macellaria* (Diptera: Calliphoridae): The possible consequences of an invasion. *Bull. Entomol. Res.* **1992**, 82, 133–137.

Wells, J. D., B. Greenberg. Effect of the red imported fire ant (Hymenoptera: Formicidae) and carcass type on the daily occurrence of postfeeding carrion-fly larvae (Diptera: Calliphoridae, Sarcophagidae). *J. Med. Entomol.* **1994**, 31, 171–174.

Wells, J. D., J. R. Stevens. Application of DNA-based methods in forensic entomology. *Annu. Rev. Entomol.* **2008**, 53, 103–120.

Wells, J. D., F. J. Introna, G. Di Vella, C. P. Campobasso, J. Hayes, F. A. Sperling. Human and insect mitochondrial DNA analysis from maggots. *J. Forensic Sci.* **2001**, 46, 685–687.

Whitworth, T. Keys to the genera and species of blow flies (Diptera: Calliphoridae) of America north of Mexico. *Proc. Entomol. Soc. Wash.* **2006**, 108. 689–725.

Wilder, S. M., D. Raubenheimer, S. J. Simpson. Moving beyond body condition indices as an estimate of fitness in ecological and evolutionary studies. *Funct. Ecol.* **2016**, 30, 108–115.

Zajac, B., J. Amendt, M. Verhoff, R. Zehner. Dating pupae of the blow fly *Calliphora vicina* Robineau-Desvoidy 1830 (Diptera: Calliphoridae) for postmortem interval estimation: Validation of molecular age markers. *Genes* **2018**, 9, 153.

Zehner, R., J. Amendt, R. Krettek. STR typing of human DNA from fly larvae fed on decomposing bodies. *J. Forensic Sci.* **2004**, 49, 337–340.

Zhang, M., H. Yu, Y. Y. Yang, C. Song, X. J. Hu, G. R. Zhang. Analysis of the transcriptome of blowfly *Chrysomya megacephala* (Fabricius) larvae in responses to different edible oils. *PLoS One* **2013**, 8(5), e63168.

PART IV
Company Innovations

CHAPTER 15

Getting the Most Information from Every Sample: Improved Length-Based and Sequence-Based Analysis

ROHAIZAH I. JAMES

Promega Corporation, 2800 Woods Hollow Road, Madison, WI 53711, USA
E-mail: Rohaizah.james@promega.com

ABSTRACT

Forensic DNA analysts have relied on the ease and accuracy of short tandem repeat (STR) genotyping technology for many years. To further improve this trusted technology, Promega is developing 8-dye capillary electrophoresis and STR systems that allow genotyping of up to 35 loci in one amplification; thus saving samples, time, and cost. Additional time saving can be achieved by rapid processing of casework samples, where DNA can be accurately quantified and amplified without purification - a step that could compromise the DNA yield. As the future of STR analysis will include sequence-based analysis, Promega has also developed multiple massively parallel sequencing-based products for sequencing both STR loci (46 autosomal and Y) and mitochondria.

15.1 INTRODUCTION

Forensic DNA analysis has advanced tremendously in the 25 years since Promega launched the first commercial multiplex short tandem repeat (STR) genotyping kit in 1994 (Budowle et al., 1997). Over this time, STR genotyping progressed from a triplex silver stain system to the current 5-dye and 6-dye fluorescence STR amplification systems. Many aspects of the forensic DNA laboratory workflow also improved along the way. Promega has invested in laboratory workflow improvements, including developing

STR amplification kits that are compatible with both casework and direct amplification samples and a quantification kit that assess the quality of casework samples to allow quick and accurate workflow decisions (Ewing et al., 2016; Lin et al., 2018).

Further improvements in the forensic DNA laboratory workflow could be achieved by eliminating the DNA purification step altogether, whenever appropriate (Cavanaugh and Bathrick, 2018). Combining its experience in developing DNA purification reagents and STR amplification reagents that are compatible with direct amplification, Promega developed the Casework Direct Kit, a cell lysis system that is compatible with DNA quantification and STR amplification, thus removing the need for DNA purification in the workflow. This direct amplification approach could be beneficial for casework samples that are expected to have low DNA amounts and where there is a risk of DNA loss during the purification process (Cavanaugh and Bathrick, 2018). Additionally, it could be used as a quick and simple screening tool for determining the next best step for analysis, such as whether to perform autosomal STR analysis or Y-STR analysis.

New DNA genotyping technologies such as rapid DNA (discussed elsewhere in this book) and massively parallel sequencing (MPS) that offer many advantages to forensic DNA genotyping have also emerged in the last few years. However, capillary electrophoresis (CE) technology will continue to be used for many years, as it provides the best time-to-answer with limited hands-on time and cost. Promega is committed to maximizing the genotype information that can be revealed from each STR amplification and CE analysis. This will be accomplished by developing an 8-dye capillary electrophoresis (CE) instrument that will enable analysis of 8-dye fluorescence STR amplification systems. In an 8-dye system, more loci will be smaller than in a 6-dye system so that genotypes from degraded samples will be more complete and informative, thus reducing the need to repeat assays with a secondary STR system. In addition to autosomal STR markers, multiple Y-STR markers can be included in 8-dye STR systems, providing both autosomal and Y-STR information from one amplification. The Y-STR information will become more useful as more relationship-based searches in both criminal and genealogical databases are performed.

Finally, Promega is developing multiple MPS reagents to further maximize the genotype information that can be obtained from each forensic sample processed. Without the technical constraints of a finite number of dye channels on a CE, MPS reagents can be developed to sequence larger genetic marker panels. This enables analysis of more STR loci, as well as combining autosomal and Y-STR, in each amplification and revealing more information from each STR locus sequence. Mitochondrial DNA sequencing is also simplified with the PowerSeq CRM Mito, which reduces multiple labor-intensive steps in MPS.

15.2 IMPROVING LENGTH-BASED SHORT TANDEM REPEAT ANALYSIS BY INCREASING MULTIPLEXING CAPABILITIES

DNA genotyping for forensic applications is routinely performed by analyzing fluorescently labeled PCR amplicons generated in a multiplexed STR amplification reaction. The performance of commercial STR genotyping kits has significantly improved over the last decade. Modifications to amplification master mixes have reduced the time needed for PCR amplification and significantly improved tolerance to common amplification inhibitors (e.g., heme, humic acid, and tannic acid), even facilitating direct amplification protocols that eliminate the need for DNA purification. Additionally, the complexity of STR genotyping kits has increased significantly in response to requests from the forensic community for additional loci. In 2006, the European forensic community expanded and standardized the number of STR loci used (Gill et al., 2006). There is consensus on the core loci except for SE33, where some countries prefer to include the locus, others decided against its adoption. In 2017, the US forensic community expanded its core loci from 13 to 20, with additional optional loci (Hares, 2012). As a result, the most commonly used STR genotyping kits simultaneously co-amplify 17–27 loci. To accurately separate and detect 27 loci, the kits utilize six fluorescent dye labels, the maximum that can be detected by commercially available CE instruments such as the Applied Biosystems 3500 Genetic Analyzer. Five of the color channels are used to detect the fluorescently labeled amplicons and the last color channel is used to detect the Internal Lane Standard (ILS). The ILS is co-injected with every sample to help determine the size of the amplicons.

Accompanying the increased use of STR kits is the growth in DNA databases over the years (Forensic Genetics Policy Initiative, 2017), resulting in the inevitable increase of potential adventitious matches with existing STR panels used up to 2017. To reduce this potential, larger panels of STR markers started to be used. These large STR panels can result in some performance limitations with challenging samples from the use of a broad range of amplicon size. With detection using six dyes, an amplicon size range of approximately 70 to 500 bp is necessary to include all the required loci. For example, Figure 15.1 is an electropherogram of the allelic ladder provided with the PowerPlex® Fusion 6C System. This ladder contains the most

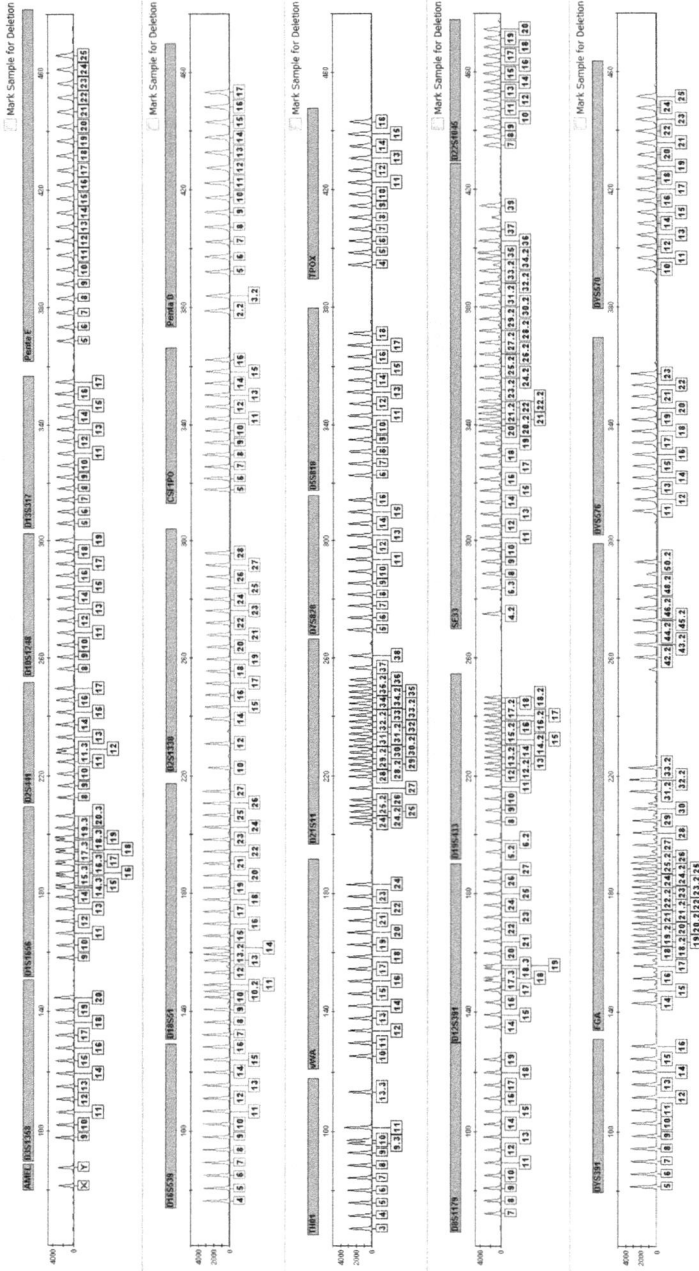

FIGURE 15.1 PowerPlex® Fusion 6C Allelic Ladder. The PowerPlex® Fusion 6C Allelic Ladder Mix was analyzed using an Applied Biosystems® 3500xL Genetic Analyzer and a 1.2 kV, 24-s injection. The sample file was analyzed with the GeneMapper® ID-X software, version 1.4, and PowerPlex® Fusion 6C panels and bins text files. (A) The FL-labeled allelic ladder components and their allele designations. (B) The JOE-labeled allelic ladder components and their allele designations. (C) The TMR-labeled allelic ladder components and their allele designations. (D) The CXR-labeled allelic ladder components and their allele designations. (E) The TOM-labeled allelic ladder components and their allele designations.

commonly encountered alleles in the human population; 431 ladder fragments in total. Additionally, almost 300 virtual bins are used to call alleles that are not represented by a ladder fragment (Promega Corporation, 2017). The use of long amplicons becomes problematic while genotyping highly degraded DNA, as commonly recovered from a crime scene, because they would be the first to "drop out." Additionally, these longer amplicons would also be more likely to dropout in the presence of amplification inhibitors. Consequently, the loci with the long amplicons provide less information with challenging forensic samples.

To address the limitation of a six-dye CE, Promega Corporation is developing a new eight-dye CE instrument, the Spectrum CE System, and accompanying eight-dye STR amplification systems. By increasing the number of fluorescent dyes that the CE instrument can detect, PCR amplicons can be generated in seven color channels; the last color channel, which is eight, will be used for the ILS. The two additional color channels enable the design of STR multiplex systems that both generate smaller amplicons and contain more loci. This is exemplified by comparing the difference between the configurations of the 6-dye PowerPlex® Fusion 6C System (Figure 15.2) with the 8-dye PowerPlex® 35GY 8C System (Figure 15.3). In the 8-dye system, alleles for 22 autosomal loci are smaller than 325 bp, compared to only 16 autosomal loci being smaller than 325 bp in the 6-dye system. The smaller loci in the 8-color system will reduce the occurrence of dropout and provide maximal information from amplification of degraded or inhibited samples.

In addition to the expanded ability to detect eight dyes, the Spectrum CE system maintains the ability to separate fragments of up to 500 bp. As Penta D is the only locus that extends beyond 325 bp in the PowerPlex® 35GY 8C System, Promega included 10 Y-STR loci in the 325–500 bp range of the other six dye channels. To provide the most information from each crime scene sample, the Y-STR loci are selected based on their high gene diversity (Ballantyne et al., 2010; Purps and Roewer, 2014). The use of 35 STR loci potentially increases the possibility of more accurately identifying the minimal number of contributors in a mixture.

Additionally, the Y-STRs could potentially provide an opportunity to simplify the familial DNA searching process. Currently, familial searching is a two-step process (Maguire et al., 2014). The first step is to search for potential male relatives of the offender in an autosomal database. The second is to exclude false potentials by matching Y-STR haplotypes. To minimize potential complications due to mutations in familial searching, as well as kinship analysis, rapidly mutating Y-STR's (Ballantyne et al., 2010) are not included in the PowerPlex® 35GY 8C System.

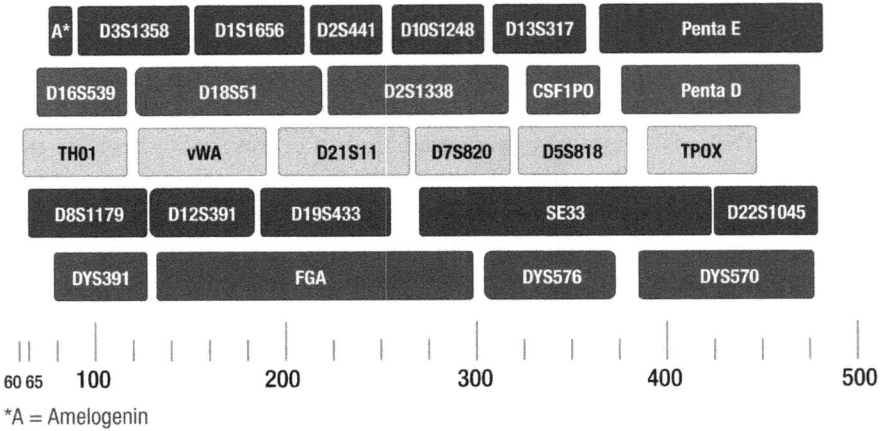

FIGURE 15.2   Configuration of the PowerPlex® Fusion 6C System.

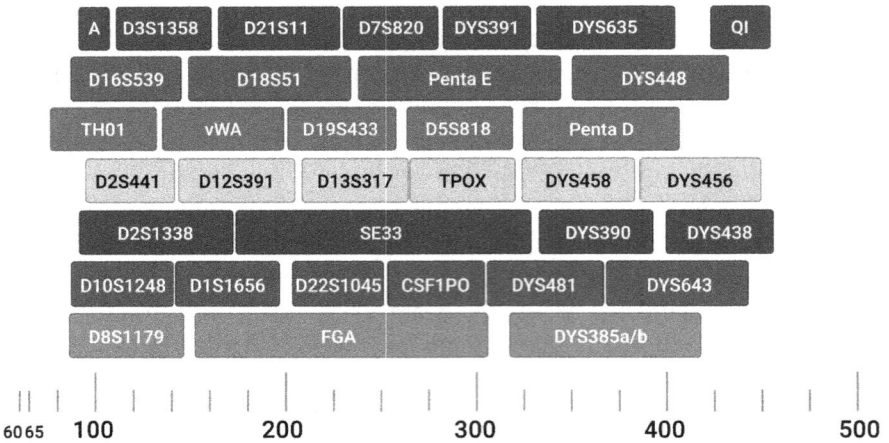

FIGURE 15.3   Configuration of the PowerPlex® 35GY 8C System.

The PowerPlex® 35GY 8C System has 35 loci, making it the largest CE-based commercial forensic DNA genotyping multiplex system. To further maximize the information from each sample, Promega included a quality indicator (QI) as the largest peak in the blue channel. The QI is designed to be sensitive to commonly found PCR inhibitors and could confirm indication of inhibitors during quantification. When direct amplification of single source reference and database samples are performed without DNA quantification, where there would be no indication of inhibitor presence, absence of STR peaks accompanied by low QI peak will indicate inhibition of the amplification reaction. However, the absence of STR peaks accompanied by high QI peak indicate the absence of DNA in the reaction. Finally, inhibited samples can be distinguished from degraded samples by the low or high QI peak heights, respectively.

This 8-dye STR system, together with the Spectrum CE system, has the potential to generate more information from each forensic crime scene and database sample than current CE-based assays. In addition to significantly enhancing the quality of STR analysis with 8-dye technology, the Spectrum CE system was designed to significantly improve efficiency with simplified sample setup and operation. It has four 96-well plate positions that are continuously accessible, allowing scientists to load and unload plates while the instrument is running. This will improve the productivity of the forensic laboratory by allowing partially full plates to be run and reducing instrument scheduling conflicts without sacrificing time or efficiency. Rush cases can be prioritized to run first even when the plate was added to the queue later. Additionally, four plate positions will increase overnight and weekend throughput without increasing the number of CE instruments.

15.3 IMPROVING LABORATORY EFFICIENCY WITH RAPID PROCESSING OF CASEWORK SAMPLES

As STR amplification systems have become more and more sensitive, forensic DNA scientists have been asked to generate data from increasingly lower amounts of input DNA, especially from touch samples gathered from property crime scenes. One way of maximizing the amount of DNA from these casework samples is the elimination of DNA purification that normally includes multiple wash steps where DNA could be lost. Instead of purifying the DNA, casework samples can be processed in one simple cell lysis step before used for STR amplification. Like direct amplification of reference and database samples, the right combination of cell lysis reagent and PCR master mix is vital for successful direct amplification of casework samples. In the case of reference and database buccal swab samples, the amount of DNA is normally high and only a small volume of cell lysate is added to the amplification reaction. This means that the effect of the cell lysis reagent on the amplification reaction is minimal. However, for touch and cutting samples where the amount of DNA on the substrate is low, the maximum volume of the cell lysate is usually added to the amplification reaction. Therefore, the cell lysis reagent has more impact on the amplification efficiency for touch samples than for reference or database samples. An additional complication is the stipulation in most countries to quantify DNA from casework samples, making it necessary that the touch or cutting sample cell lysate be compatible with a forensic DNA quantification method. Additionally, the cell lysate needs to be compatible with a DNA purification reagent, such that it could be further extracted if a high level of inhibitors is detected during quantification.

To meet all these requirements and compatibility needs, Promega developed the Casework Direct Kit that enables simple, rapid, and efficient casework sample analysis (Promega Corporation, 2016; Graham et al., 2018). Figure 15.4 shows the rapid protocol (Steps 1–4) for preparing cell lysates with the Casework Direct Solution from swabs or cuttings that can be directly used for quantification and subsequent STR amplification.

Only 2 µL of the lysate is needed for quantification using the PowerQuant® System. The information gathered at this step can determine the most efficient downstream analysis path for the sample (Figure 15.5). The autosomal-to-Y ratio of the DNA can help forensic scientists decide if an autosomal STR or Y-STR analysis would be most informative. Similarly, if the quantification indicates that the DNA is degraded, a higher amount of DNA input could be added to the amplification reaction. Alternatively, a different evidence sample altogether could be selected, if available. Finally, if the quantification indicates the presence of inhibitors, the lysate could be diluted (if the DNA concentration is sufficiently high) or the DNA could be purified using a compatible DNA purification system, such as the DNA IQ™ chemistry. This combination of rapid cell lysis followed by quantification provides forensic scientists with DNA quantity and quality information that guides the best use of precious casework samples. These data-driven decisions result in fewer repeats, thus saving forensic laboratories time and money while increasing laboratory throughput without compromising quality.

15.4   INCREASING GENOTYPE INFORMATION WITH SEQUENCE-BASED SHORT TANDEM REPEAT ANALYSIS

In addition to improving length-based STR analysis by increasing multiplexing capabilities with an 8-dye CE instrument and 8-dye STR chemistry, Promega is also developing MPS systems for human genotyping. MPS provides multiple potential advantages over length-based CE technology. MPS technology is not limited by the number of dyes or the length of the amplicon resolvable by the CE instrument. As such, MPS does not require each STR allele to be of a unique size with a unique fluorescence label (discussed elsewhere in this book). Without these constraints, MPS can generate data for more STR markers than length-based CE technology in each analysis. The PowerSeq™ 46GY System combines the 22 autosomal STR loci in the 8-dye PowerPlex 35GY System with Amelogenin and the 23 Y-STR loci in the PowerPlex Y23 System (Montano et al., 2018). The small amplicons generated by this system makes it particularly advantageous when analyzing degraded DNA.

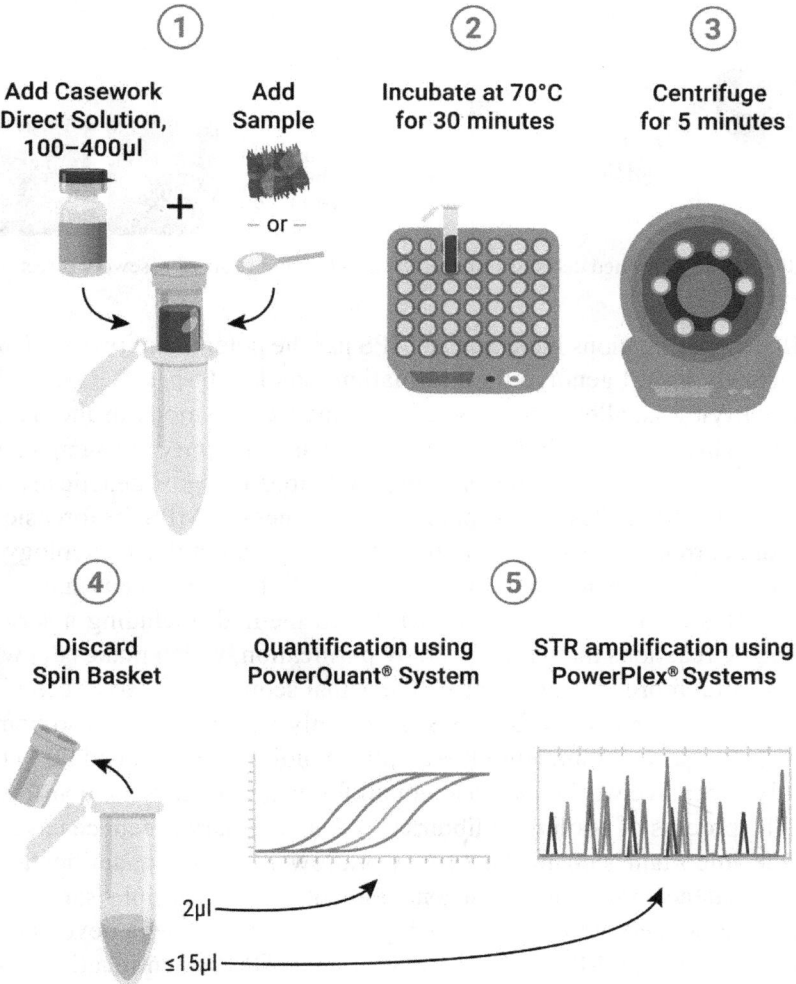

FIGURE 15.4 Rapid processing of casework samples. Sample is incubated in a spin basket assembly with Casework Direct Solution at 70 °C for 30 min and centrifuged for 5 minutes at 16,000*g*. The lysate (2 µL) can be quantified using the PowerQuant® System. Up to 15 µL of the same lysate can be used for PowerPlex® STR amplification.

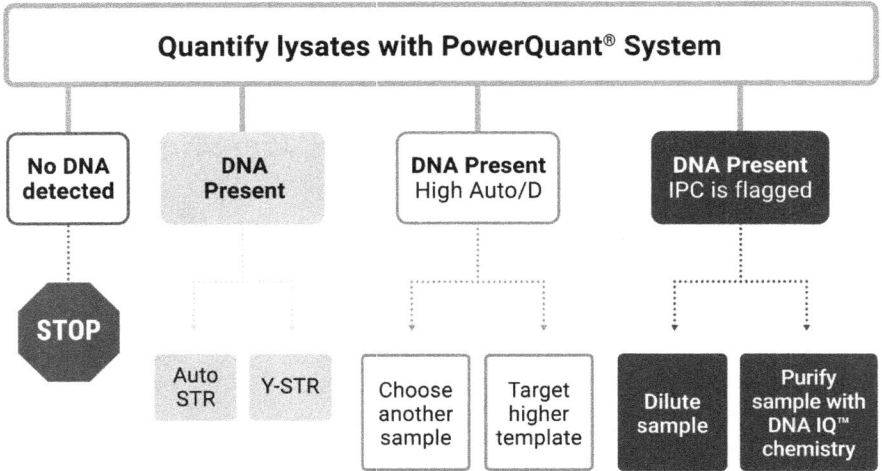

FIGURE 15.5   Informed decisions from DNA quantification data of casework direct lysate.

Recent publications indicate that MPS has the potential of revealing more forensically useful genotyping information than length-based STR analysis by identifying isoalleles and revealing sequence variations in the flanking regions. This is especially beneficial when analyzing mixture samples (van der Gaag et al., 2016) or samples from populations with low genetic diversity (Silva et al., 2018). Despite the potential advantages of MPS for forensic use, there are currently practical limitations to incorporating this technology into routine use in forensic laboratories. First of all, there are many more steps in the MPS workflow than in the CE-based method, including a series of enzymatic reactions that is followed by purification, which makes the whole process total more than 30 h before the actual sequencing starts Second, the amount of data generated by MPS is not only very large but also complicated and requires significant investments in bioinformatics in addition to an already expensive workflow. Last, not all forensic scientists are comfortable with the process of pooling of libraries that is necessary to reduce cost.

One important step in the MPS workflow is library quantification, to ensure that accurate and consistent amounts from multiple samples are pooled and loaded onto the sequencing instrument. Promega developed the PowerSeq™ Quant MS System, a qPCR-based DNA quantification system to accurately determine the concentration of MPS libraries compatible with Illumina MiSeq® platforms (Promega Corporation, 2018b). This system uses the BRYT Green® dye to achieve sensitive and reproducible DNA quantification using commonly used qPCR instruments.

15.5 SIMPLIFYING MITOCHONDRIAL DNA SEQUENCING

One area where the use of MPS technology improves the workflow over traditional methods is mitochondrial DNA analysis. This technology is frequently used to analyze samples with highly degraded DNA where it is not possible to generate an autosomal DNA profile. Mitochondrial DNA sequencing using the traditional Sanger method has been routinely used for forensic purposes for many years (Wilson et al., 1995). This method requires many individual amplification reactions, resulting in a tedious and labor-intensive process with many sample manipulations. Because MPS can sequence multiple amplicons in one reaction, it increases the throughput of mitochondrial sequencing. This increased sequencing capacity makes routine sequencing beyond the traditional control region to the sequencing of the whole genome a practical effort.

Although the MPS workflow in general improves on the traditional Sanger sequencing workflow, it is still a long process and includes multiple amplification steps: first to amplify target sequences (which in some cases takes two amplification reactions) and followed by amplification to incorporate indexing and adapter sequences. To simplify the workflow for the mitochondrial control region sequencing, Promega developed the PowerSeq™ CRM Nested System that combines the two amplifications steps in one so-called nested amplification; thus saving time and cost (Promega Corporation, 2018a). Primer pairs for the 10 small target amplicons for the HV1, HV2, and HV3 mitochondrial control region are combined with a unique combination of one of twelve index forward primers and one of eight index reverse primers in each amplification. This allows up to 96 samples to be pooled and sequenced, depending on sample type. Using this system, up to 3 h of hands-on time and 5 h of total time can be saved by eliminating multiple enzymatic and purification steps, making it possible to complete the amplification and library preparation steps in one day as opposed to two days (Figure 15.6). Gallimore et al. (2018) illustrated the functionality of this system by using it to investigate varying levels of heteroplasmy in hair relative to buccal and blood cells.

15.6 CONCLUDING REMARKS

The forensic DNA analysis field has made significant technological advances in the last 25 years, from silver-stained 3-loci STR multiplex to fluorescent 27-loci STR genotyping in about an hour. We can now look forward to another big leap to where MPS is a widely used complementary

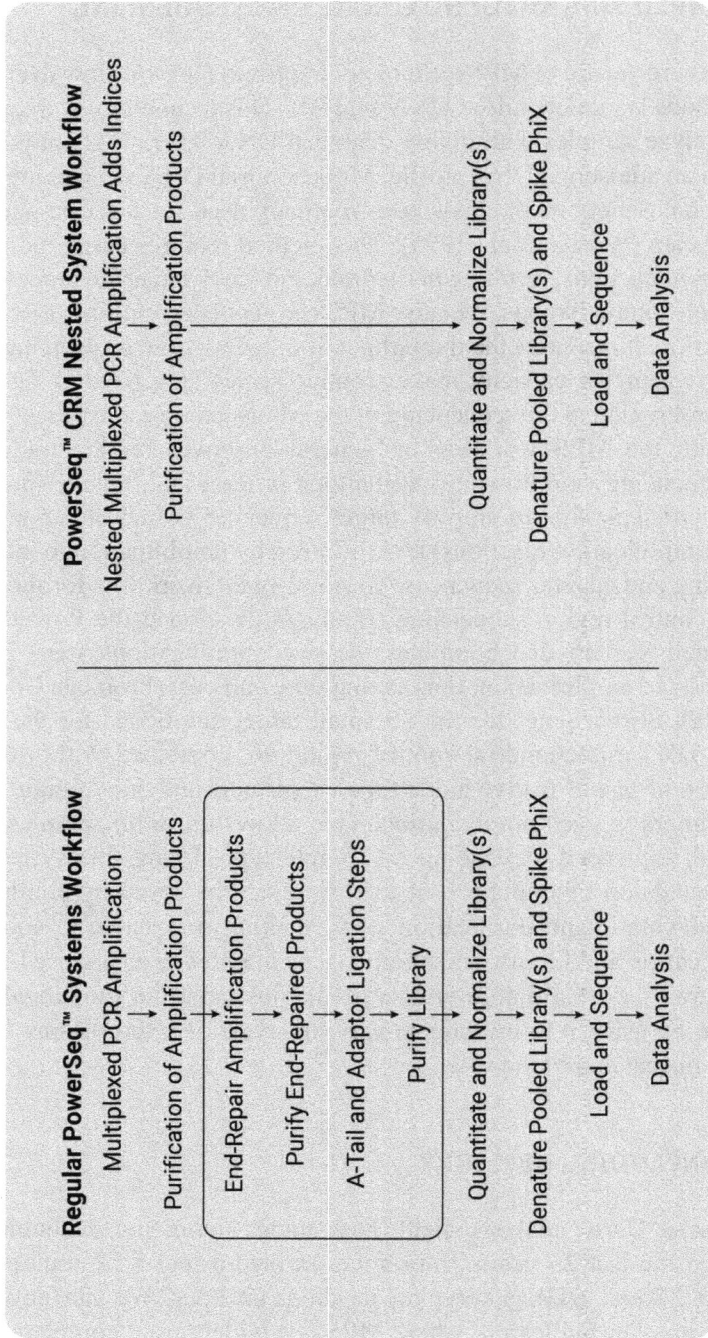

Regular PowerSeq™ Systems Workflow

Multiplexed PCR Amplification

Purification of Amplification Products

End-Repair Amplification Products

Purify End-Repaired Products

A-Tail and Adaptor Ligation Steps

Purify Library

Quantitate and Normalize Library(s)

Denature Pooled Library(s) and Spike PhiX

Load and Sequence

Data Analysis

PowerSeq™ CRM Nested System Workflow

Nested Multiplexed PCR Amplification Adds Indices

Purification of Amplification Products

Quantitate and Normalize Library(s)

Denature Pooled Library(s) and Spike PhiX

Load and Sequence

Data Analysis

FIGURE 15.6   Simplified library preparation workflow with the PowerSeq™ CRM Nested System.

technology to CE-based analysis. While the advantages of more information revealed through MPS are clear, the infrastructure surrounding the use of MPS as the primary forensic DNA genotyping technique still needs to be built. The forensic DNA community needs to agree on the nomenclature and type of data to be used, and forensic scientists will need training and proficiency testing on the new technology. Finally, the time needed for MPS analysis needs to be reduced. All these, as well as the acquisition of expensive equipment and data handling software, will take significant time and financial investment. Until the community is ready to use MPS for routine analysis, CE-based STR analysis will continue to be the main technology for forensic DNA analysis and will be used for years to come. During these years though, the number of samples to be analyzed will continue to grow as well as the number of DNA profiles in databases. Combined with the increased need to obtain more information from a crime scene sample, it is clear that continued innovation of CE technology is important. Workflow improvements and introduction of 8-dye STR technology will ensure that the use of established CE-based STR analysis combined with highly accurate quantification systems and rapid sample processing workflow will meet the need to perform the analysis quickly and at a low cost.

KEYWORDS

- **STR multiplex**
- **MPS**
- **mitochondria sequencing**
- **rapid processing**

REFERENCES

Ballantyne, K. et al.; Mutability of Y-chromosomal microsatellites: Rates, characteristics, molecular bases, and forensic implications. *American Journal of Human Genetics* **2010**, 87(3), 341–353.

Budowle, B. et al.; Validation studies of the CTT STR multiplex system. *Journal of Forensic Sciences* **1997**, 42, 701–707.

Cavanaugh, S. E. and Bathrick, A. S.; Direct PCR amplification of forensic touch and other challenging DNA samples: A review. *Forensic Science International: Genetics* **2018**, 32, 40–49.

Ewing, M. M. et al.; Human DNA quantification and sample quality assessment: Developmental validation of the PowerQuant system. *Forensic Science International: Genetics* **2016**, 23, 166–177.

Forensic Genetics Policy Initiative; *Establishing Best Practice for Forensic DNA Databases* **2017** [Online] Available at: [accessed on August 26, 2018].

Gallimore, J. M., McElhoe, J. A., and Holland, M. M.; Assessing heteroplasmic variant drift in the mtDNA control region of human hairs using an MPS approach. *Forensic Science International: Genetics* **2018**, 32, 7–17.

Gill, P., Fereday, L., Morling, N., and Schneider, P. M.; New multiplexes for Europe— Amendments and clarification of strategic development. *Forensic Science International* **2006**, 163(2), 155–157.

Graham, E. K. et al.; *Developmental Validation of the Casework Direct Kit, Custom: A Method for the Rapid Processing of Casework Samples* **2018** [Online] Available at: [accessed on February 20, 2019].

Hares, D. R.; Addendum to expanding the CODIS core loci in the United States. *Forensic Science International: Genetics* **2012**, 6(5), e135.

Lin, S.-w., Li, C., and Ip, S. C.; A performance study on three qPCR quantification kits and their compatibilities with the 6-dye DNA profiling systems. *Forensic Science International: Genetic* **2018**, 33, 72–83.

Maguire, C. N., McCallum, L. A., Storey, C., and Whita, J. P.; Familial searching: A specialist forensic DNA profiling service utilising the National DNA Database® to identify unknown offenders via their relatives—The UK experience. *Forensic Science International: Genetics* **2014**, 8(1), 1–9.

Montano, E. A. et al.; Optimization of the Promega PowerSeq™ Auto/Y system for efficient integration within a forensic DNA laboratory. *Forensic Science International: Genetics* **2018**, 32, 26–32.

Promega Corporation; *Rapid Processing of Swabs from Casework Samples Using Casework Direct Kit, Custom* **2016** [Online] Available at: [accessed on August 28, 2018].

Promega Corporation; *PowerPlex® Fusion 6C System for Use on the Applied Biosystems® Genetic Analyzers* **2017** [Online] Available at: [accessed on August 27, 2018].

Promega Corporation; *Massively Parallel Sequencing of Mitochondrial Control Region Using the PowerSeq™ CRM Nested System, Custom* **2018a** [Online] Available at: [accessed on July 24, 2018].

Promega Corporation; *PowerSeq™ Quant MS System Techincal Manual* **2018b** [Online] Available at: [accessed on July 28, 2018].

Purps, J. and Roewer, L.; A global analysis of Y-chromosomal haplotype diversity for 23 STR loci. *Forensic Science International: Genetics* **2014** 12, 12–23.

Silva, D. S. et al.; Genetic analysis of Southern Brazil subjects using the PowerSeq™ AUTO/Y system for short tandem repeat sequencing. *Forensic Science International: Genetics* **2018**, 33, 129–35.

van der Gaag, K. J. et al.; Massively parallel sequencing of short tandem repeats—Population data and mixture analysis results for the PowerSeq™ system. *Forensic Science International: Genetics* **2016**, 24, 86–96.

Wilson, M. R. et al.; Validation of mitochondrial DNA sequencing for forensic casework analysis. *International Journal of Legal Medicine* **1995**, 108(2), 68–74.

CHAPTER 16

ParaDNA® Technology: A Tool for Rapid Identification of DNA and Body Fluids

LAURA DODD[1*], STEPHANIE REGAN[2] and TOBIAS HAMPSHIRE[3]

[1]*Foster + Freeman Ltd, Vale Park, Evesham, Worcestershire, United Kingdom, WR11 1TD.*

[2]*Kauai Police Department, 3990 Kaana Street, Suite 200, Lihue, HI 96766, United States*

[3]*ParaDNA, LGC Ltd, Queens Road, Teddington, Middlesex TW11 0LY, United Kingdom*

Corresponding author. E-mail: lauradodd@hotmail.com

ABSTRACT

The development of new technologies and their applications within forensic science are crucial for the advancement of this discipline. The use of rapid DNA profiling and confirmatory body fluid identification are two such areas of research which have evolved based on a requirement from law-enforcement agencies to have access to rapid forensic intelligence, as an investigation progresses, in real time. This novel analysis technique is a nondestructive process which now permits investigators the ability to perform rapid screening, triaging, and forensic intelligence gathering at the laboratory or directly at the scene, even in the most challenging of operational environments. The multifunctional aspect of this technology provides forensic practitioners with the ability to use a single system to perform a range of different forensic tests, all of which have been designed to be practical, user friendly, and without the requirement for expert review of the results. The ParaDNA Screening Test was created to provide investigators with a more reliable approach to the triaging of evidence by delivering the ability to ascertain which crime stains contain DNA and therefore represent which are the likeliest samples to deliver probative evidential results. The ParaDNA Intelligence Test adds additional power to the ability to triage crime stains by delivering a DNA profile, providing investigators the capacity to facilitate victim exclusions, suspect identifications, or support them with the capability to link crime scenes together. The ParaDNA Body Fluid ID Test can be used for rapid confirmatory analysis of six different body fluid types commonly encountered by forensic practitioners. It also has the ability to determine whether a sample contains multiple body fluids in a single stain and is the first commercial tool to specifically identify the presence of vaginal fluids. This chapter outlines the research, development, validation, and implementation of the ParaDNA® System including its range of applications within the forensic field and a case study of its integration and utilization into the forensic workflow by a US police department.

16.1 INTRODUCTION

Since the implementation of forensic DNA profiling, the development and utilization of biometric data by police forces and scientists worldwide has revolutionized the ability to conduct forensic investigations. However, these developments all add cost to the process of bringing criminals to justice, and although many forensic service suppliers have made great strides to reduce this cost, provision is still generally restricted to being delivered from a laboratory environment requiring highly trained scientists using complex instrumentation.

In some geography's, those investigating a case may have to wait for long periods of time before the return of DNA results vital to the further progression of their case (National Institute of Justice, 2017). Likewise, many investigations may hang on gaining a result from evidence only containing minute, trace levels of DNA and it is often impossible for scene-going personnel to know how much DNA, if any, is present on a piece of forensic evidence prior to submission to a laboratory. A similar scenario occurs when scene attending personnel are overwhelmed with the number of choices available to them for collection, with investigations then experiencing delays associated with the sheer number of samples requiring processing to uncover the required evidence.

The identification of the types of body fluid found at a scene, or on a piece of evidence, can also be crucial to an investigation. Body fluid identification allows officers to reconstruct crime scenes or a version of events provided by the involved parties (Virkler and Lednev, 2009). Historically utilized methods are low cost but can be time-consuming and are often prone to cross-reactivity (Zubakov et al., 2008), plus many types of these more traditional presumptive tests only offer the option to search and identify a single target body fluid at a time (Virkler and Lednev, 2009). Analysis using these techniques can often be exposed to and fraught with subjective interpretation of the data including the potential for the introduction of cognitive bias by the analyst (White, 2016).

The ParaDNA® System is a rapid screening, triage, and early intelligence system capable of both DNA analysis and body fluid identification via a unique instrument platform containing independent thermocycler heads and fluorescent detection capability (French et al., 2008). The system is operated using the ParaDNA Software which controls the instrument and applications specific to each test, analyzes the data and displays the results, while simultaneously adding the data to an internal database of results. The system uses a patented ParaDNA® Sample Collector (Debenham and Moore, 2011), a pen-like tool consisting of four plastic tips which are brought together to form a single sampling nib to collect material from evidence items (see Figure 16.1). The nibs are expanded after sampling of an item or swab and are inserted into a custom-designed four well test plate which contains the necessary reagents required for the specific forensic assay (see Figure 16.2). The process of inserting the nibs seals the test, following which the handle of the ParaDNA Sample Collector is broken off, leaving a test plate closed to the external environment that can then be loaded onto the ParaDNA Instrument for short tandem repeats (STR) analysis or body fluid identification. A key feature of the sampling process is that it is a *nondestructive technique*, in that, sampled swabs and crime stains are still perfectly amenable to further forensic analysis in a laboratory setting, as the approach leaves behind the majority of available genetic material. For this reason, the ParaDNA System is considered to be a complementary approach to current forensic STR processes including Rapid-DNA technologies (Federal Bureau of Investigation, 2017a, 2017b, 2017c). The ParaDNA System can be and has been used prior to analysis on Rapid-DNA instrumentation as a method of determining whether a sample contains an appropriate starting amount of template DNA to make it a suitable sample for profiling on this latter type of equipment (APCC, 2018).

16.2 ParaDNA INSTRUMENTS

The ParaDNA System can currently operate on two key instruments available in the forensics sector, which can perform the same type of analysis in different scenarios or locations; the ParaDNA® Screening Instrument and the ParaDNA® Field Portable Instrument.

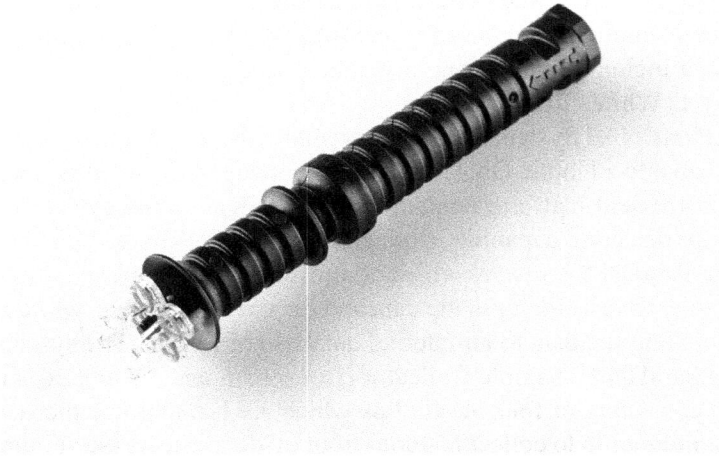

FIGURE 16.1   ParaDNA Sample Collector.

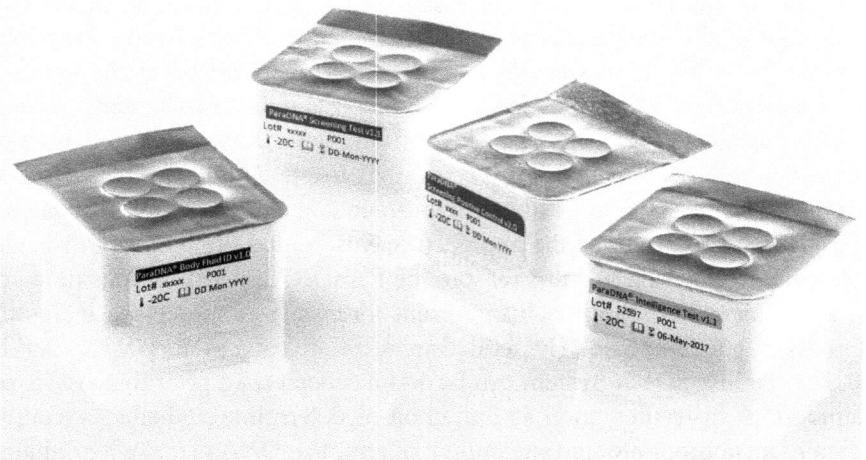

FIGURE 16.2   Forensic ParaDNA Test Plates.

The ParaDNA Screening Instrument (see Figure 16.3) is a fully integrated laboratory-based system with four independent thermal cyclers capable of running four separate samples simultaneously. This instrument was designed to be most suitable for use within indoor environments such as police screening suites, forensic submissions or screening/triage units, and DNA crime laboratories. The ParaDNA Screening Instrument is the smaller of these two options, weighing approximately 6 kg, and is simple to operate in combination with a basic desktop or laptop computer.

The ParaDNA Field Portable Instrument (see Figure 16.3) is a completely self-contained and fully mobile device which is housed in a ruggedized carry case with a built-in touch screen PC. What makes this instrument unique is that it contains two lithium-ion batteries which can be charged via a standard mains connection in around 3 h. When fully charged users can rely on up to 7 h of use without the need for a mains power source, for processing of up to 20 samples, perhaps representing multiple crime scenes visited throughout a day. It also comes equipped with two USB ports allowing for quick transfer of encrypted DNA profile data from the internal database, for use by investigators as rapid intelligence or to search an external DNA database. Offering the option to both gain DNA intelligence and screen for/identify unknown body fluids while still at scene is a major advantage to certain police and military investigators, especially when considering that many government bodies and forensic regulators are initiating activities relating to the transition of more forensic investigational work to "near-scene" locations (National DNA Database Ethics Group, 2017).

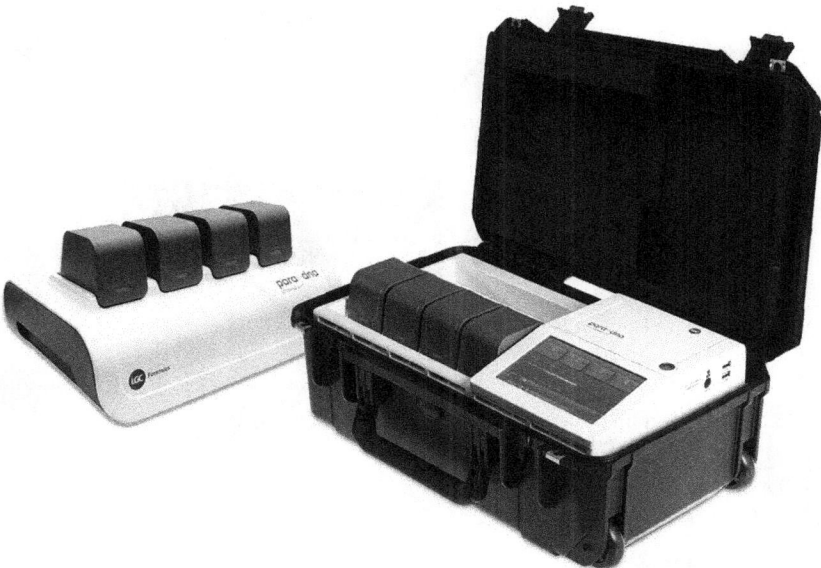

FIGURE 16.3 ParaDNA Screening Instrument and ParaDNA Field Portable Instrument.

16.3   ParaDNA SAMPLE COLLECTION

A vital component of ParaDNA Systems is a collection tool that is central to the unique approach of processing genetic material direct from source, without the requirement for any purification steps. The ParaDNA Sample Collector is a patented tool used to sample biological material recovered from a crime scene, evidence items, or even directly from individuals (see Figure 16.4) (Debenham and Moore, 2011). This pen-like design includes a handle and a detachable sampling "nib" with four points (4-nib) that is pushed together when the outer collar of the handle is slid forward to form a single sampling "nib." The collector design makes recovery of biological material a relatively simple process, regardless of whether sampling from a swab or directly from an item or surface area. Users are provided the ability to utilize an inimitable sampling technique which only removes a small percentage of the total available material, ensuring that the sample is not destroyed and is suitable for further forensic analyses, when required. Each collector is treated to remove the presence of human DNA and individually packaged for single use. Once sampling is completed, the 4-nib is reopened and loaded into the test plate via a turning mechanism that simultaneously seals and detaches the handle from the nibs, creating a sealed test that is ready to insert into the instrument for analysis.

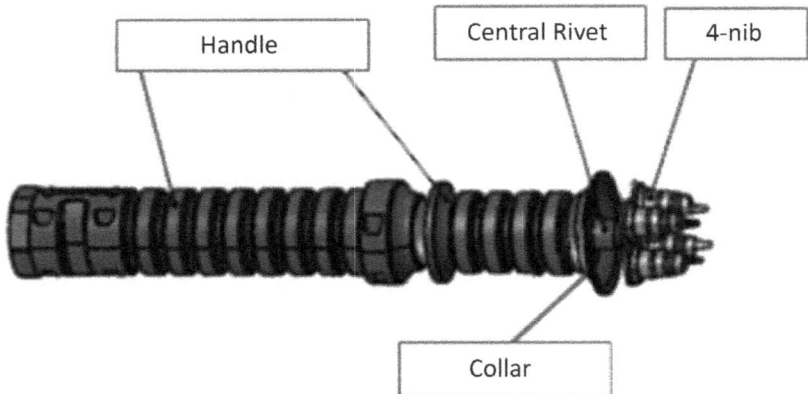

FIGURE 16.4   Diagram of the ParaDNA Sample Collector parts.

16.4   ParaDNA TESTS

The ParaDNA System currently has three different forensic test types available, all of which are designed to be accessible, simple to use, and offer the option for immediate action use without the need for expert review. System results are analyzed automatically and displayed to the user in a simple to interpret format via the standard software interface.

The ParaDNA® Screening Test was the first test to be developed histori- cally, primarily to provide forensic evidence recovery and submissions departments with a more scientific and reliable approach to the triaging of evidence collected at the crime scene but also, to ascertain which crime stains contain sufficient DNA to generate a useful profile using standard STR profiling methods (Raymond et al., 2009). In approximately 75 min, the ParaDNA Screening Test can determine the presence of human DNA, indicate the likelihood of obtaining a usable STR result, and where there is sufficient DNA to generate an Amelogenin call will display the sex of the major contributor. The test result provides users with an easily interpretable "DNA percentage score" relative to the quality and quantity of DNA in a sample. The DNA score is a qualitative measurement of the amount of DNA that was calibrated via testing conducted during the development of the ParaDNA Screening Test. As part of the internal validation, the sensitivity and precision of the DNA detection score were assessed using a range of DNA input amounts with known concentrations verified using Plexor-HY quantification. Purified DNA was added directly into the four wells at input amounts equivalent to 4 ng, 3 ng, 1 ng, 500 pg, 250 pg, and 62.5 pg of DNA per test. The dynamic range of the DNA detection score was finalized using this set of DNA concentrations, with the score declining as the input amount decreases. A sample that supports collection of 4 ng of input DNA generates a screening score of 90%–100%, and samples supporting collection of 62.5 pg of DNA generates a score of approximately 20%. Data published on the validation of the screening test demonstrated a strong correlation between the DNA detection score and the Plexor DNA quantification data, highlighting the test can deliver reliable results without the need for expert interpretation of quantitative data (Dawnay et al., 2014).

These features are useful for triaging samples effectively prior to STR analysis, in order to exclude progression of samples containing no DNA, or effectively remove low level DNA samples when better more DNA rich items are also available (Raymond et al., 2009). Forensic service providers often focus on the cost of reagents alone but more often than not, it is the suboptimal utilization of staffing resource that has the most profound effect on efficiencies and turn around times (Federal Bureau of Investigation, 2017a, 2017b, 2017c). Increased focus on reducing evidence backlogs ensures that key evidence is identified and included whether sent through a laboratory for full DNA STR profiling or through a Rapid-DNA instrument that consumes the entire sample (National Criminal Justice Reference Service, 2010). By providing a quick and simple presumptive test for DNA, the ParaDNA Screening Test augments and improves today's existing forensic processes, supporting law enforcement and forensic scientists in efforts to concentrate resources on the most probative investigative leads, and it is a particularly useful tool for recovered crime scene samples where unknown amounts of DNA are present.

The ParaDNA® Intelligence Test was later designed to provide an Amelogenin call, plus five STR loci common to the majority of worldwide forensic DNA profiling systems. Loci targeted are TH01, D3S1358 (D3), D8S1179 (D8), D16S539 (D16), and D18S51 (D18), representing core loci found in the UK National DNA Database and Combined DNA Index System (CODIS) (Crown Prosecution Service, 2017; Federal Bureau of Investigation, 2017a, 2017b, 2017c). In combination with sampling guidelines bespoke to a diverse range of crime or reference exhibits, the test delivers profile data, without the need of a DNA extraction step, within 75 min. The output from the ParaDNA Intelligence System is held on an internal database on the instrument, with the accompanying software offering options to quickly include or eliminate suspect(s) from an investigation, exclude victim DNA from an inquiry, rapidly link individual's DNA to a scene, or even link crime scenes together. The derived intelligence information can support investigators to follow and progress lines of enquiry before results are generated in a forensic laboratory but can also represent a central source of forensic information if placed within resource limited or tough operational environments. A recent development has been the utilization of ParaDNA Intelligence Test profiles to speculatively search national DNA databases allowing the generation of a list of potential suspects for investigators to target within hours of the crime scene being examined. The ParaDNA Intelligence Test results also feature a relative percentage DNA score, thus retaining the option offered by the ParaDNA Screening Test to triage and prioritize associated groups of samples (Dawnay et al., 2014) However, the wider array of allelic data generated from each item sampled enables the additional feature of identifying mixtures of DNA when multiple contributors are apparent (Blackman et al., 2015).

The ParaDNA Body Fluid ID Test® was created to simultaneously provide confirmatory testing for the presence of six different body fluid types; blood, menstrual blood, sperm cells, seminal fluid, vaginal fluid, and saliva, in around 90 min and is the first commercially available test capable of detecting and confirming the presence of vaginal fluid material (Blackman et al., 2018). Accurate identification of biological fluids can be important in aiding crime scene reconstructions during an investigation and offers further support to forensic submissions in identifying the most probative samples for full DNA analysis (Virkler and Lednev, 2009). The majority of current body fluid identification methods are time-consuming, laboratory-based processes. Further to this, current techniques do not permit the identification of all body fluids in one test and are often cross-reactive with many other potential sources likely to be present at a crime scene (Virkler and Lednev, 2009; Zubakov et al., 2008). The format of the test makes it useful in an increasingly diverse set of scenarios, for instance, sexual assault investigators may wish to rapidly determine if samples contain semen, with the added security of being able to detect seminal fluid separately to sperm cells being vital in identifying secretions from vasectomized males. This test also offers a crucial advantage in investigations involving oral sexual assault samples, whereby some current methods can have cross-reactivity between saliva and vaginal fluid material (Virkler and Lednev, 2009; James and Norby, 2003) making it difficult to identify what body fluids are present and corroborate claims made by victims and suspects during an investigation.

16.5 ParaDNA SOFTWARE

ParaDNA Software is designed to be user friendly; allowing nonforensically trained individuals to generate a DNA profile or identify body fluids without the need for any expert interpretation of the data, yet below the surface is a complex and unique operating system with additional functionality that enables more experienced users to take advantage of a variety of additional applications to support interpretation.

The ParaDNA Screening System Software outputs a simple-to-understand percentage score, situated in either a green (presence of DNA) or red (absence of DNA) window. This relative quantitative assessment of the amount of DNA loaded into the test plate yields information about the potential for the sample to deliver a full profile when submitted for subsequent STR analysis. If enough DNA is detected, the ParaDNA Software will also indicate whether the DNA obtained is of male or female origin (see Figure 16.5) (Dawnay et al., 2014).

The ParaDNA Intelligence System Software outputs a 5-STR profile, plus Amelogenin call for gender identification, alongside a DNA percentage score equivalent to that seen in the ParaDNA Screening Test (see Figure 16.5) (Dawnay et al., 2014; Blackman et al., 2015). In some territories, speculative searches of national databases have been carried out even though the obtained DNA profile might not meet the loading criteria of that database,

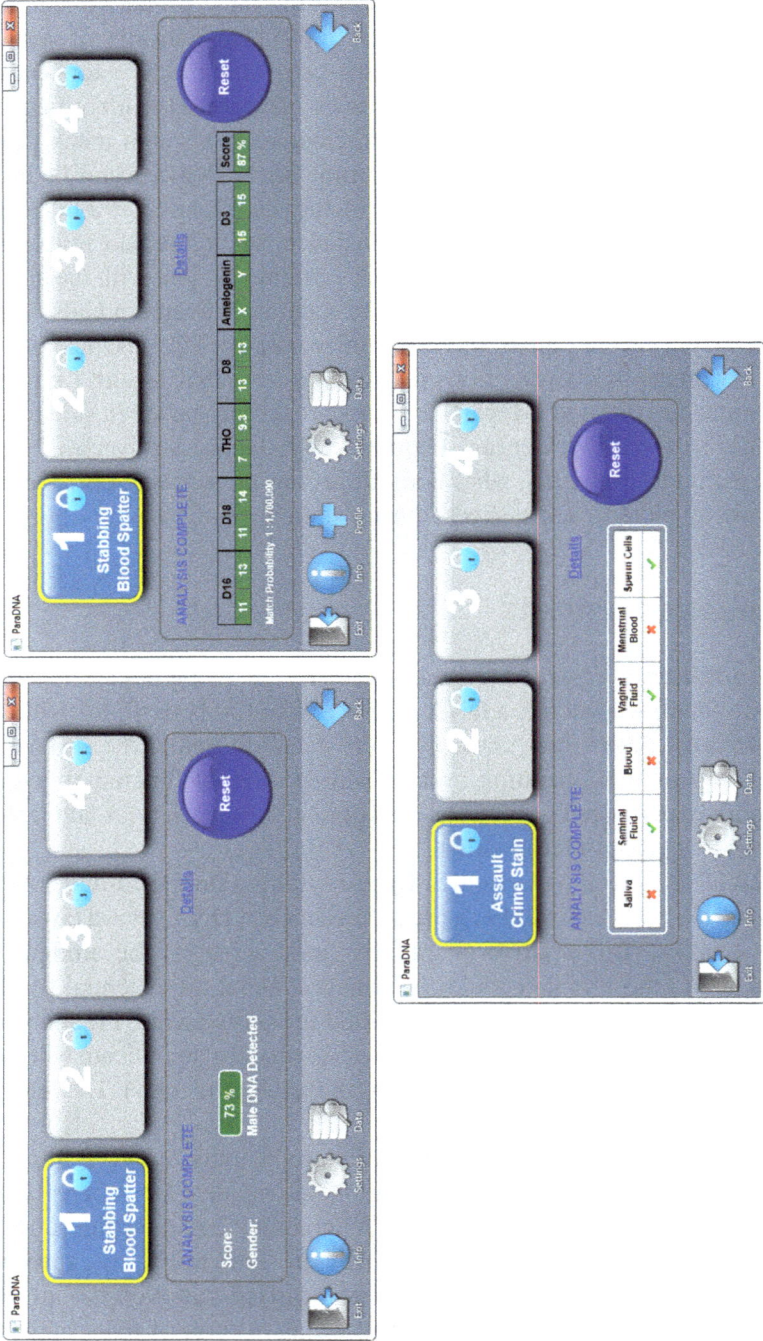

FIGURE 16.5	ParaDNA Software displaying the easily interpretable results output for the ParaDNA Screening, Intelligence, and Body Fluid Identification Tests.

with results being used solely for intelligence purposes. The ability to carry out a speculative search delivers potential new leads to an investigation, in addition to offering real-time inclusion/exclusion possibilities of existing suspects, normally in a much shorter time frame to that offered by a forensic service provider. This method has been utilized by agencies searching against ParaDNA Intelligence Test profiles on international DNA databases, including the UK National DNA database, often with the support of bespoke additional software developed for the project at no additional cost.

The ParaDNA Body Fluid ID System Software outputs a table containing each of the six targeted body fluid markers with an associated green tick or a red cross indicating the presence or absence of each specific body fluid in the tested sample (see Figure 16.5) (Blackman et al., 2018).

In general, the ParaDNA Software is easy to use and maintains a high level of accuracy, without the need for any form of complex interpretation, as rules and thresholds set within the software only allow confident calls to be displayed.

ParaDNA Data Analysis Software has also been developed for use in conjunction with ParaDNA Systems to empower experienced users to perform a more in-depth review of sample results generated from either the Intelligence Test or Body Fluid ID Test, by facilitating analysis of the raw melt curve data (see Figure 16.6). This additional software suite was created with the intention to supply users who have experience of DNA interpretation or body fluid identification, with supplementary data detailing how the software assigned data to achieved calls but also reduced confidence calls, as opposed to background noise. The software applies a fluorescence model to the observed melt curve data for each sample, resulting in quantitative data for every potential allele or body fluid call, and displays this in a Bar Chart Panel. Quantitative data is compared to a series of thresholds to decide whether an allele or body fluid should be called confidently, called with reduced confidence or confidently rejected as not detected. A reduced confidence call is produced when the software detects that an allele or body fluid could be present in the sample, but it does not meet all of the required thresholds to be confidently called.

Once trained and proficient with the Data Analysis Software, users may choose to reinstate allele or body fluid calls under appropriate circumstances, to support improvements in the outcomes potentially achievable from individual test results. The interpretation of DNA profiles and body fluid calls using Data Analysis Software should always be approached with caution and due consideration but can provide experienced users with further enhanced and timely case intelligence.

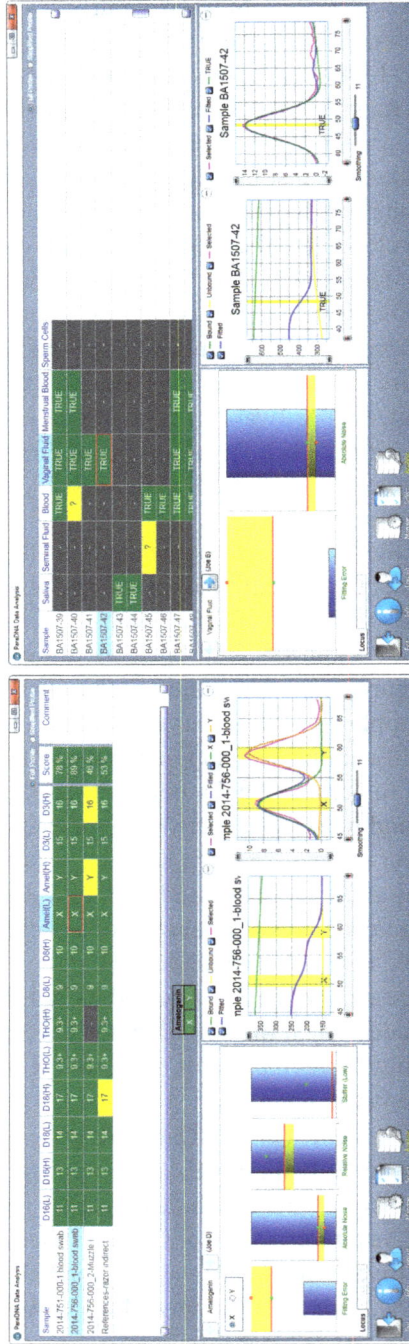

FIGURE 16.6 ParaDNA Data Analysis Software displaying the raw melt curve data for the ParaDNA Intelligence and Body Fluid Identification Tests.

16.6   THE SCIENCE BEHIND ParaDNA - APPLICATION OF HYBEACON® PROBE TECHNOLOGY

In 2001, LGC Ltd developed and patented HyBeacon® Probe Technology (French et al., 2001, 2008) which has been adapted for use as part of ParaDNA Systems. HyBeacon probes are short lengths of synthesized DNA which can be labeled with one or more fluorescent dyes, and a single probe is capable of detecting multiple allelic variations, facilitating increased options for multiplexing. Following a DNA amplification process via polymerase chain reaction (PCR) (see Figure 16.7), HyBeacon probes can be employed in a fluorescent melt curve analysis, not only to detect amplified target product but also to determine variations in the genetic sequence including Indels, SNPs, or even highly repeatable elements such as STRs.

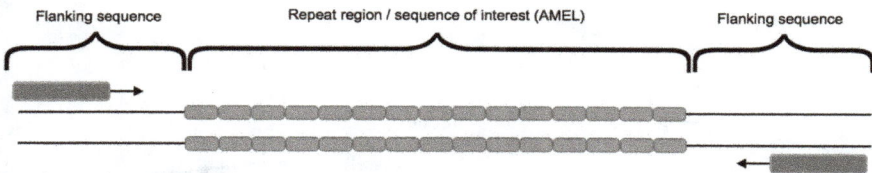

FIGURE 16.7   PCR amplification of a single tandem repeat region.

The melt curve analysis is achieved by cooling the finalized reaction components to facilitate each HyBeacon Probe hybridizing to its target DNA sequence (see Figure 16.8), at which point a measurable amount of fluorescence is emitted at a wavelength corresponding to the bound dye. The assay is then gradually heated in a controlled and staged approach until each probe dissociates from its target DNA sequence.

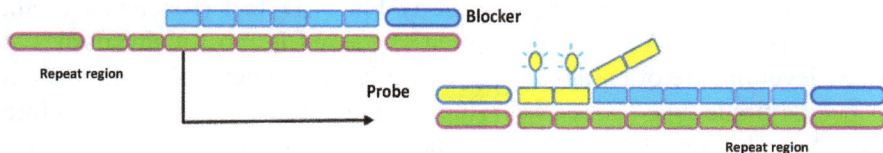

FIGURE 16.8   Hybridization of a HyBeacon probe and blocker molecule to target STR region.

A corresponding decrease in fluorescence is measured by the ParaDNA Instrument as each probe dissociates, and this change in fluorescence is analyzed to determine the genetic variation within any amplified product (see Figure 16.9). HyBeacon Probe Technology can also work in tandem with a blocker molecule designed to anneal to the DNA repeat sequence in combination with the fluorescent dye-labeled probe. Blocker molecules ensure clear separation of melt temperatures between different probes bound to DNA strands of similar sizes, resulting in clearer resolution between the genetic variations in an STR region and more successful interpretation of data by the analysis software.

HyBeacon probes have been applied to target human specific STRs in the ParaDNA Screening and Intelligence Tests. The STRs that are targeted in both the ParaDNA Screening Test and the ParaDNA Intelligence Test are present in all commonly used STR Multiplex kits, as recommended by the European Network of Forensic Science Institutes and the CODIS (European Network of Forensic Science Institutes, 2017; Federal Bureau of Investigation, 2017a, 2017b, 2017c).

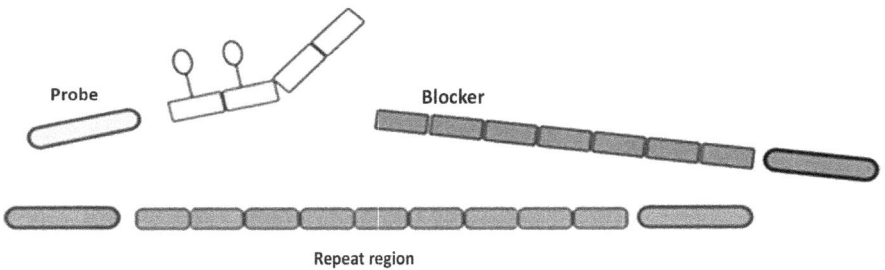

FIGURE 16.9 Dissociation of a HyBeacon probe from a target STR region. Fluorescence will decrease when the dye-labeled probe melts away from the target DNA region. The change in fluorescence in conjunction with temperature allows for determination of the appropriate genetic variation.

HyBeacon probes are utilized to target human-specific Messenger RNA (mRNA) markers in the ParaDNA Body Fluid ID Test (Blackman et al., 2018). These mRNA markers are often expressed in most major tissues at a low level but are often only expressed in large and detectable amounts in a specific tissue type (GeneCards Human Gene Database, 2017). Therefore mRNA can be considered as being particularly useful for body fluid identification as it is unique to specific proteins and so a distinct marker connected to a precise body fluid type (Haas et al., 2011; Hanson and Ballantyne, 2013). RNA can be amplified in a similar way to DNA, but the PCR technique cannot use RNA as a template directly so an initial process known as reverse transcription is carried out first. Reverse transcription employs the enzyme reverse transcriptase to convert RNA into complementary DNA (cDNA). The PCR process is able to then utilize the transcribed cDNA for amplification in an identical method to that applied by the ParaDNA Screening and Intelligence Test types.

16.7 VALIDATIONS OF ParaDNA SYSTEMS

Comprehensive internal validations have been completed and published by the manufacturer on all commercialized test options and were specifically designed to address guidelines laid out by the Scientific Working Group on DNA Analysis Methods (SWGDAM, 2017). A variety of international institutions, including academic, forensic, police, and military establishments have also completed independent validations that ultimately focused on forensic evidence types relevant to their specific operational environments. The success of these pilots has led to routine implementation for a steadily increasing number of users, with some law enforcement entities extending their current accreditation of ISO 17025 to include triaging of live casework samples prior to or in some cases post-full DNA analysis.

The ParaDNA Screening Test developmental validation study considered multiple parameters such as sensitivity, reproducibility, accuracy, inhibitor tolerance, and test performance on a range of mock evidence items. This work established that the ParaDNA Screening Test was able to detect the presence of human DNA from a range of commonly encountered sources including blood, saliva, and touch/cellular DNA. The data further demonstrated that the system is able to identify the presence of DNA from purified DNA samples, a variety of swabs types, and prevalent evidence items with similar sensitivity to that seen with standard STR profiling techniques (Dawnay et al., 2014). Positive DNA scores were also achieved from a variety of substrates containing known and common PCR inhibitors, including humic acid, tannic acid, and hemin. The accuracy of the test was a crucial parameter to ensure that samples can be correctly identified as being suitable for further forensic analysis by end users. The DNA detection score was assessed by comparison to known DNA concentrations obtained using the Plexor-HY quantification technique, with the derived screening scores displaying a strong correlation with the more established approach (Dawnay et al., 2014).

The ParaDNA Intelligence Test developmental validation considered many parameters similar to that for the Screening Test and demonstrated DNA profiles are achievable when directly sampling a variety of evidence items including blood, saliva, and even semen samples, without the requirement for

any prior extraction technique. With the additional allele information generated by the intelligence test arose the necessity to assess additional factors such
as specificity, robustness (especially in relation to degraded samples/touch
DNA samples), and the capacity to detect mixtures of multiple contributors.
Sensitivity testing highlighted allele calls could be delivered from inputs of as
little as 31.25 pg of DNA (Blackman et al., 2015); the equivalent of a sample
containing approximately 5–6 human cells (Butler, 2011) equivalent to levels
expected from touch/cellular DNA. Importantly, alleles called by the test were
compared to calls achieved using the AmpFlSTR® SGM Plus PCR test kit on
a set of replicate evidence items, with no discordant alleles observed between
the two approaches (Blackman et al., 2015). A similar and more extensive
study on concordance observed more than 99.8% of allele calls produced by
the ParaDNA Intelligence Test were concordant with the allele calls produced
using the SGM Plus assay (Ball et al., 2015). This high level of concordance is
comparable to levels observed when other STR profiling products have been
assessed, such as the published concordance of 99.7% between allele calls
made by the AmpFlSTR® Identifiler and AmpFlSTR® Minifiler assay kits (Hill
et al., 2007) establishing that the ParaDNA Intelligence Test can be considered
to have a high level of concordance with standardized STR typing assays.

DNA profiles were also achieved from a variety of directly sampled
substrates (see Figure 16.10 and 16.11), even in the presence of commonly
encountered inhibitors, without prior extraction or purification. The performance of the ParaDNA Intelligence Test was consistent when sampling from
items expected to contain high amounts of DNA, with blood and semen
samples delivering seven or more alleles in 100% of samples tested. Saliva
samples including buccal swabs, FTA cards, and drinks bottles also delivered
seven or more alleles 100% of the time, with cigarettes delivering profiles
of seven or more alleles in approximately 80% of replicates tested. Items
designated as "touch DNA," such as fingerprints, screwdrivers, and mobile
phones, generated profiles of seven or more alleles in 38% of samples tested
(Blackman et al., 2015).

The performance of the ParaDNA Intelligence Test on aged samples was
assessed using blood and saliva deposited on glass and left at room temperature for 18 months (Blackman et al., 2015). Additionally, work completed
by the University of Central Florida included blood and saliva samples aged
on cotton for one year at 37 °C, and additional samples exposed to environments thought to represent crime scene scenarios. No significant loss of test
performance was observed for all aged samples, including items stored for
two weeks in the trunk of a car, or items left outside exposed to varying
sunlight, temperature, and humidity (Blackman et al., 2015).

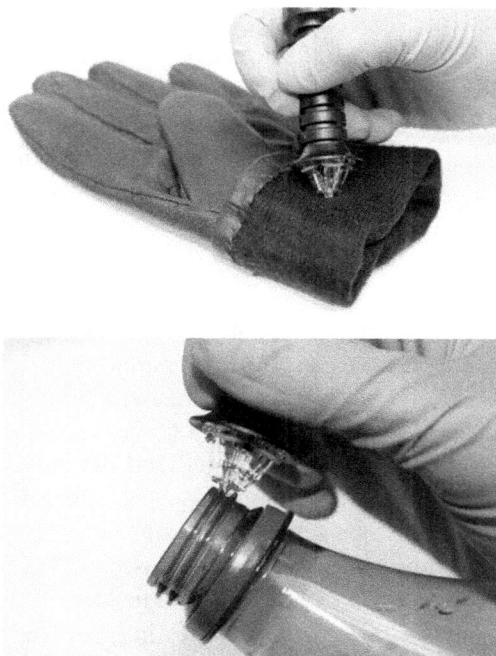

FIGURE 16.10 and 16.11 Direct sampling of common forensic evidence items with the ParaDNA Sample Collector.

The developmental validation of the ParaDNA Body Fluid ID System performed at LGC was based on the revised SWGDAM guidelines (2017) and specifically designed to address the requirements of end users and performance on a range of common mock evidence items. Although requiring no prior lysis, or any other processing steps, probative results were obtained within 90 min from a variety of stain types commonly assessed by more traditional serological approaches but with the added advantage that multiple stains could be detected simultaneously, and without the need for time-consuming manual processing. The test was also shown to be robust when analyzing stains exposed to various relevant inhibitors such as condom lubricants (Blackman et al., 2018), or substances known to be visually mistaken for commonly encountered bodily fluids such as rust and motor oil and those in particular that can result in false positives with more traditional presumptive tests such as rust that can lead to positive identification of blood with the Kastle–Meyer test (National Criminal Justice Reference Service, 2011a, 2011b).

The sensitivity of the ParaDNA Body Fluid ID Test was assessed using a dilution range of purified total RNA, different volumes of body fluids applied to specific, case-specific, substrates and dilutions of body fluids at fixed volumes (in order to mimic fluids being washed off a surface, or a person). A key finding was the demonstration that the test can detect all six target body fluids down to 1 µL stain sizes, as this was considered to be the smallest forensic stain size that forensic practitioners would attempt to apply traditional serology techniques to. The sampling approach was also demonstrated not to affect the ability to obtain a DNA profile from the remaining material (Blackman et al., 2018).

A comparison between standard STR processing and the ParaDNA Body Fluid ID Test results when processing mixtures on swabs, indicated the latter may be slightly more sensitive, particularly in relation to detection of smaller amounts of male-specific fluids, where standard STR profiling failed to identify a mixed profile. In a separate time since intercourse study, postcoital samples from volunteer donors were tested and demonstrated detection of components of semen on lower vaginal swabs. There was also detection of vaginal fluid on penile swabs taken from consenting partners up to 36 h post-intercourse, in some cases even after washing. Taken together, these points indicate potential applications specific to identifying male DNA, or identifying when more informative DNA testing, such as Y-STR profiling, may be appropriate (Blackman et al., 2018).

16.8   ParaDNA APPLICATIONS

As users of this new technology begin to diversify, so too do the number of environments instruments are housed. Forensic submissions units, and DNA crime laboratories represented some of the first placements but the development of the Field Portable Instrument has increased this reach further, with more recent examples including adaptions made to crime scene going vehicles to facilitate near-scene operations in "mobile laboratory" type scenarios. Removing the need for a direct power source has also encouraged adoption by military factions that value the opportunity to gain forensic intelligence, regardless of the operational environment.

The obvious and immediate users of ParaDNA Instruments are law enforcement and forensic professionals that value the ability to carry out immediate DNA and body fluid screening, to support more rapid identification of individuals, their potential links to scenes of interest, or a likely sequence of events, as well as to prioritize the most suitable samples for further forensic analysis. The ability to assess evidence from crime scenes in this way can also be used to exclude victim's DNA samples, which may often represent the majority of those collected. The exclusion of victim samples is particularly relevant in supporting blood pattern analysis via source identification. Exclusions ultimately improve sample submission success rates, support backlog reductions, and positively impact investigational timelines by creating intelligence information useful for progressing lines of enquiry (LGC 2017a, 2017b, 2017c, 2017d).

Established military users are likely taking advantage of the ParaDNA Intelligence System to conduct Identity Intelligence (I2) Operations and Site Exploitation to provide personnel with the capacity to verify the presence of persons of interest at specific locations. The onboard software database containing search and compare capabilities also offers the option to preload "watch lists" for immediate comparisons of individual reference samples against recovered materials even when operating in diverse and challenging environments. The ability to track known or unknown targets in theater, without the time delays associated with reach-back support functions could offer important advantages to some operations.

At the time of writing, discussions are underway with prominent human identification organizations as well as individuals involved with national public security, for the placement of devices at national borders or check-points known to be hotspots for criminal activities including terrorism, people trafficking, and travelling under a false identity. The rapid generation of DNA Intelligence profiles offers the option to quickly assess an individual's identity without the requirement to detain for extended periods of time. With growing issues surrounding the trafficking of people this approach would also allow nonforensically trained individuals, with relatively little training to verify certain claimed close familial relationships. This approach offers a low cost alternative to Rapid-DNA instrument usage that would still facilitate the identification of a high enough percentage of criminal activity to dissuade further attempts.

Users are already deploying ParaDNA System to support the identification of missing persons via comparisons against reference samples, or through searching of missing person databases. Materials as diverse as blood and cellular fluid on FTA card or direct sampling of sacral ileum have generated usable profile information which in some cases supported closure of active investigations into missing persons. In some instances, poor or degraded material can be sampled and tested several times to support building a composite profile with satisfactory match probabilities to draw conclusions. Such an approach could also support smaller scale disaster victim identification approaches if applied appropriately.

The ParaDNA Body Fluid ID Test can be used across a broader scope of users, in particular for sexual assault casework. The test is designed to identify body fluid sources, which may often be mixtures of multiple fluid types, when dealing with sexual assault cases, particularly when dealing with intimate samples recovered directly from the victim. Many nations are experiencing or have recently experienced issues arising from sexual assault kit (SAK) backlogs, the consequences of which can result in recovered SAK samples remaining in evidence storage facilities, in some cases for decades without being progressed for forensic analysis (Campbell et al., 2017). Utilization of the Body Fluid ID Test now delivers the capability to rapidly screen these types of samples for the body fluid types relevant to the case circumstances. Ultimately, this may support victims in receiving supportive information earlier, as well as delivering a new tool to investigators to assess forensic evidence quickly, in order to determine how to progress individual cases. At time of press, health facilities with forensic medical examiners or sexual assault nurse examiners are being assessed as potential resources to perform analysis *in situ*, almost immediately after recovering samples from the victim. The introduction of a rapid screening process may be a quick and cost-effective process for reducing the SAK backlog, with the critical objective of eradicating this issue entirely for future generations.

An early study of applicability of the Body Fluid ID Test to forensic casework examinations highlighted positive results could be generated by directly adding retained supernatants to the test plate. Supernatants, in this instance, are created as a by-product of a widely adopted swab extraction process aimed at concentrating sperm heads but this approach gained positive identifications of vaginal fluid, as well as seminal fluid and sperm cells (Doole, 2017). This would provide forensic scientists an alternative method for detecting body fluids during swab elution processes essentially using a waste product created during that procedure. The Body Fluid ID Test is also being employed to confirm which body fluids are the sources of DNA contributions post-DNA analysis, prior to completion of the forensic case report and before the presentation of the evidence in court. The ability to identify specific body fluids, in the context of the case circumstances, increases the evidential value of relevant exhibits. Determination of the type of biological evidence present can also be a conduit useful for reconstructing events alleged to have occurred within the case, while providing support in corroborating or even disproving claims made by the involved parties. Some current body fluid identification techniques can prove problematic when attempting to address this objective; particularly in sexual assault cases where there is a necessity to determine the presence of vaginal fluid and/or saliva. For example, when investigating oral sexual assault cases, there can be a requirement to identify saliva from sexual assault swabs or on underwear where vaginal fluid is also likely to be present. Traditional methods for identifying saliva do not have sufficient specificity and can be cross-reactive with vaginal fluid material (Virkler and Lednev, 2009; James and Norby, 2003), generating inaccurate results and making it challenging for analysts to interpret the evidence. Other similar difficulties can be faced where the requirement is to prove the identification of vaginal fluid on digits/ items used to penetrate the victim or to verify the presence of saliva in cases where victims claim to have been bitten or licked where consent was not given. Equally, sexual assault cases where the male perpetrator is vasecto-mized can make it harder to identify the presence of semen. The Body Fluid ID Test represents an important new tool in these types of case scenarios for confirming the provenance of DNA contributions which have historically been challenging to achieve, particularly when attempting to authenticate the presence of mixtures of multiple body fluid types, potentially including a previously undetectable vaginal fluid component.

Finally, a subset of Universities around the globe are also utilizing the system as an alternative for teaching DNA profiling and body fluid identifica-tion techniques to their students, with the technology being incorporated into research projects and studies being conducted that include how the system can be better employed for specific targeted applications in forensic casework.

16.9   ParaDNA USER CASE STUDY

The Kauai Police Department (KPD) began validation of the ParaDNA System in November 2015. Their validation confirmed that the instrument purchased performed similarly, in their hands, as compared to the develop-mental and external validations performed prior. KPD's validation of the ParaDNA System included both the Screening and Intelligence Tests.

KPD found the performance of the ParaDNA Screening Test matched expectations based on validation findings from other users. High level DNA samples produced positive screening results, low level DNA samples produced variable ParaDNA Screening Test results and 1:100 saliva dilutions in water were detected on some occasions. All negative controls showed no evidence of contamination. All gender calls made were concordant with the donor profiles.

KPD also evaluated the ParaDNA Intelligence Test for precision, accuracy, inhibition, sensitivity, mixture detection, and mock casework. Performance of mock evidentiary samples was consistent with developmental validation studies, with 99.31% allele calls concordant with the expected STR profile.

Sensitivity studies showed the ability to call low numbers of alleles down to a 1:100 dilution of saliva in water and improved sensitivity through user experience with the system. While the system is not designed to target mixture deconvolution, the ParaDNA Intelligence Test in combination with Data Analysis Software detected 81% of mixtures run including 50% of 9:1 ratio mixtures. The ParaDNA System does not include a DNA purification process and therefore is more susceptible to decreased performance due to PCR inhibitors than standard bench methods. Based on this, the system was evaluated on samples with varying degrees of rust, a known PCR inhibitor. While increases in the level of rust showed the expected gradual decrease in number of alleles called, 50% of samples designated as "medium inhibition" and "heavy inhibition," due to documented level of rust on item sampled, still provided >7 allele calls.

After internal validation, KPD began utilizing the ParaDNA System on live case work in May 2016 (see Figure 16.11). Prior to utilizing the ParaDNA System, KPD like many departments was limited in its utilization of DNA analysis due to large state lab backlogs and high prices for outsourcing. In fact, DNA was utilized on only around ten cases per year. In contrast, in the last year and a half, KPD has run just under 100 samples. In this time, they also estimate a cost savings of around $50,000 versus blind submission of samples without prior screening.

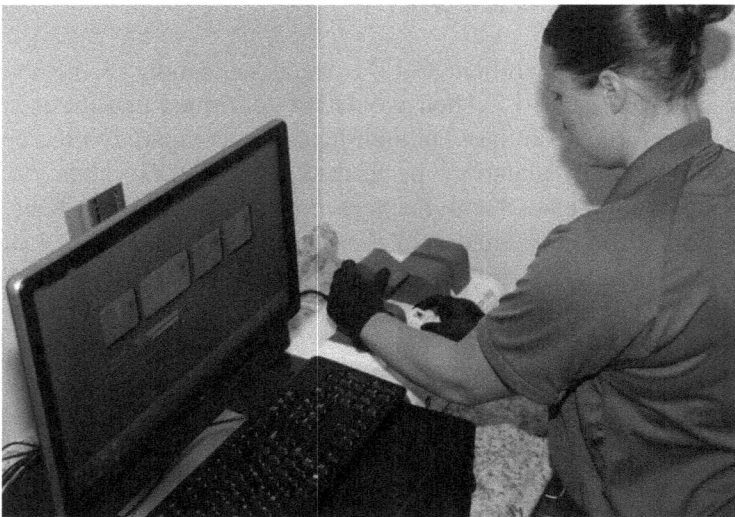

FIGURE 16.12 A crime scene specialist from Kauai Police Department utilizing the ParaDNA system for live casework testing.

Where the department had not previously exploited DNA analysis for property crimes, over half of all samples run were utilized for these types of cases. This includes a business burglary where the use of the ParaDNA Intelligence System added confidence to the identification of the suspect within hours of the incident occurring. The system has also aided in the identification of unidentified human remains, allowing department resources to be focused elsewhere while awaiting confirmation of the results. In one sexual assault case, the presumptive profile generated by the ParaDNA Intelligence Test from a cigarette that the suspect was seen smoking earlier in the evening was found to match that of one found near to the entrance of the primary scene. This information aided in obtaining a search warrant for the suspect's buccal sample for further comparison to the rest of the case evidence.

Additional highlights over this period include the saving of over $5000 on a single homicide case, in which a multitude of cigarettes were screened with a combination of the Screening and Intelligence Tests. This allowed for the identification of just two cigarettes that would be pushed forward for confirmatory analysis against the suspect and victim's profiles. Another $1400 was saved on a single-attempted murder case when the blood sample recovered in the suspects residence was found to not be case relevant and therefore did not need further processing by an external lab.

The KPD has begun validation work on the ParaDNA Body Fluid Identification Test. The department already sees great potential for this test including use in a suspected serial sexual offender case where the differentiation between saliva and vaginal fluid as well as peripheral blood and menstrual blood will add tremendous case detail.

16.10   CONCLUDING REMARKS

Around the globe, crime rates remain a key social issue (United Nations Office on Drugs and Crime, 2016) and yet public-sector budgets seem to be under increasing pressure to deliver more with less, putting pressure on law enforcement agencies' abilities to conduct and conclude investigations. The ParaDNA System represents an innovative new tool designed to assist the modern investigator with an additional array of forensic applications that decentralize forensic practice, support more rapid investigational progression, and in many instances strengthen outcome, all delivered with the ultimate goal of achieving measurable time and cost savings. The

ParaDNA System provides an augmentative tool which can be used to train and empower forensically trained or *nonforensically trained* individuals to screen samples for the presence of DNA, generate DNA intelligence profiles, and identify the presence of specific bodily fluids, all without the need for the relatively high capital expenditure associated with providing a forensic service. The recent development of the ParaDNA Body Fluid ID Test, however, makes a stronger case than ever that ParaDNA Instruments also have a place within forensic laboratories, adding a further tool to support rapid confirmation of the bodily fluids present on evidence items, and the first commercial tool to specifically identify the presence of vaginal fluids. A single test provides accurate identification of multiple biological fluid types associated with crimes, and specifically sexual assault crimes, whether present single source or mixtures. Reducing reliance on time-consuming laboratory-based serology, a technique known to be prone to cross-reactivity with other bodily fluids, represents a key new tool to the modern laboratory.

Where applicable, users of the ParaDNA Screening Test can preferentially target which items from an available set should be submitted for full STR analyses, based on sound scientific rationale, and represent the likeliest to deliver probative evidential value. This screening approach delivers improved profiling success rates, increased investigational successes and takes pressure off any associated laboratory backlogs. The ParaDNA Intelligence Test adds additional power to the ability to triage crime stains, facilitating victim exclusions, suspect identification, and ultimately the option to compare profiles against a "watch-list" (uploaded onto the instrument software), local or even national databases, in order to identify suspects. The immediate nature of the supplied intelligence information supports accelerated investigational outcomes, in tandem with improvements in efficiencies associated with resource allocations. Despite the reduced discriminatory power the profiles generated by the ParaDNA Intelligence Test have compared to modern lab-based STR kits (Blackman et al., 2015), the speed and ease with which results are achieved can be pivotal to successes in numerous operational environments. The technology was not designed to replace existing forensic processes but to support direct testing from crime scene samples using a nondestructive technique and to specifically gather actionable forensic intelligence as an investigation develops in real time, in some situations before these samples even reach a laboratory.

KEYWORDS

- **ParaDNA**
- **HyBeacon® probe technology**
- **field portable instrument**

REFERENCES

APCC—The Association of Police and Crime Commissioners. *APCC—The Association of Police and Crime Commissioners, Specialist Capabilities.* **2018**. [online] Available at: http://www.apccs.police.uk/our-work/police-reform/specialist-capabilities/. [Accessed January 30, 2018].

Ball, G.; et al.; Concordance study between the ParaDNA® Intelligence Test, a rapid DNA profiling assay, and a conventional STR typing kit (AmpFlSTR® SGM Plus™). *Forensic Sci Int Genet.* **2015**, *16*, 48–51.

Blackman, S.; et al.; Developmental validation of the ParaDNA Intelligence System—A novel approach to DNA profiling. *Forensic Sci Int Genet.* **2015**, *17*, 137–148.

Blackman, S.; et al.; Developmental validation of the ParaDNA Body Fluid ID System. *Forensic Sci Int Genet.* **2018**, *37*, 151–161.

Butler, J.M.; *Advanced Topics in Forensic DNA Typing: Methodology*, Elsevier Academic Press, **2011**.

Campbell, R.; et al.; The national problem of untested Sexual Assault Kits (SAKs): Scope, causes, and future directions for research, policy, and practice. *Sage Journals.* **2017**, *18*(4), 363–376.

Crown Prosecution Service. *DNA-17 Profiling.* [online] Available at: https://www.cps.gov.uk/legal-guidance/dna-17-profiling. **2017**. [Accessed September 15, 2017].

Dawnay, N.; et al.; Developmental validation of the ParaDNA Screening System—A presumptive test for the detection of DNA on forensic evidence items. *Forensic Sci Int Genet.* **2014**, *11*, 73–79.

Debenham, P.G.; Moore, D.J. Methods for direct PCR using a polymeric material as sample carrier. GB. World Patent WO/2011/158037, **2011**.

Doole, S. An investigation into the use of the ParaDNA® Body Fluid Identification System in forensic examinations. *Forensic Sci Int Genet.* **2017**, *6*, e492–e493.

European Network of Forensic Science Institutes, DNA Working Group. *DNA Database Management Review and Recommendations.* [online] Available at: https://enfsi.eu/wp-content/uploads/2017/09/DNA-databasemanagement-review-and-recommendatations-april-2017.pdf. **2017**. [Accessed November 15, 2017].

Federal Bureau of Investigation. *Combined DNA Index System (CODIS).* [online] Available at: https://www.fbi.gov/services/laboratory/biometric-analysis/codis. **2017a**. [Accessed September 15, 2017].

Federal Bureau of Investigation. *Forensic Science Communications, Critical Human Resource Issues: Scientists Under Pressure.* [online] Available at: https://archives.fbi.gov/archives/about-us/lab/forensic-science-communications/fsc/april2007/research/2007_04_research02.htm. **2017b**. [Accessed September 15, 2017].

Federal Bureau of Investigation. *Rapid DNA.* [online] Available at: https:// www.fbi.gov/about-us/lab/biometric-analysis/codis/rapid-dna-analysis. **2017c**. [Accessed July 15, 2017].

French, D.J.; et al.; HyBeacon probes: A new tool for DNA sequence detection and allele discrimination. *Mol Cell Probes.* **2001**, *15*(6), 363–374.

French, D.J.; et al.; Interrogation of short tandem repeats using fluorescent probes and melting curve analysis: A step towards rapid DNA identity screening. *Forensic Sci Int Genet.* **2008**, *2*(4), 333–339.

GeneCards® Human Gene Database. *SEMG1 Gene Expression.* [online] Available https://www.genecards.org/cgi-bin/carddisp.pl?gene=SEMG1&keywords=semg1#expression. **2017**. [Accessed November 1, 2017].

Haas, C.; et al.; Collaborative EDNAP exercises on messenger RNA/DNA co-analysis for body fluid identification (blood, saliva, semen) and STR profiling. *Forensic Sci Int Genet.* **2011**, *3*(1), e5–e6.

Hanson, E.; and Ballantyne, J.; Highly specific mRNA biomarkers for the identification of vaginal secretions in sexual assault investigation. *Sci Justice.* **2013**, *53*(1), 14–22.

Hill, C.R.; et al.; Concordance study between the AmpFlSTR® Minifiler™ PCR amplification kit and conventional STR typing kits. *J Forensic Sci.* **2007**, *52*(4), 870–873.

James, S.H.; and Norby, J.J.; *Forensic Science: An Introduction to Scientific and Investigative Techniques*, CRC Press, **2003**.

National Criminal Justice Reference Service. *Evaluation of the Impact of the Forensic Casework DNA Backlog Reduction Program.* [online] Available at: https://www.ncjrs.gov/pdffiles1/nij/grants/225803.pdf. **2010**. [Accessed October 27, 2017].

National Criminal Justice Reference Service. *Establishment of a Fast and Accurate Proteomic Method for Body Fluid/Cell Type Identification.* [online] Available at: https://www.ncjrs.gov/pdffiles1/nij/grants/236538.pdf. **2011a**. [Accessed July 14, 2017].

National Criminal Justice Reference Service. *Rapid STR Pre-Screening of Forensic Samples at the Crime Scene.* [online] Available at: https://www.ncjrs.gov/pdffiles1/nij/grants/236434.pdf. **2011b**. [Accessed October 27, 2017].

National DNA Database Ethics Group. *Notes of the 37th Meeting.* [online] Available at: https://www.gov.uk/government/uploads/system/uploads/attachment_data/file/608218/NDNAD_Ethics_Group_Minutes_-_22_02_2017.pdf. **2017**. [Accessed December 18, 2017].

National Institute of Justice. *DNA Evidence Backlogs: Forensic Casework.* [online] Available at: https://www.nij.gov/topics/forensics/lab-operations/evidence-backlogs/pages/forensic-evidence-backlog.aspx. **2017**. [Accessed November 14, 2017].

Raymond, J.; et al.; Trace DNA success rates relating to volume crime offences. *Forensic Sci Int Genet.* **2009**, *2*(1), 136–137.

Scientific Working Group on DNA Analysis Methods (SWGDAM). *Validation Guidelines for DNA Analysis Methods.* [online] Available at: https://docs.wixstatic.com/ugd/4344b0_813 b241e8944497e99b9c45b163b76bd.pdf. **2017**. [Accessed July 14, 2017].

White, P.; *Crime Scene to Court*, Royal Society of Chemistry Publishing, **2016**.

United Nations Office on Drugs and Crime. *Annual Report.* [online] Available at: https://www.unodc.org/documents/AnnualReport2016/2016_UNODC_Annual_Report.pdf. **2016**. [Accessed December 19, 2017].

Virkler, K.; and Lednev, I.K.; Analysis of body fluids for forensic purposes: from laboratory testing to non-destructive rapid confirmatory identification at a crime scene. *Forensic Sci Int.* **2009**, *188*(1–3), 1–17.

Zubakov, D.; et al.; Stable RNA markers for identification of blood and saliva stains revealed from whole genome expression analysis of time-wise degraded samples. *Int J Legal Med.* **2008**, *122*(2), 135–142.

CHAPTER 17

DEPArray™ System: Key Enabling Technology for Cell Separation from Forensic Mixtures

ROBERTA AVERSA*, FRANCESCA FONTANA, GIANNI MEDORO, and NICOLÒ MANARESI

Menarini Silicon Biosystems Spa, 40013 Castel Maggiore (BO), Italy

Corresponding author. E-mail: raversa@siliconbiosystems.com

ABSTRACT

Despite the great scientific and technological advances in recent years, mixed profiles interpretation represents a persisting challenge in forensic genetics, routinely complicating expert witness reporting in court and fostering backlogs in evidence processing worldwide. Current solutions to the complexity of mixed profiles interpretation include either the physical separation of a mixture into its biological components before genotyping (e.g., differential lysis for sperm–epithelial mixtures, laser capture microdissection, and micromanipulation) or biostatistical data analysis exploiting dedicated semicontinuous and fully continuous algorithms. Moreover, complex mixtures deriving from the contribution of the same body fluid from different individuals determine a higher level of complication since no available method allows to phenotypically distinguish the admixed biological components. DEPArray™ digital sorting technology has been reported to enable the isolation of pure single cells from forensic mixed samples also in real-casework scenarios. The advent of single-cell analysis in forensics offers a promising approach to complex mixtures interpretation enabling the identification of each contributor's profile through the collection of multiple single cells each purely representing one single contributor to the sample.

17.1   THE PROBLEM OF THE FORENSIC MIXTURES

With the latest increases in sensitivity of genotyping technologies for human identification, ever smaller biological samples can be now analyzed, and the ultimate limit of a single cell as suitable input is within reach. In this scenario, biological mixtures remain one of the major challenges in forensic biology. Biological mixtures derive from the contribution of two or more individuals to the formation of a physically inseparable forensic evidence. Standard genotyping of such evidence would result in *complex DNA profiles* where more than two alleles can be detected per locus. The number of possible allelic combinations that can be associated to each contributor thus hampers the interpretation of multiallelic genetic profiles. Increased peak imbalance (especially in heterozygous loci), augmented stutter peaks height (>15%), and drop in incidence further complicate the analysis when dealing with low-template (LT) inputs.

Genetic contribution of the two or more individuals is generally unbalanced defining one or more major and minor contributors. Indeed, because of different cell density, even when the volume of biological fluids involved is identical, DNA proportion would still be preferential for one of them. It has been demonstrated that the quantitative ratio is maintained by PCR amplification, allowing the use of peak height ratio as an indicator of the real biological material contribution (Gill et al., 2006). This point is used to statistically assign alleles to each contributor using peak height/area according to international guidelines such as that issued by SWGDAM and specifically developed software (SWGDAM, 2017). Taken to the extreme, when ratios unbalance exceeds about 1:20, sensitivity limitations or saturation by the major components (Vuichard et al., 2011) can cause the detection failure of the minor component, causing the misinterpretation as single genetic profile.

Currently, the approach to complex DNA profiles is to attempt their interpretation through statistical analysis by assessing the likelihood ratio (LR), which is the probability ratio of an event (a genetic profile) evaluated under two mutually exclusive hypotheses: the prosecution hypothesis (numerator) or the defense hypothesis (denominator) (Willis et al., 2015). This approach leads to a statistical interpretation of the profiles and involves elaborated computations, which are today operated by specifically developed and validated software packages such as LRmix Studio© and EuroForMix among the most used. The software compares the mixed DNA profile to reference profiles and returns the computed probability of profiles match or mismatch.

Besides not being an exact analysis, but rather a probabilistic assessment of profiles match/mismatch, the statistical interpretation of complex DNA profiles is often further complicated by additional factors. Electropherograms generated from mixtures often show extra peaks, which may be due to several and not always clarified factors: alleles drop in/out, stutter peaks or additional alleles due to contaminant DNA will contribute to the generated profile lowering the confidence of the result.

The forensic community has made many efforts to standardize the statistical analysis of complex profiles, but the broad combination of variables makes complex DNA profiles interpretation still an open question.

17.2 METHODS CURRENTLY APPLIED TO FORENSIC MIXTURES

Immunochromatographic assays are normally used as presumptive or confirmatory tests for the body fluid identification present in a biological evidence. Once the presence of a mixture is established, forensic scientists follow standard procedures in order to attempt the identification of each contributor.

Blood, semen but also saliva, sweat, hair, nails typically compose biological evidence. Sperms from perpetrator(s) and epithelial cells, shed from victim's vaginal, rectal, or buccal fluids, constitute the majority of mixed evidence reaching crime laboratories. This type of mixture is usually processed with the well-characterized and diffused method of *differential DNA extraction.*

Other types of mixtures cannot benefit from specific procedures for the separation of DNA and generally result in complex DNA profiles, which are then managed through statistical analysis.

To overcome this problem and achieve more robust results from forensic mixtures, a number of alternative methods have been explored to attempt the physical separation of a mixture into its biological components.

17.2.1 DNA DIFFERENTIAL EXTRACTION

From its first description by Gill et al. (1985), *differential DNA extraction* has represented the gold standard for the separation of male and female DNA fractions from forcible rape cases evidence that contain mixtures of assailant's and victim's DNA. This kind of evidence is collected and analyzed with the aim to obtain single male profiles for the perpetrator's identification.

The differential DNA extraction (or differential lysis) is a chemical extraction method used to separate the DNA from sperm cells (male fraction) and epithelial cells (female fraction). This method exploits the presence of protein disulfide bonds in sperm cells outer membrane, which makes them more resistant to extraction reagents than epithelial cells. According to this method, DNA is first released from epithelial cells using a low concentration SDS/Proteinase K treatment. Subsequently, male fraction is physically separated by pelleting the intact sperm cells, removing the victim's fraction and repeatedly washing the sperm pellet prior to lysis with the addition of dithiothreitol (DTT) to allow the reduction of disulfides bonds and the consequent release of DNA from sperm cells. Male and female DNAs can then be amplified and genotyped separately obtaining reliably interpretable profiles in the majority of cases.

The differential DNA extraction offers several advantages, such as the low cost and short time required, the efficacy and the overall good performance. However, although routinely applied, this method shows some limitations: first, it can be applied only to mixtures of sperm and epithelial cells. In the presence of azoospermic or oligospermic semen (e.g., vasectomized perpetrators), differential lysis will most likely fail due to the absence/scarcity of spermatozoa. Furthermore, in the presence of few sperm cells, the sensitivity is relatively low and the repeated pellet washes can lead to an extensive loss of material. Over time, the method has been optimized (QIAGEN, 2010; Wiegand et al., 1992), for example, with the two-step modified protocol by Yoshida et al. (1995) and more recently the Differex™ System (Promega Corporation, Madison, Wisconsin, United States). Differex™ exploits the use of an organic buffer, whose density is higher than the aqueous lysis buffer, to pellet sperm cells without the need of pellet washes. Despite the high efficiency, the method is still influenced by possible carryover between the two fractions (Tsukada et al., 2006).

17.2.2 NEXT-GENERATION SEQUENCING

In recent years, the application of the next-generation sequencing (NGS) technologies in forensic genetics has improved the ability to obtain genetic information from DNA samples. NGS analysis adds information about SNPs to STRs analysis, introducing the possibility to collect a deeper and wider set of information from the analyzed DNA (Jäger et al., 2017; Fordyce et al., 2015). NGS is starting to be adopted for the identification of phenotypical features, such as hair/eyes colors or ancestry and age determination as a potentially useful tool for investigations. Despite the broader information available and the consequent gain in robustness in data analysis, NGS still requires biostatistics computations to separate the contributors of a mixture. Therefore, although NGS represents a further analytical method to manage mixtures, it still fails to provide a complete and clear resolution of the problem.

17.2.3 METHODS BASED ON CELL SEPARATION

In principle, the upfront physical separation of the distinct cellular elements present in a mixture (e.g., sperm cells, epithelial cells, or blood cells) could provide a pure genetic source for human identification assays. Moreover, in addition to helping the resolution of mixed genetic profiles, this approach would provide information about tissue origin, which would otherwise be lost when cells are destroyed to release the DNA. Different approaches have been applied for this purpose, including laser-capture microdissection (LCM) or fluorescence-activated cell sorting (FACS), but none of them has gained a full endorsement from the forensic community.

The LCM is a clinical procedure to isolate cells of interest on a microscope slide. For forensic purposes, sperm cells can be identified from rape evidence collected on slides to confirm the happening of a sexual intercourse (Elliott et al., 2003) and obtain the perpetrator's profile through STR typing. Although LCM has gained positive endorsement by the forensic community for its capacity to operate on tiny and scarce evidence with powerful resolution, its applicability is undermined by intrinsic variability due to its laborious and highly operator dependent procedure and the lack of complete purity of the separation (Vandewoestyne et al., 2010).

The FACS is a method already implemented as medical diagnostic procedure routinely applied to sort cells based on expression of specific antigens on the cells of interest, which are detected with fluorescent probes. When applied to forensic testing, FACS has shown to have an intrinsic limit because the cell input amount needed to execute cell separation is high (Dean et al., 2015; Verdon et al., 2015) and the purity of the sorted cells is not guaranteed.

17.3 THE DEPArray™ SYSTEM

The DEPArray™ system (Menarini Silicon Biosystems, Bologna, Italy) is a highly automated, image-based digital cell sorter that combines advanced microfluidics and microelectronics with high-resolution fluorescence imaging for the isolation of pure cells of interest with single-cell precision. This technology has been extensively applied in clinical research and validated to isolate pure cells starting from a broad variety of rare cell suspensions including both fixed and live cells. The main applications include isolation of pure circulating tumor cells from enriched blood and the separation of pure tumor and stromal cell populations from Formalin-Fixed Paraffin-Embedded tissues (Peeters at al., 2013; Polzer et al., 2014; Krebs et al., 2014; Hodgkinson et al., 2014; Carpenter et al., 2014; Campton et al., 2015; Normand et al., 2016; Bolognesi et al., 2016; Carter et al., 2017; Di Trapani et al., 2018).

The DEPArray™ system is composed of an instrument and a single-use microfluidic cartridge, which constitutes the core of the technology where immunofluorescently labeled cells are specifically selected and isolated with 100% precision (Figure 17.1).

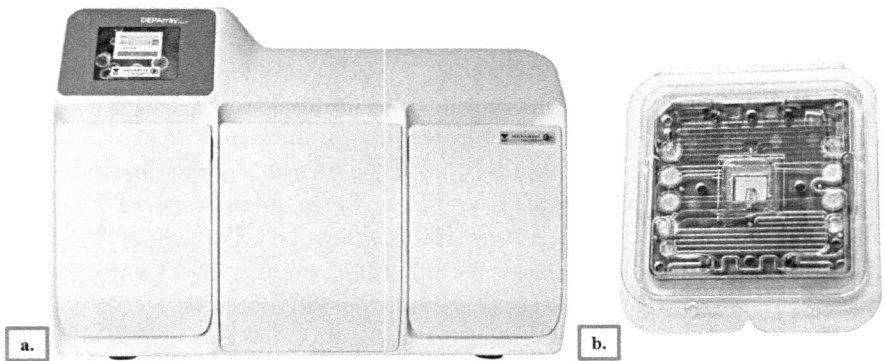

FIGURE 17.1 The DEPArray™ system. The DEPArray™ system is composed of an automated instrument (A) and a single-use microfluidic cartridge (B).

The DEPArray™ technology is based on the ability of a nonuniform electric field to exert forces on polarizable particles such as cells in liquid suspension, a physical principle known as dielectrophoresis (DEP). An array of about 300k microelectrodes integrated in a semiconductor chip at the "core" of the cartridge allows the generation of up to 30.000 "DEP cages," each one able to capture a single cell. When a single-cell suspension is loaded into the cartridge, cells are trapped in DEP cages in stable levitation through the application of gentle dielectrophoretic forces. In this configuration, if a DEP cage is moved by switching the voltages applied to the electrodes, trapped cell will move along the path defined by the software. The multi-channel fluorescence microscope (five fluorescence channels plus Bright Field visualization) and the CMOS camera integrated in the DEPArray™

system scan the chip and acquire images with high resolution. After image analysis, cells correspondent to desired criteria of morphology and fluorescence are analyzed by means of the proprietary CellBrowser™ software. Exploiting the above said principle of moving DEP cages, selected cells are independently routed from the DEPArray™ Cartridge Main Chamber into a Parking Chamber (Figure 17.2). Finally, single or homogenous pools of cells are moved to the recovery chamber from which they are eluted by means of a drop of clean buffer directly into PCR tubes (or plates) ready for downstream genetic analysis (Figure 17.2). Notably, interacting only with disposable parts, the sample never gets in contact with the machine, which prevents potential carryover between different samples.

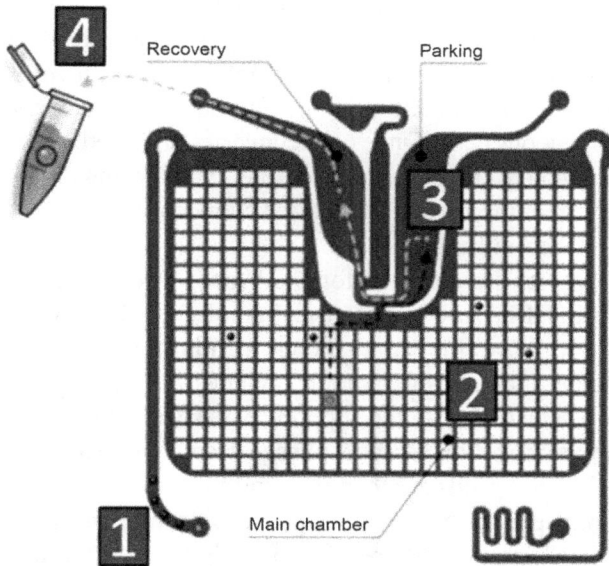

FIGURE 17.2 DEPArray™ cartridge. Cells are loaded through a microfluidic channel (A) into the main chamber area (B) and trapped singularly in DEP cages. Once analyzed, selected cells are automatically routed to the parking chamber (C) and then to the recovery chamber to be recovered single or in pools into 0.2 mL tubes or plates (D).

The benchtop instrument DEPArray™ NxT implements the third generation of DEPArray™ technology. This platform enables the execution of up to 96 single-cell recoveries and integrates high-resolution imaging for real-time visualization and image acquisition. Moreover, the system has been configured to provide a higher level of automation thanks to preset cell selection criteria that lower the hands-on time required by the operator. An external barcode reader and the generation of an all-inclusive report permit to always guarantee complete traceability of the sample.

17.4   DEPArray™ CAPABILITY TO SEPARATE FORENSIC MIXTURES

Extensively reported and validated in the oncology field, the DEPArray™ systems enable the separation of pure cells with single-cell precision from mixed samples. It appears straightforward that the same principle of cell sorting can be applied to the resolution of forensic biological mixtures.

The workflow for DEPArray™ analysis of forensic samples starts from sample preparation to obtain an immunofluorescently labeled cell suspension. This cell suspension is loaded into the DEPArray™ cartridge and, running an application-program tailored to forensic samples, cells are identified by means of their specific staining and morphology in order to be recovered single or in pools of homogeneous cells. Once cell recoveries are lysed, the lysates can be analyzed with standard forensic methods (i.e., STR typing, NGS).

A full representation of DEPArray™ workflow for forensic mixtures analysis is provided in Figure 17.3.

Forensic samples are prepared for DEPArray™ sorting using the specifically developed DEPArray™ Forensic SamplePrep Kit (Menarini Silicon Biosystems) that allows the simultaneous staining of sperm, epithelial, and white blood cells. Sample preparation includes a first phase of incubation where cells are detached from the support (e.g., swab, cloth portion, etc.) and released in solution, followed by a phase of cells collection from which a cell pellet is obtained. Cells are then immunofluorescently stained using antibodies targeting membrane or cytoplasmic specific antigens (allophycocyanin (APC)-conjugated sperm-head specific antibody for sperm cells, cytokeratin-fluorescein-5-isothiocyanate (FITC) for epithelial cells, CD45-phycoerythrin (PE) for white blood cells) and fixed. Hoechst dye is used for nuclei staining of any cell type. Each sample is washed in a specific manipulation buffer (DEPArray™ Buffer for Fixed Cells, Menarini Silicon Biosystems), which confers the appropriate electric proprieties for the sample analysis with DEPArray™ system.

A 12 µL cell suspension is finally loaded into the DEPArray™ Cartridge and pumped into the Main Chamber through a microfluidic manifold. Here, with cells kept in stable levitation in DEP cages, the chip area is scanned in multifluorescence channels and brightfield. During this step, high resolution images are acquired and cell events are simultaneously detected.

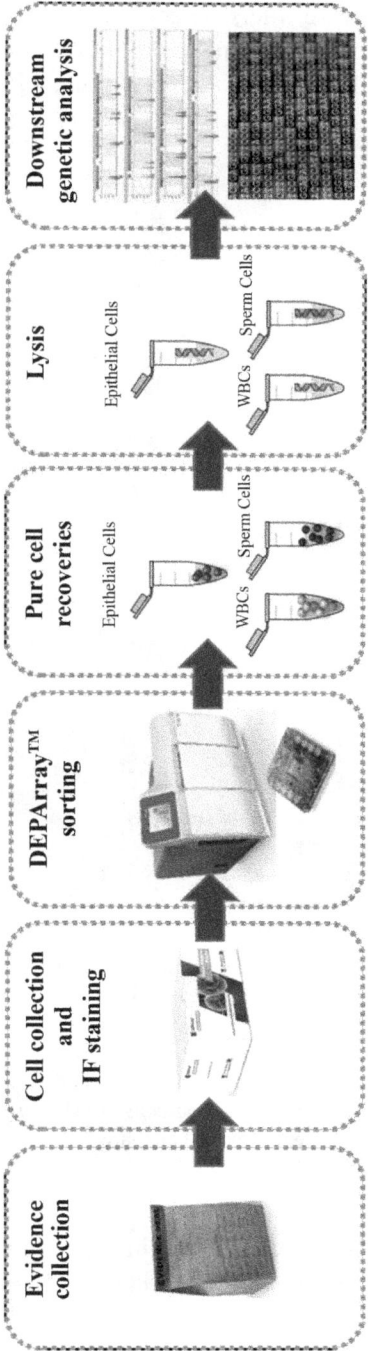

FIGURE 17.3 DEPArray™ workflow for forensic samples. Overview of the workflow used for forensic mixtures analysis with the DEPArray™ system: the principal macrosteps include evidence collection, sample preparation, DEPArray™ sorting, isolation of pure cells, lysis, and downstream genetic analysis of the recovered cells. *IF*, immunofluorescent.

The CellBrowser™ software filters detected cells to exclude by default events not falling into the desired parameters of dimension and fluorescence and creates scatter plots of the detected events (Figure 17.4).

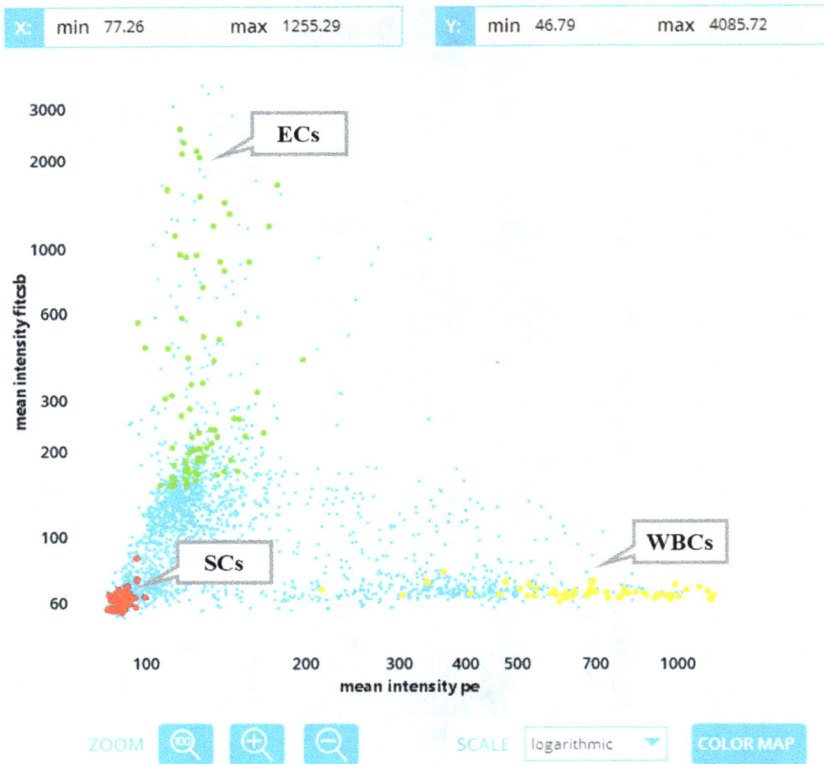

FIGURE 17.4 DEPArray™ analysis based on scatter plot distribution. The CellBrowser™ scatter plot tool allows the visualization of the detected events as distinct distributions of cell populations based on the positivity to specific fluorescence signals. The scatter plot provided represents the discrimination of three cell populations (sperm cells, epithelial cells, and white blood cells) from a mixed sample. Cytokeratin-FITC positive epithelial cells are shown as green dots; CD45-PE positive white blood cells are shown as yellow dots; Sperm Head-specific Antigen-APC positive events (sperm cells) are shown as red dots in the double negative region of the plot. Blue dots represent unselected events.

Cell images can be analyzed one by one in image galleries: only those showing the correct morphology, integrity, and specific immunofluorescent staining are assigned to their specific selection group by the operator (sperm cells, epithelial cells, or white blood cells) and recovered single or in pools of homogeneous cells (Figure 17.5). Thanks to image-based selection, only fluorescent events qualified appropriately as cells of interest are recovered.

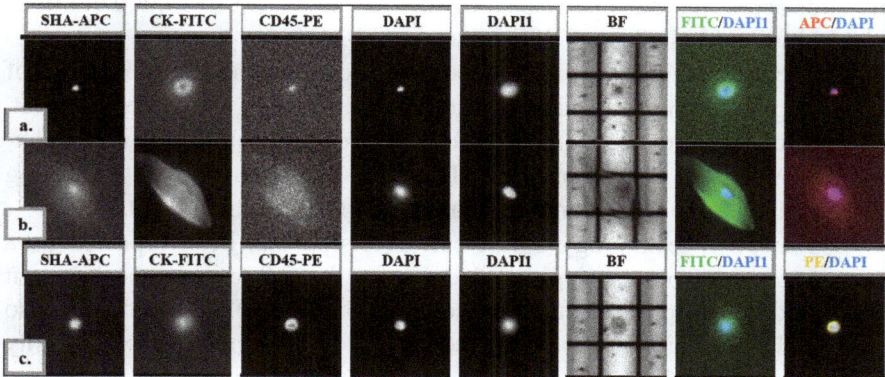

FIGURE 17.5 DEPArray™ analysis based on cell images. DEPArray™ image-galleries are shown for each cell type: (A) Sperm cell, (B) epithelial cell, and (C) white blood cell. From the left, images are reported in grayscale across the different fluorescence channels (APC, FITC, PE, and 4,6 diamidino-2-phenylindole (DAPI)) along with Bright-Field (BF). The last two images on the right represent overlays of cell specific and nuclear staining for each cell type in false colors. Two different images are provided for DAPI channel with two distinct offsets due to the different dimensions of the cells analyzed: DAPI represents the correct focus for sperm cells and white blood cells while DAPI1 is optimized for observation of epithelial cells. All images are acquired with 10× magnification.

Finally, cell recoveries are lysed to release the DNA content with a single tube method (DEPArray™ LysePrep Kit, Menarini Silicon Biosystems) with the addition of DTT to sperm cell recoveries for optimal lysis conditions. At this point, DNA released from lysed cells is available for standard analysis such as genotyping and quantification.

17.5 DEPArray™ WORKFLOW APPLICATION TO FORENSIC CASES

Widely demonstrated on simulated mixtures adsorbed on swabs, the established workflow has shown to reliably allow the precise isolation of pure cells also from real forensic evidence (Fontana et al., 2017). Studies on real casework have focused primarily on evidence samples from sexual assault cases demonstrating the ability to obtain highly complete, concordant, and uncontaminated genetic profiles from each DEPArray™ cell recovery. Remarkably, the genetic profile concordance constitutes an additional proof of DEPArray™ ability to clearly and unambiguously discriminate distinct cell types. DEPArray™ processed samples have also shown to enable increased sensitivity and specificity compared to the use of differential extraction methods across periods up to 72 h post-coitus and up to 1 to 10,000 dilutions of semen to epithelial cells (Williamson et al., 2018).

The technique has additionally been tested to assess the robustness of standard genotyping methods when using DEPArray™ recoveries as input. The exact number of recovered cells can be used to calculate the correspondent DNA content for an optimal STR amplification reaction set up, saving template needed for the quantitation assays (Fontana et al., 2017).

DEPArray™ technology single-cell precision has been reported as a new approach to obtain single molecules for the inference of peak height distribution of drop in events (Hansson and Gill, 2017). These studies also open up the possibility of using the technology as a method to assess quality standards in forensics.

As a further alternative approach, DEPArray™ technology has also been applied to clinical research for the evaluation of chimerism in allogeneic bone marrow or blood stem cell transplanted patients (Anslinger et al., 2017), demonstrating the coexistence of two different genotypes in the same individual.

The DEPArray™ workflow has proved to be effective also in the extreme scenario of cold cases samples. It has been reported that, depending on the sample preservation, intact cells can be isolated from up to 27-year-old samples. In particular, pure white blood cells from 10- to 27-years-old casework samples were identified and recovered by means of DEPArray™ system. In both cases, recovered cells provided partial but fully matching profiles and allowed a higher discriminatory power (i.e., LR) with respect to the original mixed profiles obtained from stains (Anslinger et al., 2018).

Moreover, the precision of the digital-sorting approach for the first time brings to forensic genetics the possibility to generate meaningful data even from single cells: almost complete genetic profiles can be obtained from single intact cells recovered by means of DEPArray™ platform (Figure 17.6). Indeed, a single pure cell constitutes a perfectly complete system in which the entire genetic information, from both nuclear and mitochondrial DNA, is present. In a single cell, the DNA quantity represents the extreme condition of LT DNA: any given genomic locus of a diploid cell is represented only by two double-stranded DNA molecules in a diploid cell or a single double-stranded molecule in a haploid cell, totaling about 6.6 or 3.3 pg of DNA for the entire cell, respectively. Still, the genomic representation is utterly complete, as it is unaffected by the stochastic sampling that would

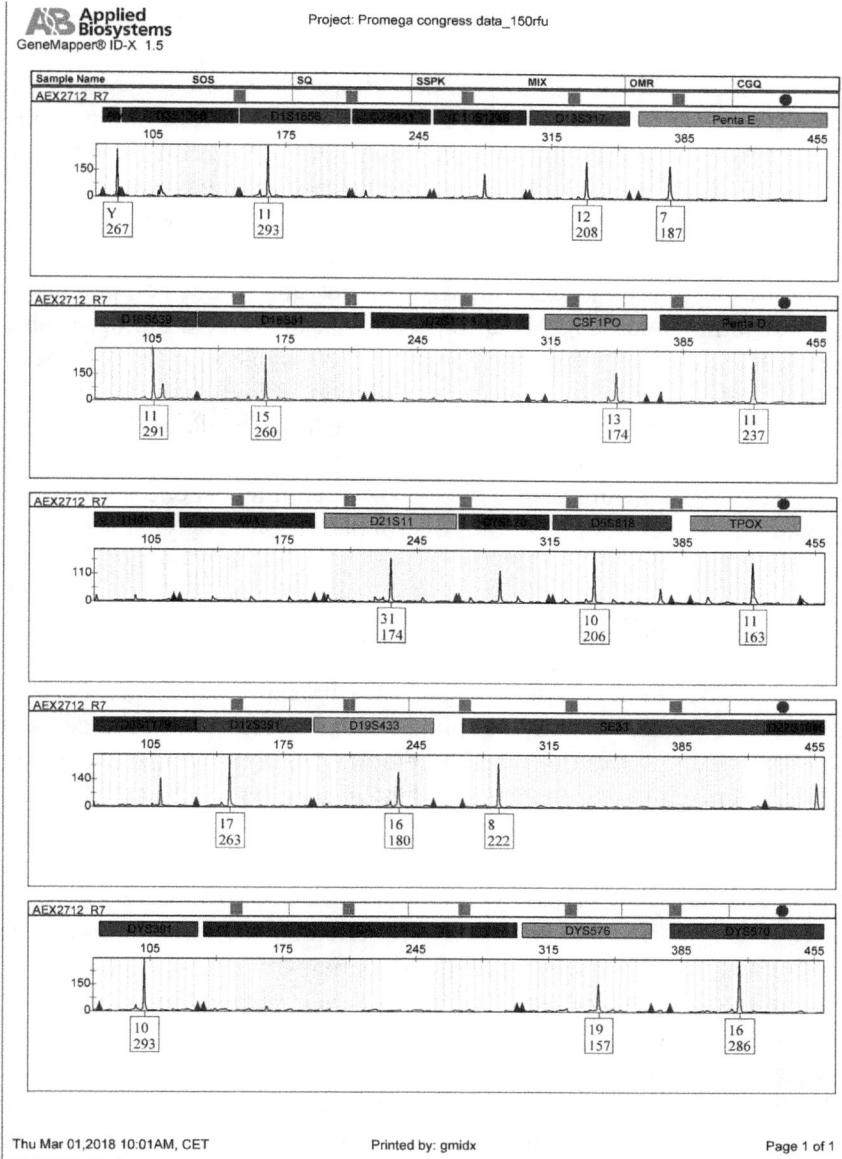

FIGURE 17.6 Single sperm cell haplotype. An example of a genetic profile obtained by the PowerPlex® Fusion 6C amplification of a single sperm cell recovery showing an almost complete haplotype. Coherently with the haploidy of male gametes, profiles obtained from single sperms may show maximum one allele for each locus. In particular, in case of sperm cells carrying the Y chromosome, Amelogenin locus shows only the Y allele and a single allele is present also for Y-mapping loci DYS391, DYS576, and DYS570.

be unavoidable when starting from an equivalent quantity of cell-free DNA molecules.

Currently, no described method can afford the separation of the same admixed body fluid from different individuals. In this respect, the application of STR profiling to single cells opens new perspectives for deducing each single contributor involved in a mixture of the same biological fluid. Moreover, this approach appears better suited to the investigation of balanced mixtures than software-based deconvolution models based on peak heights, respectively more suited when major and minor components are clearly determinable. It has been reported that the STR profiling of single white blood cells ($n = 17$) isolated from a blood–blood mixture collected on a murder case sample (knife blade) allowed obtaining single-source partial profiles of both the victim and the suspect (Anslinger et al., 2019). In consideration of the extreme LT condition of these samples, the routine application of this new discipline in forensic biology will certainly benefit of appropriate international guidelines for profiles interpretation.

17.6   CONCLUDING REMARKS

DEPArray™ technology has emerged as a breakthrough approach in the forensic field for the resolution of biological mixtures. It has been described that DEPArray™ system enables the precise separation of pure cells from different admixed biological fluids and the generation of clean profiles from each correspondent contributor.

With respect to other alternative approaches proposed so far (LCM or FACS), DEPArray™ technology has demonstrated to meet the standards of throughput, purity, and sensitivity requested by the forensic community guidelines. The upfront separation of the components of a mixture permits to combine single source genetic profiles with their correspondent precise cell phenotype information.

Cells recovered by means of DEPArray™ system are fully compatible with standard human identification methods, ensuring almost complete profiles from as little as few haploid cells. Moreover, by knowing the number of cells recovered, quantitation assays can be omitted, thus avoiding further template losses.

The studies reported so far pave the way to a wide adoption of DEPArray™ technology for its application to forensic mixture in casework evidence, also opening up new avenues in single-cell forensic genetics.

KEYWORDS

- **forensic mixtures**
- **DEPArray™**
- **digital sorting**
- **single-cell separation**
- **genotyping**

REFERENCES

Anslinger, K.; et al.; Application of DEPArray™ technology for the isolation of white blood cells from cell mixtures in chimerism analysis. *Rechtsmedizin,* **2017**, *28*, 134–137.

Anslinger, K.; et al.; Whose blood is it? Application of DEPArray™ technology for the identification of individual/s who contributed blood to a mixed stain. *Int. J. Legal Med.* **2018**, *133(2)*, 419–426.

Anslinger, K.; et al.; Deconvolution of blood–blood mixtures using DEPArray™ separated single cell STR profiling. *Rechtsmedizin* **2019***, 29*, 30–40.

Bolognesi, C.; et al.; Digital sorting of pure cell populations enables unambiguous genetic analysis of heterogeneous formalin-fixed paraffin-embedded tumors by next generation sequencing. *Sci. Rep.* **2016**, *11(6)*, 209–244.

Campton, D.E.; et al.; High-recovery visual identification and single-cell retrieval of circulating tumor cells for genomic analysis using a dual technology platform integrated with automated immunofluorescence staining. *BMC Cancer* **2015**, *6(15)*, 360.

Carpenter, E.; et al.; Dielectrophoretic capture and genetic analysis of single neuroblastoma tumor cells. *Front. Oncol.* **2014**, *31(4)*, 201.

Carter, L.; et al.; Molecular analysis of circulating tumor cells identifies distinct copy-number profiles in patients with chemo sensitive and chemo refractory small-cell lung cancer. *Nat. Med.* **2017**, *23(1)*, 114–119.

Dean, L.; et al.; Separation of uncompromised whole blood mixtures for single source STR profiling using fluorescently-labeled human leukocyte antigen (HLA) probes and fluorescence activated cell sorting (FACS). *Forensic Sci. Int.: Genet.* **2015**, *17*, 8–16.

Di Trapani; M; et al.; DEPArray™ system: An automatic image-based sorter for isolation of pure circulating tumor cells. *Cytometry* **2018**, *93A*, 1260–1266.

Elliott, K.; et al.; Use of laser microdissection greatly improves the recovery of DNA from sperm on microscope slides. *Forensic Sci. Int.* **2003**, *137*, 28–36.

Fontana, F.; et al.; Isolation and genetic analysis of pure cells from forensic biological mixtures: the precision of a digital approach. *Forensic Sci. Int.: Genet.* **2017**, *29*, 225–241.

Fordyce, S.L.; et al.; Second-generation sequencing of forensic STRs using the Ion Torrent™ HID STR 10-plex and the Ion PGM™. *Forensic Sci. Int. Genet.* **2015**, *14*, 132–140.

Gill, P.; et al.; Forensic application of DNA 'fingerprints.' *Nature* **1985**, *318*, 577–579.

Gill, P.; et al.; DNA commission of the International Society of Forensic Genetics: Recommendations on the interpretation of mixtures. *Forensic Sci. Int.* **2006**, *160(2–3)*, 90–101.

Hansson, O.; Gill, P. Characterization of artefacts and drop-in events using STR-validator and single-cell analysis, *Forensic Sci. Int.: Genet.* **2017**, *30*, 57–65.

Hodgkinson, C.L.; et al.; Tumorigenicity and genetic profiling of circulating tumor cells in small-cell lung cancer. *Nat. Med.* **2014**, *20(8)*, 897–903.

Jäger, A.C.; et al.; Developmental validation of the MiSeq FGx Forensic Genomics System for Targeted Next Generation Sequencing in Forensic DNA Casework and Database Laboratories. *Forensic Sci Int.* **2017**, *28*, 52–70.

Krebs, M.G.; et al.; Molecular analysis of circulating tumor cells—Biology and biomarkers. *Nat. Rev. Clin. Oncol.* **2014**, *11(3)* 129–144.

Normand, E.; et al.; Comparison of three whole genome amplification methods for detection of genomic aberrations in single cells. *Prenat. Diagn.* **2016**, *36(9)*, 823–830.

Peeters, D.J.; et al.; Semiautomated isolation and molecular characterization of single or highly purified tumour cells from CellSearch enriched blood samples using dielectrophoretic cell sorting. *Br. J. Cancer* **2013**, *108(6)*, 1358–1367.

Polzer, B.; et al.; Molecular profiling of single circulating tumor cells with diagnostic intention. *EMBO Mol. Med.* **2014**, *30(11)*, 1371–1386.

QIAGEN. Purification of DNA from epithelial cells mixed with sperm cells using the MagAttract® DNA Mini M48 Kit, **2010**.

Scientific Working Group on DNA Analysis Methods (SWGDAM). SWGDAM interpretation guidelines for autosomal STR typing by forensic DNA testing laboratories, **2017**.

Tsukada, et al.; Sperm DNA extraction from mixed stains using the Differex™ system. *Int. Congr. Ser.* **2006**, *1288*, 700–703.

Vandewoestyne, M.; Deforce, D. Laser capture microdissection in forensic research: A review. *Int. J. Legal Med.* **2010**, *124*, 513–521.

Verdon, T.J.; et al.; FACS separation of non-compromised forensically relevant biological mixtures. *Forensic Sci. Int. Genet.* **2015**, *14*, 194–200.

Vuichard, S.; et al.; Differential DNA extraction of challenging simulated sexual-assault samples: A Swiss collaborative study. *Invest. Genet.* **2011**, *2*, 11.

Wiegand, P.; et al.; DNA extraction from mixtures of body fluid using mild preferential lysis. *Int. J. Legal Med.* **1992**, *104*, 359–360.

Williamson, V.R; et al.; Enhanced DNA mixture deconvolution of sexual offense samples using the DEPArray™ system. *Forensic Sci. Int.: Genet.* **2018**, *34*, 265–276.

Willis, S.; et al.; ENFSI Guideline for evaluative reporting in forensic science 3.0. Strengthening the Evaluation of Forensic Results across Europe (STEOFRAE), **2015**.

Yoshida, K.; et al.; The modified method of two-step differential extraction of sperm and vaginal epithelial cell DNA from vaginal fluid mixed with semen. *Forensic Sci. Int.* **1995**, *72*, 25–33.

CHAPTER 18

Rapid DNA by ANDE Corporation: A Useful Tool for Disaster Victim Identification

ROSEMARY TURINGAN WITKOWSKI and RICHARD F SELDEN*

ANDE Corporation, 266 Second Avenue, Waltham, MA 02451, USA

Corresponding author. E-mail: rfs4n6@ande.com

ABSTRACT

The application of the ANDE Rapid DNA Identification System to disaster victim identification (DVI) and familial reunification has the potential to dramatically improve the response to natural and human-made disasters. The ability of first responders, primarily individuals without backgrounds in laboratory-based forensic DNA analysis and genetics, to perform automated short tandem repeat (STR) and kinship analyses eliminates the interval between the disaster and receipt and analysis of samples at a laboratory. The benefits of processing DVI and family reference samples and performing database searching on site include reduction in the deterioration of sample quality, reduction in time to result, and increase in the number of samples that can be processed. These advantages are amplified by the ability of the ANDE system to process challenging samples including degraded bone and tissue, with data quality that is at least as good as and often superior to those generated by conventional laboratory methodologies. Most importantly, the fully automated Rapid DNA Identification System can bring timely closure to grieving family members.

18.1 INTRODUCTION

ANDE's vision is to expand the power of DNA identification by bringing it from the laboratory to everyday use in the field, including at the police station, disaster sites, the battlefield, embassies, and borders and ports. In a sense, just as information technology moved from supercomputer laboratories to smartphones, ANDE envisions DNA technology becoming part of the fabric of everyday life. ANDE defines "Rapid DNA Identification" as the real-time identification of an individual by short tandem repeat (STR) analysis as performed by nontechnical users outside the laboratory. The purpose of this paper is to describe ANDE's work in one of the most important applications of Rapid DNA: disaster victim identification (DVI). The work discussed herein is also directly applicable to unidentified human remains (HR) that are commonly encountered in the battlefield and by coroners and chief medical examiners.

The most powerful and reliable tool available today in human identification is DNA fingerprinting. Following Jeffreys' recognition that variable loci are transmitted by simple Mendelian rules of inheritance and might be harnessed to identify individuals (Jeffreys et al., 1985), a series of major advances propelled this fundamental observation to widespread societal use. The application of the polymerase chain reaction to the amplification of variable repeat-loci-enabled DNA fingerprinting to be performed on smaller quantities of DNA template, and the analysis on polyacrylamide gels (as opposed to agarose gels) improved resolution of the resulting amplicons (Weber and May, 1989; Litt and Luty, 1989). As the analysis of variable repeats improved, the selection of loci appropriate for human identification evolved in parallel. Rassmann et al. (1991) and Edwards et al. (1991) pioneered the use of trimeric and tetrameric STRs, ultimately leading to the selection of a standard set of 20 tetrameric STR loci used in DNA fingerprinting in the USA as of January 2017 (Hares, 2015). The sensitivity and reliability of STR technology led law enforcement agencies to develop databases of DNA IDs from individuals and forensic samples. Originally, these techniques were employed primarily to match criminal suspects with evidentiary samples to investigate crime, exonerate the innocent, and provide evidence in judicial proceedings. The success of the approach has led to its expansion to DVI, military, counterterrorism, and homeland security applications.

Although DNA fingerprinting has been established for more than two decades, current STR analysis techniques demand numerous manual procedures and decision/interpretation points by expert analysts and require a sophisticated laboratory infrastructure with specialized instruments. Even with semiautomated sample batching and processing, a substantial sample backlog (https://obamawhitehouse.archives.gov/the-press-office/2015/03/16/fact-sheet-investments-reduce-national-rape-kit-backlog-and-combat-viole) has developed, generally requiring weeks to months to obtain DNA IDs. The combination of prolonged processing times, sample backlogs, and new applications has inspired a desire to accelerate and simplify the generation of DNA IDs.

Development of a rapid, fully integrated system for the automated generation of DNA IDs has the potential to address this growing need. Fundamentally, a field-forward Rapid DNA Identification System provides substantial control to agencies, allowing samples to be assessed and data to be generated in real time on site. Ideally, a Rapid DNA Identification System should have the following properties:

- *Rapid time to result:* In order to have a practical impact on individual processing in field-forward settings such as the police booking desk, time to result should be approximately 2 h or less.
- *Ease-of-use for nontechnical operators:* To allow DNA analysis to be performed by a nontechnical operator outside of the laboratory (thereby reducing time to obtain and take action on the result), the system should not require the operator to perform any manual processing steps, reagent loading, assembly, or maintenance.
- *Minimal space and environmental requirements:* All processes should be performed in a single instrument, avoiding the need for separate centrifuges, thermal cyclers, and electrophoresis instruments, and the system should not require a controlled laboratory environment.
- *Ruggedization:* The system must withstand transport and be operable "out-of-the box" without the requirement for any recalibration.
- *Unitary consumable:* To minimize operator time, training, and potential for error, a single chip containing all necessary materials and reagents should be utilized. The chip should be closed and disposable to minimize both sample contamination and user exposure.
- *Data and sample security:* As the results of STR analysis can have profound impact on the individuals being tested, it is critical that privacy rights are adhered to and that the samples are used only for their approved purposes.
- *Data utility:* To maximize the generation of actionable results in the field, the system must allow nontechnical operators to use the data. For example, database search and match and kinship analyses should be seamlessly integrated into the system.
- *Platform technology:* Many sample types and assays will be required as out-of-laboratory uses of Rapid DNA Identification expand. Accordingly, a platform technology with modular elements to enable

product modification and customization should form the basis of the system.

- *Performance:* Finally, and most importantly, DNA ID quality must be at least as good as those generated conventionally, and profiles must adhere to established acceptance guidelines (Adams and Lothridge, 2000).

Identifying individuals and body parts *post-mortem* can be challenging, even in the best of circumstances. Depending on the cause of death, some biometrics are of limited utility soon after time of death, and most are of limited utility as the body decomposes. Conventional identification of bodies includes (Technical Working Group for Mass Fatality Forensic Identification, 2005) the following:

- *Forensic anthropology*: Determination of condition of remains, including fragmentation, comingling, decomposition, and degradation (e.g., by fire, trauma, chemicals, and explosives). Determination of age, sex, race, and stature.
- *Forensic pathology*: Identification of tattoos, body piercings, surgical interventions, nonsurgical amputations, and signs of disease.
- *Radiography*: Identification of healed fractures, diseases, and surgical implants and comparison of antemortem and *post-mortem* X-rays.
- *Conventional biometrics*: Fingerprints, palm prints, and footprints.
- *Odontology*: Identification of missing teeth, restorations, and appliances and comparison of identified antemortem documentation with *post-mortem* documentation of unknown remains.

All the features noted above may be destroyed or altered beyond recognition by explosions, fire, caustic chemicals, projectiles, decay, or combinations of these factors. In contrast, DNA is better able to survive physical and chemical insults and is of enormous value in identifying the deceased. DNA typing in a conventional laboratory has become a standard tool for identification of victims from mass casualty events including the World Trade Center attack (Brenner and Weir, 2003; Biesecker et al., 2005), natural phenomena (Deng et al., 2005; Donkervoort et al., 2008; Hartman et al., 2011), plane crashes (Hsu et al., 1999; Leclair et al., 2004), and terrorist attacks (Sudoyo et al., 2008). Typically, the longer the body has decayed, the lower the likelihood that a buccal (cheek) swab will generate a useful DNA ID. Instead, tissues such as bone and teeth (optimal for protecting DNA) and muscle (reasonably stable following exposure) can be effective for performing STR analysis.

Conventional DNA processing of DVI samples requires sophisticated equipment, highly skilled technical operators, complex data interpretation, and kinship analysis - all of which require significant time. Local laboratories may be rendered nonfunctional by the disaster, and other laboratories may be overwhelmed by the volume of samples to be analyzed. Accordingly, even a relatively small disaster such as a commercial plane crash can take years for body parts to be identified by conventional processing. When large mass disasters occur, bodies may be unidentified for years or decades - frequently, thousands of bodies are disposed of in mass graves (Why dead body management matters, 2012). The 2004 Indian Ocean earthquake and tsunami is a tragic example—more than a decade later, approximately 10% of victims remained unidentified (Tsunami anniversary: 10 years after disaster, 2004).

Rapid DNA Identification offers the potential to supplement the armamentarium for dealing with natural and human-made disasters. What follows is a summary of the ANDE system and its ability to quickly and accurately process a wide range of sample types in the field.

18.2   OVERVIEW OF THE ANDE SYSTEM

The ANDE Rapid DNA Identification System consists of five major components:

- The instrument (see Figure 18.1) is ruggedized and can be operated by nontechnical users outside the laboratory.
- The Chip (see Figure 18.2) is a single-use consumable that integrates all steps performed in DNA identification, including DNA purification, STR amplification, and electrophoretic separation and detection. The chips are stable at room temperature for six months, and two types are available: the A-Chip for buccal swabs and the I-Chip for all other sample types, including DVI samples.
- The Swab. The swab cap contains an embedded RFID chip, critical for maintaining evidence chain of custody and minimizing sample mix-up.
- Expert System Software automatically performs data processing and analysis to generate a DNA ID.
- FAIRS software is an integrated package of analytical software, including database generation and management, search and match, and kinship determination functionalities.

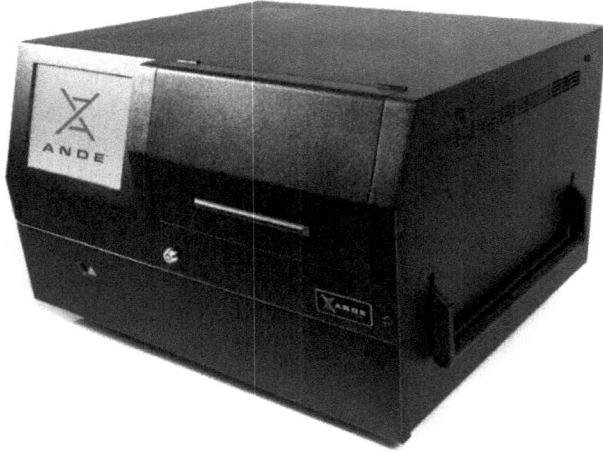

FIGURE 18.1   The ANDE instrument. Ruggedized and certified to US MIL STD 810G for shock and vibration, the instrument can be transported to a disaster site and operated outside the laboratory by nontechnical users.

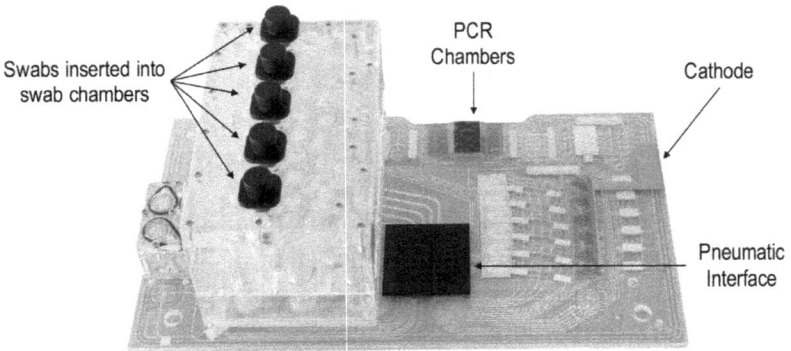

FIGURE 18.2   The ANDE A-Chip. The single-use plastic consumable processes up to five buccal samples per run. Buccal swabs from family members of unidentified disaster victims would typically be run at a Family Assistance Center and matched against victim tissue samples processed on an I-Chip located elsewhere. The FAIRS software module imports both sets of data, creates family member and victim databases, and performs kinship analysis.

The ANDE system utilizes a multiplexed assay that interrogates 27 STR loci simultaneously (23 autosomal, 3 Y-chromosomal, and Amelogenin). Also termed FlexPlex27, this six-color assay is modeled after Promega's PowerPlex® Fusion 6C with the main difference being the substitution of

D6S1043 in place of Penta D. The assay contains all expanded CODIS, UK, Interpol, European Standard, German, and Australian core loci, and D6S1043, an important STR marker broadly used in China. Accuracy, concordance, precision, resolution, peak height ratio, sensitivity, species specificity, and all other relevant measures meet or exceed required metrics (Grover et al., 2017).

ANDE's 16-locus predecessor (Della Manna et al., 2016; Tan et al., 2013) (also known as ANDE 4C) received National DNA Index System (NDIS) approval in March 2016 for use with buccal swabs, the first and only Rapid DNA system to receive NDIS approval. Developmental validation of the ANDE 6C system based on the FlexPlex assay is in progress and was designed to follow essentially the same studies as the initial approval. NDIS approval is particularly important in light of the unanimous passage in the US House and Senate of the Rapid DNA Act of 2017 (https://www.congress.gov/bill/115th-congress/house-bill/510). This critical new law will permit police stations to use NDIS-approved Rapid NDA Systems, with DNA IDs from arrestees generated at the booking desk and immediately ported to the Federal DNA database for search and matching - all without any human review. Furthermore, ANDE has been shown to successfully type forensic and DVI samples, including minute amounts of blood, tooth, and bone (Turingan et al., 2016). In fact, the State of Massachusetts Office of the Chief Medical Examiner in Boston has identified HR using ANDE and is the first and only AABB-accredited Rapid DNA laboratory in the world to date.

18.3 RAPID DNA IDENTIFICATION OF BONE SAMPLES

There are challenges to efficient DNA purification and DNA ID generation from bone and teeth, major sample types of relevance to DVI, and the processing of unidentified remains. Bone is a good source of DNA under scenarios where the biological evidence has been exposed to a variety of environmental conditions. The extensive mineralization within the bone provides a barrier to protect against both DNA degradation and microbial decomposition, but this same barrier also interferes with standard DNA purification protocols. Current methods of DNA purification from bone generally require hours or even days to obtain material suitable for analysis. Bone and tooth purification protocols are based on extraction and purification of DNA from bone or tooth powder pulverized by a freezer mill or blending cup and related protocols. The need to initiate the process with powder requires cumbersome equipment and limits the techniques to sophisticated laboratories. In addition, pulverization equipment and dental cutting discs can cause the production of airborne biological material and, without proper containment, pose health risks to operators as well as risks of sample-to-sample contamination. Furthermore, extensive demineralization of the bone powder or bone slices, often requiring special reagents and processing at elevated temperatures with agitation, is time-consuming and requires sophisticated equipment (Arismendi et al., 2004). Taken together, it is no wonder why the time to generation of DNA IDs from bone and teeth is a major problem in forensic laboratories, coroners' offices, and offices of chief medical examiners.

Many forensic laboratories send out bone and tooth processing to highly specialized laboratories that can take several months or years to return DNA IDs and have limited capacity to do even that. As a result, it is estimated that 40–80,000 unidentified corpses are now in US medical examiners' and coroners' offices, and many are buried or cremated before they are identified (Ritter, 2007). ANDE's approach to address the problems inherent in bone and tooth processing and to enable such processing in the field includes the following:

- Eliminating the need for pulverizing bone or tooth powder. We have demonstrated that a few blows of a hammer or scraping with a heavy-duty nail clipper macerate the sample sufficiently for further processing. The surface area generated by hammering is sufficient to enable efficient demineralization while avoiding the generation of airborne bone particles or need of a cryogenic grinder/freezer mill.
- Depending on the quality and type of bone or tooth, the process of demineralization can be significantly reduced to a few minutes.
- The demineralization volume has been reduced, and the overall process accelerated and simplified.

A small fragment of bone, typically ranging from one to a few hundred milligrams, is sufficient for the rapid procedure. Figure 18.3 shows representative photographs of bone samples submitted for analysis in ANDE. The fragment is cleaned, air dried, and hammered. Figure 18.4 summarizes the hammering protocol. The resulting sample is subjected to demineralization. After the demineralization solution is added, an ANDE swab is then utilized to collect the supernatant (see Figure 18.5), and the swabs are run on an I-Chip. Figure 18.6 shows a typical DNA ID generated from a bone sample processed, as described earlier.

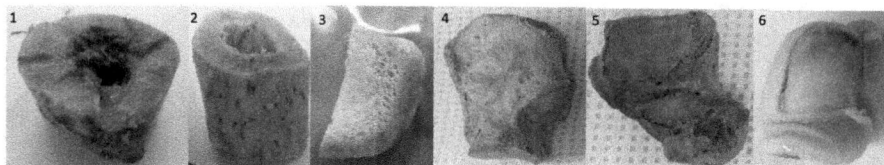

FIGURE 18.3 Selected bones utilized for Rapid DNA analysis. 1—femur; 2—humerus; 3—aged femur; 4—aged calcaneus; 5—aged talus; 6—fresh distal phalanx

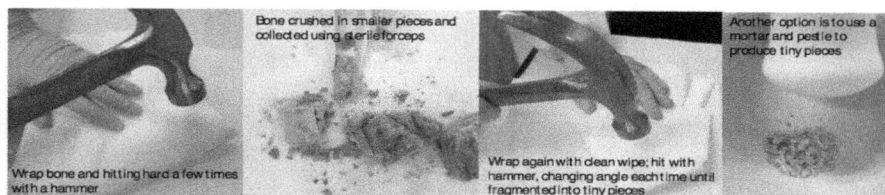

FIGURE 18.4 Hammering protocol. By eliminating the need for a cryogenic grinder/freezer mill, this simplified approach enables bone and tooth processing in field-forward settings.

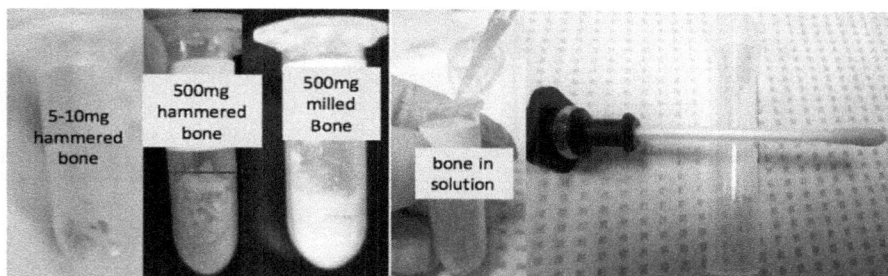

FIGURE 18.5 Typical bone quantities used for Rapid DNA processing. Bone solution is collected onto swab for processing. Milled bone photograph included for comparison.

The simplified protocol not only reduces reagent and material cost but also substantially decreases processing time and potential for sample loss during extensive manipulation. Critically, the work can be performed by nontechnical users outside the laboratory, a major benefit in DVI scenarios.

18.4 RAPID DNA IDENTIFICATION OF MUSCLE, LUNG, LIVER, AND OTHER TISSUES

The ability to perform Rapid DNA Identification using a wide range of relevant sample types is critically important for supporting DVI activities.

The ability to rapidly process muscle, lung, liver, and brain, among others, will significantly reduce the time gap between sample collection, sample analysis, and generation of actionable identification and kinship results. Accordingly, developing the ANDE system to enable processing a wide range of sample types was a major priority.

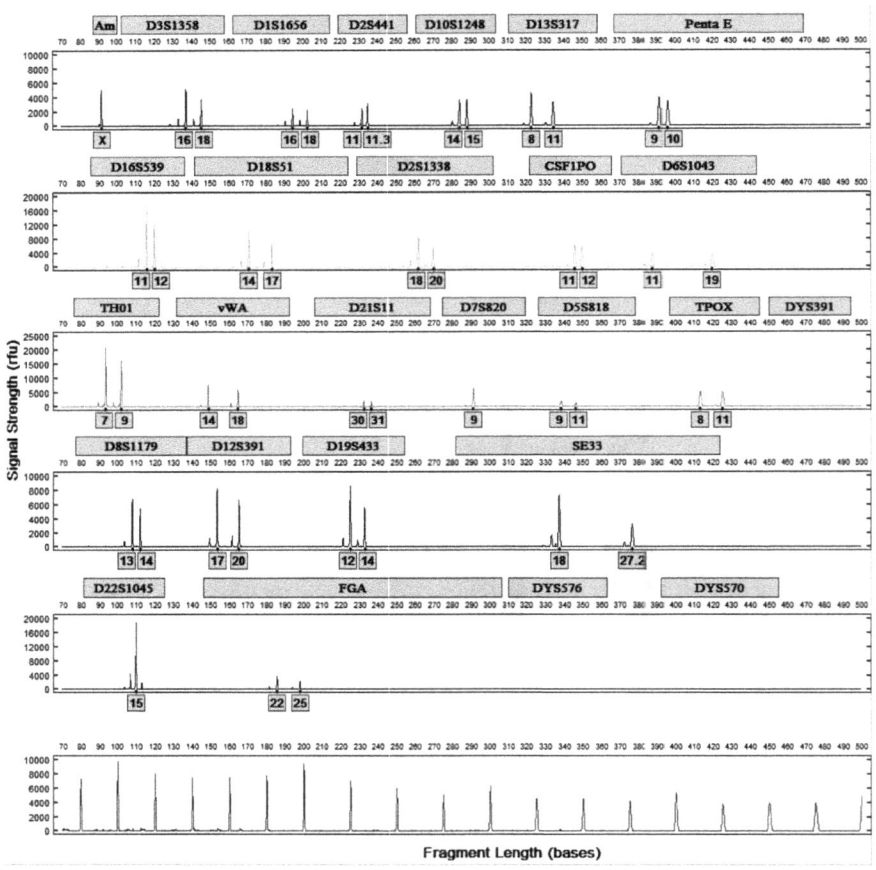

FIGURE 18.6   Representative DNA ID generated from bone using the rapid procedure described above.

Although bone and teeth require brief preprocessing steps prior to ANDE runs, as described earlier, the remaining DVI sample types do not. The ANDE chip was designed to accept a swab as the sample source, and most tissues can be processed in ANDE by either (1) swabbing the tissue itself or (2) placing a small tissue fragment on the swab. The swabs are then processed on an A-Chip or an I-Chip. Figure 18.7 shows tissue samples being prepared both ways. Figure 18.8 shows a DNA ID generated by a muscle swab using an A-Chip, Figure 18.9 by a muscle fragment, and Figure 18.10 by a lung tissue fragment both processed using an I-Chip.

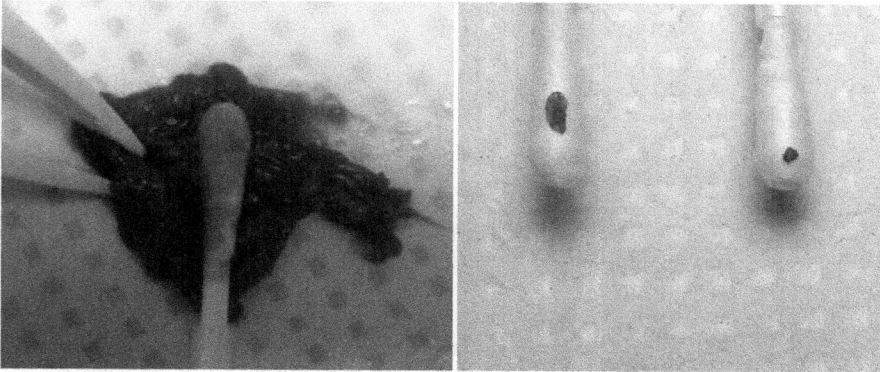

FIGURE 18.7 Two approaches to processing tissue. For swabbed muscle tissue, (L) a disposable sterile forceps was used to hold the sample. The ANDE swab was rubbed over the surface of the tissue while rotating to cover the entire cotton head. For muscle tissue fragments (R), each sample was cut in small pieces using a sterile razor blade and placed onto the swab.

18.5 ANDE IN FIELD-FORWARD DVI APPLICATIONS

ANDE is being used by military, law enforcement, and Office of the Chief Medical Examiner (OCME) agencies in the United States and around the world. To illustrate the use of ANDE in DVI applications, an exercise conducted in Vermont, Vigilant Guard 16 (VG16), will be described.

18.5.1 OVERVIEW

ANDE participated in the VG16 Exercise at Camp Ethan Allen Training Site (CEATS) in Jericho, VT, USA. The exercise was a large-scale disaster response event sponsored by NORTHCOM (US Northern Command) and the National Guard. It involved over 5000 emergency responders at 50 Vermont locations, including state and local agencies, 16 hospitals, the Burlington International Airport, and the Vermont National Guard Camp Johnson and CEATS. Other participating organizations were US Customs and Border Protection Laboratories and Scientific Services Directorate (CBP LSSD),

Department of Homeland Security Science & Technology, Massachusetts OCME, and Massachusetts Task Force 1 Urban Search and Rescue (MA-TF 1 US&R). Figure 18.11 shows the Rapid DNA operations site. The ANDE system was placed inside a mobile van provide by US CBP LSSD. The mobile van provided standard electrical power and was used to run ANDE in three locations during the exercise.

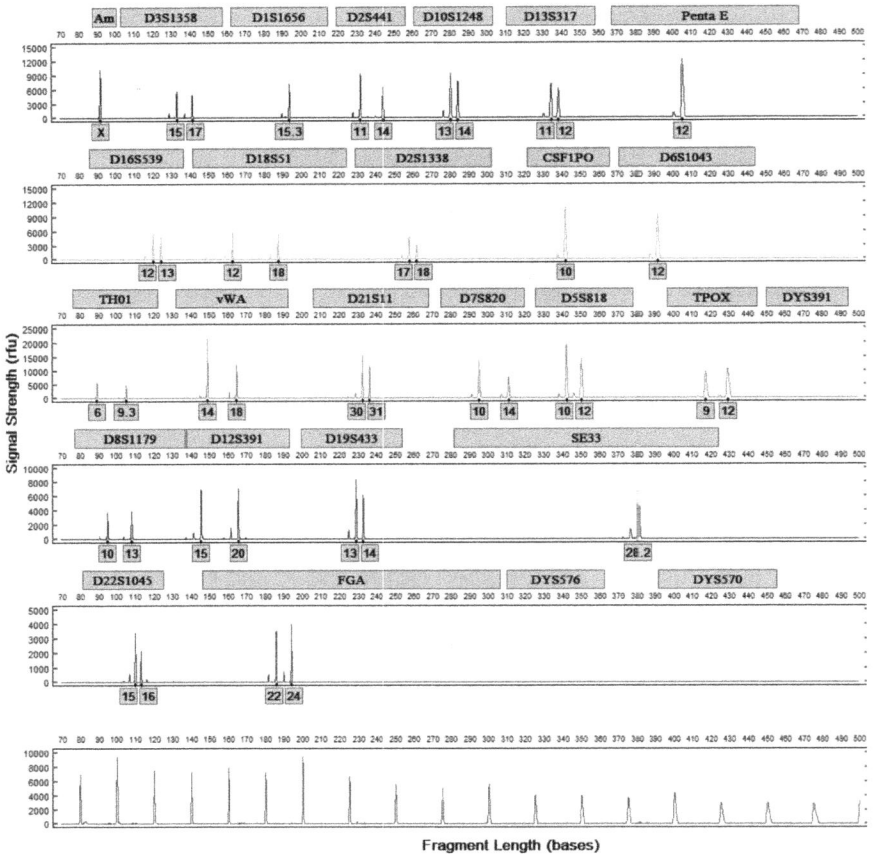

FIGURE 18.8 Representative DNA ID generated from a muscle swab.

The VG16 exercise involved multiple mock disasters (pneumonic plague, radioactive incident, bus accident, and an earthquake) that resulted in multiple mass fatalities that involved fragmentation of HR with no known manifest of victims. The exercise demonstrated that ANDE could identify critical or mass casualty victims even prior to body recovery, including settings in which HR are contaminated and cannot be immediately transferred to a morgue. The DNA IDs can be matched to family member or reference DNA samples collected in a Family Assistance Center, permitting rapid and high-confidence victim identification and reunification of families.

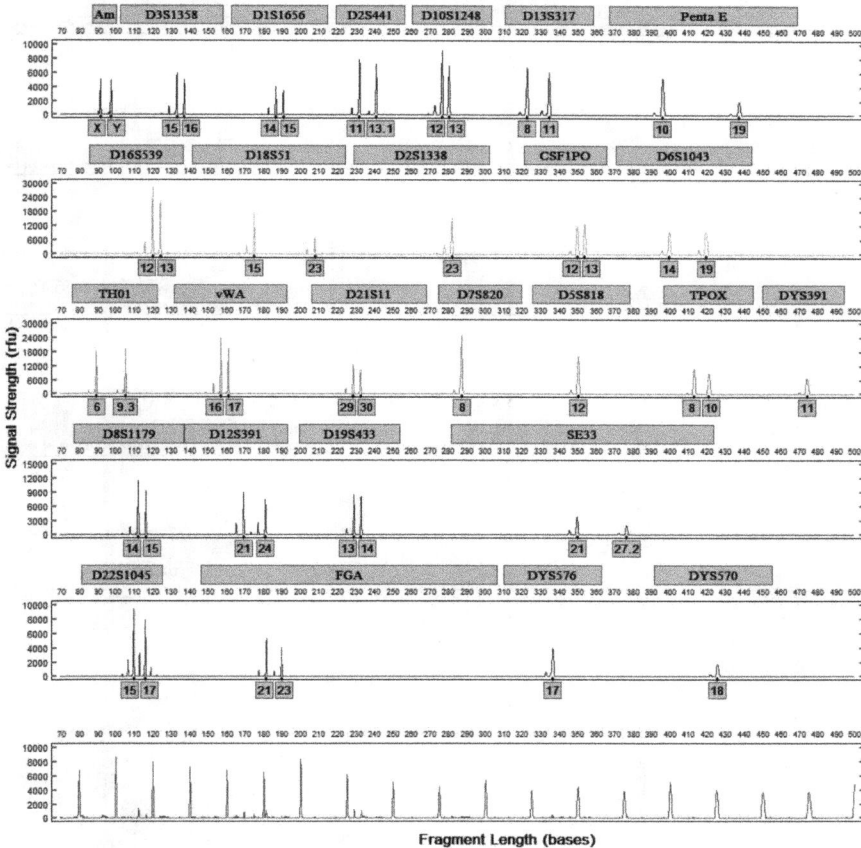

FIGURE 18.9   Representative DNA ID generated from a muscle tissue fragment.

18.5.2   *EXERCISE PURPOSE AND DESIGN*

Following a mass fatality, HR must be identified and returned to their legal next of kin. Historically, DNA testing has been used as a last resort for the identification of HR because it is time-consuming and requires unique, specialized laboratory facilities staffed with highly trained DNA analysts. Rapid DNA can now be used to quickly generate DNA IDs from HR that, if not immediately processed in the morgue, might decompose, making traditional identifications more difficult. The advent of Rapid DNA technology is changing how DNA can be used to identify HR following a mass fatality.

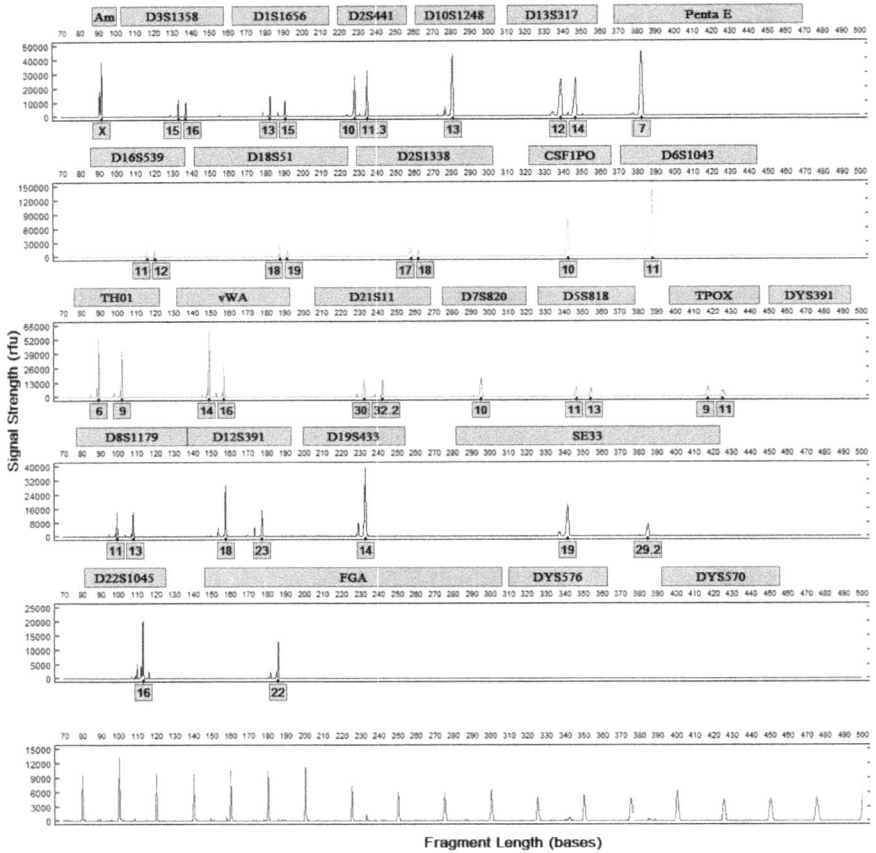

FIGURE 18.10   Representative DNA ID generated from lung tissue fragment.

The purpose of the exercise was to conduct a proof-of-concept demonstration of the identification of HR by Rapid DNA in the field prior to body recovery. This particular approach to identification will be useful in situations when HR are contaminated and cannot be immediately processed in the morgue or whenever expedited identification is required.

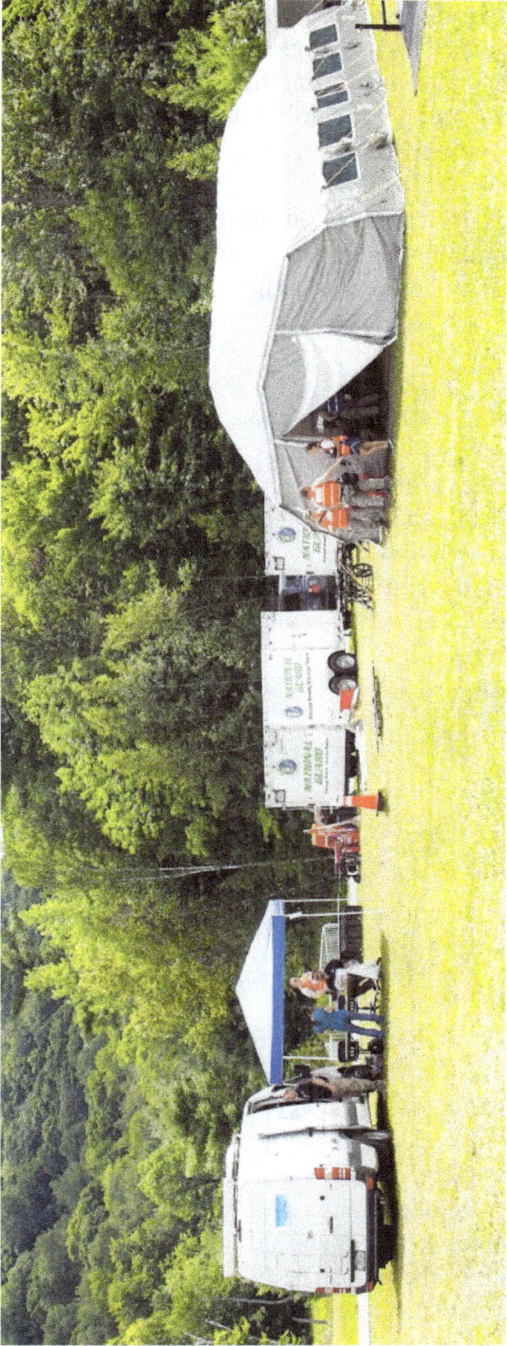

FIGURE 18.11   Rapid DNA operations site, located in the white van and blue tent on left.

The design of the mock disaster scenario involved having an HR dog locate hidden remains. "Just-in-time" training was provided to sample collectors who collected swabs from the HR (muscle and placenta tissues) and human bone fragments hidden in the disaster area. The samples were documented, labeled, and transferred to the Incident Command Center. Samples were processed on ANDE, and the paperwork was examined to determine if the "just-in-time" training was effective and if proper chain of custody was maintained. Rapid DNA IDs were compared to those previously obtained by conventional laboratory testing to assess accuracy of the system.

18.5.3   LOCATING HUMAN REMAINS

At least 1 h prior to the start of search and rescue operations, MA-TF 1 US&R placed four biological samples (bone, muscle, and two placentas) in four different mock disaster areas exposed in heat at CEATS. The HR dog was tasked with locating the remains, and time to find and locate the HR was recorded. The HR dog located the remains in 2–5 min (see Figure 18.12).

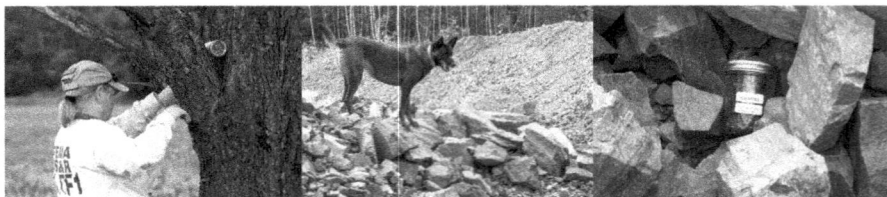

FIGURE 18.12   Sample placement and HR dog locating the samples. The HR dog averaged approximately three minutes to find and locate the four biological samples.

18.5.4   SAMPLE PROCESSING FOR RAPID IDENTIFICATION IN ANDE

The ANDE is equipped with a barcode reader (1D/2D) and RFID reader to easily track the samples and associate with their identities as written on the Sample Collection Forms (see Figure 18.13). Small fragments (approximately the size of a sesame seed to a grain of rice) from muscle and placenta tissue samples were cut and placed with gentle pressure on a swab for direct insertion into the chip. The bone was fragmented with a hammer and approximately 5–10 mg was processed by demineralization for 1 min at room temperature and then placing the solution onto a swab for analysis. All swabs were inserted into the I-Chip, which was then inserted into the ANDE instrument for fully automated processing and generation of DNA IDs.

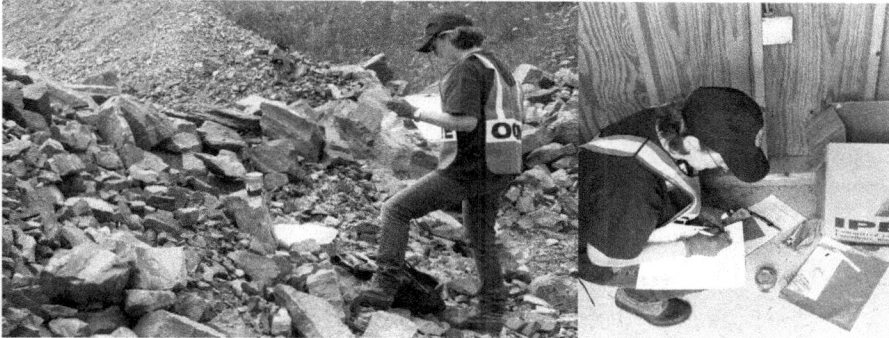

FIGURE 18.13 Sample collector documenting location, description, and condition of the recovered HR.

18.5.5 RESULTS AND CONCLUSIONS FROM EXERCISE

DNA IDs were obtained from all samples. Full profiles were obtained from bone (see Figure 18.14), muscle (see Figure 18.15), and placenta 1. Placenta 2 generated a mixed profile, not surprising as placental samples, depending on the collection site, may contain DNA from both mother and child. All Rapid DNA IDs contained sufficient data to identify the source of the samples. Finally, all ANDE DNA IDs were concordant with those generated conventionally.

Several conclusions were drawn from the exercise, including the following:

- The ANDE system played a significant role in the exercise, demonstrating that Rapid DNA can process and generate DNA IDs from tissues and bone samples in the field. All samples gave accurate DNA IDs and could be tracked back to the correct HR.
- The DNA operations site was relocated three times during the exercise. The ANDE system worked well following transport and when using generator power.
- Nontechnical users were trained to operate the system. During the exercise, volunteers simply followed prompts on the touchscreen after all the swab collections were completed.

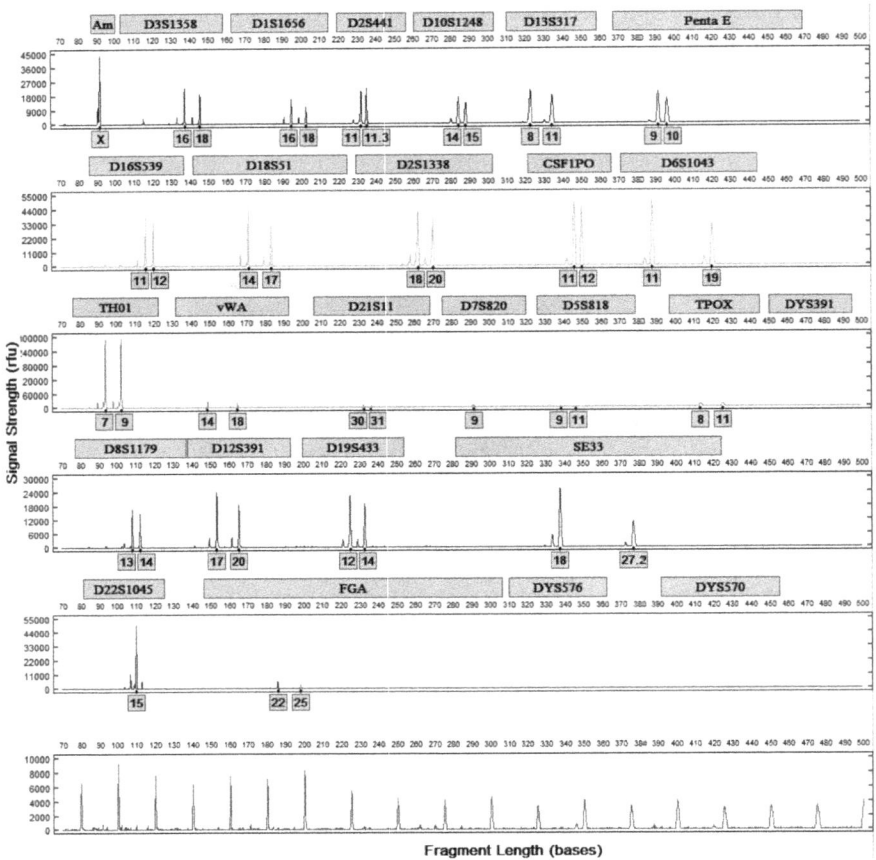

FIGURE 18.14 DNA ID generated in the field from bone fragment during VG16.

18.6 CONCLUDING REMARKS

In summary, ANDE enables rapid identification of HR and kinship identification in field-forward settings. The ability of first responders, primarily individuals without backgrounds in laboratory-based forensic DNA analysis and genetics, to generate DNA IDs and perform sophisticated kinship analysis offers the potential to change the current paradigm in DVI. In particular, by eliminating the interval between the disaster and receipt and analysis of samples at a laboratory, the deterioration of sample quality and time to DNA ID generation are minimized. Furthermore, mass disasters often inundate local medical examiner offices and forensic laboratories, and Rapid DNA offers the potential for significant near-term increases in processing capacity and data analysis. Most importantly, these advantages offer the potential to expedite familial reunification and to bring closure to grieving family members.

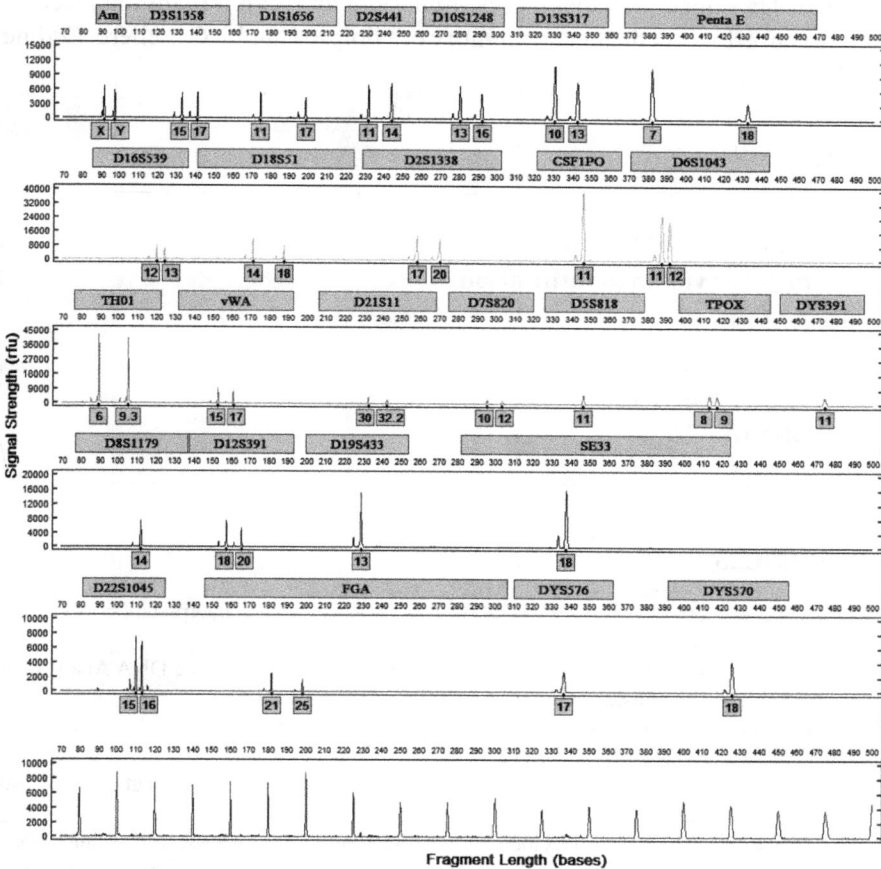

FIGURE 18.15 DNA ID generated in the field from muscle tissue fragment during VG16.

DVI represents one of many applications of Rapid DNA Identification. The ANDE system is capable of generating DNA IDs from a broad range of sample types, including blood stains, oral epithelial samples (e.g., drinking cups, soda cans, water bottles, and chewing gum), FTA and untreated paper, hair, semen, and sexual assault kits. Rapid DNA Identification is in its infancy, but major progress over the past decade suggests that Rapid DNA will have a profound impact on DVI, law enforcement, military, counterterrorism, immigration, homeland security, and countless other applications.

ACKNOWLEDGMENTS

We thank Dr. Eugene Tan for helpful discussions and review of the manuscript. This manuscript is dedicated in memory of Giorgio Cambi, Cavaliere, Ordine al Merito della Repubblica Italiana.

KEYWORDS

- **rapid DNA identification**
- **disaster victim identification**
- **A-Chip**
- **I-Chip**
- **short tandem repeat (STR)**
- **DNA ID**

REFERENCES

Adams, D. E. and Lothridge, K. L.; FBI—Short Tandem Repeat (STR) Interpretation Guidelines by SWGDAM. *Forensic Sci. Commun. FBI* **2000**, *2* (3).

Arismendi, J. L.; et al.; Effects of Processing Techniques on the Forensic DNA Analysis of Human Skeletal Remains. *J. Forensic Sci.* **2004**, *49* (5), 930–934.

Biesecker, L. G.; et al.; Epidemiology. DNA Identifications after the 9/11 World Trade Center Attack. *Science* **2005**, *310* (5751), 1122–1123.

Brenner, C. H.; and Weir, B. S.; Issues and Strategies in the DNA Identification of World Trade Center Victims. *Theor. Popul. Biol.* **2003**, *63* (3), 173–178.

Della Manna, A. D.; et al.; Developmental Validation of the DNAscan™ Rapid DNA Analysis™ Instrument and Expert System for Reference Sample Processing. *Forensic Sci. Int. Genet.* **2016**, 25, 145–156.

Deng, Y.-J.; et al.; Preliminary DNA Identification for the Tsunami Victims in Thailand. *Genomics. Proteomics Bioinform.* **2005**, *3* (3), 143.

Donkervoort, S.; et al.; Enhancing Accurate Data Collection in Mass Fatality Kinship Identifications: Lessons Learned from Hurricane Katrina. *Forensic Sci. Int. Genet.* **2008**, *2* (4), 354–362.

Edwards, A.; et al.; DNA Typing and Genetic Mapping with Trimeric and Tetrameric Tandem Repeats. *Am. J. Hum. Genet.* **1991**, *49* (4), 746–756.

Grover, R.; et al.; FlexPlex27—Highly Multiplexed Rapid DNA Identification for Law Enforcement, Kinship, and Military Applications. *Int. J. Legal Med.* **2017**, *131* (6), 1489–1501.

Hares, D. R.; Selection and Implementation of Expanded CODIS Core Loci in the United States. *Forensic Sci. Int. Genet.* **2015**, *17*, 33–34.

Hartman, D.; et al.; The Contribution of DNA to the Disaster Victim Identification (DVI) Effort. *Forensic Sci. Int.* **2011**, *205* (1–3), 52–58.

Hsu, C. M.; et al.; Identification of Victims of the 1998 Taoyuan Airbus Crash Accident Using DNA Analysis. *Int. J. Legal Med.* **1999**, *113* (1), 43–46.

Jeffreys, A. J.; et al.; Individual-Specific 'Fingerprints' of Human DNA. *Nature* **1985**, *316* (6023), 76–79.

Jeffreys, A. J.; et al.; Positive Identification of an Immigration Test-Case Using Human DNA Fingerprints. *Nature* **1985**, *317* (6040), 818–819.

Jeffreys, A. J.; et al.; Hypervariable 'Minisatellite' Regions in Human DNA. *Nature* **1985**, *314* (6006), 67–73.

Leclair, B.; et al.; Enhanced Kinship Analysis and STR-Based DNA Typing for Human Identification in Mass Fatality Incidents: The Swissair Flight 111 Disaster. *J. Forensic Sci.* **2004**, *49* (5), 939–953.

Litt, M. and Luty, J. A.; A Hypervariable Microsatellite Revealed by in Vitro Amplification of a Dinucleotide Repeat within the Cardiac Muscle Actin Gene. *Am. J. Hum. Genet.* **1989**, *44* (3), 397–401.

Rassmann, K.; et al.; Isolation of Simple-Sequence Loci for Use in Polymerase Chain Reaction-Based DNA Fingerprinting. *Electrophoresis* **1991**, *12* (2–3), 113–118.

Ritter, N.; Missing Persons and Unidentified Remains: The Nation's Silent Mass Disaster. *NIJ J.* **2007**, *256* (7).

Sudoyo, H.; et al.; DNA Analysis in Perpetrator Identification of Terrorism-Related Disaster: Suicide Bombing of the Australian Embassy in Jakarta 2004. *Forensic Sci. Int. Genet.* **2008**, *2* (3), 231–237.

Tan, E.; et al.; Fully Integrated, Fully Automated Generation of Short Tandem Repeat Profiles. *Investig. Genet.* **2013**, *4* (1), 16.

Technical Working Group for Mass Fatality Forensic Identification; *Mass Fatality Incidents: A Guide for Human Forensic Identification: US Department of Justice,* National Institute of Justice, Office of Justice Programs. **2005**.

Tsunami anniversary: 10 years after disaster, victims' relatives learn bodies weren't lost; CBS News https://www.cbsnews.com/news/10-years-after-tsunami-victims-relatives-learn-bodies-werent-lost/ (accessed Mar 11, 2019).

Turingan, R. S.; et al.; Rapid DNA Analysis for Automated Processing and Interpretation of Low DNA Content Samples. *Investig. Genet.* **2016**, *7* (1), 2.

Weber, J. L. and May, P. E.; Abundant Class of Human DNA Polymorphisms Which Can Be Typed Using the Polymerase Chain Reaction. *Am. J. Hum. Genet.* **1989**, *44* (3), 388–396.

Why dead body management matters; IRIN Why dead body management matters http://www.irinnews.org/report/96673/analysis-why-dead-body-management-matters (accessed Mar 11, 2019).

CHAPTER 19

Massively Parallel Sequencing as an Operational Forensic Tool: Current and Future Perspectives—Improving Results for Current Applications and Paving the Way for Expanded Capabilities

NICOLA J. OLDROYD CLARK* and CYDNE L. HOLT

Verogen Inc., 11111 Flintkote Ave, San Diego, CA 92121, USA

Corresponding author. E-mail: noldroyd-clark@verogen.com

ABSTRACT

Advances in genomic technologies underpin the practical and powerful application of massively parallel sequencing (MPS) to forensic science. MPS provides the highest resolution of targeted, forensic PCR amplicons, harnessing the full power of genomic technology. Illumina Sequencing By Synthesis (SBS) provides the core sequencing technology of the MiSeq FGx™ Forensic Genomics System and ForenSeq® chemistries, provided exclusively by Verogen (www.verogen.com). MiSeq FGx-generated short tandem repeat (STR) allele calls are fully compatible with current database formats, providing a seamless link between capillary electrophoresis (CE)-based and MPS data, such that laboratories may transit from legacy to contemporary data with minimum disruption to existing training and infrastructure. Unlike CE-based STR typing systems, forensic MPS approaches are not limited to dye channels and size restrictions, as genetic markers may occupy the same "real estate" by length such that 100s of polymorphisms of different categories can be analyzed simultaneously. The ForenSeq DNA Signature Prep Kit is the first commercially developed and validated assay to combine 27 autosomal STRs, 24 Y-STRs, and 7 X-STRs with a dense SNP set in a single test, which can reduce iterative testing, redundant quality assurance and quality control procedures, and training programs for increased efficiencies. Targeting the smallest forensic amplicons possible (<150 bases), identity SNP amplicons aid in data recovery from partially degraded DNA samples, phenotypic SNPs enable analysis of visible traits such as hair and eye color and biogeographic ancestry is estimated using a third class of SNPs. These data may arm investigators with actionable genetic intelligence as opposed to CE-based genetic clues which are effectively limited to whether or not DNA originated from a male or female. Because alleles are resolved at the nucleotide level using MPS, more conclusive results can be reached, especially in complex mixtures. Although not as powerful (in statistical terms) as nuclear DNA, mitochondrial DNA (mtDNA) is important for specific forensic scenarios and has been hampered by the limitations of Sanger sequencing on CE platforms. MPS-based mtDNA analysis is quicker, simpler and, for some methods, less expensive than Sanger. MPS also extends mtDNA variant analysis capabilities beyond the control region to the entire mtGenome sequence in a practical way. ForenSeq mtDNA Control Region and ForenSeq mtDNA Whole Genome kits spare laboratories of the need to QC in house ("home brew") reagent formulations, while ForenSeq software flattens analysis and interpretation time such that onsite bioinformatics expertise is not required. This chapter clarifies some of the misperceptions associated with MPS and highlights milestones that have been reached in the global forensic community. MPS allows exploration of a variety of forensic analyses that have not been in the forensic realm historically. Laboratories that are expert in MPS are future proofing their operations for the "omics" era that encompass the transcriptome, nuclear genome, epigenome, and microbiome. Investigative intelligence that incorporates genetic data, including but not limited to the use of GEDmatch for long-range familial searching, is on the rise and expected to become part of the mandate and day-to-day affairs of crime lab systems. Strategic planning in forensic infrastructure should anticipate advanced workflows that answer more forensic questions than ever before, extending capabilities of the contemporary forensic laboratory to truly exploit the power of "omics."

19.1 INTRODUCTION

Genetic typing may be considered as a cornerstone of contemporary forensic science. Today, most forensic DNA testing utilizes polymerase chain reaction (PCR) and capillary electrophoresis (CE) to detect fragment length (size) variation in fluorescently labeled short tandem repeat (STR) markers.

These tests form the basis of more than 125 million profiles stored on at least 60 investigative DNA databases worldwide (DNA Resource Forensic DNA Policy, 2019). A smaller percentage of forensic investigations also use CE-based Sanger sequencing to determine each nucleotide of specific regions of mitochondrial DNA (mtDNA); an even smaller percentage invoke the use of CE-based single-nucleotide polymorphism (SNP) detection in genomic DNA (gDNA) to assist where other methods fail to yield a result. Despite the undoubted success of traditional STR analysis in propelling DNA to the center of forensic investigations, inherent technical limitations of fluorescent, CE-based analysis, whether size-based or Sanger sequencing, leaves gaps in the armory available to forensic scientists to fully evaluate questioned material and deliver a comprehensive result. In the "CE era," additional limitations result in the need for multiple, different workflows and analytical components to drive toward comprehensive genetic data and mean that easy-to-use commercial solutions for mtDNA and SNP analysis have not been readily available.

Advances in genomic technologies have long outpaced the methods that were first introduced into forensic DNA testing laboratories over 20 years ago. As the number of forensic samples profiled has increased dramatically, the fundamentals of CE-based testing have remained relatively static. Measurable demonstration of the value of national DNA databases in aiding investigations or solving cases by leading to the identification of perpetrators encouraged more countries to establish criminal intelligence databases. As a result, the number of casework samples requiring DNA processing continues to increase. In parallel, the critical role DNA testing plays in the identification of missing persons, kinship testing, ancestry investigations, and other complex human identification applications continues to drive interest in more powerful, modern analysis methods that, in turn, place increasing demand and strain on the fixed capabilities of CE-based forensic analyses.

Massively parallel sequencing (MPS) is a powerful approach for the highest resolution of targeted, forensic PCR amplicons. MPS allows forensic scientists worldwide to improve results from the current range of analyses performed (e.g., STR casework and databasing, mtDNA sequencing, etc.), to expand capabilities to fully harness the power of genomic technology and to explore a variety of forensic analyses that have not been in the forensic realm historically. With the highest yield of error-free reads, best performance in repetitive sequence regions such as STRs, and lowest base-by-base price, Illumina sequencing by synthesis (SBS) is the most widely adopted chemistry in the MPS industry (Bentley et al., 2008; Liu et al., 2012;

Loman et al., 2012; Nakazato et al., 2013; Sebastian et al., 2013; Quail et al., 2012). SBS provides the basis of the MiSeq FGx™ Forensic Genomics System and ForenSeq® chemistries, provided exclusively by Verogen (www. Verogen.com). Using Verogen systems, examiners can generate data that span targeted, forensic loci across human nuclear and mitochondrial genome (mtGenome) to address more forensic questions than can ever be possible with the size and color-based limitations of the CE-based systems of the past. Moreover, MiSeq FGx-generated STR allele calls are fully compatible with current database formats, providing a seamless link between CE-based and MPS data, such that laboratories may transition from legacy to contemporary data with minimum disruption to existing training and infrastructure. Adoption of Verogen workflows for forensic applications continues to accelerate as an increasing number of laboratories recognize the value of generating more conclusive results for the smallest, most compromised, and highly mixed evidentiary samples with a powerful, flexible, reliable, and easy-to-use workflow.

19.2   SIMULTANEOUS ANALYSIS OF FORENSIC STR AND SNP LOCI

Due to a reliance on amplicon size and fluorescence, CE-based STR typing systems are inherently limited by the number of dye channels and the requirement to space loci out sufficiently to enable identification of each individual marker by length and color alone. This restricts the number of markers to effectively four to five times the number of dye channels, meaning that it will only ever be possible to analyze 10s of markers simultaneously. Given that some current international marker sets already contain >20 commonly used autosomal STRs (Hares, 2012) and with laboratories increasingly looking to analyze other classes of STRs for sexual assault and relationship testing, this limitation on locus number is becoming ever more restrictive. Forensic laboratories are thus driven to validate and maintain multiple PCR-based systems and conduct multiple rounds of testing. Such iterative workflows can be either impossible on limited or poor-quality material or may yield insufficient information and lead to an inconclusive result. Laboratories are then left with the burden of maintaining redundant procedures, each requiring its own quality assurance/quality control, training, and proficiency programs, and with samples that could be better resolved at the nucleotide level for more conclusive results.

Forensic MPS approaches amplify DNA with the same, basic PCR technology that historical STR assays relied upon but then identify markers by actual base sequence, not by size/location on an electropherogram. As forensic MPS systems are not limited by the available number of dye channels and size restrictions, markers may occupy the same "real estate" by length such that 100s of polymorphisms of different categories can be simultaneously analyzed. The ForenSeq DNA Signature Prep Kit is the first commercially developed and validated assay to combine 27 autosomal STRs, 24 Y-STRs and 7 X-STRs with a dense SNP set in a single test (Jaeger et al., 2017, England et al., 2019). The STR primers are designed to target forensic amplicons of the smallest length possible such that the majority of the most valuable markers reside around or less than 200 bases. Furthermore, the 94 identity SNP amplicons are all less than 150 bases in length, improving data recovery from degraded samples, where longer DNA regions are lost (Guo et al., 2017). A further set of 78 SNPs, selected from established, forensically characterized marker sets enable phenotypic analysis of visible traits such as hair and eye color (Walsh et al., 2013) and biogeographic ancestry (Kidd et al., 2013). These data may arm investigators with actionable genetic intelligence. As opposed to CE-based genetic clues, which are effectively limited to gender, did DNA originate from a male or female?

A clear advantage of MPS in forensic genomics is the ability to resolve alleles that are identical by size, but different by sequence. Intra-STR SNPs are revealed at the nucleotide level. Precise allele recognition is thus reportable for casework and complex human identification. Multiple studies illustrate the increased level of variation visible at the sequence level (Devesse et al., 2018; Gettings et al., 2018; Phillips et al., 2018), which leads to reduced sharing of contributions by the different donors in complex mixtures. This facilitates number of contributor estimation in mixed DNA samples and assists with deconvolution of individual contributor genotypes. The ForenSeq Universal Analysis Software (UAS), part of the Verogen Forensic Genomics portfolio, clearly and easily visualizes where alleles of the same length but different sequence coincide within the same sample, allowing the analyst to leverage that information in mixture interpretation (see Figure 19.1).

Another benefit of MPS for forensic analysis is that, unlike CE-based systems that produce analog metrics such as peak color, size, shape, and height, MPS systems deliver precise digital data (i.e., discrete read counts). The digital nature of the data generated by the MiSeq FGx system and the ability to tune the sensitivity of an experiment by increasing or decreasing coverage level supports a dynamic range with no relevant limitations. Digital read counts and deep sequencing provide high sensitivity for quantitative evaluations such as minor DNA contributor detection in complex mixtures, which can be missed or only partially detected using CE-based methods.

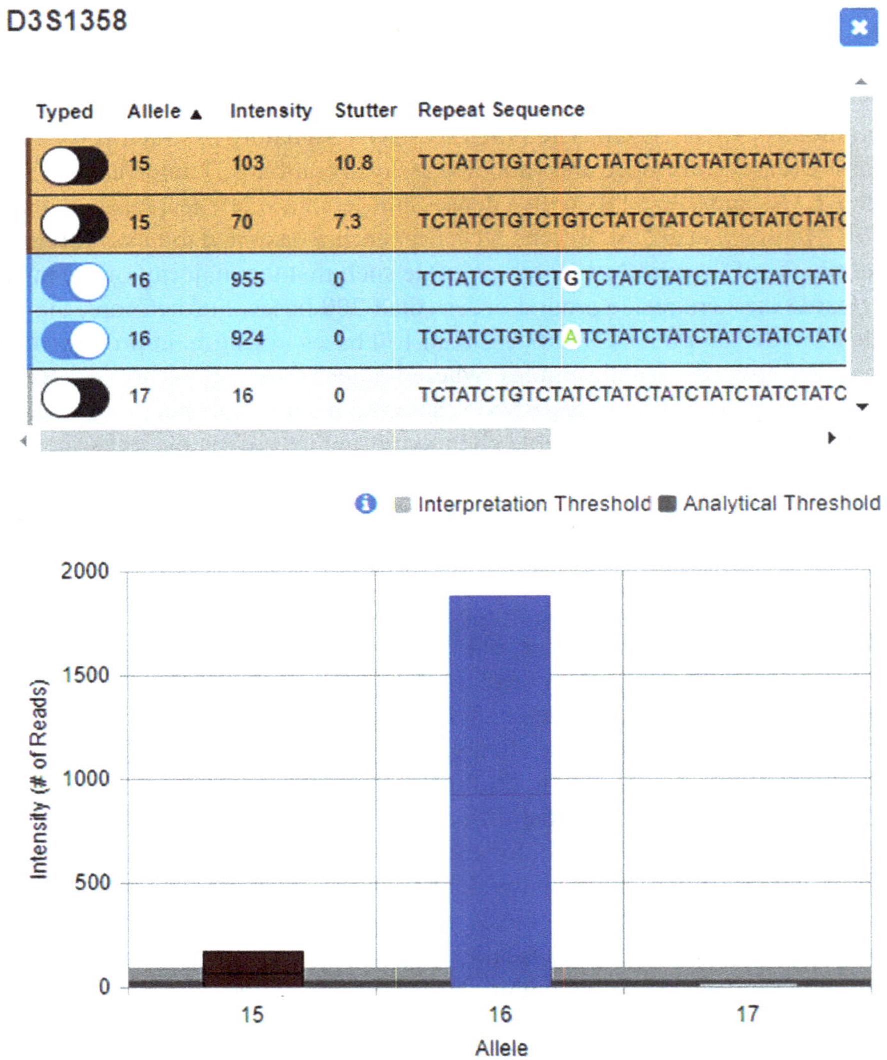

FIGURE 19.1 Example of how sequence-level variation within STR markers is displayed within the ForenSeq UAS v1.3. Allelic data are displayed as histograms (blue) representing the read count of each contribution. Contributions in brown represent data, which have been filtered according to predefined criteria such as stutter. The data shown for D3S1358 would display as a homozygote, represented by a single fluorescent peak, on a CE electropherogram. When sequenced, two distinct alleles of different sequence are revealed, as depicted by the black line delineating the precise read counts of each contribution for allele 16. Two separate stutter contributions are also visible.

The interpretation of mixed profiles from DNA evidentiary material continues to pose challenges for forensic scientists. Traditionally, analysts have used a "binary" approach to interpretation, where inferred genotypes are either included or excluded from the mixture using a variety of criteria such as stochastic threshold, heterozygote balance, mixture ratio, and stutter ratios. The sensitivity of STR multiplexes and associated CE instrument has improved over the last two decades, which, when combined with the change in the type of evidence being submitted for analysis from high-quality/ quantity (often single-source) to low-quality/quantity (often mixed) samples, means the complexity of DNA profile interpretation has also increased over time. This has prompted efforts to move from binary to probabilistic methods of interpretation, which focus either on semicontinuous (e.g., LR Mix Studio; Gill and Haned, 2013) or continuous (e.g., EuroForMix; Bleka et al., 2016) models, which are increasingly becoming a validated part of the forensic laboratory's arsenal of tools to address mixtures. Studies have already shown that MPS SNP mixture can be analyzed effectively using a fully continuous model (Bleka et al., 2017), and this capability is expected to be extended to include MPS STR mixture data. The increased amount and resolution of data produced by MPS assays such as the ForenSeq DNA Signature Prep kit combined with probabilistic genotyping models can only enhance the interpretation of complex mixtures going forward. Likewise, the richer and more quantitative nature of MPS data surely assists ProbGen models and algorithms to perform more effectively.

One benefit of CE-based methods is the short amount of time required to achieve a result. Blood or saliva samples on FTA® card or similar substrates can be directly amplified and run on a CE platform in as little as 2 h (Flores et al., 2014), which contrasts with the longer overall workflow of most MPS assays. Due to the requirement for library preparation instead of one round of PCR and the longer sequencing runtime compared to a CE fragment analysis run, MPS assays do take longer than the simple, CE-based STR analyses. This time penalty is compounded if multiple individual MPS assays are required to generate a comprehensive result (e.g., separate panels for individual marker types). However, CE analysis times increase linearly if more than one analysis are required per sample. When comparing the analysis time required for a complex casework sample analyzed with two or three different CE-based assay systems with the overall workflow time for the expanded marker set contained in a single ForenSeq DNA Signature Prep kit reaction, the difference is likely to be negligible. Analyst-ready data for the ForenSeq DNA Signature Kit are generated within a total workflow time of less than 40 h for all supported sample batch sizes, which arguably offers a more efficient workflow option than multiple rounds of CE testing, which may still ultimately fail to yield the conclusive results to move a case forward.

Considering the inherent limitations of CE-based analyses of size and color and the multiple benefits to be gained by combining analyses of higher marker numbers and different marker types, the ForenSeq DNA Signature Prep Kit represents a new era of analyses, offering new possibilities to laboratories to improve workflow efficiency and analysis outcomes.

19.3   FLEXIBLE, RELIABLE mtDNA ANALYSIS

Forensic scientists have long faced the challenge of analyzing severely degraded samples in which nuclear DNA, recognized as the most powerful source for identification of individuals, may be undetectable. Human remains exposed to the environment for extended periods can be compromised due to erosion; DNA samples from bone fragments or hair shafts can be highly degraded or present in very small quantities. While not as powerful (in statistical terms) as nuclear DNA due to its uniparental inheritance, mtDNA can offer an attractive and viable option for analysis of severely degraded samples due to enhanced copy number relative to nuclear DNA (100s–1000s of copies per cell, depending on cell type and function, compared to a single copy of the nucleus) and its circular construction, which enables it to survive in environments where nuclear DNA does not (Butler and Levin, 1998).

In the past, forensic laboratories analyzing mtDNA used Sanger sequencing on CE platforms and focused on analysis of part or all of the control region only, due to the high density of mutations in a relatively short expanse of DNA (approximately 1200 bases for the entire control region), and the substantial labor required to sequence the entire mtGenome. Despite Sanger sequencing being an invariably manual process and not particularly pleasant, such a short segment as the control region can be practically interrogated. MPS is quicker, simpler, and, for some methods, less expensive for mtDNA analysis and extends capabilities to the entire mtGenome sequence (Parson et al., 2015), something that can be a soul-destroying and intractable task using CE-based Sanger sequencing, deterring most laboratories from attempting mtGenome analysis using this method. Given the 16.5-kb extent of the mtGenome represents a mere snack for most MPS systems and can be analyzed in approximately the same amount of time as the control region, and for larger number of samples simultaneously, mtDNA analysis becomes not just a niche tool to be reserved for rare circumstances where all else fails, but a complementary one that can be analyzed and interpreted in a fraction of the time required using CE.

Most Sanger sequencing-based methods are home-brewed by laboratories, requiring them to order the numerous primers needed to amplify the target and perform the sequencing reactions. This causes challenges with quality control, reproducibility, and laboratory efficiency. With the emergence of MPS technologies and the greater ability to interrogate mtDNA more easily, a number of commercial solutions are now available. Each could be perceived to have limitations in terms of the completeness of known variant data used to generate the design, the workflow employed, or the bioinformatics required to analyze the data. mtDNA variant databases have increased in size, data quality, and in our ability to mine them in recent years (Huber et al., 2018). mtDNA systems designed prior to this data explosion, therefore, cannot reflect the current state of our sequencing knowledge regarding the mtDNA genome and may, therefore, fail to detect some of the variants now known to exist. In July 2019, Verogen released the first installment in a mtDNA portfolio designed to take advantage of the very latest knowledge and to harness the proven advantages of MPS technology for mtDNA analysis. Based on the same simple, efficient ForenSeq library prep workflow as the DNA Signature Prep kit, the ForenSeq mtDNA Control Region kit (Verogen Inc., 2019) interrogates the entire mtDNA control region using two primer pools of nine amplicons. Designed against mtDNA database data current as of December 2018, 18 primary amplicons are generated by >120 primers, representing a high degree of degeneracy and, therefore, engineered to detect the maximum number of known variants. The largest amplicon is approximately 150 bases in length, with the vast majority being less than 100 bases for best in class design and maximized performance, even on much degraded samples. All amplicons overlap by at least three bases, accounting for bioinformatic trimming and ensuring complete coverage of the entire control region. By leveraging the same workflow as the DNA Signature Prep kit, with the exception of two amplifications per sample for PCR1 and PCR 2 instead of one, laboratories already using the DNA Signature Prep kit can easily adopt the mtDNA assay with the bare minimum of additional training. A new module for the UAS offers a rapid data review capability, aligning data to the revised Cambridge reference sequence (rCRS), and has been reported to support analysis of up to 48 mitochondrial control regions generated in a single MiSeq FGx run with the MiSeq FGx Reagent Micro kit in less than 1 h (test site feedback, personal communication). A simple user interface allows the analyst to review run metrics and control results, check variants against the rCRS, and compare up to eight control region sequences simultaneously (see Figure 19.2).

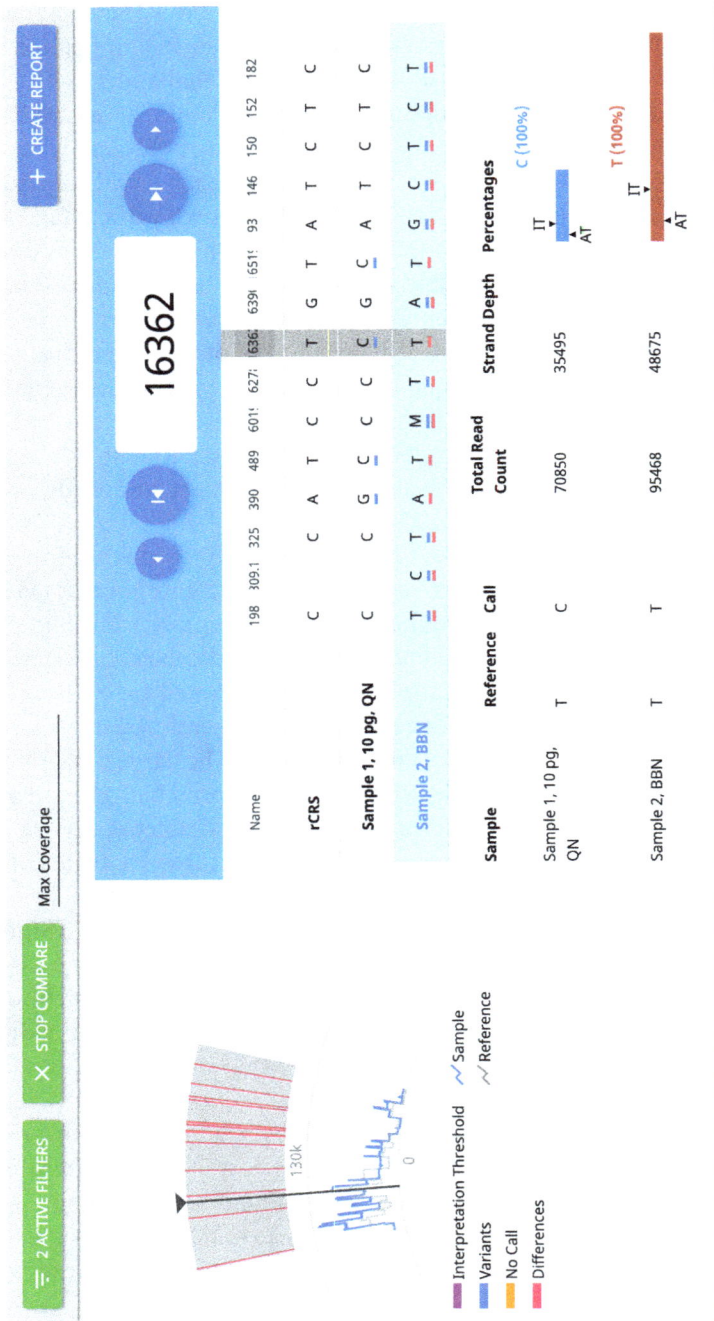

(A)

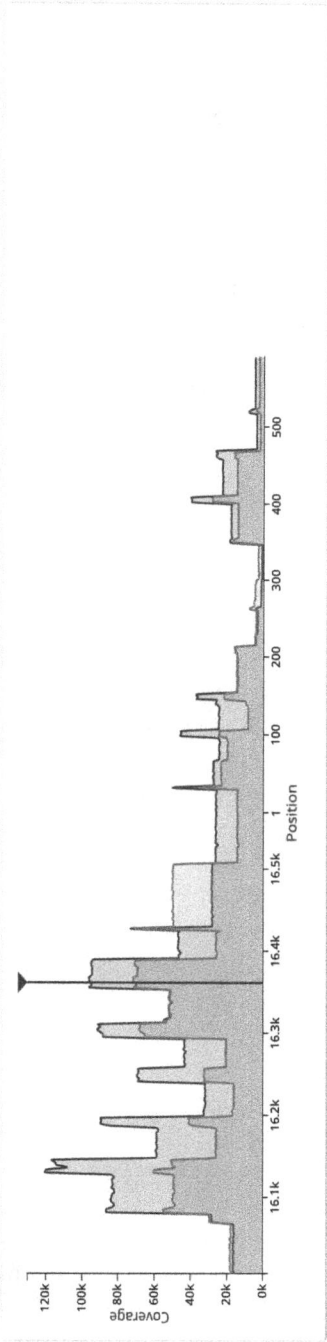

(B)

FIGURE 19.2 Example interface from ForenSeq UAS v2 showing comparison of mtDNA control regions from two different samples analyzed by the ForenSeq mtDNA Control Region Kit. The display is filtered to show only the differences compared to the rCRS and between the two samples. (A) The top pane of the sample display interface showing the condensed coverage plot on the left and the list of mutations for each sample relative to the rCRS and the positions where the two samples differ highlighted by red underlines on the right. The red lines on the condensed coverage plot show the differences between each sample, and the position indicator can be moved by the user to interrogate the various differences. Information on depth of strand coverage and total read count is provided. (B) The bottom pane of the sample display interface showing the expanded coverage plot and the position indicator, which moves to orient the analyst to the sequence as each individual mutation is selected in either the left or right sections of the top pane of the display.

The bioinformatics associated with circular genome analysis can be complex, so Verogen leveraged in-house bioinformatic expertise to create UAS v2, which offers a simple and user-friendly software experience so that the analyst may focus on reviewing the data and deciding the outcomes instead of being distracted by analysis complexities. By concurrently developing a chemistry kit that includes all required components and is based on a familiar workflow, prewritten instrument protocols for ease of use, and fast efficient data review tools, laboratories are spared the need to QC in-house reagent formulations, can adopt the workflow with minimal requirement for additional equipment, reagents, or training, and leverage the workflow to successfully interrogate the mtDNA control region. The portfolio was recently enhanced by the addition of the ForenSeq Whole Genome mtDNA Kit, which offers the benefits of the control region kit, extended to the entire mtGenome.

19.4   MPS MYTHS

Whenever methods are introduced to the forensic sciences, there is a period of education and evaluation as forensic analysts explore the technicalities and expand their knowledge of the given technology. It is perhaps unsurprising that general myths surrounding the design and use of MPS may arise, since there are a number of MPS technologies available for laboratories to investigate, an extended range of applications for which those technologies may be applied, and different levels of experience surrounding these different methods (within both the commercial and laboratory sections of our industry). It is important to address these myths so that forensic analysts are armed with the maximum amount of information with which to draw comparisons between different techniques and make informed decisions regarding which is best suited to their individual laboratory and application needs. Here is just a brief overview of some of the common myths that surround MPS methods for forensic applications and the reality as it pertains to Verogen solutions:

Library prep is a long and laborious process: More so historically, but also for some current techniques, library prep methods can take a few days to complete. In general, the amount of time required is related to protocol complexity, which is, in turn, determined by the capabilities of the specific MPS technology and the nature of the sample type and/or application. Library prep workflow times have steadily decreased, with some methods (e.g., Nextera-XT, Illumina Inc., 2012) taking as little as 90 min total time for a simple, tagmentation-based prep. This prep type is not suitable for the generation of forensic STR amplicons, given that it fragments the DNA, interrupting the repeat regions that require sequencing in an uninterrupted read in order to generate accurate allele calls. The ForenSeq Library Prep process was, specifically designed to address this requirement and generate complete forensic amplicons, minimizing the steps and tube changes required to create a targeted forensic amplicon library. It consists of four major steps - two rounds of PCR followed by cleanup and normalization (see Figure 19.3) - taking less than 8 hours total time for a batch size of 96 samples if performed manually (Verogen Inc. 2018-2) or approximately 12 h for batches of 96 samples using automated options (Hollard et al., 2019).

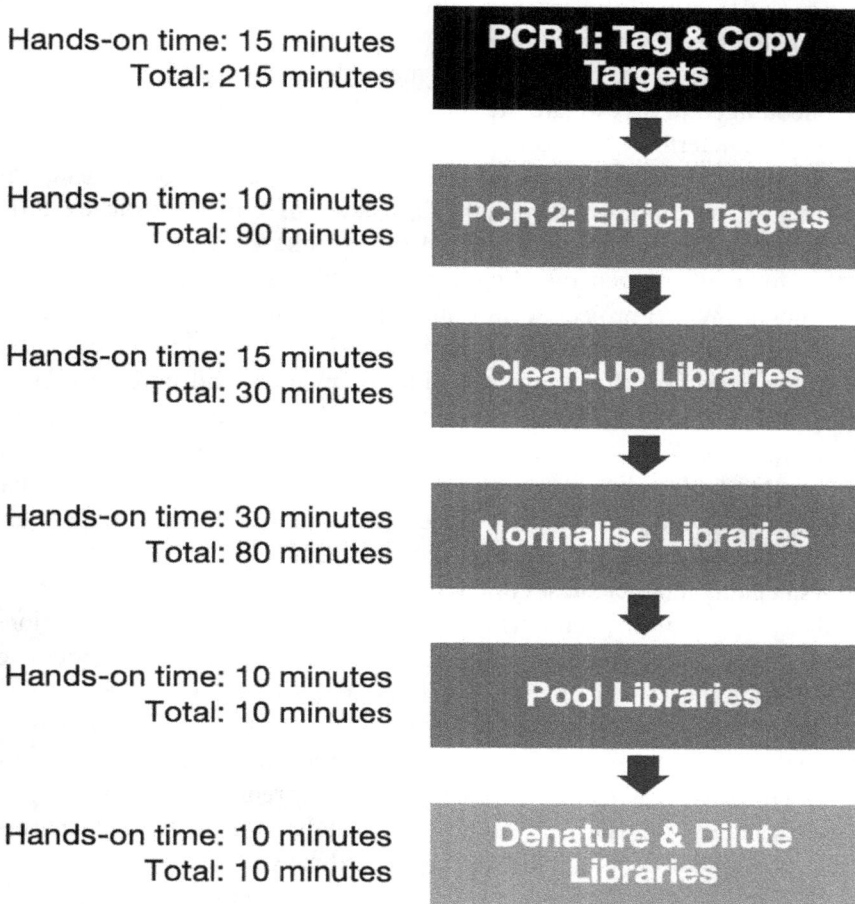

Hands-on time: 15 minutes Total: 215 minutes	**PCR 1: Tag & Copy Targets**
Hands-on time: 10 minutes Total: 90 minutes	**PCR 2: Enrich Targets**
Hands-on time: 15 minutes Total: 30 minutes	**Clean-Up Libraries**
Hands-on time: 30 minutes Total: 80 minutes	**Normalise Libraries**
Hands-on time: 10 minutes Total: 10 minutes	**Pool Libraries**
Hands-on time: 10 minutes Total: 10 minutes	**Denature & Dilute Libraries**

FIGURE 19.3 Workflow illustration for the ForenSeq DNA Signature Prep Kit.

Amplicons from PCR 1 are generated using unlabeled, target-specific primers tailed with priming sites for the second round of PCR. Amplicons from PCR 1 are loaded straight into PCR 2 without cleanup, where the adapters necessary to sequence the library on an Illumina sequencing platform, such as the MiSeq FGx, are attached. Enriched amplicons from PCR 2 are cleaned up and normalized using either a bead-based or manual quant method. The workflow can be performed manually, for laboratories with low to medium throughput, or automated for those with higher sample number requirements. Automation of the steps from PCR 2 onward is possible on a range of common liquid handling platforms, which preserves integrity of laboratory spaces designated for pre-PCR and post-PCR work to make best use of existing infrastructure, obviating the need for specific, method-dependent automation investments.

Given the diversity of library prep methods available, forensic scientists are encouraged to investigate the specific methods available for their applications and determine the exact amount of time that will be required.

You need to be a bioinformatician to handle data analysis: The vast majority of perceptions surrounding the level of bioinformatic expertise required to manage the analysis of MPS data likely arises from the high-profile focus of the general scientific and public media on whole genome sequencing (WGS) projects of all nuclear DNA (nontargeted sequencing). WGS reveals all the differences between individuals across the whole genome, including variations that occur in coding, regulatory, and intronic regions. While WGS is immensely valuable in the biological study of humans and other organisms and delivers the most comprehensive genomic data, it also requires the largest data management and data analysis efforts. Rather than taking such a broad genomic view, forensic scientists typically require and perform more focused or "targeted" sequencing of forensically relevant loci. By sequencing a target subset of the genome, casework and database efforts are directed toward the genomic regions that best answer forensic questions. This approach relieves privacy concerns, produces manageable amounts of data, and simplifies data analysis - a common bottleneck in current forensic DNA workflows. The ForenSeq UAS offers two user-friendly modules for the analysis of data generated by the ForenSeq kits for nuclear SNP and STR analysis and mtDNA. Designed by and for forensic scientists, the UAS system enables forensic analysts to easily analyze, manage, and interpret forensic amplicon data without the need for extensive bioinformatic training.

MPS analysis for forensic applications is cost-prohibitive: Due to the increased complexity of the process necessary to generate the enhanced amounts of data generated, MPS methods will sometimes incur a higher cost compared to CE-based STR fragment analysis. In addition, the cost per sample of MPS analyses is also dependent on the number of samples in each batch, given that the sequencing consumables for many MPS systems are single use and, therefore, cost the same regardless of how many samples are multiplexed. These basic cost increases are inherent to MPS technology; however, the differential between the costs per sample for CE and MPS will also vary significantly depending on the application and the exact technology being used. Verogen assays are designed to fall within the cost per sample range usually expected for the analysis of complex casework samples based on batch sizes of 24–32 samples, where repeat or multiple analyses of the same sample may be necessary to generate a result using comparable CE technology. Every additional CE analysis incurs additional time, resource, and financial costs, all of which can be consolidated into a single analysis with a larger MPS multiplex such as the DNA Signature Prep kit resulting in a cost per sample, which is roughly equivalent to, and a cost per data point that is significantly below, CE-based methods (Verogen internal cost comparison). Forensic scientists are encouraged to look critically at the total cost per result and at the value of the resulting data set in the context of the investigation to determine the real cost and ultimate value of each test to each laboratory.

MPS workflows are complicated: Similar to the other myths explored here, this perception is likely based on a genericization across methods and not individual assessments of each individual workflow to determine the specific level of expertise required and how easy it may be to adopt. As with any technology introduced to forensic science, there will be a requirement for training, education, and a building of experience. These need not be a significant barrier to introduction. The MiSeq FGx Forensic Genomics system was specifically designed to slot into the current forensic DNA laboratory layout and workflow, with a minimal specification for additional equipment or change to upstream processes. In addition to the standard laboratory equipment required for CE-based STR analysis, the MiSeq FGx system and ForenSeq chemistries require only a heated shaker capable of reach 1800 RPM and a specific magnetic stand (Thermo Fisher Scientific, part # AM10027). The ForenSeq kits contain all required library prep reagents of the kit-prescribed number of samples (96 or 384 for the DNA Signature Prep kit; 48 for the mtDNA kits) with the exception of water and ethanol. The MiSeq system, on which the MiSeq FGx system is based, could be considered one of the easiest MPS systems to use, and the ForenSeq UAS is designed to make complex bioinformatics simple to manage, presenting data in such a way that forensic scientists with prior STR, SNP, or mtDNA experience on CE platforms can leverage that existing expertise to easily interact with, and perform interpretation of, MPS-generated forensic data. As is often the case in life, things are generally perceived as difficult when they are unknown. With the relevant training, guidance, and support, which Verogen offers to all users of our technology, MPS technology need not be daunting or unreachable but a functional, operational tool with the demonstrated ability to enhance the analysis of complex forensic samples.

19.5   MPS MILESTONES

Forensic methods undergo rigorous testing, evaluation, and validation in order to gain acceptance and adoption into routine use, and MPS methods are no different. In 2017, the DNASEQEX project published the results of a survey conducted of European laboratories (Alonso et al., 2017). The information gathered provided data about the accessibility of MPS technology, future trends, and expectations in the participating institutes, including the identified scientific and legal challenges for the implementation of MPS in their jurisdictions. The perceived barriers to introduction of MPS methods for forensic analysis included a lack of nomenclature and reporting standards, the inability of National DNA Databases to accommodate MPS data, insufficient population data to support the interpretation, lack of adequate national legislation frameworks, the lack of specific validation guidelines available, no specific proficiency tests available, and generally not yet demonstrated to be reliable. Move forward just two years to 2019 and the situation was entirely different with all but one of these areas already addressed and significant progress made against the remainder.

Databases in France and the Netherlands already accept MPS data, and in May 2019, the MiSeq FGx System, ForenSeq DNA Signature Prep Kit, and ForenSeq UAS became the first SNP/STR system to achieve NDIS approval for upload onto the US CODIS database. Multiple population studies, many of which harness the capabilities and resources of multiple collaborative laboratories, have been published describing concordance and sequence-level variation compared to CE-based STR results and detailing the sequenced based allele frequencies essential to allow full exploitation of the more powerful statistics possible with sequence-based variation (Devesse et al., 2018; Gettings et al., 2018; Churchill et al., 2017; Phillips et al., 2018). In December 2016, the Scientific Working Group on DNA Analysis Methods (SWGDAM) updated their validation guidelines to include a section on MPS technologies—a reassuringly brief addition focusing mainly on the impact of sample multiplexing on sensitivity and the verification of the integrity of the indexing process (SWGDAM, 2016). This effectively illustrated the similarity of validation studies required for MPS methods versus CE-based genotyping by amplicon size alone. This was followed in April 2019 by the release of the "Addendum to SWGDAM Interpretation Guidelines for Autosomal STR typing by Forensic DNA Testing Laboratories to Address Next Generation Sequencing" (SWGDAM, 2019). With regard to proficiency testing, Collaborative Testing Services, Inc. have offered proficiency testing services for the ForenSeq DNA Signature Prep kit for several years, and MPS data, including that generated by the DNA Signature kit, have been submitted to the GEDNAP proficiency trials. With regard to reliability, the complete MiSeq FGx Forensic Genomics System, which includes the ForenSeq DNA Signature Prep kit, the MiSeq FGx instrument, and the ForenSeq UAS, is at time of publication still the only MPS system for which a comprehensive developmental validation has been published (Jaeger et al., 2017). Multiple internal validation studies have been completed and published (e.g. Moreno et al., 2018; Hollard et al., 2019), the MiSeq FGx has been accredited for mtDNA analysis in the Netherlands (Annex to declaration of accreditation, 2018), and the first criminal conviction using MPS-based STR methods on a MiSeq platform was secured in January 2019 (ECL:NL:GHAMS:2019:98) in the Netherlands courts. The only area still outstanding from the original list is the question of standardized nomenclature. Since 2016, two collaborative papers have been published discussing this issue (Parson et al., 2016; Phillips et al., 2018), and in May 2019, the Strand Working Group met in London for face-to-face discussions that advanced the conversation further. Laboratories are continuing to evaluate, validate, and operationalize MPS methods to take advantage of the many benefits offered; agreement on nomenclature standards is expected to benefit this landscape in due course.

19.6 FUTURE PROOFING FORENSIC LABORATORIES FOR THE ERA OF "OMICS"

The majority of this discussion around forensic MPS methods has focused on traditional disciplines of STR and mtDNA, and the increasing benefit SNP markers for identity and phenotyping purposes offer to the forensic industry. Commercially supplied dedicated kits and reagent systems and analytical software are available for these forensic marker types. These solutions will continue to be adapted to suit sample types, laboratory needs, and the rapidly growing body of scientific information that informs the applied forensic sciences. Currently, details pertaining to allele calling of the entire forensic amplicon, not just the STR repeat regions, are well on the way to becoming approachable for mainstream laboratories, to include SNPs in STR flanking regions (Gettings et al., 2018; Navroski et al., 2016; Wendt et al., 2017; Woener et al., 2019) and additional SNPs that reside on targeted SNP amplicons, thus comprising microhaplotypes (Bulbul et al., 2018; Oldoni et al., 2019; Wendt et al., 2017). These data are especially important in mixed and/or partial DNA profiles, where genetic polymorphisms may assist to resolve a mixture and lead to the ability to render a conclusion relative to a known sample(s).

The power of genomics in forensic science has only partially been unlocked, and our work here is far from complete. An emerging suite of applications, already in development by the forensic research community, leverages a range of approaches for generating and analyzing data from the transcriptome, nuclear genome, epigenome, and microbiome (Kayser and Parson, 2018; Kayser, 2019). As these "omics" mature and integrate into the operational forensic laboratory, the community stands to gain more precise, conclusive test results, with a lower investment of cost and labor time. Investigative intelligence that incorporates genetic data is on the rise and expected to continue to become more informative and part of the mandate and day-to-day affairs of forensic laboratory systems.

When desired, conventional serology is used by crime laboratories to classify or identify body fluids encountered in investigations. Primary reasons for these tests are (1) to "screen" biological items for merit and probability of obtaining DNA typing prior to expending time and resources, and (2) to better understand or establish crime context which could afford probative value. Conventional serological testing includes light microscopy and various enzymatic and immunological tests that may assist to support or refute claims made by suspects, survivors of sexual assault, or to reconstruct events in sexually motivated homicides, or in shooting incidents. The limitations of conventional serology include (1) the need to train analysts, (2) quality control of varied reagents, kits and assays, (3) low sensitivity levels mean that interpretable DNA typing results can sometimes be obtained from a "serology negative" sample, (4) the inconclusive nature or low specificity of some test results, and (5) evidence sample consumption. Targeted mRNA analysis of transcripts that are highly specific to body fluids and tissues of forensic interest may be considered as "molecular serology." Strong beginnings of molecular serological testing have been available for some body fluids for some time, using multiplex PCR-based analysis of targeted mRNA (Lindenbergh et al., 2013). MPS-based approaches are poised to allow analysis of multiple body fluids or tissues simultaneously (Dørum et al., 2019; Hanson et al., 2018; Ingold et al., 2018; Albani and Fleming, 2018; Wang et al., 2019) to supply conclusive results, based on differential mRNA expression or levels, even between fluids such as menstrual blood and circulatory blood. MPS data may be able to eliminate subjective body fluid interpretation via meaningful and robust internal controls and improved quantitative data. Coextraction of DNA and RNA followed by targeted sequencing, of specific forensic gDNA or mtDNA amplicons, and cDNA from mRNA transcripts, may in future reduce evidentiary material consumption for efficient, semiautomated, and simultaneous high-resolution genotyping and conclusive molecular body fluid/tissue identification, all on one MPS platform in a single run.

As forensic genomics matures, forensic laboratories that previously focused mostly on human identification (source attribution) may experience increased demand for deeper and routine investigative intelligence. Historically, genetic intelligence was limited to the genetic sex of the DNA contributor via fragment-based typing of the commonly used marker, Amelogenin. Familial searching using Y-STR profiles of known samples on law enforcement databases can provide genetic clues (investigative intelligence) about male relatives of a suspected perpetrator in an unsolved crime, necessitating collection of a reference sample directly from the implicated individual and direct comparison to the crime scene sample(s) for confirmation. Use of X-STRs in familial searching could be considered in order to provide additional familial links, as maternal and paternal lineages each pass down X haploblocks to female offspring. These X-STR data can serve to improve Y haplotype-based resolution among male relatives in law enforcement databases.

Recently, long-range familial searching, known as "forensic genetic genealogy" (FGG) has emerged in the public domain. FGG arose as a large number of consumers have purchased and shared their own personal genetic data online. In the past few years, unidentified human remains and crime samples have been traced to origin through use of the GEDmatch website, followed by manual research of varied documents such as census records, birth, marriage, death certificates, and so on (sometimes a cumbersome task). Unknown samples must be analyzed for SNPs that are held in common among the typical "direct to consumer" DNA sequencing services such as ancestry.com and 23andMe. Time-consuming workflows, such as microarray analysis and Whole Genome Sequencing approaches, are used today to generate GEDmatch-compatible data, which can require bioinformatic resources for SNP imputation as partial call rates are experienced from small quantities of DNA available from crime scene samples (Lord, 2019). These types of methods and workflows are not available today in crime laboratories. Targeted MPS offers a more sustainable approach and is anticipated to provide built for purpose assays and simple software that interrogates SNPs, curated for higher order kinship detection, and designed for small, partial, and mixed forensic DNA samples. Targeted MPS-based forensic solutions for forensic genealogy have the potential to reduce price, sample preparation burdens, and data analysis complexities. By building reverse family trees and mining genealogical records, we may be able to identify virtually any evidence sample once a threshold number of human SNP profiles are available. The value of forensic genealogy to the public good is being discussed, relative to real and perceived privacy concerns. Multiple cases have already gone to trial, and ended in criminal conviction including one where the defendant was identified through reverse genealogy for a case that had gone unresolved for 32 years (Hutton, 2019).

One of the most anticipated types of investigative leads is the genetic witness or molecular photofit, where a person's physical appearance, what they look like, is estimated from DNA alone. Most human visible traits of interest are controlled by multiple genes (multigenic) and thus require knowledge about interactions and pathways, which can then provide the capability to target specific SNPs that influence the way a person physically appears. Facial morphology estimation from DNA evidence (usefully accurate "mugshots" for identification of perpetrators linked to violence, terrorism, national security, etc.) is confounded by the lack of fundamental understanding of genetic architecture of facial variation. Genome-wide association studies provide craniofacial trait/morphogenesis insights; data indicate that with proper scientific investigation, advanced facial projections via sequencing select DNA targets will be achieved. Exhaustive, controlled exploration of DNA elements has already brought accurate investigative leads for sex, pigmentation (eye, hair, and skin), ancestry, and familial inference. Furthering this type of high-quality work using MPS will advance the ability to generate actionable facial renderings from crime scene DNA alone (Sero et al., 2019). Improved data outputs could, in the long term, enable facial image database queries and searches of static images, such as mugshots, which at the very least narrow the suspect pool and may return close, actionable identifications.

DNA modifications can also assist in providing investigative information when a suspect has not been identified through traditional means (Vidaki and Kayser, 2018). DNA experiences dynamic modifications as a result of environmental factors, where the deoxyribonucleic acids themselves are not altered. These modifications and their ramifications are studies in epigenetics and can provide genetic clues of forensic relevance. Foremost currently is the ability to estimate the chronological age of a person who is the source of an unknown sample within a range of years (Aliferi et al., 2018; Jung et al., 2019; Peng et al., 2019). In future, the epigenome may afford the ability to predict, from DNA alone, lifestyle attributes such as tobacco use, illicit drug or alcohol abuse, diet, and level of physical exercise/activity and aggregate data that inform socioeconomic status. We expect to see MPS-based data routinely generated in forensic laboratories regarding the methylation state of specific CpG sites and potentially of the up or down regulation of transcription, mediated by methylation in promoter regions of genes of forensic interest, which could provide actionable intelligence.

Nonhuman DNA analysis is another area of forensic research and application that has garnered attention and in which we anticipate continued advancements and refinement. The human microbiome, the compliment of nonhuman species that reside on and in every individual, may be useful directly in human identification. Our skin microbiomes may be somewhat similar to those with whom we cohabit but differs from others and could assist to narrow suspect pools and/or to strengthen other genetic and nongenetic leads (Schmedes et al., 2018). The human gut and nasal microbiomes may provide a vast array of information such as antibiotic use, disease states, geographical area of habitation, and recent travel. In death investigations, estimation of time of death (*post-mortem* interval) is aided by analysis of insect DNA and of the entirety of bacterial and other organisms that live in and on a decedent, known as the necrobiome (Metcalf, 2019).

Diagnostics and clinical research are advancing global efforts to improve human health outcomes at a rapid rate. A primary goal is to provide precision medicine, based on the individual genetic makeup of a patient, to prevent disease and for customized, smart medical treatment. In the hunt for genetic disease associations, whole genome sequences of millions of healthy individuals and of individuals with health problems are being generated, studied, and curated. Modern genetic marker discovery will continue to assist forensic genomics, spanning genetic elements in the nucleus, the epigenome, the transcriptome, and ramifications of nonhuman species with living and deceased persons. Strategic planning in government and private forensic infrastructure today should anticipate advanced workflows that answer more forensic questions than ever before, extending capabilities of the contemporary forensic laboratory to truly exploit the power of "omics."

19.7 CONCLUDING REMARKS

Legacy forensic workflows artificially truncate the power of genomics, using techniques that predate the Human Genome Project and require multiple rounds of analysis to produce complete genetic profiles. With MPS, forensic scientists have access to a greater number of informative loci, superior analysis of degraded samples, higher resolution sequencing, and greater overall throughput with library multiplexing. DNA database organizations are expanding marker sets to enable more efficient and collaborative work with global and regional law enforcement. For databases that seek to house X-and Y-STRs in addition to aSTRs, the ForenSeq DNA Signature Prep Kit brings the ability to type all loci of interest in one reaction. Research efforts are evaluating phenotypic SNPs that provide association with an even wider range of attributes than currently possible. These and other advances not only aid or help solve more cases in a shorter amount of time for human identification, but also produce investigative leads for cases that would have reached dead ends when a suspect is not produced from traditional investigations.

Using systems specifically designed and validated for forensic genomic applications today, forensic scientists are leveraging streamlined efficient and user-friendly tools and workflows to supplement and ultimately replace legacy CE. Research teams around the world continue to develop new capabilities using MPS technology in forensic case work and complex human identity testing. Transforming existing laboratories into MPS workspaces sets up the criminal justice system for the future. Sample processing using MPS platforms, such as the MiSeq FGx, positions the forensic laboratory environment and analysts' knowledge and skills in line with our ability to benefit from integrated capabilities and expanded options. The age of "omics" in the forensic sciences is just starting to reveal itself. Today, WGS has already been employed to investigate forensic questions, including the ability to differentiate between monozygotic twins. As diagnostics and clinical research deepen and accelerate, advanced methods and our ability to estimate human traits will emerge and flow over into the applied sciences, including forensic genomics. Precise capabilities that empower more and more conclusive forensic answers are already on our immediate horizon. Further into the future, strategies to fully leverage genetic information to positively impact public safety in responsible ways are sure to materialize. As forensic genomic methods continue to evolve, Verogen is dedicated to both supporting and advancing these efforts.

KEYWORDS

- **MPS**
- **MiSeq FGx**
- **ForenSeq**
- **STR**
- **SNP**
- **mtDNA**
- **epigenetics**
- **phenotyping**
- **forensic genomics**
- **investigative intelligence**

REFERENCES

Albani, P. and Fleming, R. Novel messenger RNAs for body fluid identification. *Sci. Justice* **2018** 58:145–152.

Aliferi, A., Ballard, D., et al. DNA methylation-based age prediction using massively parallel sequencing data and multiple machine learning models. *Forensic Sci. Int. Genet.* **2018** 37: 215–226.

Alonso, A., et al. European survey on forensic applications of massively parallel sequencing. *Forensic Sci. Int. Genet.* **2017** 29:e23–e25.

Annex to declaration of accreditation (scope of accreditation). Normative document: EN ISO/IEC 17025:2005. Registration number: L 146. of Nederlands Forensisch Instituut Defined departments (KvK: 50384511). [Online] Available at https://www.rva.nl/system/scopes/file_ens/000/000/079/original/L146-sce.pdf?1518051623

Bentley, D. R., Balasubramanian S., Swerdlow H. P., et al. Accurate whole human genome sequencing using reversible terminator chemistry. *Nature* **2008** 456(7218):53–59.

DNASEQEX. DNA-STR Massive Sequencing & International Information Exchange. https://dnadatabank.forensischinstituut.nl/binaries/dnaseqex-letter-160531_tcm127–629975_tcm37–209493.pdf

Bleka, Ø., Eduardoff, M., Santos, C., Phillips, C., Parson, W., and Gill, P. Open source software EuroForMix can be used to analyse complex SNP mixtures. *Forensic Sci. Int. Genet.* **2017** 31:105–110.

Bleka, Ø., Storvik, G., Gill, P. EuroForMix: An open source software based on a continuous model to evaluate STR DNA profiles from a mixture of contributors with artefacts. *Forensic Sci. Int. Genet.* **2016** 21:35–44.

Bulbul, O., Pakstis, A. J., et al. Ancestry inference of 96 population samples using microhaplotypes. *Int J Legal Med.* **2018** 132:703–711.

Butler, J. M., Levin B. C. Forensic applications of mitochondrial DNA. *Trends Biotechnol.* Apr. **1998** 16(4):158–62.

Churchill, J. D., et al. Population and performance analyses of four major populations with Illumina FGx Forensic Genomics System. *Forensic Sci. Int. Genet.* **2017** 30:81–91.

Claes P., Hill H., and Shriver M. D. Toward DNA-based facial composites: preliminary results and validation. *Forensic Sci. Int. Genet.* **2014** 13:208–216.

Devesse, L. et al. Concordance of the ForenSeq system and characterization of sequence-specific autosomal STR allele across two major population groups. *Forensic Sci. Int. Genet.* **2018** 34:57–61.

DNA Resource Forensic DNA Policy **2019** [Online] Accessible at: http://www.dnaresource.com/

Flores, S., Suna, J. King, J., Budowle, B. Internal validation of the GlobalFiler™ Express PCR Amplification Kit for the direct amplification of reference DNA samples on a high-throughput automated workflow. Forensic Sci. Int. Genet. **2014** 10:33–39.

Dørum G., Ingold S., et al. Predicting the origin of stains from whole miRNome massively parallel sequencing data. Forensic Sci. Int. Genet. **2019** 40:131–139.

England R., Harbison S. A review of the method and validation of the MiSeq FGx™Forensic Genomics Solution. *WIREs Forensic Sci.* **2019** e1351, [Online] Available at https://doi.org/10.1002/wfs2.1351

Gettings, K. et al. Sequence-based US population data for 27 autosomal STR loci. *Forensic Sci. Int.: Gen.* **2018** 37:106–115.

Gill, P. and Haned, H. A new methodological framework to interpret complex DNA profiles using likelihood ratios. *Forensic Sci. Int. Genet.*, **2013** 7(2):251–263.

Guo, F., Yu, J., Zhang, L., Li, J. Massively parallel sequencing of forensic STRs and SNPs using the Illumina® ForenSeq™ DNA signature prep kit on the MiSeq FGx™ forensic genomics system. *Forensic Sci. Int. Genet.* **2017** 31:135–148.

Hanson, E., Ingold, S., *et al.* Messenger RNA biomarker signatures for forensic body fluid identification revealed by targeted RNA sequencing. *Forensic Sci. Int. Genet.* **2018** 34: 206–221.

Hares, D. R. Addendum to expanding the CODIS core loci in the United States. *Forensic Sci. Int. Genet.* **2012** 6(5):e135.

Hoger beroep materieel strafrecht – 21 Januari 2019 ECLI:NL:GHAMS:2019:98 [Online] Accessible at https://www.uitspraken.nl/uitspraak/gerechtshof-amsterdam/strafrecht/materieel-strafrecht/hoger-beroep/ecli-nl-ghams-2019–98

Hollard, C., *et al.* Automation and developmental validation of the ForenSeq() DNA Signature Preparation kit for high-throughput analysis in forensic laboratories. *Forensic Sci. Int. Genet.* **2019** 40:37–45.

Huber, N., Parson, P., Dür, A. Next generation database search algorithm for forensic mitogenome analyses. **2018** 37:204–214.

Hutton C. SeaTac man guilty of 1987 murders solved with DNA technique. Seattle Weekly [online as of 29 July 2019] https://www.seattleweekly.com/news/seatac-man-guilty-of-1987-murders-solved-with-dna-technique/

Illumina (**2012**) By digging deeper into the genome, next-generation sequencing may yield more forensic clues. Interview. (applications.illumina.com/content/dam/illumina-marketing/documents/products/other/interview_budowle.pdf).

Illumina Inc. Nextera EXT DAN Library Preparation Kit **2012**. [Online] Available at: https://www.illumina.com/content/dam/illumina-marketing/documents/products/datasheets/datasheet_nextera_xt_dna_sample_prep.pdf

Ingold S., Dørum G., et al. Body fluid identification using a targeted mRNA massively parallel sequencing approach—Results of a EUROFORGEN/EDNAP collaborative exercise. **2018** *Forensic Sci. Int. Genet.* 34:105–115.

Jager, A. C., et al. Developmental validation of the MiSeq FGx forensic genomics system for targeted next generation sequencing in forensic DNA casework and database laboratories. *Forensic Sci. Int. Genet.* **2017** 28:52–70.

Jung, S. E., Lim, S. M., et al. DNA methylation of the ELOVL2, FHL2, KLF14, C1orf132/MIR29B2C, and TRIM59 genes for age prediction from blood, saliva, and buccal swab samples. **2019** *Forensic Sci. Int. Genet.* 38:1–8.

Kayser, M. and Parson, W. Special Issue Guest Editors. Transitioning from Forensic Genetics to Forensic Genomics. *Genes* **2018** 9:3.

Kayser, M., Special Issue Guest Editor. Trends and perspectives in forensic genetics 2018. *Forensic Sci. Int. Genet.* **2019** 38.

Kidd, K. K., Speed, W. C., Pakstis, A. J, et al. Progress toward an efficient panel of SNPs for ancestry inference. *Forensic Sci. Int. Genet.* **2013** 10:23–32.

Lindenbergh, A., Maaskant, P., Sijen, T. Implementation of RNA profiling in forensic casework. *Forensic Sci. Int. Genet.* **2013** 7(1):159–166.

Oldoni, F., Kidd, K. K., and Podini, D. Microhaplotypes in forensic genetics. *Forensic Sci. Int. Genet.* **2019** 38:54–69.

Parson, W. et al. Massively parallel sequencing of complete mitochondrial genomes from hair shaft samples. *Forensic Sci. Int. Genet.* **2015** 15:8–15.

Parson, W. et al. Massively parallel sequencing of forensic STRs: Considerations of the DNA commission of the International Society for Forensic Genetics (ISFG) on minimal nomenclature requirements *Forensic Sci. Int.* **2016** 22:54–63.

Peng, F., Feng, L., et al. Validation of methylation-based forensic age estimation in time-series bloodstains on FTA cards and gauze at room temperature conditions. *Forensic Sci. Int. Genet.* **2019** 40:168–174.

Phillips, C. et al. Global patterns of STR sequence variation: Sequencing the CEPH human genome diversity panel for 58 forensic STRs using the Illumina ForenSeq DNA signature prep kit. *Electrophoresis* **2018**, 39(21):2708–2724.

Phillips, C. et al. "The devil's in the detail": Release of an expanded, enhance and dynamically revised forensic STR sequencing guide. *Forensic Sci Int Genet.* 34 (**2018**):162–169.

Phillips C, Prieto L, Fondevila M, et al. Ancestry analysis in the 11-M Madrid bomb attack investigation. *PLoS One.* **2009** 4(8):e6583.

Quail, M. A., Smith, M., Coupland, P., et al. A tale of three next generation sequencing platforms: Comparison of Ion torrent, pacific biosciences, and illumina MiSeq sequencers. *BMC Genomics* **2012** 13:341.

Sanchez, J. J., Phillips, C., Børsting C., et al. A multiplex assay with 52 single nucleotide polymorphisms for human identification. *Electrophoresis* **2006** 27(9):1713–1724.

Schmedes, S. E., Woerner, A. E., et al. Targeted sequencing of clade-specific markers from skin microbiomes for forensic human identification. *Forensic Sci. Int. Genet.* **2018** 32:50–61.

Scientific Working Group on DNA Analysis Methods Validation Guidelines for DNA Analysis Methods (**2016**) [Online] Available at: https://docs.wixstatic.com/ugd/4344b0_91f2b89538844575a9f51867def7be85.pdf

Scientific Working Group on DNA Analysis Methods – Addendum to "SWGDAM Interpretation Guidelines for Autosomal STR Typing by Forensic DNA Testing Laboratories" to Address Next Generation Sequencing (**2019**) [Online] Available at https://docs.wixstatic.com/ugd/4344b0_91f2b89538844575a9f51867def7be85.pdf

Sebastian, J., Fritz, J. S., Karola, P., et al. Updating benchtop sequencing performance comparison. *Nat. Biotechnol.* **2013** 31:294–296.

Sero, D., Zaidi, A., et al. Facial recognition from DNA using face-to-DNA classifiers. *Nat. Commun.* **2019** 10:2557.

Strand Working Group **2019** [Online] Available at: https://www.researchgate.net/project/STRAND-Working-Group

Verogen Inc. ForenSeq DNA Signature Prep Kit data sheet (**2018–1**) [Online] Available at: https://verogen.com/wp-content/uploads/2018/08/ForenSeq-prep-kit-data-sheet-VD2018002.pdf

Verogen Inc. ForenSeq DNA Signature Prep Reference Guide (**2018–2**) [Online] Available at: https://verogen.com/wp-content/uploads/2018/08/ForenSeq-DNA-Prep-Guide-VD2018005-A.pdf

Verogen Inc. ForenSeq Universal Analysis Software User Guide (**2018–3**) [Online] Available at https://verogen.com/wp-content/uploads/2018/08/ForenSeq-Univ-Analysis-SW-Guide-VD2018007-A.pdf

Verogen Inc. ForenSeq mtDNA Control Region Kit Data Sheet (**2019**) [Online] Available at: https://verogen.com/wp-content/uploads/2019/07/ForenSeq-mtDNA-Control-Region-data-sheet-VD2019003_June2019.pdf

Vidaki, A. and Kayser, M. Recent progress, methods and perspectives in forensic epigenetics. *Forensic Sci Int Genet.* **2018** 37:180–195.

Walsh, S., Liu, F., Wollstein A., et al. The HIrisPlex system for simultaneous prediction of hair and eye colour from DNA. *Forensic Sci. Int. Genet.* **2013** 7(1):98–115.

Wang, S., Wang, Z., et al. The potential use of Piwi-interacting RNA biomarkers in forensic body fluid identification: A proof-of-principle study. *Forensic Sci. Int Genet.* **2019** 39: 129–135.

Wendt, F., King, J. L., et al. Flanking region variation of ForenSeq™ DNA signature prep kit STR and SNP Loci in Yavapai Native Americans *Forensic Sci. Int. Genet.* **2017** 28:146–154.

Woener, A., King, J. L. and Budowle, B. Compound stutter in D2S1338 and D12S391. *Forensic Sci. Int. Genet.* **2019** 39:50–56.

Index

For Product Safety Concerns and Information please contact our EU
representative GPSR@taylorandfrancis.com
Taylor & Francis Verlag GmbH, Kaufingerstraße 24, 80331 München, Germany